Extra Diet Guides & Counters

BOOK DISCLAIMER ~ PAGE 24

Weight Control Tips

✅ Eat Sensibly

- Avoid fad diets. Eat 3 sensible meals daily with adequate fruit and vegetables.
- Limit portion size. Limit fats and high-fat foods, sugar, soda and alcohol. *(Sample Meal Plan ~ Page 11)*

✅ Exercise Daily

- Get active and exercise every day!
- Include muscle-strengthening exercises. You'll lose more fat and keep it off. You'll also feel and look better, and you can eat a little more! *(Exercise Guide ~ Page 12)*

✅ Reshape Eating Behaviors

- Be aware of eating habits and behaviors that lead to overeating.
- Also focus on social and emotional situations that lead you to snack compulsively. *(Extra Notes ~ Page 14)*

✅ Keep a Food & Exercise Journal

- A journal helps you see exactly what you eat and drink, and how much you exercise. *(Extra Notes ~ Page 15)*
- An excellent motivator and proven weight loss aid. Keeps you honest!

✅ Arrange Moral Support

Gain the support of family and friends. Get extra professional help if required, from your doctor, dietitian, psychologist, exercise trainer, or slimming group. Beware of family saboteurs who discourage you from adopting a healthier lifestyle!

DOCTOR CHECK-UP

Ask your doctor to check your blood pressure, blood sugar and blood cholesterol levels.

HEALTHY WEIGHTS
~ MEN & WOMEN ~
(Over 18 Years)

Based on weights with least risk of disease or death from heart disease, diabetes, stroke and cancer.

Based on Body Mass Index of 20-25

BMI calculated as: $\dfrac{\text{Weight (kg)}}{\text{Height (m)}^2}$

Height (No Shoes) Ft Ins		Healthy Weight Range (Pounds)
4'7"	~	86-108
4'8"	~	88-110
4'9"	~	92-114
4'10"	~	97-121
4'11"	~	99-123
5'0"	~	101-127
5'1"	~	105-132
5'2"	~	110-136
5'3"	~	112-140
5'4"	~	114-145
5'5"	~	119-149
5'6"	~	123-156
5'7"	~	127-158
5'8"	~	129-162
5'9"	~	134-167
5'10"	~	138-173
5'11"	~	143-178
6'0"	~	145-182
6'1"	~	149-187
6'2"	~	156-193
6'3"	~	158-198
6'4"	~	162-202
6'5"	~	170-211
6'6"	~	172-215
6'7"	~	175-220

Body Fat Distribution & Health

Moderate amounts of body fat do not compromise health. However, excess fat above the hips carries a far greater health risk than fat on or below the hips - better to be a 'pear-shape' than an 'apple-shape'.

Abdominal obesity greatly increases the risk of developing diabetes, heart disease, high blood fats, hypertension, stroke, sleep apnea, arthritis and some cancers. So-called '**cellulite**' carries no extra health risk.

Waist Circumference directly reflects the increased health risk of abdominal obesity. Waist size associated with a high health risk:
Men ~ Over 40 inches **Women** ~ Over 35 inches

Body Mass Index (BMI)

BMI is a general (but not specific) indicator of body fatness. Although BMI alone is not diagnostic, the higher the BMI, the greater the health risk of developing diabetes, high blood pressure and heart disease. BMI does not apply to heavily muscled persons. BMI is used in a different way for children.

Abdominal obesity greatly increases the risk of ill-health and earlier death.

Check Your BMI: Find your height (no shoes) - look across the row to the weight nearest your own. Then track down to BMI.

Ht	WEIGHT (LBS) ~ ADULTS													
5'1"	100	106	111	116	122	127	132	137	143	148	153	158	185	211
5'2"	104	109	115	120	126	131	136	142	147	153	158	164	191	218
5'3"	107	113	118	124	130	135	141	146	152	158	163	169	197	225
5'4"	110	116	122	128	134	140	145	151	157	163	169	174	204	232
5'5"	114	120	126	132	138	144	150	156	162	168	174	180	210	240
5'6"	118	124	130	136	142	148	155	161	167	173	179	186	216	247
5'7"	121	127	134	140	146	153	159	166	172	178	185	191	223	255
5'8"	125	131	138	144	151	158	164	171	177	184	190	197	230	262
5'9"	128	135	142	149	155	162	169	176	182	189	196	206	236	270
5'10"	132	139	146	153	160	167	174	181	188	195	202	207	243	278
5'11"	136	143	150	157	165	172	179	186	193	200	208	215	250	286
6'0"	140	147	154	162	169	177	184	191	199	206	213	221	258	294
6'1"	144	151	159	166	174	182	189	197	204	212	219	227	265	302
6'2"	148	155	163	171	179	186	194	202	210	218	225	233	272	311
6'3"	152	160	168	176	184	192	200	208	216	224	232	240	279	319
6'4"	156	164	172	180	189	197	205	213	221	230	238	246	287	328
BMI	19	20	21	22	23	24	25	26	27	28	29	30	35	40

BMI Classification:

BMI Below 19
Underweight

BMI 19-24.9
Healthy Weight
(Low Health Risk)

BMI 25-29.9
Overweight
(Moderate Health Risk)

BMI 30-40
Obese (High Health Risk)

BMI Over 40
Morbid Obesity
(Very High Risk)

Interactive BMI Calculator
www.calorieking.com

Calories & Weight Loss

Calories in Food

Calories in food are derived from protein, fat and carbohydrate. Alcohol also provides calories. Vitamins, minerals and water provide no calories.

Calorie Values Per Gram	
Fat/Oil	~ 9 Calories
Carbohydrate	~ 4 Calories
Protein	~ 4 Calories
Alcohol	~ 7 Calories

Note that fats have over double the calories of protein and carbohydrate. The higher the fat content of food, the higher the calories.

Sample Calculation

**QUARTER POUNDER®
WITH CHEESE
has 510 calories
derived from:**

26g Fat (x 9 cals/gram)	= 234
40g Carbohyd.(x 4 cals/gram)	= 160
29g Protein (x 4 cals/gram)	= 116
Total Calories	= 510

Calorie Levels for Weight Loss

Start with a calorie-controlled diet that allows a moderate weight loss of ½ - 1 pound per week. Weight loss is usually much greater in the first few weeks due to extra fluid losses.

Note: It is better to increase exercise rather than lessen food calories too drastically.

Suggested Calories for Weight Loss	
Women: Non-active	1000 - 1200
Active	1200 - 1500
Men: Non-active	1200 - 1500
Active	1500 - 1800
Teenagers:	1200 - 1800

The MyPyramid symbol represents the recommended proportion of foods from each food group and focuses on the importance of making smart food choices in every food group, every day. Daily physical activity is also important. *(More info: www.MyPyramid.gov)*

Examples of Single Serving Sizes

Grains (Eat 6 servings per day):
- 1 slice wholegrain bread (1 oz)
- ½ bun, small bagel or English muffin
- 4 small crackers or 1 tortilla
- 1 oz ready-to-eat wholegrain cereal
- ½ cup cooked cereal, rice or pasta

Vegetable (Eat 3-5 servings per day):
- 1 cup raw leafy vegetables
- 1½ cups raw chopped vegetables
- ½ cup cooked vegetables
- ½ - ¾ cup vegetable juice

Fruits (Eat 3-5 servings per day):
- 1 medium apple, orange, banana
- ½ cup canned fruit (in own juice)
- ¼ cup dried fruit
- ¾ cup fruit juice (unsweetened)
- ¼ medium avocado

Milk (2-3 servings per day):
- 1 cup (8 fl.oz) milk/soy (enriched)/yogurt
- 1½ oz cheese or ½ cup cottage cheese

Meat & Beans (Eat 2-3 servings per day):
- 2-3 oz (cooked) lean meat/poultry/fish
- 2 eggs **or** 7 oz tofu **or** ¼ cup nuts
- 1 cup (cooked) dried beans **or** chickpeas
- 4 Tbsp peanut butter **or** ½ cup nuts/seeds

Portion Size Counts!

Food portion size is critical to controlling calorie intake for weight control.

Super-sized food servings have become more common when eating out and in the home. This can mean a day's worth of calories being consumed in one meal; or a snack being equivalent to a full meal.

It is easy to underestimate portion size of foods and drinks, and unwittingly consume excess calories – even if the fat content is low or even zero!

To more accurately estimate portion size of different foods, weigh and measure your food with food scales, measuring spoons and cups. Better control of calories will result.

For a visual idea of portion sizes, visit www.CaloricKing.com. See examples (fries and cola) on this page.

Allow for Extra Calories in Packaged Food

The actual weight of packaged foods is usually 5-10% more than the label net weight (the minimum legal weight) - and in some cases up to 50% more. However, manufacturers calculate the calories based on the net weight. For actual calories, weigh the product and calculate the extra calories. **For extra details see www.CalorieKing.com**

Basic 'Tools of the Trade'

Fries	Cal	Fat	Carb
Small	250	13	30
Medium	380	20	47
Large	570	30	70

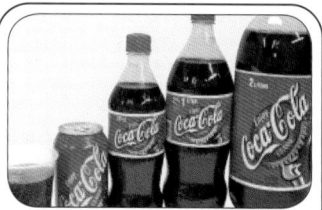

Cola	Cal	Fat	Carb
8 fl.oz Cup	100	0	25
12 fl.oz Can	150	0	37
20 fl.oz Bottle	250	0	63
1 Liter Bottle	400	0	100
2 Liter Bottle	800	0	200

Recommended Fat Intake

Recommended Fat Intake

Americans consume too much fat with many getting over 40% of total calories from fat – either as fat or oil, or as fat in foods and drinks. A range of 20-30% is healthier.

Fat Intake - Healthy Ranges

Children	~	30-60g
Teenagers (Active)	~	40-80g
Women	~	30-60g
Men: Active	~	40-80g
Heavy Activity/Athlete	~	80-120g

MAXIMUM DESIRABLE FAT INTAKE (Daily)

Calories	Fat	% Fat Cals
1200 cals	30g fat	23%
1500 cals	40g fat	24%
1800 cals	50g fat	25%
2000 cals	60g fat	27%
2200 cals	70g fat	28%
2500 cals	80g fat	29%
3000 cals	100g fat	30%
4000 cals	135g fat	30%

Percentage Fat Calories Formula:

$$\frac{\text{Grams of Fat Per Serving} \times (900)}{\text{Total Calories Per Serving}}$$

Fat Percent Content

(Grams of fat per 100 grams of food)

Don't be fooled by promotion of foods claiming to have a low percentage of fat. It's serving size and total grams of fat that count.

Examples: Whole Milk with 3.5% fat sounds low (3.5g fat/100ml) but an 8 fl.oz cup contains 8g fat; and 2 cups contain 16g fat.

Ice cream with 10% fat seems high, yet a regular scoop (3 fl.oz) has only 5g fat.

(Low-fat ice cream has less than 2g fat/serving.)

3 Cookies: 140 calories

6 oz Muffin: 450 calories

Reduced fat & fat-free foods are not necessarily low calorie. Portion size is still important.

It is a mistake to think that eating low-fat or fat-free foods allows you to eat double the quantity. You can end up with even more calories than eating smaller amounts of regular fat products.

Also fat-free but high in calories are soda drinks, fruit juices, beer, alcoholic spirits, sugar and candy. Bread, rice and pasta also have negligible fat.

Total Calories Count!

Ultimately, it is food portion size and total calories that count whether from fat, carbohydrate or protein. Remember, cows get fat on grass!

FOOD LABEL MEANINGS

FDA Nutrition Claim Definitions
(All are on a Per Serving Basis)

Low Calorie: 40 Calories or less
Light or Lite: One third fewer calories or, 50% or less fat than regular product
Fat-Free: Less than half a gram of fat
Low-Fat: 3 grams or less of fat
Reduced Fat: 25% less fat than regular product
Fewer or Less Calories: At least 25% fewer calories than regular product

Hints to Reduce Fat

Meats, Poultry, Fish

- Choose **lean cuts** of meat with little marbling. **Trim all visible fat** from meat and remove the skin from poultry. Removal of fat after cooking, is okay (to prevent dryness). Choose 'extra lean' ground beef.
- **Avoid high-fat meat products** such as salami, bacon, sausage and franks.
- **Broil or bake. Avoid frying in oil.** Allow casseroles to cool and skim off surface fat.
- **Avoid fried fish**, frozen fish in batter and canned fish in oil.

Fats & Oils

- **Use minimal amounts** of all types of fat and oil. All are high in calories.
- **Choose** 'light' and 'reduced fat' spreads but still use sparingly.
- Use minimal amounts of oil when stir-frying. Use no-stick sprays like Pam.

Salad Dressings & Sauces

- **Avoid regular mayonnaise and oil dressings.** Choose 'light', 'reduced fat' or 'fat-free' brands.
- **Choose** low-fat or fat-free sauces (mainly tomato-based). Avoid 'pesto', 'alfredo', 'cheese' and 'creamy' sauces.

Milk, Cheese

- **Choose** low-fat or nonfat milks and yogurts. **Avoid** full-cream milk, cream, Half & Half.
- **Cheese:** Choose fat-free, and low-fat cheese. Part-skim ricotta is still high in fat. Low-fat cottage cheese is a good choice. Cheese substitutes can still be high in fat.

Snacks, Cookies, Candy

- **Avoid** high-fat snacks such as potato chips, corn/tortilla chips, cheesy balls, buttered popcorn, chocolate and carob bars.

Desserts/Sweets

- **Avoid high-fat desserts**, such as cake, pie, pastries, cheesecake, full-fat puddings.
- **Choose** fresh fruits, fresh fruit salad, canned fruit in water pack, low-fat ice cream. Use low-fat yogurt in place of cream.

Fast-Foods & Take-Out

Check the Fast-Foods Section of this book for actual fat and calorie counts.

- **Avoid deep-fried chicken**, french fries, and onion rings.
- **Pizzas:** Avoid sausage/pepperoni. Choose vegetarian topping and modest quantity of cheese. Eat a moderate serving. Eat extra salad and fresh fruit.
- **Hamburgers:** Choose medium size, lower fat burgers. Avoid bacon. Have a side salad (with fat-free dressing).
- **Delis:** Choose sandwiches/bread rolls, pitas with low-fat fillings and plain salad. Limit meat/cheese to small portions.
- **Coffees:** Avoid large sizes of latte and frappuccino. Request nonfat milk and no whipped cream. Avoid cookies and pastries.

Extra Information: www.CalorieKing.com

FRYING ADDS FAT!

The greater the surface area of potato exposed to fat or oil, the higher the fat content and calories.

Whole Potato (3 oz)
0g Fat, 65 Cals

Roast Potato (3 oz)
5g Fat, 155 Cals

Fries (Large cut, 3 oz)
12g Fat, 220 Cals

Fries (Small, 3 oz)
15g Fat, 265 Cals

Potato Chips (3 oz)
30g Fat, 450 Cals

Carbohydrates ~ Friend or Foe?

Naturally Friendly Carbs

- **Carbohydrate foods in their more natural forms** (not overly processed) are essential to good health. They are the main source of fuel for the body, and also provide important vitamins, minerals, antioxidants and fiber – all of which help protect against heart disease, diabetes, hypertension, constipation-related ailments and many other diseases.

- Carbohydrates even help the body produce serotonin, the 'feel good' brain chemical that helps control appetite and overeating. Too little serotonin can lead to mood swings and depression.

Carbohydrates are found in different forms in food as:

- Sugars in fruit, sugar cane, milk
- Starches in whole grains, legumes, nuts, seeds and vegetables
- Dietary fiber (See Fiber Guide ~ Page 276)
Glycemic Index & Diabetes ~ Page 20

Low carb diets only work if total calories are reduced.

FAT MATTERS ~ CARBS COUNT ~ BUT CALORIES ARE KING!

Low Carbohydrate Diets

- Popular low carbohydrate diets are extreme in their recommendations to initially cut carb intake to as little as 20 grams per day – the amount in 1 thick slice of bread, or 1 medium apple, or 1 small potato.

  This greatly increases the risk of nutritional deficiencies and compromises health, particularly if fat intake is excessive through fatty meats, high-fat dairy products, and fried foods.

- While overweight Americans do need to reduce carbohydrate intake, it should be done **sensibly as part of reducing portion size and total calories.**

- Simply eating 'low carb' food products without regard to portion size, calories or fats, will do little to promote weight loss or good health.

- **Low carb diets (and indeed any diet) only work if total calories are reduced.**

- Refined sugars should be one of the first targets in moderating carb intake.
Extra Info ~ www.CalorieKing.com

RECOMMENDED CARBOHYDRATE INTAKE

Calories (Daily)	Carbohydrate (Grams)	Percent Carbohydrate Calories
1200 cals	120g	40%
1500 cals	170g	45%
1800 cals	210g	47%
2000 cals	250g	50%
2500 cals	345g	55%
3000 cals	450g	60%

How Much Do We Need?

- As shown in the chart, well-balanced diets above 2000 calories contain 50-60% of total calories from carbohydrate.
- At lower calorie levels used for weight control (1200-1500 calories), carbohydrates account for as little as 40% of total calories. This is because protein calories have nutritional priority.
- Carbohydrate & Diabetes ~ *See Page 20*

CarbSmart

Lower carbohydrate products may still be high in calories and fat.

- Many overweight, inactive people consume over 500 calories of refined sugars per day either self-added or as part of food products. This is equivalent to over 30 level teaspoons - a significant amount in weight control terms. Halving this amount would be reasonable and worthwhile.

  Note: Naturally occurring sugars in fruits, vegetables and milk are fine when consumed in normal recommended amounts. These foods are also rich in other nutrients.

  Refined sugar is referred to as having 'empty calories' because it supplies calories but negligible nutrients and no fiber.

- Most sugar in our diet is 'hidden' in processed foods such as soft drinks, fruit drinks, candy, cookies, cake, jam, sauces, ice cream, desserts, canned foods, and breakfast cereals.

  Certainly enjoy moderate quantities of these foods, but for serious weight control, look for 'low calorie', 'diet' or 'sugar-free'.

  However, be careful not to substitute sugar-rich foods with high-fat foods which might boost calories even more!

- Be aware that sugar comes in different forms such as sucrose, glucose, fructose, malt, high-fructose corn syrup, molasses, honey and maple syrup. Check the label.

- **Sugar alcohols** such as sorbitol, mannitol and maltitol are carb-based and have $1/2 - 3/4$ the calories of regular sugar. While not counted as sugar on food labels, they do add to the carb count. Excess amounts can cause bloating, gas and diarrhea.

- **Sugar-free sweeteners** such as *Equal, DiabetiSweet, NutraSweet, Splenda, Sweet'n Low* and *Stevia* make it easy to reduce sugar in drinks and recipes. Use only in moderation.
  Note: Most recipes can be adapted to contain less sugar with little effect on taste or quality.

Extra Info ~ www.CalorieKing.com

Sugar-free snacks and foods may be higher in fat and calories than the regular product.

Example ~ Creme Wafers (3):
Regular ~ 115 cals, 6g fat
Sugar-Free ~ 160 cals, 10g fat

SUGAR CONTENT OF SOME COMMON FOODS

	Teaspoons of Sugar
Coca Cola or *Pepsi,* 12 fl.oz	10
20 fl.oz size	17
Iced Tea, sweetened, 12 fl.oz	8
Chocolate Milk, 12 fl.oz	6
Honey Smacks Cereal, 1 oz	4
Popcorn, caramel, 1 cup	3.5
Chocolate Bar, 1.5 oz	6
M&M's 1.7 oz pkg	7
Muffin, large, 4 oz	6
Choc Chip Cookie, 1 oz	2
Donut, iced	6
Apple Pie, 1 piece	7
Jell-O, $1/2$ cup	4.5
Jam, 1 Tbsp, 20g	2.5
Syrup, maple, 1 Tbsp	3

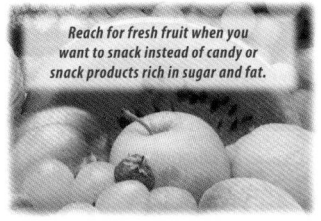

Reach for fresh fruit when you want to snack instead of candy or snack products rich in sugar and fat.

Tips For Overweight Kids & Parents!

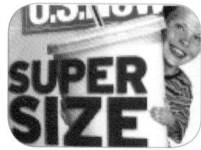

The XL Generation

Some 15% of American kids and adolescents are overweight; and childhood obesity has doubled over the last 20 years. Diabetes, high blood pressure and high cholesterol are major problem areas for overweight children and adolescents, as are depression, low self-esteem, sleep apnea and bone joint problems.

To address this problem, cooperation is required between kids, parents, schools and government. Weight control is a family and community affair.

Five Simple Tips To Get Started:

❶ Watch Soda Intake

Limit soda and sugary drinks to one serving on the weekends. Soda should not be an everyday beverage – water should be. When at restaurants or using a soda fountain, choose small servings with ice or choose diet soda instead. Schools should provide water and restrict access to soda as should parents when eating out or in the home!

❷ Cut back on Fast-Foods and Eating Out

Many more calories are consumed when you eat out. Healthy meals prepared at home are best for the whole family.

❸ Say "No" to Super-Sizing

When meals are upsized, loads more calories are consumed. Choose sensible portion sizes when eating out and at home. Use smaller plates and choose smaller packages.

❹ Limit Between-Meal Snacking

Watch out for high-fat and high-calorie snacks – they can have more calories than a meal! Keep your eye on portion sizes and limit salty snack foods and candy to parties and special occasions. Choose fresh fruit, vegetables and low-fat milk instead.

❺ Get Moving ~ Watch Less TV

Kids need at least 60 minutes of physical activity every day. It's critical for their fitness, and greatly lessens the risk of obesity.

Encourage kids to be active out of school hours. Wearing a pedometer can be highly motivational for kids to move more – as can playing dance video games such as *Dance Dance Revolution* (which is becoming popular in schools).

Limit TV and non-active computer games to just one hour per day. Also limit the accompanying snacks! Include exercise in family activities.

Extra information and tips ~ www.CalorieKing.com

Sample Meal Plan - 1400 Calories

For Healthy, Overweight Persons ~ Not for Persons With Any Medical Condition
~ Please Check With Your Doctor & Dietitian ~

 Breakfast (approx. 300 cal)

	1 Small Fruit or ½ oz Dried Fruit
Plus	Cereal: 1½ oz Dry (high fiber)
	or 1 cup cooked Oatmeal
Plus	½ oz Almonds/Seeds
Plus	Milk (from daily allowance) or Yogurt (low-fat)

 Breakfast ~ Choice 2

	1 Small Fruit
Plus	2 Eggs (no added fat)
	or 2 oz Cheese (low-fat)
	or 4 oz Cottage Cheese (low-fat)
	or 2 oz Lean/Canadian Bacon
Plus	1 Tomato
Plus	1 Slice Whole-Grain Toast

Daily Milk Allowance (approx. 160 calories)
2 cups Non-Fat Milk or 1½ cups Low-fat (1%) Milk
or equivalent Soy Drink, Yogurt, Cheese, Tofu

Fat Allowance (140 calories; 15g Fat)
4 tsp Fat or 6-8 tsp Diet Margarine or 3 tsp Oil
or 1½ Tbsp Mayonnaise or ½ medium Avocado
or 1½ Tbsp Peanut Butter or 30g Nuts/Seeds

 Lunch (approx. 440 calories)

	2 slices Whole-Grain Bread (2 oz)
	or 4 Crispbreads/Crackers or 6" Pita
Plus	2 oz lean Meat, Chicken or Turkey
	or 3½oz Tuna (in water) or 2½ oz Salmon
	or 1 oz Cheese or ½ cup (4 oz) Cottage Cheese
	or ½ cup (4 oz) Ricotta Cheese (low-fat)
	or ½ cup (4 oz) Fruit Yogurt (low-fat)
	or ½ cup (4 oz) Bean Salad
Plus	Large Salad (Oil-free dressing)
Plus	1 small Fruit or ½ oz Dried Fruit

 Dinner (approx. 360 calories)

	Soup (fat-free)
Plus	3 oz lean Meat (cooked weight)
	or 4 oz Chicken Breast (no skin)
	or 3 oz Chicken Thigh/Leg (no skin)
	or 5 oz Fish (grilled, no fat)
	or ¾ cup (6 oz) Beans (Soy, Kidney, Pinto etc)/Lentils
	or Low-fat Entree (e.g. Lean Cuisine)
Plus	1 small Potato or ½ cup Rice/Pasta/Sweet Corn
	or 1 slice Whole-Grain Bread
Plus	2-3 servings Vegetables/Salad
Plus	1 small Fruit + Diet Gelatin Dessert

 Between Meals Water, Coffee, Tea, Diet drinks,
Fruit from main meals; Raw vegetable pieces, Milk from Daily Allowance

Exercise & Weight Control

- Persons who exercise regularly lose more weight and keep it off longer than non-exercisers.

- Exercise also improves general health and well-being. Mood, confidence and self-esteem are enhanced by a sense of control and accomplishment.

- **Exercise increases the metabolic rate** of the body even for hours after exercise - a good way to 'wake up' a sluggish metabolism and burn extra fat. Exercise compensates for any decrease in metabolic rate with increasing age and also in some heavy smokers who stop smoking.

- **Strength training** further builds muscle and aids body reshaping. You can also eat a little more food! Note: Each extra pound of muscle burns an extra 50 calories daily ~ even while you sleep! Weight from exercised muscles is okay. It is surplus fat (particularly abdominal fat) that is potentially harmful to health.

- **Avoid injury** by beginning with walking, low impact aerobics, or weight-supported exercise (e.g. swimming, cycling). Avoid competitive sports.

- **How Much?** Start with 10 - 20 minutes/day and progress to 30 - 60 minutes/day.
  Also walk up stairs instead of using elevators. Take a brisk walk at lunch. Use an exercise bike, treadmill or stair machine while watching TV. Walk the dog.

- **How Often?** While aerobic fitness requires only 3 - 4 sessions weekly, **weight control is a daily event which requires daily exercise.**

Be Active Every Day!

Brisk walking each day is a safe and effective way to keep trim and fit. Try it – you'll like it!
Strength-training with light weights helps to retain or rebuild muscle tissue. It enhances weight control.

FATNESS VS FITNESS

An overweight but fit person can be healthier than a thin, unfit person.

TV CAN BE FATTENING!

- Many adults and children spend over 20 hours per week watching TV or at the computer (playing games or 'surfing') – at the same time as eating high calorie snacks and drinks.

- Are you a TV couch potato or computer addict? Limit your TV and computer hours and plan healthy physical activities.

- At home, limit kids to just one hour daily for TV and computers. Kids need at least 60 minutes of physical activity every day.

Too little exercise and too much food are the main contributors to middle-age spread.

Daily exercise and sensible eating can minimize middle-age spread. Include some strength-training to retain or build muscle.

Calories Used in Exercise

LIGHT	MODERATE	HEAVY
130 lbs ~ 3 Cals/Min	130 lbs ~ 5 Cals/Min	130 lbs ~ 8 Cals/Min
170 lbs ~ 4 Cals/Min	170 lbs ~ 6 Cals/Min	170 lbs ~ 10 Cals/Min
220 lbs ~ 5 Cals/Min	220 lbs ~ 7 Cals/Min	220 lbs ~ 12 Cals/Min

LIGHT	MODERATE	HEAVY
Walking, slow	Walking, brisk	Walking (power), Jogging
Cycling, light	Cycling, moderate	Cycling (vigorous), Spinning
Gardening light	Swimming, crawl	Swimming, strenuous
Golf, social	Weight-training, light	Weight-training, heavy
Tennis, doubles	Tennis, moderate	Wrestling/Judo, advanced
Housework, cleaning	Racquetball, beginners	Racquetball, advanced
Calisthenics, Yoga	Aerobics, light	Tae Bo, Kick Boxing
Bowling	Football, touch	Football, training
Ping-pong, social	Basketball, Baseball	Basketball (Pro)
Ice Skating	Walking Downstairs	Climbing Stairs
Aquarobics, light	Snow Skiing (downhill)	Skipping Rope
Skate Boarding	Shovelling snow	Skiing (cross country)
Line/Square Dancing	Dancing (ballroom)	Aquarobics, advanced
		Dancing (strenuous), Zumba

Note: Only those sports or activities that are sustained over a period of time (e.g running) qualify for heavy exercise. Stop-start sports such as tennis are considered 'moderate'.

Interactive Calculations ~ www.CalorieKing.com/tools

WALKING PROGRAM

USE DISTANCE, STEPS OR TIME

Weeks	Distance	Steps Pedometer	Time
1-2	1 mile	2000	20 mins
3-5	1.5 miles	3000	18 mins
6-8	2 miles	3500	35 mins
9-10	2.5 miles	4500	45 mins
11+	3.5 miles	6000	60 mins

10,000 STEPS PER DAY

A pedometer can motivate you to be more active. It clips to your belt or waist band and registers each step.

Aim for 8,000 - 10,000 steps per day, instead of an average of only 3,000 - 4,000 steps.

For Extra Information:
www.CalorieKing.com

Order Details ~ Page 303

Reshaping Eating Behaviors

• Eating is a behavior that is largely controlled by people with whom we live or socialize, places in which we carry out our lives, and our emotions. Become aware of those situations that commonly lead to extra food being eaten.

• We may also be unaware of 'bad' eating habits that can lead to excess calorie intake; e.g. eating quickly, large mouthfuls, eating when tense or bored, finishing a large serving of food when not hungry.

Tips to help uncover and correct those 'bad' eating habits:

• **Don't eat while engaged in other activities;** for example, watching TV, reading. Eat only at the table, not at the fridge or while standing.

• **Don't eat quickly.** Chewing slowly allows time to register a feeling of fullness. Don't use fingers, only utensils. Cut food into smaller pieces. Don't load your fork until the previous mouthful is finished.

Practice saying 'NO' politely but assertively.

• **Don't purchase problem high calorie foods.** Shop from a set list to prevent impulse buying. Avoid shopping with children.

• **Buy snack foods** in the smallest package. The larger the serving size or package, the more you are likely to eat or drink.

• **Plan meals in advance. Stick to a set menu.**

• **Plan a strategy to avoid uncontrolled eating** and drinking at social events, or when your emotions urge you to binge.

Rehearse repeatedly in your mind exactly what you will do in such situations. Remind yourself several times each day that you are in charge of your actions and that you can be strong-willed. Seek counseling or coaching on various strategies.

• **Promise yourself** that when you feel the urge to snack, you will engage in some activity that will distract you away from food (e.g. go for a walk, brush your teeth, phone a friend.)

If you eat out of boredom, find some new hobby or interest that gets you out of the house. Even enroll in an adult education class.

Do you use food as an emotional crutch? If so, professional counseling may be helpful.

The Value of a Food Journal

The food journal is the most powerful proven aid for dieters. Persons who keep a food and exercise journal not only lose more weight, they also keep it off. Here are some of the reasons:

- **Recording your eating and exercise habits** jolts you into realizing just what you do eat and drink each day; and also whether you exercise sufficiently.

- **Helps you identify problem foods** and drinks with excessive calories and fat.

- **Helps identify moods,** situations and events that lead to excessive eating of unwanted calories. You can then plan to overcome or avoid them.

- **Prevents 'calorie amnesia',** the forgetfulness that leads to rebound weight gain after successful weight loss. Recording puts you back on the right track.

- **Helps you develop greater self-discipline.** You will think twice about overindulging if you have to record it - especially if someone checks your journal regularly. It certainly keeps you honest!

- **Motivates you** to carefully plan your meals and to exercise each day.

- **Serves as a check system** for your doctor, dietitian or counselor to assess your progress and make recommendations.

Write It Down!

"Keeping a journal gives me feedback on exactly what I eat and drink each day.

It helps prevent 'calorie amnesia' and reminds me to exercise each day.

It's a must for successful weight control!"

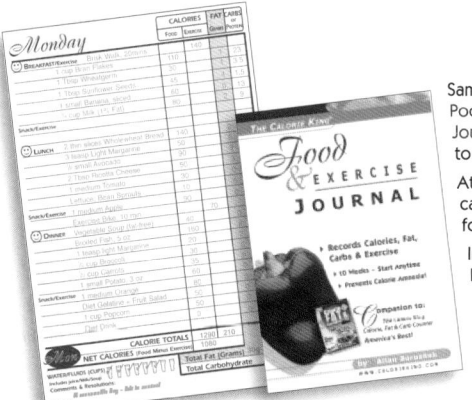

Sample Page from The Pocket Food & Exercise Journal, a 10-week journal to record food and exercise.

At day's end, exercise calories are deducted from food calories.

Includes Weekly Summary Page & Progress Checklist.

EXTRA DETAILS

~ SEE PAGE 302

Diabetes Guide
(In Association with Joslin Diabetes Center)

What is Diabetes?

Diabetes is a disorder whereby the body cannot use carbohydrates (sugar and starches) properly.

- **After digestion**, sugar and starches are changed into **glucose** – the simplest form of sugar vital for body energy and growth.
- **Insulin** is the hormone which acts like a key that opens the door to body cells and allows glucose to enter.
- **Without enough insulin**, glucose builds up in the blood and passes into the urine. High blood glucose levels lead to frequent urination, extreme thirst, and tiredness.
- **Untreated diabetes increases the risk of damage to nerves and blood vessels.** This, in turn, increases the risk of heart disease, stroke, blindness, kidney damage, foot ulcers and gangrene (with amputation), impotence and other complications.

Insulin acts like a key. It opens the door to body cells and allows glucose to enter.

People with type 1 diabetes and some with type 2 have too few or no keys and require insulin injections.

Others (primarily type 2) make enough insulin but the body doesn't use it as well as it should – particularly if obese and inactive.

SYMPTOMS OF DIABETES

- Frequent urination
- Extreme thirst
- Unusual hunger
- Rapid weight loss
- Extreme fatigue
- Blurred vision
- Skin infections that are slow to heal
- Tingling/numbness in feet

DON'T IGNORE DIABETES
It's A Serious Disease!

Note: Diabetes can be present even with no symptoms.

TYPE 2 DIABETES

- Occurs in 90% of diabetes cases
- Occurs mainly in adults - particularly in overweight and inactive persons
- Insulin is produced but body cells resist its action and glucose cannot enter cells
- Usually treated with meal planning and physical activity. Sometimes requires medication (pills or insulin)

TYPE 1 DIABETES

- Occurs in 10% of diabetes cases
- Usually in children and young adults
- Pancreas produces little or no insulin. Daily insulin injections (or use of an insulin pump or inhaled insulin) are necessary, as well as:
  - Matching pre-meal insulin to the amount of carbohydrate eaten
  - Weight control and regular physical activity

GESTATIONAL DIABETES

- Occurs in some women during pregnancy
- Usually disappears after the baby's birth
- Women who have had gestational diabetes still have a high risk of developing type 2 diabetes within 5 to 10 years
- Requires weight control, a healthy lifestyle and regular medical checks

Are You At Risk for Diabetes?
Pre-Diabetes ~ An Early Warning!

Pre-diabetes means that your blood glucose levels are higher than normal, but not high enough to be called diabetes.

If you have pre-diabetes, you have a higher risk for getting diabetes later on.

The good news is that you can start taking steps to prevent diabetes by making healthy lifestyle changes – such as losing weight if overweight, and being more physically active

BLOOD GLUCOSE CLASSIFICATION OF DIABETES	
Normal:	Below 100 mg/dl*
Pre-Diabetes:	100-125 mg/dl*
Diabetes:	Over 125 mg/dl*

(*Fasting Blood Glucose)

KNOW YOUR BGL
(Blood Glucose Level)
Everyone over the age of 45 should have a blood glucose test every three years

WHAT'S YOUR RISK?

Find out if you're at risk for diabetes by answering the following questions:

☐ I have been told I have pre-diabetes

☐ I have a family history of diabetes

☐ I am African American, Latino American, Asian American, Native American or a Pacific Islander

☐ I have had gestational diabetes (diabetes during pregnancy)

☐ I am over age 65

☐ I am overweight

☐ I get little or no physical activity

☐ My waist is larger than: 35 inches (for a woman) or 40 inches (for a man)

☐ My blood pressure is higher than 130 over 85

☐ My HDL (good cholesterol) is too low

☐ My triglycerides (blood fats) are too high

✓ CHECK YOUR RESULT

• **If you've put a check mark in two or more of the boxes,** you may be more likely to develop type 2 diabetes.

• **Talk with your healthcare provider** to see if you should have a blood test for diabetes.

Importance of Weight Control

• **Type 2 diabetes** is more common in people who are overweight.

• **Being overweight** means that your insulin doesn't work as well to control blood glucose levels.

• **Losing just 10 to 20 pounds** can help you better manage your diabetes and lower your risk for heart disease.

• **Keys to weight control include:**
  • Following a healthy eating plan
  • Controlling food portions
  • Being physically active most days of the week
  • Keeping food records
  • Setting realistic goals

• **Work with a registered dietitian** who can help you reach a weight that's good for you.

KEEP MOVING!

Everyday, do at least 30 minutes of moderate intensity exercise.
(even in 5-minute sets)

It's the key to improving insulin action. Add muscle strength training 3-4 times a week to double the benefits.

Diabetes Guide ~ (Cont)

Managing Diabetes

Don't battle diabetes alone. Establish a partnership with your doctor, dietitian, certified diabetes educator, and pharmacist.

Extra Support: • *Joslin Diabetes Center*
  • *American Diabetes Association*
  • *American Association of Diabetes Educators*
  • *Juvenile Diabetes Research Foundation*
  • *National Diabetes Education Program*

Hints to keep blood glucose within safe limits:

• **Control your food intake.** Know what and when you will eat. Seek referral to a dietitian for expert advice.

• **Exercise regularly.** It assists weight control and can improve sensitivity of body cells to insulin. Plan physical activity into your daily routine.

• **Monitor your blood glucose** at home and work with a blood glucose meter. It will help you become familiar with your blood glucose patterns, and the effects of food, activity and medication.

• **Take insulin or oral medication as prescribed.** If on insulin, know what action to take if hypoglycemia (low blood glucose) occurs. Also educate your family and friends.
More Info: www.joslin.org

Be Heart Smart ~ Know Your ABC's

If you have diabetes, you are at a higher risk for heart attack and stroke than someone without diabetes. But you can fight back!

Be smart about your heart!
Take control of the ABC's of diabetes and live a long and healthy life. Talk to your healthcare provider about your ABC targets.

Be Smart About Your **Heart**
Control the **Diabetes**
ABCs of
— A1C
— Blood Pressure
— Cholesterol
National Diabetes Education Program

A **is for A1C**
The A1C (A-one-C) test – short for hemoglobin A1C – measures your average blood glucose (sugar) over the last 3 months.
Suggested target: below 7%

B **is for Blood Pressure**
High blood pressure makes your heart work too hard. **Suggested target: below 130/80**

C **is for Cholesterol**
Bad cholesterol, or LDL, can build up and clog your arteries. **Suggested target: below 100**

(U) **Joslin Diabetes Center**
RESEARCH • EDUCATION • CARE

Joslin Diabetes Center, an affiliate of Harvard Medical School, is the world's largest diabetes research center, diabetes clinic and provider of diabetes education.

MORE INFORMATION
www.joslin.org or call 800-344-4501

Blood glucose meters and insulin pumps can greatly improve control of diabetes

BLOOD GLUCOSE METERS (EXAMPLES)

INSULIN PUMPS (EXAMPLES)

Guidelines for choosing a healthy diet apply equally to people with or without diabetes. Eating a wide variety of foods that are mainly low in fat and refined sugars, and high in fiber, is recommended.

However, actual food quantities, as well as when you eat, will also influence control of blood glucose. Your dietitian will individualize a meal plan to suit your food preferences, lifestyle and medical status. Here are a few tips:

- **Maintain a healthy weight.** If overweight, even a modest weight loss plus daily physical activity can help manage blood glucose in type 2 diabetes.

- **Don't skip meals.** If you take insulin or an oral hypoglycemic agent, regular meals are important.

- **If on insulin**, eat meals at the same time each day. Eat a similar amount of food at each meal. Eating about the same amount of carbohydrate over the day will make best use of insulin and prevent wide variations in blood glucose levels.

  Note: Take your rapid-acting insulin no more than 15 minutes before eating. Regular and combination insulins are best taken about 30 minutes before the meal.

- Know how much carbohydrate you should eat at your meals and snacks each day.

- **Choose whole-grain breads, cereals and pasta.** Eat fresh fruits, vegetables and legumes. These foods contain more fiber and slow the release of glucose into your blood after a meal.

- **Limit foods high in saturated fat, trans fat and cholesterol.** Enjoy fish, soy foods, and other foods rich in omega-3 fats. *(Extra Notes: Page 271)*

- **Limit sugars and foods high in added sugar** particularly if overweight. Small amounts of sugar as part of a meal may occasionally be okay. Check with your dietitian. *(Extra Notes: Page 9)*

- **Read the Nutrition Facts label** on foods. Check the serving size, total fat and total carbohydrate.

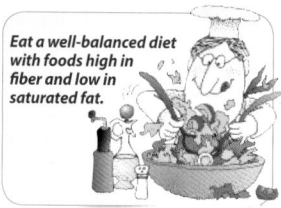

Eat a well-balanced diet with foods high in fiber and low in saturated fat.

The Plate Method is an easy way to eat healthfully. (See next page)

Vegetables & Salad Greens

Bread · Starch · Grain

Meat · Protein

ALCOHOL TIPS

- **If you drink alcohol, have only moderate amounts:**
  Men ~ 1-2 drinks/day
  Women ~ 1 drink/day
  For some people, safe drinking will mean no alcoholic drinks at all.
  (Also see Alcohol Guide ~ Page 166)

- **Drink along with your food** – especially if you use insulin or diabetes pills.

- **Do not omit any carb food** in exchange for an alcoholic drink. However, non-alcoholic beers (12 fl oz) count as one carb exchange.

- **Alcohol increases the risk of hypoglycemia** (low blood sugar) and drug interactions if you take insulin and certain types of diabetes pills.

- **Check with your doctor and dietitian.**
  Extra Info: www.joslin.org

Diabetes Guide ~ The Plate Method

The Plate Method — An Easy Way to Eat Healthfully

The plate method is a helpful tool to guide your food choices until you see a dietitian for your own meal plan.

For a healthy meal:

- **Fill half of your plate** with non-starchy vegetables (broccoli, green beans, carrots).
- **Fill a quarter of your plate** with carbohydrate (whole-grain bread, pasta, potato, brown rice).
- **Fill the other quarter of your plate** with 3-4 ounces of lean meat, poultry, or fish.
- **Use 1-2 teaspoons of tub margarine** or a heart-healthy vegetable oil.
- **Add** a small piece of fruit or 8 ounces of skim/low-fat milk or yogurt.

MAIN MEAL

Vegetables & Salad Greens

Bread · Starch · Grain | **Meat · Protein**

PLUS ONE CHOICE

Milk, Fruit, Dessert or other Carb Food

How Much Carbohydrate Should You Eat?

A dietitian can best determine how much carbohydrate you need at each of your meals, based on your lifestyle, food preferences, and overall diabetes control.

Until you see a dietitian, aim to keep the amount of carbohydrate you eat the same at each of your meals.

CARB CHOICES MEAL PLAN
One Carb Choice = 15 Grams of Carb

The amount in: 1 slice Bread **or** ¾ cup Cereal (unsweetened) **or** 1 small Potato **or** 1 small Fruit

 Breakfast
- Eat 2-3 carb choices (30-45 grams)
- Include a low-fat protein source such as egg whites or skim milk.

Lunch and Dinner
- Eat 3-4 carb choices (45-60 grams carb)
- Include fruit and non-starchy vegetables. Choose small portions of low-fat protein foods.

Snacks: If needed, eat 1-2 carb choices (15-30 grams carb).

Diabetes ~ Carbs & Glycemic Index

Carb Type Affects Blood Glucose

The various forms of carbohydrate affect blood glucose levels in different ways. It is difficult to predict the effect of particular foods, sugars, or meals, simply by their carbohydrate content.

Thus the same amount of carbohydrate from different foods may affect blood sugar levels very differently. Many factors affect the rate of digestion and absorption – particularly the type of sugar, starch, and fiber; the degree of processing and cooking (which increases digestion rate); and the amount of protein and fat (which slow stomach emptying and digestion).

Glycemic Index (GI)

The GI is a method of ranking carbohydrate foods on a scale (0-100) according to how they affect blood glucose levels. (See next column). The higher the GI value, the greater the food's ability to rapidly raise blood glucose levels, and the more insulin needed by the body (not desirable).

Eating low-GI foods may lead to better control of blood glucose and insulin levels (which in turn lowers the risk of damage to blood vessels and nerves). The slower digestion of low-GI foods may also help to delay hunger pangs and benefit weight control.

Note: Choosing low-GI foods is not a license to eat unlimited amounts. Calorie restriction and portion control for weight control is of prime importance.

- GI is not meant to be used by itself without regard to portion size, and other dietary recommendations for healthy eating. Foods are not good or bad on the basis of their GI.

- While GI may be a helpful tool for some people with diabetes, what is most important is to control the total amount of carbohydrate that you eat.

Extra Info: www.joslin.org
www.glycemicindex.com

LOWER-GLYCEMIC FOODS

Slower-Acting Carbohydrates

These foods are more slowly digested and absorbed. They help maintain more even blood glucose levels, as long as excessive amounts are not eaten. Use these foods regularly but still limit portion size for weight control.

Examples:

- Dried beans, peas, lentils
- Nuts and seeds
- Whole-grain breads
- Bran cereals, oats
- Sweet corn, barley, buckwheat
- Whole-grain pasta, basmati rice
- Fresh fruit: apples, avocados, bananas (firm), cherries, grapefruit, grapes, olives, oranges, peaches, pears, plums. Fresh juices.
- Vegetables: broccoli, yam, sweet potatoes, salad greens
- Milk, yogurt, soy drinks
- Dark chocolate
- Sugar alcohols (sorbitol, maltitol)

HIGHER-GLYCEMIC FOODS

Quicker-Acting Carbohydrates

These foods more rapidly raise blood glucose levels. Eat only in moderation.

- White bread, rice cakes, bagels, croissants, doughnuts
- Low-fiber cereals: Cornflakes, *Rice Krispies, Froot Loops*
- White potatoes, white rice
- Watermelon, ripe bananas, cantaloupe, pineapple
- Soda, sugar-sweetened sports and energy drinks
- Sugar, candy, popcorn (plain)
- Ice cream (low-fat), frozen yogurt

High-GI fruits and potatoes are still healthy choices when eaten in moderate amounts.

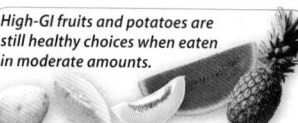

Calcium & Osteoporosis Guide

Calcium's Role in the Body

Calcium plays a vital role in nerve and muscle function, clotting of blood, enzyme regulation, insulin secretion and overall bone strength. Bones and teeth store 99% of the body's calcium.

The calcium level in blood is kept at a steady level by the continual exchange of calcium between blood and bone. When insufficient calcium is obtained from food the body draws calcium out of the bones.

This bone loss over a period of years may lead to **osteoporosis** – thinning of the bones (porous bones).

The bones become weak, brittle and easy to fracture, particularly the bones of the wrist, hips and spine. Loss of height and curvature of the spine may also result, as may periodontal disease - the deterioration of the jaw bones that support the teeth.

Common in Women & Men

While osteoporosis also occurs in men, women are particularly vulnerable (1 in 4 by age 60). They have about 30% less bone than men, and a greater bone loss at menopause when oestrogen levels drop. Slender framed women are at greater risk. (A woman in her eighties can have lost up to two thirds of her skeleton.)

Insufficient dietary calcium during pregnancy and breastfeeding will see bone reserves drawn upon, increasing the risk of osteoporosis in later years.

Hip fractures account for 300,000 hospitalizations each year. One in 5 older Americans with hip fracture die within a year – and 1 in 5 end up in a nursing home.

Causes of Osteoporosis

The major factors associated with the bone loss of osteoporosis appear to be:

- hormone changes of menopause
- inadequate dietary intake of calcium and other bone nutrients such as magnesium, vitamin D, zinc and protein
- insufficient exercise (weight bearing - such as walking, cycling ~ 30-60 minutes daily)
- family history of osteoporosis

Other contributing factors may include:

- excessive cola (regular or diet) and alcohol intake
- cigarette smoking
- some drug medications (e.g. steroids, thyroid)

As osteoporosis progresses after menopause, vertebrae may collapse causing the spine to curve and shoulders to hunch.

RECOMMENDED DAILY INTAKE OF CALCIUM

Children:		
	1-3 yrs	~ 500mg
	4-8 yrs	~ 800mg
	9-12 yrs	~ 1300mg
Teenagers:		
	13-18 yrs	~ 1300mg
Adults:		
	19-50 yrs	~ 1000mg
	51+ yrs	~ 1200mg
Women:		
Pre-menopausal		~ 1000mg
Menopausal (beginning)		~ 1200mg
Post-menopausal		~ 1500mg
Pregnant & Breastfeeding		
	14-18 yrs	~ 1300mg
	19+ yrs	~ 1000mg

Calcium & Osteoporosis Guide

Early Prevention Important

Gradual loss of bone begins in the thirties after maximum bone mass is reached. The stronger the bones at that time, the less trouble is likely to occur later. The earlier that prevention or treatment begins the greater the benefit. **The key to prevention is to build strong, dense bones early in life. By age 16, some 80% of peak bone mass is already reached.**

Young women may lessen the risk by:

- eating high calcium foods as well as adequate fruits, vegetables, wholegrains and nuts
- drinking less soda, and more milk
- not engaging in extreme dieting that results in menstrual period cessation (via less estrogen)
- taking regular exercise and not smoking

▲ Osteoporotic   ▲ Healthy
Fragile Bone   Dense Bone

Good Dietary Sources of Calcium
(Eat 3-4 servings a day of calcium-rich foods)

- Milk, Yogurt, Cheese
- Flavored Milk Drinks & Fruit Smoothies
- Ice Cream (low-fat), Frozen Yogurt (low-fat)
- Soy Drinks (calcium-enriched)
- Orange Juice (calcium-fortified)
- Tofu (with calcium coagulant), Miso, Tempeh
- Canned Salmon or Sardines (with edible bones)
- Breakfast Cereals (calcium-enriched): *Total, Wheaties*
- Broccoli, Dried Beans, Baked Beans
- Almonds, Brazil nuts, Hazelnuts, Seeds

GOOD SOURCES OF CALCIUM (MILLIGRAMS)

MILK
8 fl.oz
250

YOGURT
6 oz
200

CHEESE
1 oz
200

RICOTTA CHEESE
Part Skim ½ cup

160

SOY DRINK
Calcium Enriched
8 fl.oz
250

SALMON
w. Bones 3 oz
220

ALMONDS
1 oz
70

BROCCOLI
1 Cup
100

BAKED BEANS
½ cup

70

> ### Calculating Calcium From Food Labels
>
> The calcium content of packaged foods and drinks is shown in the Nutrition Facts label as a percentage of the DRI (dietary reference intake) of 1000 mg calcium.
>
> To convert this percentage into milligrams of calcium, simply multiply the percent figure by 10 (or add a zero). Examples: 5% = 50 mg calcium; 35% = 350 mg calcium.
>
> **Food Calcium Counter ~ www.CalorieKing.com**

Calcium Supplements

Because absorption of dietary calcium decreases with age, prescribed high doses of calcium (1500-2000mg/day) may benefit persons with osteoporosis - as well as vitamin D (preferably in D3 form, not D2), vitamin K, magnesium and zinc. Check with your doctor.

Notes, Abbreviations, Disclaimer

>> **Calorie and fat values have been rounded off.**
Calories ~ to the nearest 5 or 10 calories.
Fat ~ to nearest half gram. **Note:** Trace amounts of fat (less than 0.3 grams) have been treated as zero.

>> **Carbohydrate figures** in this book are for total carbohydrate, and not **Net Carbs** (which deducts fiber, polydextrose and sugar alcohols from total carbs).

>> Because manufacturers' figures on labels are rounded off, figures in this book may differ slightly from the label. Serving sizes may also vary.

IMPORTANT DISCLAIMER

* The authors and publishers of this book are not physicians and are not licensed to give medical advice. This book is not a substitute for professional advice. Users should consult their medical professional before making any health, medical or other decisions based on the material contained herein.

* This book is a compilation of original material from other sources intended for educational purposes only. Users should consult the source material before making any health, medical or other decisions based on the material contained herein. As food manufacturers constantly change their products, only they are an authoritative source for food's most current nutritional information.

* As nutrition data for food products are subject to change, users should consult the latest publication of this book and the author's website www.calorieking.com.

* Use of the information herein for any medical purposes, such as by persons with diabetes to match insulin dosage to carbohydrate intake, should not rely on the accuracy of figures herein, and should independently check food labels or contact the food manufacturer for the latest data.

* **WARRANTY DISCLAIMER:**
THE AUTHOR AND PUBLISHER DISCLAIM ANY LIABILITY ARISING DIRECTLY OR INDIRECTLY FROM THE USE OF THIS BOOK. THE INFORMATION HEREIN IS PROVIDED "AS IS" AND WITHOUT ANY WARRANTY EXPRESSED OR IMPLIED. THE IMPLIED WARRANTIES OF MERCHANTABILITY AND FITNESS FOR PARTICULAR PURPOSE ARE EXPRESSLY DISCLAIMED. ALL DIRECT, INDIRECT, SPECIAL, INCIDENTAL, CONSEQUENTIAL OR PUNITIVE DAMAGES ARISING FROM ANY USE OF THIS INFORMATION IS DISCLAIMED AND EXCLUDED.

This information is also provided subject to Family Health Publications' Terms and Conditions found at the website, www.calorieking.com/terms and incorporated herein.

C ~ Calories
F ~ Fat (grams)
Cb ~ Carbohydrate (grams)

Abbreviations

tsp = teaspoon
Tbsp or T = Tablespoon
oz = ounce(s)
c = cup
fl.oz = fluid ounce(s)
g = gram(s)
avg = average
pkg = package

Volume Measures

(All measures are level)
3 tsp = 1 Tbsp
2 Tbsp = 1 fl.oz
½ cup = 4 fl.oz
1 cup = 8 fl.oz
2 cups = 1 Pint
2 Pints = 1 Quart

Note: 8 oz weight is not the same as 8 fl oz volume (space occupied). Dense foods weigh more per set volume. Examples:

1 cup popcorn weighs ½ oz
1 cup milk weighs 8½ oz
1 cup pudding weighs 10 oz

Metric Conversion

½ oz = 14 grams
1 oz = 28.4 grams
2 oz = 57 grams
3½ oz = 100 grams
1 fl.oz = 30 mls
1 cup (8 fl.oz) = 240 mls
33 fl.oz = 1 liter (volume)

INFORMATION SOURCES

• U.S. Dept. of Agriculture
• Food Manufacturers
• Food Industry Boards & Councils
• Author extrapolations

FEEDBACK WELCOME!

Please contact the author with your queries and suggestions.
feedback@calorieking.com

Quick Guide

	C	**F**	**Cb**
Cow Milk ~ *Average All Brands*			
Whole (3.25% fat):			
2 Tbsp, 1 fl.oz	20	1	1.5
1 Glass, 6 fl.oz	110	6	8.5
1 Cup, 8 fl.oz	150	8	12
1 Pint, 16 fl.oz	295	16	22
1 Quart, 946 ml	590	32	44
Reduced-Fat (2% fat):			
2 Tbsp, 1 fl.oz	15	0.5	1.5
1 Glass, 6 fl.oz	90	4	8.5
1 Cup, 8 fl.oz	120	5	12
1 Pint, 16 fl.oz	245	10	23
1 Quart, 946 ml	490	20	46
Light/Low-Fat (1% fat):			
2 Tbsp, 1 fl.oz	13	0.3	1.5
1 Glass, 6 fl.oz	75	2	9
1 Cup, 8 fl.oz	100	2.5	12
1 Pint, 16 fl.oz	205	5	25
1 Quart, 946 ml	410	10	49
Light/Low-Fat (½ % fat):			
2 Tbsp, 1 fl.oz	12	0.1	1.6
Fat Free/Skim:			
2 Tbsp, 1 fl.oz	10	0	1.5
1 Cup, 8 fl.oz	90	0.5	13
1 Pint, 16 fl.oz	180	1	26
w. Replace (Oatrim Fiber): 1 cup	85	0	12
Buttermilk: *Average All Brands*			
Reduced-Fat (2%), 1 cup	120	5	10
Low-Fat (1%): 1 cup	100	2.5	12
Lactose-Reduced:			
Whole Milk, *Dairy Ease*, 1 cup	150	8	12
Reduced-Fat: *Lactaid*, 1 cup	130	5	12
Dairy Ease 100, 1 cup	130	5	12
Low-Fat, *Lactaid*, 1 cup	110	2.5	13
Fat-Free: *Lactaid/Lucerne*, 1 cup	80	0	13
Fat-Free: *Lactaid/Lucerne*, 1 cup	80	0	13
Lower Carb Dairy Drinks: *Per 8 fl.oz Cup*			
Calorie Countdown (Hood): Whole	130	8	3
2% Reduced-Fat, 1 cup	90	5	3
Fat-Free, 1 cup	45	0	3

Goat/Sheep Milk, Kefir

	C	**F**	**Cb**
Goat's Milk (Meyenberg):			
Whole, 1 cup, 8 fl.oz	140	7	11
Light/Low-Fat (1%), 8 fl.oz	100	2.5	11
Evaporated, reconst., 1 cup	150	8	11
Kefir: *Nancy's*, Plain Kefir, 1 cup	110	3	14
Nancy's, fruit flavors, avg, 1 cup	180	2.5	34
Sheep's Milk: Whole, 1 cup	265	17	13

Canned & Dried Milk

	C	**F**	**Cb**
Condensed: Reg. 2 Tbsp, 1 fl.oz	130	3	23
Low-Fat (Eagle), 2 Tbsp	120	1.5	23
Fat-Free (Eagle), 2 Tbsp	110	0	24
Evaporated: Whole, 2 Tbsp	40	3	3
Whole, ½ cup	170	10	13
Low-Fat (Carnation), 2 Tbsp, 1 oz	25	0.5	3
½ cup, 4 fl.oz	115	2.5	14
Fat-Free, 2 Tbsp, 1 oz	25	0	4
Dried: Whole, ¼ cup, 1 oz	160	9	12
Skim/Non Fat, ⅓ cup	80	0	12
Made-up, 1 cup, 8 fl.oz	80	0	12
Buttermilk sweetcream, 1 oz	110	2	14
Non-Fat, 1 Tbsp	25	0	3
Malted (Carnation), dry, 1 Tbsp	30	0.5	6

Chocolate Milk & Shakes ~ See Next Page

Soy/Non-Dairy Drinks ~ See Page 27

*For Full Nutritional Data including Saturated Fat, Cholesterol, Protein, Calcium and Sodium
~ See www.CalorieKing.com*

'What ever happened to sensible portion size?!'

Flavored Milk Drinks

 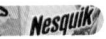

Quick Guide

Chocolate Milk
C **F** **Cb**

Average All Brands: *Per Cup (8 fl.oz)*

	C	F	Cb
Whole Milk (3.3%): 1 cup	210	8	26
1 Pint	415	17	52
Reduced-Fat (2%), 1 cup	190	5	30
Low-Fat (1%), 1 cup	160	2.5	26

Brands ~ Flavored Milk

Ready-To-Drink: Per 8 fl.oz Cup Unless Indicated

	C	F	Cb
Albertson's, low-fat, 1 cup	200	3	32
Alta Dena: Chocolate, 1 cup	260	9	37
Low-Fat Chocolate, 1 cup	200	3	32
Bravo!: Slim Slammers, 1 cup	110	3	14
Blenders Dble Choc., 11 fl.oz	180	4	20
Dominick's Low-Fat, 1 cup	170	2.5	28
Golden Guernsey, 1 cup	130	2.5	15
Grocers Pride Choc D'Lite, 1 cup	120	3	22
Hershey's			
Chocolate, 1% No Sugar Added, 1 c.	120	2.5	15
Chocolate, Reduced-Fat, 1 cup	200	5	31
Drink Box: Chocolate Drink, 1 box	130	1	29
Chocolate Reduced-Fat, 1 box	200	5	30
Chocolate Shake, 1 box	230	4.5	42
White Reduced-Fat, 1 box	130	5	12
MilkShake: Creamy Choc., 14 fl.oz	470	14	75
Strawb., Cookies'N'Crm, 14 fl.oz	490	12	78
Van. Crm; York Mint, avg., 14 fl.oz	560	12	96
Strawberry, Red-Fat, 14 fl.oz	350	9	52
Hood: Low-Fat (1%), Chocolate	170	3	28
Chocolate	230	9	31
Horizon Organic: Smoothies, 6 fl.oz	120	0	25
Chocolate, Low-Fat, 1 cup	170	3	27
Reduced-Fat flavors, avg., 1 cup	180	5	27
Kroger/Ralphs, Low-Fat, 8 fl.oz	200	2.5	34
Muscle Milk, (Hi Prot.), avg., 17 fl.oz	350	17	17
Nesquik: Chocolate,16 fl.oz bottle	400	10	64
Banana, 16 fl.oz	400	10	60
Choc. Fat Free, 16 fl.oz bottle	320	0	64
Double Choc., 16 fl.oz bottle	400	10	60
Very Vanilla, 16 fl.oz	400	10	60
Quaker Milk Chillers, 14 fl.oz bottle	250	9	32
Skinny Cow, Chocolate, 1 cup	150	0	26
Slammers: Starburst, 8 fl.oz	170	8	21
3 Muskateers, 8 fl.oz	140	3	17
Milky Way, 8 fl.oz	170	5	22
Starbucks, Strawb. & Creme, 12 fl.oz	320	2	66
Yoo Hoo Choc Drink, 6½ fl.oz	110	1	24

Bottled Coffee

See Coffee Section: *Page 164*

Shakes & Smoothies

Smoothies
C **F** **Cb**

Made Up Ready-To-Drink
(8 fl. oz Milk/Soy + Fruit): Per 12 fl.oz

	C	F	Cb
Average all types w. Whole Milk	300	8	50
+ Ice Cream, 1 scoop	400	13	62
with Non-Fat Milk	240	0	50

Fruit Smoothies ~ See Page 152
Freshens; Jamba Juice; TCBY: See Fast-Foods

Shakes

	C	F	Cb
Regular: Chocolate, 10 fl.oz	340	8	60
Vanilla/Strawberry, 10 fl.oz	320	9	51

Nutrition/Meal Shakes ~ See page 158
Burger King; McDonald's: See Fast-Foods

Cocoa-Chocolate Mixes

Add extra cals/fat/carbohydrate for milk
Carnation Breakfast Drinks: See Page 158

Ghirardelli	C	F	Cb
Choc Mocha, 4 Tbsp, 1.4 oz	130	1.5	33
Double Chocolate, 4 Tbsp, 1.4 oz	140	0.5	34
White Mocha, 2 Tbsp, 0.8 oz	90	0	23
Hershey's, Dutch Choc., 1 Env.	200	3	41
Horlicks, Malt Extract, 1 oz	90	1	18
Land O' Lakes: Per 1¼ oz Pkg			
Choc.Mint/Raspb./Supreme	140	3.5	26
Nestle: French Vanilla, 1 envelope	120	3	22
Milk Chocolate, 2 Tbsp	80	2.5	15
Fat-Free Hot Cocoa, 1 envelope	25	0	1
w. Marshmallows, 1 envelope	35	0	8
Rich Chocolate, 1 pkg	80	3	15
No Added Sugar, 1 pkg	50	0	10
Dble Choc Meltdown, 1 pkg	140	3.5	28
Nesquik Powder *(Nestle): Per 2 Tbsp*			
Choc.; Dble Choc; Strawberry	60	0	15
Chocolate, No Added Sugar	40	1	7
Ovaltine Cocoa Mixes, avg., 4 tsp	80	0	20
Swiss Miss: Cocoa Mixes			
Milk Chocolate, 1 oz pkg	120	2.5	23
w. Marshmallows, 1 oz pkg	120	2	24
Choc. Sensation, 1.2 oz pkg	150	3.5	28
Hot Cocoa Diet, 1 pkg	25	0	4
Fat-Free, 0.6 oz	50	0	10
Marshmallow Lovers, 1 pkg	140	2.5	29
Mocha Cappuccino, 1 pkg	110	1.5	24
Vending Machine, 1.34 oz pkg	145	2	24

Soy ~ Ready-To-Drink

Per 1 Cup Serving (8 fl.oz)	C	F	Cb
Eden Blend, 1 cup	120	3	18
Edensoy: Original, 1 cup	140	5	14
Vanilla, 1 cup	150	3	24
Light: Original	100	2	15
Vanilla	110	1	22
Extra Original; Unsweetened	130	4	13
Carob; Chocolate, average	175	4	28
8th Continent: Chocolate, 1 cup	140	3	23
Light Chocolate, 1 cup	90	1.5	12
Original: 1 cup	80	3	8
Fat-Free	60	0	8
Light	50	2	2
Vanilla: 1 cup	100	3	11
Fat-Free	70	0	11
Light	60	2	5
Smoothie, 1 cup	100	1	18
Hansen's Soy Smoothies: See Page 153, 159			
Lifeway: Slim 6 Kefir, 8 fl.oz	110	2	8
SoyTreat, 8 fl.oz	160	4	23
Naked Juice: See Page 155			
Naturally Preferred (Ralph's/Kroger)			
Low-Fat: Plain; Vanilla, 8 oz	100	2.5	11
Odwalla: Plain, 1 cup	110	4	11
Choc-ahh-lot	150	2.5	27
Vanilla Being	100	3	13
O Organics (Safeway): Plain, 8 oz	90	3.5	10
Chocolate	150	4	23
Vanilla Soy	100	3	9
Pacific: Select Plain, Low -Fat	70	2.5	9
Select Vanilla, Low-Fat	80	2.5	9
Organic, Original Unsweetened	90	4.5	4
Ultra (Extra Protein/Calcium): Plain	120	4	12
Pearl			
Orig., Vanilla, Green Tea, avg., 8 fl.oz	110	3.5	12
Chocolate, 8 fl.oz	150	4.5	21
Tropical Delight, 8 fl.oz	110	3.5	14
Unsweetened, 8 fl.oz	90	4.5	6
Power Dream (Imagine Foods):			
Java Jolt; Soy High Chai, avg., 11 fl.oz	245	4.5	42
X-Treme Choc, 11 fl.oz	260	5	48
Vanilla Blast, 11 fl.oz	240	5	39
Silk (White Wave): Plain, regular	100	4	8
Plain, unsweetened	80	4	4
Light: Plain	70	2	8
Vanilla	80	2	10
Chocolate	120	1.5	22
Chai, 1 cup	130	3.5	19
Chocolate; Mocha, average, 1 c.	140	3.5	23
Coffee Soylatte, 1 cup	150	3.5	25
Enhanced, 1 cup	110	5	8
Live! Smoothie, avg., 10 oz	220	4	39
Spice Soylatte, 11 oz bottle	190	5	27
Vanilla Plus Fiber, 8 fl.oz	100	3.5	14

	C	F	Cb
Slim-Fast: Easy to Digest	180	5	26
Nutritional Drinks: See Page 160			
SoyDream: Orig./Enriched 8 fl.oz	100	4	8
Chocolate Enriched	150	4	21
Classic Vanilla	120	4	14
Vanilla Enriched	140	4	14
SoyCoffee, 5.5 fl.oz prepared	5	0	0
Soy Fusion: Berry, 1 cup	120	1.5	24
So Nice: Natural, 1 cup	80	4	3
Original, 1 cup	80	3	7
Chocolate, 1 cup	150	3	24
Vanilla, 1 cup	100	3	11
Green Tea, 1 cup	110	1.5	19
Sun Milk: Healthy Heart, 8 oz	120	2	15
Vitasoy: Smooth Vanilla	120	4	13
Creamy Original	110	4	11
Classic Original	120	4.5	11
Green Tea Soy Drink	120	4	13
Rich Chocolate	160	4	24
Unsweetened Original	90	4.5	5
Vanilla Delight	120	4	13
Light: Original	60	2	7
Chocolate	100	2	17
Vanilla Soy Drink	70	2	10
WestSoy			
Smoothies: Banana Berry, 1 cup	140	1.5	28
Lite: Plain, 1 cup	90	1.5	15
Vanilla	110	1.5	19
Low-Fat: Plain, 1 cup	90	1.5	19
Vanilla	120	1.5	21
Non-Fat: Plain, 1 cup	70	0	10
Vanilla	80	0	12
Organic: Original, 1 cup	130	3.5	18
Unsweetened	90	4.5	5
Plus: Plain, 1 cup	130	3	17
Vanilla	130	3	19
Soy Shakes: Chocolate, 1 cup	170	3.5	30
Vanilla	170	3	28
Soy Slender: Plain	60	3	4
Other varieties, avg., 1 cup	70	3	4
Unsweetened: Almond, 1 cup	90	4.5	5
Chocolate; Vanilla, avg.	100	4.5	6
Vitamite 100: 1 cup, 8 fl.oz	110	5	14
Wild Oats: Plain, 1 cup, 8 fl.oz	100	2	10
Vanilla, 1 cup, 8 fl.oz	110	3.5	13
Zen Soy: Plain, 8 fl.oz	90	3.5	14
Chocolate	170	4	27
Cappuccino	150	3.5	22
Vanilla	110	3.5	14

Rice & Cereal Drinks ◆ Yogurt

Soy Powder Mix	C	F	Cb
1 oz (⅛ cup) mix makes 1 Cup (8 fl.oz)			
Soy Protein Isolate, 1 oz dry	95	1	0
Better Than Milk: Original, 2 T.	100	2.5	16
Chocolate, 3 Tbsp	110	1.5	22
Vanilla, 2½ Tbsp	80	2	18
Light, 8 oz	75	2.5	7
Joy Soy, Soy Melk, avg., 1 oz	90	2.5	10
Now Soy, ¼ cup, 22g	95	4.5	6.5
Revival Soy Shakes: *Per Packet*			
Plain; Unsweetened	130	2.5	3
Flavors, average: with Fructose	240	2.5	37
Unsweetened or Splenda	120	2.5	6
Soy Quik *(Ener-g)*, 1 oz dry	100	4.5	8

Rice & Cereal Drinks			
Amazake, Original, 1 cup, 8 fl.oz	150	0	34
Blue Diamond Natural			
Almond Breeze: Original, 8 fl.oz	60	2.5	8
Chocolate, 8 fl.oz	120	3	22
Vanilla, 8 fl.oz	90	2.5	16
Cacique, Horchata; Strawb., avg., 8 oz	160	3.5	31
Don Jose: Horchata, 8 fl.oz	140	4	25
Cereal Match, 1 cup	100	3	17
Eden Blend, Rice & Soy, 1 cup	120	3	18
Lundberg: Rice Drink, 8 oz	120	2.5	20
Vanilla Rice Drink, 8 oz	120	2.5	23
Pacific			
Rice Drinks: Multigrain, 8 fl.oz	160	2	30
Low-Fat Plain/Vanilla, 8 fl.oz	130	2	27
Organic Oat: Original, 8 fl.oz	130	2.5	24
Vanilla	130	2.5	25
Nut Drinks: Hazelnut Orig., 8 fl.oz	110	3.5	18
Almond: Original Low-Fat, 8 fl.oz	80	2.5	11
Almond, Vanilla, 8 fl.oz	100	2.5	13
Rice Dream: Carob, 1 cup, 8 fl.oz	150	2.5	30
HeartWise, 1 cup	170	3	36
Vanilla/Vanilla Enriched, 1 cup	130	2.5	27
Original/Original Enriched, 1 cup	120	2.5	24
Westbrae Rice, 8 fl.oz	110	2.5	20
WestSoy: Plain Rice, 1 cup, 8 fl.oz	110	2.5	20
Vanilla Rice, 8 fl.oz	110	2.5	20
Wild Oats: Vanilla, 1 cup, 8 fl.oz	130	2	25
Original, 1 cup, 8 fl.oz	130	2	25

Rice/Nut Drink Mixes			
Better Than Milk			
Original, 2 Tbsp powder	70	1	16
Vanilla, 2 Tbsp powder	75	2	15

Quick Guide	C	F	Cb
Yogurt			
Average All Brands: Per 8 oz Cup			
Plain Yogurt: Whole, 8 oz	140	8	10
Low-Fat	145	3.5	16
Fat-Free	125	0.5	17
Fruit Flavored: Whole, 8 oz	225	8	32
Low-Fat	230	3	43
Fat-Free, regular	215	0.5	43
Fat-Free, no sugar added	80	0	15
Goat's Milk Yogurt ~ Same as Regular Yogurt			

Yogurt ~ Brands	C	F	Cb
Alex Rod: Fat-Free, all flav., 8 oz	70	0	12
Albertson's (Low-Fat): Plain, 8 oz	140	2	19
Swiss, avg. all flavors, 8 oz	240	2	49
Fruit on the Bottom (low-fat):			
Average all flavors, 8 oz	230	2	45
Alta Dena			
Low-Fat: Plain, 8 oz	170	4.5	20
Average other flavors, 8 oz	220	2	41
Non-Fat: Fruit Flavors, avg., 8 oz	190	0	38
Plain, 8 oz	110	0	16
Vanilla, 8 oz	160	0	30
America's Choice: Swiss Style	210	2.5	41
Non-Fat, all flavors, 8 oz	100	0	15
Blue Bunny: Lite85, 6 oz	80	0	14
Sweet Freedom: Avg., all flav., 6 oz	90	3	5
Smoothie, 7 oz	70	1.5	5
Breyers: Fruit On The Bottom, 8 oz	240	2	46
Light varieties, 8 oz	110	1.5	16
Creme Savers, 8 oz	240	3.5	45
Smart! (w. DHA Omega-3), 6 oz	170	1.5	34
Smooth & Creamy, avg., 8 oz	240	2	48
Brown Cow			
Cream Top: Plain, 6 oz	130	7	9
Chocolate, 6 oz	200	7	31
Creamy Coffee, Vanilla, 6 oz	160	7	19
Fruit Flavors, average, 6 oz	170	6	27
Whole Fruit & Grains, avg., 6 oz	150	2.5	23
Low-Fat: Plain, 8 oz	130	3	15
Flavors, average, 8 oz	150	2	27
Non-Fat: Plain, 8 oz	110	0	16
Fruit Flavors, average, 8 oz	130	0	26
Smoothie: Original, 8 oz	150	2	25
Strawberry, 8 oz	170	2	31
Cabot: Plain, 8 oz	100	0	19
Flavors, 8 oz	130	0	24
Cascade Fresh: Low-Fat, 6 oz	140	2	23
Fat-Free, all flavors, 6 oz ctn	110	0	20
Whole Milk: Plain, 8 oz	170	8	12
Flavored, 8 oz	200	7	24

Yogurt ~ Brands (Cont)

	C	F	Cb
Colombo			
Light, all flavors, 8 oz	120	0	21
Classic, avg. all types, 8 oz	220	2	42
Fat-Free, Plain, 8 oz	100	0	16
Continental: Vanilla, 8 oz ctn	190	0	38
Plain, 8 oz	130	0	17
Crowley: Low-Fat Blueberry, 8 oz	240	2.5	48
Dannon: Plain (Natural), 8 oz	160	8	12
Activia, avg. all flavors, 4 oz	110	2	19
All Natural: Flavors, average, 6 oz	160	2.5	26
Non-Fat, Plain, 6 oz	80	0	12
Danimals: Super Creamy, 4 oz	90	2	14
XL, 5.75 oz	130	1	27
Smoothie, 3.1 fl.oz	70	0.5	15
Sprinkl'ins, 4.1 oz ctn	120	1.5	21
Fruit Blends, avg., 6 oz	170	1.5	33
Fruit on the Bottom, avg.,6 oz	150	1.5	28
Frusion Smoothie, 10 fl.oz bottle	260	3.5	50
la Creme: Regular, avg., 4 oz	140	5	19
Mousse, all flavors, 2.6 oz	110	5	14
w. Choc Pieces, 4 oz	170	7	22
Light 'n Fit (0% Fat): Avg., 6 oz	60	0	11
Carb + Sugar Control Smoothie, 4 oz	60	3	3
Crave Control, 4 oz	70	0	13
Smoothie, 7 fl.oz bottle	70	0	13
Dominick's: Low-Fat, 8 oz	230	2	40
Fruit on the Bottom, avg, 8 oz	230	2	40
Fat-Free 80 Calories, 8 oz	80	0	13
Plain: Low-Fat, 8 oz	130	2.5	15
Non-Fat, 8 oz	120	0	17
Friendship: Plain, 6 oz	150	3	18
Grocer's Pride: Low-Fat, 4.4 oz	140	1.5	28
Hellios: Kefir Organic, 1 cup	120	4.5	13
Horizon Organic			
Whole Milk, Plain Vanilla, 8 oz	220	6	32
Low-Fat: Blended, 6 oz cup	160	1.5	30
Tubes (1)	70	1	12
Fat-Free, all varieties, 6 oz	140	0	27
32 oz Carton, Plain, 8 oz	110	0	15
Yo Yo's, 4 oz	110	1	20
Jewel: *8 oz Ctn (Low-Fat)*			
Fruit On The Bottom, average	240	2.5	46
Swiss, average	200	2	38
Vanilla	210	2	40
32 oz Tubs: Plain, 1 cup, 8 oz	170	3	20
Plain, Non-Fat, 1 cup, 8 oz	130	0	19

	C	F	Cb
Kemps: '100 Calories' (Non-Fat), 5 oz	100	0	22
Light '80 Calories', 6 oz ctn	80	2	16
Yo Stix, average, 2.25 oz tube	80	2	13
Yo-J Drink, average, 8 fl.oz	150	0	35
Knudsen: 70 Calories, 6 oz	70	0	11
Free, average, 6 oz	170	0	33
Kroger: Active Lifestyle, 6 oz	80	0	12
Carb Master, 8 oz	80	1.5	4
Lite (Non-Fat) avg. all flavors, 8 oz	100	0	16
Low-Fat: Plain, 8 oz	150	4	17
Blended, average, 8 oz	250	2.5	47
Fruit on the Bottom, 8 oz	220	3	41
La Yogurt: Original, average, 6 oz	150	2	30
Light, average, 6 oz	90	0	15
Rich & Creamy, 6 oz	160	2	30
Enriched, average, 6 oz	160	2	30
Fruit 'N' Cream, avg., 8 oz	200	2	39
Fruit on the Bottom, avg., 8 oz	220	2.5	43
Sabor Latino: Dulche De Leche, 6 oz	190	1.5	36
Fruit Flavors, average, 6 oz	170	2	34
Lala			
Reduced-Fat: Fruit Flav., avg., 8 oz	200	4	36
Light n' Lively			
Fruit Flavors, average, 4.4 oz	135	1	27
Lucerne			
Low-Fat: Plain, 8 oz	150	3.5	18
Fruit flavors, average, 8 oz	240	2.5	45
Vanilla	240	2.5	44
Fat-Free: Plain, 8 oz	120	0	20
Light Fat-Free, fruit, 8 oz	130	0	19
Smoothie: Strawberry, 11 oz	300	4	57
Berry; Peach, avg., 11 oz	335	4	64
Light: Peach, 11 oz	190	0	42
Other flavors, avg., 11 oz	155	0	30
YoCups, avg all flavors, 4 oz	130	1	27
Yo On The Go: 2.25 oz tube	80	2	13
Smoothie, 8.25 oz	180	3	31
Meadow Gold, avg., 6 oz ctn	90	2.5	10
Mountain High			
Original Style, plain, 8 oz	180	8	17
European Delight, all flavors, 4 oz	110	2	19
Low-Fat: Plain, 8 oz	140	2.5	18
Classic, avg., 8 oz	175	2.5	18
Fat-Free, Plain, 8 oz	120	0	18
Mystic Lake Dairy (Goat Milk Yogurt)			
Plain, 1 cup, 8 oz	120	6	9

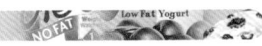

Brands (Cont)

	C	F	Cb
Nancy's: *Per 8 oz Serving*			
Whole Milk: Honey, plain, 8 fl.oz	180	8	16
w. Fruit Cup, avg, 9.5 oz	230	5	41
Low Fat: Plain/Lemon/Vanilla, avg	150	3	15
Other flavors, average	180	3	27
Non-Fat: Plain, 8 oz	120	0	17
Maple, Vanilla (8 oz ctn)	160	0	27
w. Fruit Cup, avg, 9.5 oz	150	0	27
Vanilla (32 oz ctn), swtn'd, 8 oz	220	0	40
Soy Cultured: (6 oz ctn): Plain	150	3	25
Berry flavors, average	140	3.5	24
Vanilla	120	3	19
O Organics (Safeway), avg., 6 oz	150	2.5	25
Publix: Fat-Free, Plain, 8 oz	140	0	23
Swiss Style, Low-Fat, 8 oz	240	2.5	41
Redwood Hill Farm (Goat Milk Yogurt)			
Vanilla; Fruit flavors, avg., 6 oz	140	4	23
Plain, 6 oz	100	4.5	11
Silk (Soy): Plain, 1 cup, 8 oz	150	4	22
Vanilla, 6 oz ctn	150	3	25
Other flavors, average, 6 oz	150	2	30
Stater Bros: Plain, 8 oz	140	2	15
Fruit on the Bottom, avg., 8 oz	220	2	44
Blended Low-Fat, avg., 8 oz	240	2	48
Non-Fat, avg., 8 oz	130	0	25
Stonyfield Farm (Organic)			
All Natural Fat-Free: Plain, 6 oz	80	0	14
Chocolate Underground, 6 oz	170	0	37
Other varieties, 6 oz	130	0	26
All Natural Fat-Free Light, 6 oz	100	0	28
Low-Fat: Caramel	190	1.5	38
Plain	90	1.5	13
Other varieties, average	130	1.5	25
Whole Milk Yogurt: Vanilla Truffle	210	5	37
French Vanilla, 6 oz	190	6	27
Other varieties, avg.	170	6	24
O'Soy: Choc.; Vanilla, avg., 6 oz	160	2	26
Fruit on Bottom, average, 6 oz	170	2	32
Yo Kids: all flavors, 57g	60	1	11
Cups, 4 oz	110	1	21
Stop & Shop: Light (0% Fat), avg., 8 oz	110	0	20
Fruit on the Bottom, avg., 8 oz	220	2.5	42
32 oz Tub: Low-Fat, Plain, 8 oz	140	3	16
Non-Fat: Plain, 8 oz	130	0	18
Vanilla, 8 oz	190	0	34
Trader Joe's: Low-Fat, 8 oz	220	3	40
Non-Fat: Regular 8 oz	170	0	34
French Village, Vanilla, 6 oz	130	0	26
Organic Vanilla, 8 oz	160	0	40
Organic Low-Fat, average, 6 oz	150	2.5	25
Cultured Soy, average all, 6 oz	150	3	28
Fruit on the Bottom, Crm Top, 6 oz	170	6	23

	C	F	Cb
Wallaby (Organic), avg., 6 oz	150	2.5	26
Weight Watchers, all flav., 6 oz ctn	100	0.5	17
Wildwood: Soyogurt Plain, 6 oz	90	3.5	11
Other varieties, avg., 6 oz	130	3	23
Smoothie, average, 10 oz	210	4	40
Whole Soy & Co: Plain, 6 oz ctn	150	3	27
Other flavors, avg., 6 oz	160	3	30
YoCrunch: *Low-Fat w. Toppings, 6.5 oz Cup*			
Oreo Cookies	190	3.5	34
Peach/Strawb./Rasp. w. Granola	190	2	38
Average other varieties	210	4.5	35
Yoplait			
Original, average all flavors, 6 oz	170	1.5	33
99% Fat-Free Original Flavors, 4 oz	110	0	20
Light: Fruit Flavors, 6 oz	100	0	19
Indulgent Flavors, 6 oz	110	0	20
Thick & Creamy, Light, 6 oz	100	0	20
Thick & Creamy Custard Style, 6 oz	190	3.5	32
Go-Gurt!, Fruit Flavors, 2.2 oz tube	80	2	13
Grande!: Fat-Free Plain, 8 oz cup	130	0	19
99% Fat-Free Plain, 8 oz cup	250	2.5	44
Trix, Fruit Flavors, 4 oz	120	1.5	23
Whips!: Chocolate Flavors, 4 oz	160	4	26
Fruit Flavors, 4 oz	140	2.5	25
Yoplait Kids, 4 oz	100	2	17

Yogurt Drinks & Probiotics

	C	F	Cb
Actimel *(Dannon)* Probiotic, 3.3 fl.oz	95	1.5	17
Activia *(Dannon):* Regular, 4 oz	110	2	19
Light (Fat-Free), 4 oz	70	0	13
Biokult, 2.1 oz bottle	40	0	8
Dannon: Danimals, 3.4 fl.oz bottle	90	1.5	15
Danimals XL, 5.7 fl.oz	170	3	29
DanActive, 3.4 fl.oz	95	1.5	17
Glen Oaks, all flavors, avg., 1 cup	240	3.5	45
Nouriche, Regular, 11 fl.oz	260	0	55
Silk Live! 10 oz	230	4	33
Stonyfield Farm			
Smoothies, avg., 10 oz	250	3	49
Light, all flavors, 10 oz	130	0	41
Weight Watchers, Smoothie, 7 oz	80	0	13
WholeSoy, 12 fl.oz bottle	230	4.5	36
Yo Soy, 8 fl.oz	80	4	4
Yonique: Pina Colada, 6 fl.oz	190	4	30
Peach; Banana; Guava, 6 fl.oz	170	2	30
Yoplait Go Gurt, 5 fl.oz	120	0.5	23
Yoplait: Smoothie, 8 fl.oz	220	2.5	44
Light Smoothie, 8 fl.oz	90	0	16

Quick Guide   Ⓒ Ⓕ Ⓒb

Ice Cream

Vanilla: *Average All Brands*
Other flavors ~ See Brand Listings.
Regular Ice Cream (10% fat):
Examples: *Borden/Hood*

	C	F	Cb
3 fl.oz scoop	105	5	12
½ cup, 4 fl.oz	140	7	17
1 Pint, 16 fl.oz	560	28	68
½ Gallon (4 Pints)	2240	112	272

Rich (16% fat):
Example: *Hood (Red Sox)*

	C	F	Cb
3 fl.oz scoop	135	7.5	15
½ cup, 4 fl.oz	180	10	20
1 Pint	720	40	80

Super-Rich (20% fat): *Haagen-Dazs/Ben & Jerry's*

	C	F	Cb
3 fl.oz scoop	200	13	18
½ cup, 4 fl.oz	270	17	24
1 Pint	1080	68	96

Reduced-Fat/Light (6% fat):
Breyer's Light/Hood Light

	C	F	Cb
3 fl.oz scoop	95	3	15
½ cup, 4 fl.oz	125	4	20
1 Pint	500	16	80

Fat-Free: *Baskin-Robbins FF/Borden FF/ Breyers FF/Dreyers FF/Hood FF*

	C	F	Cb
3 fl.oz scoop	70	0	16
½ cup, 4 fl.oz	90	0	21
1 Pint	360	0	84

Soft Serve: Regular, ½ cup

	C	F	Cb
Regular, ½ cup	190	11	19
1 cup	380	22	38
Light, ½ cup	110	2	19
1 cup	220	4	38

Quick Guide

Frozen Yogurt   Ⓒ Ⓕ Ⓒb
Average All Brands

		C	F	Cb
Hard:	Low-Fat, ½ cup	110	3	19
	Non-Fat, ½ cup	110	0	24
Soft:	Low-Fat, ½ cup	120	4	17
	Non-Fat, ½ cup	100	0	30

Brands: *See Ice Cream & Ices Section*

Quick Guide   Ⓒ Ⓕ Ⓒb

Gelato/Ices/Frozen Custard

Gelato: *Per ½ Cup*

	C	F	Cb
Milk base: Vanilla	160	6	25
Choc. Hazelnut	230	15	21
Water base, ½ cup	100	0	26

Frozen Custard: *Per ½ Cup*

	C	F	Cb
Chocolate	140	6	18
Orange Sherbet	105	2	21
Vanilla	130	6	16

Ice (Milk base): Average all flavors

	C	F	Cb
Hard (4% fat), ½ cup	100	3	15
Soft Serve (3% fat), ½ cup	110	2	19
Shaved Ice: Average, 12 fl. oz	160	0	40
Sherbet: Avg., ½ cup	110	1.5	22
Sorbet: Fruit (no fat), ½ cup	70	0	19
Fruit Ice Pops	80	0	20

Tofu Frozen Desserts: *See Page 35*

Sundaes   Ⓒ Ⓕ Ⓒb

Denny's: Sundaes,

	C	F	Cb
Single Scoop, no topping	190	14	14
Double Scoop, no topping	375	27	29
Banana Split	895	43	121
Toppings: Cherry, 3 oz	85	0	21
Chocolate, 2 oz	135	0.5	34
Fudge, 2 oz	200	10	30
Strawberry, 2 oz	80	1	17

McDonald's: Sundaes,

	C	F	Cb
Hot Fudge Sundae	330	10	54
Strawberry Sundae	280	6	49
Toppings: Peanuts, ¼ oz	45	3.5	2

Ice Cream Bars & Pops

See Pages 36-38

Ice Cream, Cones & Cups

Average All Brands	C	F	Cb
Wafer Cone/Cup, average	20	0	4
Sugar Cone, average	50	0	14
Waffle Cone:			
Small	50	1	10
Large	90	0.5	19
Brands:			
Oreo Chocolate Cone	50	1	10
Comet Sugar Cone	50	0	11
Keebler Sugar Cone	50	0	10

Ice Cream & Frozen Yogurt (Cont)

Brands | C | F | Cb

	C	F	Cb
Atkins: Per ½ Cup			
Endulge, average all flavors	155	13	14
Baldwin: Per ½ cup			
Blacksweet Cherry	160	8	19
Butter Pecan	180	11	16
Extreme Moose Tracks	200	12	20
Neopolitan	150	8	17
New York Cherry	160	8	19
Vanilla	160	9	16
Baskin-Robbins: See Fast-Foods Section			
Ben & Jerry's: Per ½ Cup			
Body & Soul: Cherry Garcia	170	9	22
Chocolate Chip Cookie Dough	190	9	26
Chocolate Fudge Brownie	180	7	25
Half Baked	190	8	29
Singles: Per Container (3.6 oz)			
Cherry Garcia	200	12	22
Chocolate Fudge Brownie	220	11	27
Cookie Dough	220	12	26
Vanilla	190	12	18
Original: Butter Pecan	280	21	20
Cherry Garcia	240	14	26
Chocolate	250	16	25
Chocolate Chip Cookie Dough	270	15	32
Chocolate Fudge Brownie	260	13	32
Chubby Hubby	330	20	31
Chunky Monkey	300	18	30
Coffee	230	14	21
Coffee Heath Bar Crunch	290	18	29
Everything But The...	310	19	30
Half Baked	280	14	34
Karamel Sutra	280	15	32
Mint Choc Chunk	270	17	26
New York Super Fudge Chunk	310	20	29
Oatmeal Cookie Chunk	270	15	31
Peanut Butter Cup	340	23	29
Phish Food	270	12	39
Pistachio Pistachio	260	17	21
Smores	290	16	36
Turtle Soup	280	15	30
Vanilla	230	14	21
Vanilla Heath Bar Crunch	290	17	29
Vermonty Python	310	19	30
Frozen Yogurt: Per ½ Cup			
Phish Food	210	6	37
Ligten-Up!: Black Raspberry	140	1.5	28
Cherry Garcia	160	3	31
Chocolate Fudge Brownie	170	2.5	34
Half Baked	180	3	35
Strawberries & Cream	150	3.5	29
Sorbet: Average all flavors	115	0	30
Bars/Pops: See Page 36			

	C	F	Cb
Blue Bunny			
Fat-Free, No Added Sugar: Per ½ Cup			
Brownie Sundae; Burgundy Cherry	90	0	23
Average other flavors	80	0	19
Reduced-Fat, No Added Sugar: Per ½ Cup			
Banana Split; Butter Pecan, avg.	125	5	18
Rocky Road	130	6	21
Turtle Sundae	140	7	20
Other flavors, avg.	120	5	17
Hi Lite: Butter Pecan; Fudge Nut	120	4.5	17
Caramel Pecan	130	4	21
Cookies & Cream; Vanilla, avg.	130	3.5	21
Other varieties, avg.	110	3	18
Personals (Light): Bunny Tracks	130	5	21
PB Fudge	130	5	18
Super Fudge Brownie	120	3	22
Other varieties, average	100	2.5	18
Frozen Yogurt, ½ cup	100	0	21
Bars/Pops: See Page 36			
Breyers: Per ½ Cup			
CarbSmart: Rocky Road	130	10	12
Chocolate	120	10	8
Vanilla	110	8	10
All Natural: Butter Pecan, avg.	160	10	14
Cherry Vanilla	140	8	17
Cookies & Cream; Rocky Road	160	8	19
Fried Ice Cream	140	4.5	22
Fruit Sherbet, average	130	1.5	26
Lactose Free Vanilla	130	7	14
Vanilla & Choc. & Strawberry	130	7	16
Other varieties, avg.	160	8	17
Creamery Style: Per ½ Cup			
Chocolate Caramel Brownie	150	4.5	23
Cookies & Cream	140	5	21
Creamy Vanilla; Extra Creamy Choc.	120	4	18
Cyclone Soft Serve: Per ½ Cup			
Average all varieties	150	7	20
Double Churn Fat-Free:			
Chocolate; Vanilla, average	90	0	22
Cappuccino Choc Chunk	110	0	26
Caramel Swirl	120	0	29
Light: Butter Pecan, ½ cup	120	5	16
Choc. Mocha Silk; Mint Choc. Chip	130	5	19
Rocky Road	130	4.5	22
Vanilla, Chocolate, Strawberry	100	3.5	16
Other varieties, average	120	4	19
No Sugar Added: Butter Pecan	110	6	14
Chocolate Fudge Brownie	90	1.5	20
Peanut Butter; Triple Choc., avg.	115	4	17
Other varieties, avg.	85	4	14
Wild Flavors: Peanut Butter Tracks	170	9	19
Very Chocolate Cherry	140	4.5	21
Other varieties, avg.	160	8	20

Brands (Cont)

	C	**F**	**Cb**
Brigham's: *Per ½ Cup*			
Ice Cream: Big Dig	210	12	24
Chocolate/Chip; Vanilla, avg.	195	13	19
Mocha Almond	210	15	18
Raspberry Lime Rickey Sherbert	130	2	27
Other varieties, avg.	190	11	21
Bruster's			
Frozen Yogurt: Chocolate, ½ cup	150	4.5	24
Vanilla, ½ cup	220	6.5	34
No Added Sugar Ice Cream: *Per ½ Cup*			
Chocolate; Vanilla, avg.	210	12	24
Choc. Caramel Swirl/Fudge Ripple	120	0	31
Cinnamon; Coffee	100	0	24
Other varieties, average	110	0	30
Carvel Ice Cream: *See Fast-Foods Section*			
Coldstone Creamery: *See Fast-Foods Section*			
Colombo: *Per ½ Cup*			
Frozen, Soft Serve: Non-Fat, avg.	105	0	22
Slender Sensations, average	60	0	15
Low-Fat, Old Worlde; Cookies	120	2	21
Sorbet, all varieties	100	0	25
Costco: Frozen Yogurt, 12 oz	270	0	57
CremaLita (Soft Serve)			

Calories will vary with density (air in product) and serving size. Best to weigh product and calculate on 25 cals per 1 oz weight.

	C	**F**	**Cb**
Vanilla: Small (4 fl.oz cup),			
If 2½ oz weight	60	0	14
If 4 oz weight*	100	0.5	23
If 6 oz weight*	150	1	35
(*) Most common weights			
Medium (8 fl.oz cup), 11 oz wt	275	1.5	63
Chocolate: Small, 6 oz weight	160	1	36
Dairy Queen/Brazier: *See Fast-Foods Section*			
Dippin' Dots			
Dots 'n Cream: *Per ½ Cup*			
Banana Split; Vanilla	170	10	16
Butter Pecan	180	10	18
Chocolate	165	10	15
Mint Chocolate Chip	200	9	25
Dove: *Per ½ Cup*			
Beyond Vanilla	240	15	23
Caramel Pecan Perfection	300	18	30
Chocolate & Brownie Affair	300	19	30
Irresistibly Raspberry	240	13	29
Unconditional Chocolate	290	17	21
Other varieties, avg.	300	19	30
Miniatures: All varieties, avg., 5 pcs	300	20	30

	C	**F**	**Cb**
Dreyers/Edys: *Per ½ Cup*			
Grand: Almond Praline	150	7	20
Chocolate; Vanilla Bean, avg.	150	8	17
Coffee; Neapolitan, avg.	140	8	15
Fudge Tracks; Peanut Butter Cup	180	11	18
Nestle Drumstick Sundae Cone	180	10	19
Real Strawberry	130	6	16
Toffee Bar Crunch	160	8	21
Vanilla	150	10	14
Other flavors, avg.	160	9	18
Slow Churned: Neopolitan	100	3	15
Cherry Choc Chip	120	4	18
Other varieties, average	110	4	18
Yogurt Blends, average	110	3	17
Sherbet, avg. all flavors	130	1.5	28
Friendly's: *Per ½ Cup Unless Indicated*			
Ice Cream: Butter Crunch	150	7	19
Chocolate Alm. Chip	160	10	17
Forbidden Chocolate	160	9	17
Hunka Chunka PB Fudge	240	16	21
Vanilla Choc. Strawberry	140	7	16
Vienna Mocha Chunk	180	9	20
Light: Purely Pistachio	120	5	16
Chocolate PB Swirl	150	7	18
Frozen Yogurt: *Per ½ Cup*			
Fudge Berry Swirl	150	4	24
Mint Chocolate Chip	130	4	21
Sundaes: *Per 3 Scoops*			
Apple Pie	1040	62	118
Royal Banana Split	940	37	136
Jim Dandy	1130	48	159
Reese's Peanut Butter Cup	930	54	90
Friend-Z's: Oreo Cookies, 12 fl.oz	750	23	120
Frostline (Soft Serve): Chocolate	90	1	19
Vanilla, ½ cup	100	1	20
Gelati-da			
Gelato: *Per ½ Cup (4 oz)*			
Amaretto Chocolate	150	4.5	23
Choc Mint Milano	120	2.5	22
Coffee Fudge Latte	130	2	22
Red Raspberry	130	1.5	25
Vanilla Marsala	120	2	21
White Chocolate	130	3	23

Brands (Cont)	C	F	Cb
Good Humor: *Per ½ Cup*			
Light: Cookies n' Crm	120	6	16
Choc.; Vanilla & Neopolitan, avg.	110	5	14
Strawberry Shortcake	130	4.5	23
Sherbets, all flavors	130	1	28
Haagen-Dazs			
Ice Cream, Sorbet, Frozen Yogurt: *See Fast-Foods Section*			
Bars: *See Page 37*			
Hola Fruta!: *Per ½ cup*			
Pure Fruit Sherbert: Margarita	140	1	30
Peach; Strawberry	130	1	31
Pina Colada	140	1.5	31
Pomegranate; Raspberry	140	1	32
Pomegranate & Blueberry	150	1	34
Hood: *Per ½ Cup*			
Frozen Yogurt: Mocha Fudge	120	0	27
Old Fashioned Vanilla	110	0	24
Low-Fat, Choc.Almond Pralin	140	3	23
Fat-Free, Double Raspberry	110	0	25
Ice Cream: Birthday Party	150	8	19
Chippedy Chocolaty	150	9	19
Chocolate	140	7	17
Cookie Dough Delight	160	8	20
Cookies'N Cream	160	8	19
Fudge Twister	150	7	20
Golden Vanilla	140	7	17
Holiday Egg Nog	150	8	17
Maple Walnut	150	9	17
Red Sox, Fenway Fudge	180	10	20
Light: Brownie Sundae	130	3.5	23
Other varieties, average	110	3	18
New England Creamery ~ *www.CalorieKing.com*			
Sherbet, average	110	0	27
Bars: *See Page 37*			
I Can't Believe It's Yogurt: *See Fast-Foods Section*			
Jerseymaid (Vons): *Per ½ Cup*			
Cookies & Cream	160	8	18
Choc Chip; Mint Choc Chip	150	9	16
Heavenly Hash; Nut Chunky Choc.	170	10	17
Mocha Almd Fudge; Rocky Road	155	9	17
Neopolitan; Vanilla	145	7	16
Strawberry	130	6	17
Oberweis: *Per ½ Cup*			
Chocolate	230	15	2
Chocolate Peanut Butter	280	19	21
Cookie Dough	230	13	26
Vanilla	210	14	18

Per Serving	C	F	Cb
Rice Dream (Non-Dairy): *Per ½ Cup*			
Carob Almond	180	10	26
Cocoa Marble Fudge; Neapolitan	150	6	24
Cookies N' Dream	170	8	24
Orange Vanilla Swirl	160	7	22
Strawberry	160	8	25
Supreme, avg all flavors	150	7	23
Tea Dreams, average	145	6.5	25
Vanilla	150	6	24
Vanilla Swiss Almond	190	10	24
Soy Delicious: *Per ½ Cup*			
It's Soy Delicious: Choc Almond	140	4.5	23
Choc Peanut Butter	135	3.5	24
Pistachio Almond	130	4.5	23
Other flavors, avg.	110	1.5	25
So Delicious Organic: Butter Pecan	160	7	22
Cookies'N Cream	150	4	26
Chocolate Velvet	130	3	24
Creamy Vanilla; Mocha Fudge	130	3	24
Neapolitan; Strawberry	120	3	23
Peanut Butter	150	6	23
Twisted Vanilla Orange	120	3	23
Other varieties, avg	140	4	25
Purely Decadent: PB Zig Zag	230	13	32
Swingin' Anna Bannana	230	13	31
Other flavors, avg.	200	8.5	32
Soy Dream (Non-Dairy): *Per ½ Cup*			
Butter Pecan	140	9	17
Green Tea	140	8	18
Vanilla	140	7	18
Starbucks: *Per ½ Cup*			
Caramel Cappuccino	240	12	30
Classic Coffee	230	12	26
Coffee Almond Fudge; Java Chip	250	13	29
Coffee Fudge Brownie	190	11	25
Mud Pie	240	11	32
Low-Fat Latte	170	3	30
Bars: *See Page 38*			
Stonyfield Farm (Organic)			
Ice Cream, Super Premium: *Per ½ Cup*			
After Dark Chocolate	250	17	21
Chocolate Raspberry Swirl	230	13	25
Cookies 'n Dream	270	18	27
Creme Caramel	250	14	29
Gotta Have Vanilla; Vanilla Chai, avg.	240	16	21
Javalanche	250	16	22

Brands (Cont)

	C	F	Cb
Stop & Shop: *Per ½ Cup*			
Butterscotch Ripple	140	7	19
Chocolate	140	8	18
Chocolate Chip (Reg./Chunky)	150	9	17
Country Club	130	6	19
Heavenly Hash	170	8	22
Neopolitan; Vanilla	140	8	16
Vanilla Fudge Swirl	150	8	18

TCBY

	C	F	Cb
Soft Serve Frozen Yogurt: *Average all Flavors*			
96% Fat-Free: Kids Cup	100	2	16
Junior Cup	175	4	29
Small Cup	245	5	40
Regular Cup	315	7	52
Large Cup	385	8	63
Non-Fat: Junior Cup	140	0	29
Small Cup	190	0	40
Regular Cup	250	0	52
Large Cup	300	0	63
No Sugar Added/Non-Fat: Small	160	0	35
Regular Cup	200	0	45
Large Cup	250	0	55
Low-Carb Lovers: Small	190	12	28
Regular	250	16	36
Large Cup	300	19	44
Kids	75	5	11
Hand Scooped Frozen Yogurt: *Average all Flavors*			
Kids Cup	90	3	14
Junior Cup	165	5	26
Small Cup	230	8	37
Regular Cup	300	10	47
Large Cup	365	12	58
No Added Sugar, Vanilla:			
Small Cup	140	1	33
Regular Cup	180	1	43
Large Cup	220	1.5	52

Tasti D-Lite (Soft Serve)

Calories will vary with density (air in product) and serving size
Best to weigh product and calculate on 25 cals per 1 oz weight.

	C	F	Cb
Vanilla: Small (4 fl.oz cup), 6 oz wt	180	4	35
Medium (8 fl.oz cup), 11 oz wt	330	7	64

Tofutti, Non-Dairy Dessert: *Per ½ Cup*

	C	F	Cb
Premium Pints: Better Pecan	210	13	21
Chocolate Cookie Crunch	210	11	26
Chocolate Supreme	180	11	18
Vanilla	210	13	21
Vanilla Almond Bark	240	15	24
Vanilla Fudge; Wildberry, avg.	190	9	25

Per Serving

	C	F	Cb
Turkey Hill: *Per ½ Cup*			
Premium: Black Cherry	130	6	18
Butter Pecan	160	10	15
Choc Mint	160	9	17
Chocolate Peanut Butter Cup	180	11	18
Cookies 'n Crm	150	8	19
French Vanilla	140	7	16
Rocky Road	170	8	23
Tin Roof Sundae	150	8	19
Lite: Moose Tracks	130	6	19
Peanut Butter Mania	130	5	19
Vanilla Bean	100	2.5	16
Other flavors, average	120	4	19
All Natural: Average all flavors	140	8	17
CarbIQ: PB Paradise	150	12	13
Choco Mint Chip	120	9	14
Chocolate; Vanilla Bean	110	8	11
No Sugar Added: *Per ½ Cup*			
Cherry Fudge Ripple	80	0	22
Dutch Chocolate; Vanilla	70	0	20
Peanut Brittle	120	0	16
Frozen Yogurt: Graham Canyon	160	7	21
Choc. Chip Cookie Dough	130	3.5	21
Low-Fat: Mint Cookies 'n Cream	110	1.5	21
Vanilla Bean	100	2	17
Fat-Free: Choc. Marshmallow	110	0	24
Other flavors, average	100	0	21
Smoothie, all flavors, average	100	0	21
Sherbet	120	1	26

Walgreens

	C	F	Cb
One Pint Container: *Per ½ Cup*			
Banana Split	130	5	20
Creme de Menthe	160	9	19
Homemade Vanilla	130	7	16
New York Cherry	130	6	17
Rocky Road	150	7	18
Strawberries 'n Cream	130	6	14
Toasted Butter Pecan	170	10	18
Waffle Cone	150	7	19
Scoops Orange Sherbert	120	1	26
1¾ Quart Container: *Per ½ Cup*			
Banana Split	150	6	22
Homemade Vanilla	150	8	17
New York Cherry	150	7	20
WholeSoy & Co., ½ cup (70g), avg.	120	1	25

Ice Cream Bars & Pops

Bars & Pops

Per Bar/Serving

	C	F	Cb
Barq's Root Beer & Ice Cream Float, 4 fl.oz cup	120	3	22
Ben & Jerry's			
Peace Pops: Cherry Garcia (1)	270	19	29
Almond Original	340	23	30
Cookie Dough (1)	340	16	46
Vanilla (1)	300	20	46
The Bar	360	16	46
The Cone	360	19	44
Novelties: 'Wich Ice Cream, Cookie Sandwich	350	18	45
Big Bear: *See Klondike*			
Big Ed's Super Saucer, 10 fl.oz	590	29	75
Blue Bunny: Ice Pops, avg.	120	0	24
Bomb Pops, avg.	50	0	11
Chocolate Cup, 1.7 oz	100	5	12
Choc Raspberry	270	18	25
Cookies and Cream	250	15	28
Fudge Bar, 2.7 oz	110	1.5	21
Health Smart, 2.2 oz	60	0	15
Hot Fudge Bar	370	25	33
Milk Choc Bar	300	21	25
Milk Choc with Almonds	320	23	25
Mini Mix, 4 pieces, 91g	320	19	35
Sno Cone, 200g	60	0	15
Sweet Freedom S'wich, avg.	140	1.5	32
Twin Pops	70	0	18
Turtle Bar	360	24	33
Twin Pops	70	0	18
Vanilla Brownie Cone, King Size	440	22	56
Vanilla Nutty Cone, 3 oz	250	11	34
Personals: Banana Split	170	8	22
Turtle Sundae	180	10	21
Supreme: Bunny Tracks	220	14	22
Peanut Butter Panic	230	16	19
Super Fudge Brownie	200	12	23
Bon Bons *(Nestlé):* Milk Choc., (8)	330	22	29
Dark Chocolate, 8 pces	310	22	29
Breyers			
Pure Fruit Bars: Coconut	150	2.5	31
Fruit & Cream	60	0.5	12
Fruit Swirl, all varieties, 1.7 oz	40	0	10
Goya Strawb./ Mangos & Cream	90	2	16
Lime	110	0	27
No Sugar Added Bar	25	0	5
Pineapple	100	0	26
Strawberry	100	0	25
CarbSmart Bar: Fudge Bar	100	7	9
Almond Bar; Vanilla Bar, avg.	175	15	9

Per Bar/Serving

	C	F	Cb
Breyers (Cont)			
Ice Cream Poppers: Heath (27)	410	30	32
Hershey's (27)	430	31	31
Oreo (27)	410	27	38
Reese's (27)	470	34	35
Double Churned Extra Creamy Bars: *Per Bar*			
Light: Cookies & Cream Sandwich	140	1.5	30
Vanilla Sandwich	130	1.5	28
Bars: Rocky Road	180	9	23
Vanilla	160	8	21
Vanilla & Almond	170	9	21
Blisscotti: Coffee & Milk Chocolate	280	15	34
Raspberry & Dark Chocolate	270	15	28
Vanilla & Chocolate	290	15	33
Butterfinger *(Nestle):* 52g Bar	180	13	16
King Size, 112g	310	22	26
California Natural: Mango Sorbet	130	0	33
Lemon & Strawberry Sorbet Cups	120	0	31
Carnation *(Nestle):* Sandwich, avg.	195	8	28
Sundae Cups, average	205	10	28
Chiquita: Swirls, all flavors	80	3	12
Cool Creations			
Cool Classics: Pops, average	35	0	9
Mini Sandwich	110	4	16
Vanilla Sandwich	170	6	28
Toffee/Chocolate Bar, avg.	155	11	14
Cream Pops, 61g	100	2.5	18
Fudge Pops	100	1	21
Sundae Cones	300	18	30
Creamsicle: Sugar-Free Pops (2)	40	2	10
Orange, 2.7 oz	110	2	21
Orange, 1.65 oz	70	1	13
Crunch *(Nestle):* Caramel	210	14	19
Vanilla Flavored	210	14	18
Reduced-Fat	140	8	15
Disney Magic: Orange Pop Tops	90	0	20
Chocolate & Vanilla Pop Tops	110	5	13
Dove: Original Dove	320	21	32
Milk Chocolate	330	21	31
Milk Chocolate w. Almonds	340	23	28
Triple Chocolate	340	22	35
Miniatures, 5 pces	300	20	30
Dreyers/Edys			
Dibs: With Chocolaty Coating (26 Pieces)			
Caramel	440	32	35
Chocolate; Mint; Vanilla	420	32	29
Coffee	400	29	31
Peanut Butter	510	39	32
Van. w. Nestle Crunch/Drumstick	390	29	29
Whole Fruit Bars	80	0	20
Whole Fruit Smoothie Bars	100	2	20

Bars & Pops (Cont)	C	F	Cb
Per Bar/Serving			
Drumstick *(Nestlé)*: Classic	360	23	33
Original Vanilla	340	21	33
Vanilla Caramel	360	22	36
Reduced Fat, Vanilla	280	13	36
Simply Dipped: Vanilla	320	17	38
Cookies & Cream	330	17	40
Eskimo Pie			
No Sugar Added, Van. Dark Choc	120	8	13
Milk/Dark Choc	160	11	14
Fat Boy: Ice Cream Sandwich	220	10	30
Cookies N Cream Sandwich	240	10	34
Ice Cream Sandwich Jr., 49g	120	5	17
Nut Sundae on a Stick	310	24	21
Raspberry Cheesecake Sandwich	220	8	33
FrozFruit:			
Banana; Strawb. Crm Bar, avg.	160	6	27
Fruit Bars: Pina Colada	180	10	21
Coconut	150	10	14
Superfruit Bar: Acacia	60	0	15
Cherry	80	0	19
Fruit A Freeze: Coconut	160	9	20
Lime	70	0	17
Banana; Strawberry	120	4	19
Cappuccino	140	6	21
Dark Choc-Dipped Strawberry	210	12	26
Mango	70	0	16
Fudge Bar *(Nestlé)*	110	1	23
Fudgesicle: Fudge Bar (1)	100	2	17
Fat-Free (1)	70	0	14
No Added Sugar	40	0	10
Good Humor: Oreo Bar	250	15	28
Candy Center Crunch	310	23	24
Cherry Lemonade Freeze, 10 oz	230	0	58
Chocolate Eclair	220	11	30
Premium Vanilla	260	17	24
Reese's Peanut Butter Cup	310	21	27
Toasted Almond	235	12	30
Cones: Giant King	390	21	44
King	250	13	30
Premium Sundae	260	15	29
Strawberry Shortcake, 4 oz	230	12	30
Sandwiches: Premium Vanilla	160	5	26
Cherry Lemonade Freeze, 10 oz	230	0	58
Choc Chip Cookie	280	13	41
Giant Neapolitan/Van., 6 oz	250	9	38
Swirlwind Cup, 6 oz	160	2.5	31

	C	F	Cb
Per Bar/Serving			
Haagen-Dazs: Mint & Dark Choc	290	20	23
Chocolate & Dark Chocolate	300	21	24
Coffee & Almond Crunch	310	22	23
Dulce de Leche	300	19	28
Raspberry Sorbet & Vanilla Yogurt	90	0	21
Vanilla & Almonds	320	23	22
Vanilla & Dark Chocolate	300	21	23
Vanilla & Milk Chocolate	290	21	22
Healthy Choice: Fudge Bar	80	1	13
Caramel Swirl Sandwich	150	2	30
Fudge Bar	80	1	13
Ice Cream Bar w. Fudge Coating	80	1	13
Swirls, average	90	1.5	17
Vanilla Sandwich	130	3	25
Hood: Chocolate Eclair, 1 bar	150	10	14
Fudge Bar: Chocolate	90	0.5	19
Fudge Stix	90	0	20
Nutty Royal Cone	220	12	26
Vanilla Sandwich	180	6	29
Light Sandwich	160	3	29
Hoodsie Cup Van./Choc.	100	5	12
Hoodsie Pops	60	0	16
Orange Cream Bar	90	1.5	19
Rocket, 54g	120	5	16
Sport Sundae Bar	250	16	26
Ice Cream Sandwich *(Nestle)*	240	10	34
Icee Freeze, 2.25 oz	70	0	17
Klondike: Choco Taco	290	15	36
Caramel Pretzel	260	14	30
Dark Chocolate	250	17	22
Heath Bar	250	17	22
Hershey's Almond Bar	240	15	23
Krunch Bar	250	17	22
Sara Lee Strawberry Cheesecake	290	18	29
Movie Bites	290	21	24
Nascar Bar	200	14	31
Oreo Bar	260	17	26
Original Bar	250	17	22
Reese's Peanut Butter Bar	260	16	26
Triple Chocolate	240	14	27
Whitehouse Cherry	250	17	24
Slim a Bear:			
No Sugar Added: Van. S'wich	100	2	21
Vanilla/Krunch Bar	170	10	21
100 Calories: Fudge Bar	100	2.5	19
Sandwich, 3 oz	100	1.5	21
Cones: Klondike Sundae Cone	300	16	35
Vanilla Sundae Cone	280	16	30
Sandwich: Oreo Cookie	230	9	35
Choc Chip Cookie	260	12	38
Original Vanilla	190	7	29

Per Bar/Serving	C	F	Cb
Luigi's Real Italian Ice: *Per Cup (6 fl.oz)*			
All flavors, average	130	0	33
Squeeze Tubes, 4 oz	70	0	18
M&Ms: Cookie Ice Cream S'wich	220	10	29
Cone, 79g	255	12	34
Matterhorn Cone, 10 fl.oz	510	38	19
Milky Way Ice Cream Bar	220	12	25
Minute Maid: Fruit Juice Pops	60	0	15
Soft Frozen Lemonade	70	0	19
Molli Coolz: Strawb. & Cream, 2.5 oz	90	10	7
Cookies and Cream, 2.5 oz	155	10	14
Sour Cherry, 2.5 oz	70	1	13
Nestlé: Push Up Pop, average	80	1	18
Crunch Vanilla, 3 oz bar	210	14	18
Mini Wiches	90	3	14
Rolo King Size, 4 oz	300	19	30
Drumstick: Cookies n Cream	350	19	40
Vanilla w. Choc Layers	440	24	50
Toll House Sandwich, Choc Chip	500	24	64
No Pudge: Choc Eclair Bar	110	1.5	20
Brownie Batter Swirl	130	1.5	28
Cookies and Cream	100	2.5	21
Cones, average	140	2.5	24
Fudgy Bar	60	0	18
Strawberry Shortcake	90	1	20
Oreo: Sandwich	260	11	38
Pathmark Vanilla w. choc. coat.	150	10	14
Pops (water/juice), avg., 1.75 fl.oz	40	0	10
Popsicles: Big Stick Ice Pops	60	0	15
Creamsicle Pop, 1.65 fl.oz	70	1	13
Fudgesicle Fudge Pop	100	2	17
Fat-Free	70	0	14
No Added Sugar	40	1	9
Fear Factor Pop Ups	90	0	23
Firecracker	40	0	10
Minis Ice Cream Pop (3)	40	0	9
Rainbow, 1.65 fl.oz	40	0	10
Sponge Bob Squarepants Pop Up	80	1	16
Strawberry Shortcake	170	9	21
Scribblers Pops: 2 pces	60	0	15
ACE Juice Pops, 2 pces	50	0	12
Ice Pops: 1 pce	60	0	15
Sugar-Free, 1 pce, 1.9 oz	15	0	4
Reese's Peanut Butter Ice Cream	270	18	24
Rice Dream: Pies, all flavors	330	19	40
Bars: Vanilla	230	15	24
Choc/Vanilla Nutty	320	24	27
Tea Dreams Bar	240	15	28
Safeway Select Coffee Almd Bar	270	17	26

Per Bar/Serving	C	F	Cb
Skinny Cow			
Fat-Free Chocolate Fudge Bar	100	0	22
No Added Sugar Fudge	110	2	19
Vanilla/Strawberry Sorbet Bar	110	0.5	22
Cones, average	150	3	28
Sandwiches, all flavors	145	2	30
Snapple: Snapple Flavored Stick	80	0	20
Snapple On Ice	40	0	10
Diet Snapple On Ice	15	0	1
Snickers: Ice Cream Bar, 50g	180	11	18
Cone	280	15	33
Snack Bar (1)	90	6	9
So Delicious Sugar Free: Fudge Bar	80	5	12
Vanilla Bar	150	14	15
Soy Delicious: Sandwiches, avg.	150	3	28
Minis	90	2	17
Soy Dream (Non-Dairy):			
Lil' Dreamers, Choc; Vanilla	100	4	15
Starbuck's Frappuccino Bars, avg.	120	2	22
Mud Pies Bars	320	19	32
Sweet Nothings: Fudge Bar	100	0	23
Mango Raspberry	100	0	23
Other flavors, 3 oz, average	120	0	28
Tofutti			
Cuties: Peanut Butter	165	8	20
Other varieties, avg.	125	5	17
Sticks: Fudge Treats Bar	30	0	6
Marry Me Bar	170	8	22
Mint by Mintz	170	7	7
Totally Fudge Pops	95	1.5	19
Trader Joe's Fruit Floes: Cafe Latte	130	0	26
Caribbean, 4 oz	80	0	21
Mocha Fudge	140	1.5	20
Strawberry, 4 oz	110	0	31
Trix: Pops, regular	40	0	10
Sugar Free	15	0	4
Tropicana: Fruit Wise Bar	180	0	36
Turkey Hill: Ice Cream Sandwich	190	7	30
Light Sandwich	160	3	32
Sundae Cone	320	18	33
Twix Bar	170	10	19
Weight Watchers			
English Toffee Crunch	110	6	13
Fudge Sundae Cups, average	160	1	38
Fudge Sundae Cones, average	140	4	32
Giant Cookies 'n Cream	140	5	26
Giant Fudge Bar	110	1	25
Wildberry & Orange Bar, average	110	0.5	29
Strawb., Passionfr., Lime Sorbet Bar	60	0.5	13
Sandwich: Rounds, average	140	2	33
Vanilla	120	2	28

Quick Guide

Cream

	C	F	Cb
Average All Brands			
Half & Half Cream:			
1 Tbsp, 0.5 oz	20	1.5	0.5
2 Tbsp, 1 oz	40	3	1
Light: Coffee/table (20% fat): 1 T.	30	3	0.5
2 Tbsp, 1 oz	60	6	1
Sour Cream:			
Regular: 1 Tbsp, 0.5 oz	25	2.5	1
1 cup, 8 oz	490	48	10
Low-Fat/Light: 1 Tbsp, 0.5 oz	20	1.5	1
2 Tbsp, 1 oz	40	3	2
Fat-Free: Average, 2 Tbsp, 1 oz	25	0	4
Hood, 2 Tbsp, 1 oz	25	0	4
Kroger, 2 Tbsp, 1 oz	20	0	3
Naturally Yours; Oak Farm, 2 T.	20	0	3
Knudsen, 2 Tbsp, 1 oz	30	0	5
Sour Cream Substitute:			
Albertson's, 2 Tbsp, 1 oz	60	5	2
Tofutti Sour Supreme, 2 T., 1 oz	85	7	9
Whipping Cream:			
Heavy (37% fat):			
1 Tbsp fluid/2 Tbsp whipped	50	5.5	0.5
¼ cup whipped	100	11	1
½ cup fluid/1 cup whipped	400	44	3.5
Light (30% fat):			
1 Tbsp fluid/2 Tbsp whipped	45	4.5	0.5
½ cup fluid/1 cup whipped	350	37	4

Coconut Cream/Milk

	C	F	Cb
Coconut Cream (Canned),			
Plain/unsweetened: 2 Tbsp, 1 oz	75	6.5	3
½ cup, 4 oz	285	26	12
Sweetened: *Coco Lopez,* 1 oz	130	5	21
½ cup, 4 oz	520	20	84
Coconut Milk (Canned):			
Natural Value: Reg., ¼ c., 2 fl.oz	105	10	2
Lite, ¼ fl.oz	55	5	1
Thai Kitchen: Lite, ¼ cup, 2 fl.oz	45	4	1
Premium, 2 fl.oz	120	10	4
Coconut Water (Center), 1 cup	45	0.5	9

Whipped Toppings

	C	F	Cb
Average All Brands			
Cream (Pressurized): 2 Tbsp	20	1	1
¼ cup	45	4	2
½ cup	90	8	4
Cream Topping: Lite, 2 Tbsp	20	1	3
Cool Whip: Extra Creamy, 2 T.	25	2	2
Lite, 2 Tbsp, 9g	20	1	3
Free, 2 Tbsp, 9g	15	0	3
Kraft: Dream Whip, 2 Tbsp	15	0	2
Reddi-Wip: Original, 2 T., 8g	15	1	0.5
Chocolate, 2 Tbsp, 8g	15	1	1
Extra Creamy, 2 Tbsp, 8g	15	1.5	0.5
Fat-Free, 2 Tbsp, 8g	5	0	1

Non-Dairy Coffee Creamers

	C	F	Cb
Powder:			
Coffee-Mate/Cremora/N-Rich			
Original, 1 tsp	10	0.5	1
1 heaping tsp	25	2	2
Lite, 1 tsp	10	0	2
Flavors: 4 tsps	60	3	8
Fat-Free: Average, 4 tsps	60	2.5	9
Liquid/Refrigerated: *Per Tablespoon*			
Coffee-Mate Non-Dairy Creamer			
Plain: Original/Plain, 1 Tbsp	20	1	2
Fat-Free, 1 Tbsp	10	0	2
Low-Fat, 1 Tbsp	10	0.5	1
Flavors: All flavors, 1 Tbsp	40	2	5
Fat-Free, all flavors, 1 Tbsp	25	0	5
Hood (Non-Dairy), 1 Tbsp	20	1.5	2
International Delight: 1 Tbsp	35	1.5	6
Fat-Free flavors, 1 Tbsp	30	0	7
Mocha Mix: Original, 1 Tbsp	20	1.5	1
Fat-Free, 1 Tbsp	10	0	1
Lite, 1 Tbsp	10	0.5	1
Silk (*White Wave*) Creamer, 1Tbsp	20	1	3
French Vanilla; Hazelnut, 1 T.	20	1	3

Get Moving!
Take a computer
break every hour.

Fats, Spreads & Oils

 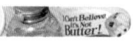

Quick Guide   **C** **F** **Cb**

Butter & Margarine
Average All Brands

	C	F	Cb
Regular: 1 tsp (5g)	35	4	0
1 Pat (5g)	35	4	0
1 Tbsp, approx. ½ oz	100	11	0
2 Tbsp, 1 oz	205	23	0
1 Stick, ½ cup, 4 oz	815	92	0
1 Pound, 2 cups, 16 oz	3260	360	0
Light (Regular) 40% Fat:			
1 tsp (5g)	25	3	0
1 Tbsp, ½ oz	75	8.5	0
2 Tbsp, 1 oz	150	16	0
Whipped Butter (Regular):			
1 tsp (4 g)	30	3	0
1 Tbsp (10g)	70	7.5	0
1 Stick, ½ cup, 2 ⅔ oz	545	62	0
Whipped Light Butter 40% Fat:			
1 tsp, 5g	25	3	0.5
1 Tbsp, 9g	45	5	1
2 Tbsp, 18g	90	10	2
Unsalted: Same as Regular			

Clarified Butter

	C	F	Cb
100% Fat: 1 tsp (5g)	45	5	0
1 Tbsp, 1 oz	180	20	0

Flavored Butter/Spread

Average All Brands

	C	F	Cb
Honey Butter (60% Fat):			
1 Tbsp, ½ oz	90	8	4
Downey's, 1 Tbsp, ½ oz	60	1	11
Garlic Butter (80% Fat):			
1 Tbsp, ½ oz	100	11	0
Macadamia Butter, 1 Tbsp	115	12	2
Sweet Cream Butter:			
Regular, 1 Tbsp	100	11	0
Stick *(Parkay)*, 70% Fat, 1 Tbsp	90	10	0
Tub *(Land O'Lakes)*, 60% Fat, 1 T.	80	8	0

Other Spreads & Fats

	C	F	Cb
Copha, Dripping, Lard, Suet, Shortening:			
1 Tbsp, ½ oz	120	13	0
Chicken, Duck, Goose Fat:			
1 Tbsp, ½ oz	115	13	0

Light & Reduced Fat Spreads

Per 1 Tbsp, ½ oz (Unless Stated)   **C** **F** **Cb**

	C	F	Cb
Albertson's: Country (48%), 1T.	60	7	0
Butter Blend, 1 Tbsp	80	9	0
Benecol: Spread, 1 Tbsp, 14g	70	8	0
Light, Spread, 1 Tbsp, 14g	50	5	0
Blue Bonnet, Homestyle (48% Veg Oil)	60	7	0
Brummel & Brown, Spread, 1 T.	45	5	0
Country Crock *(Shedd's)*: Regular	80	7	0
Light; Calcium & Vitamins	50	5	0
Spreadable Butter, 1 Tbsp	80	9	0
Downey's, Honey Butter, 1 Tbsp	60	1	11
Fleischmann's: Soft Spread	70	8	0
Original Stick, 1 Tbsp	100	11	0
Light Spread, 1 Tbsp	40	4.5	0
'I Can't Believe It's Not Butter': Reg.	80	8	0
Light; Sweet Cream	50	6	0
Imperial: Stick, 1 Tbsp	80	9	0
Tub, 1 Tbsp	60	7	0
Land O'Lakes: Buttery Taste, 1 T.	80	8	0
Honey Butter, 1 Tbsp	90	8	4
Light Butter Whipped, 1 Tbsp	45	5	0
Light Butter, 1 Tbsp	50	6	0
Parkay: Squeeze, 1 Tbsp	70	8	0
Light Stick, 1 Tbsp	50	5	0
Original Stick, 1 Tbsp	80	9	0
Original, 1 Tbsp	60	7	0
Promise: Buttery, 1 Tbsp	80	8	0
Fat-Free, 1 Tbsp	5	0	0
Buttery Light, 1 Tbsp	45	5	0
Smart Balance: 67% Buttery, 1 T.	80	9	0
Light (37%), 1 Tbsp	45	5	0
Smart Beat, Fat-Free, 1 Tbsp	50	0	1
Smart Squeeze, 1 Tbsp	5	0	1
Take Control: Regular, 1 Tbsp	80	8	0
Light Spread, 1 Tbsp	45	5	0

Canola Margarine contains beneficial omega-3 fats.
(Extra Notes ~ Page 272)

Butter Substitutes C F Cb

	C	F	Cb
Butter Buds: 1 serving, ½ tsp	5	0	2
Sprinkles, 1 tsp	5	0	0
Earth Balance, Non GMO,1 Tbsp	100	11	0
Molly McButter, ½ tsp	5	0	1
Shedd's Willow Run, Soy, 1 T.	100	1	0
Sunsweet: Baking Butter, 1 Tbsp	35	0	9
Lighter Bake, 1 Tbsp	35	0	9

Spreads Comparison

	C	F	Cb
Mayonnaise: Regular, 1 Tbsp	100	11	0
Light, average, 1 Tbsp	50	5	1
Fat-Free, 1 T.	10	0	2
Miracle Whip (Kraft):			
Regular, 1 Tbsp	40	3.5	2
Light, 1 Tbsp	25	1.5	3
Free, 1 Tbsp	15	0	3
Smart Beat Dressing: 1 Tbsp	10	0	2.5

Extra Listings for Mayonnaise & Dressings
~ See Page 89 ~

	C	F	Cb
Avocado, mashed, 1 Tbsp	45	4	2.5
Peanut Butter, 1 Tbsp	100	8	3.5
Nutella, 1 Tbsp	100	5.5	12

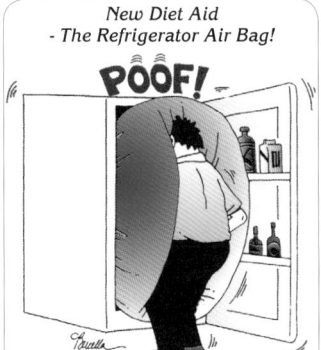

New Diet Aid
- The Refrigerator Air Bag!

POOF!

Animal Fats/Lards C F Cb

Average All Types
Beef Tallow/Drippings, Lard (Pork),
Chicken, Duck, Goose, Turkey.

	C	F	Cb
1 Tbsp (13g)	115	13	0
2¼ Tbsp, 1 oz	255	28	0
1 cup, 7¼ oz	1850	205	0
½ pound, 8 oz	2040	227	0
Ghee/Butter Oil: 1 Tbsp, 13g	110	13	0
2¼ Tbsp, 1 oz	250	28	0

Vegetable Shortening

Average All Types (example, Crisco)

	C	F	Cb
1 Tbsp, 0.44 oz	113	13	0
2¼ Tbsp, 1 oz	250	28	0
1 cup, 7¼ oz	1810	205	0

Vegetable Oils

Includes almond, avocado, canola, corn, coconut, flaxseed, grapeseed, linseed, mustard, olive, palm, peanut, rice-bran, safflower, sesame, sunflower, soybean, wheatgerm. Note: Oil is 100% fat.

	C	F	Cb
1 tsp, 5g	45	5	0
1 Tbsp, ½ oz	120	14	0
2 Tbsp, 1 oz	250	28	0
1 cup, 7¾ oz	1930	205	0

Fish Oils

Average All Types (Includes cod liver, herring, salmon, sardine):

	C	F	Cb
1 Tbsp, ½ oz	125	14	0

Cooking Sprays/Squeezes

Cooking Sprays (Pam, Mazola, I Can't Believe It's Not Butter, Weight Watchers, Wesson):

	C	F	Cb
Per serving	2	0	0
1-3 second spray	6	1	0
I Can't Believe It's Not Butter	0	0	0
Parkay Buttery Spray	0	0	0
Squeeze (Parkay), 1 Tbsp, 0.5 oz	70	8	0

Olestra (Olean)

	C	F	Cb
Olestra *(Olean)*	0	0	0

Olean is Proctor & Gamble's brand name for olestra – a no-calorie cooking oil that gives snacks (like potato chips, tortilla chips and crackers) taste and texture without adding fat or calories.

Cheese

Quick Guide   C F Cb

Firm/Hard Cheeses
(American, Cheddar, Colby, Coon, Swiss)

Regular Cheese:

	C	F	Cb
Thin Deli slice, ¾ oz	90	7	0
1 oz slice/piece	115	9	0.5
8 oz package	915	75	3
16 oz (1lb) package	1830	150	6
Cubes: 1" cube, ¾ oz	85	7	0.5
1¼" cube, 1 oz slice	115	9	0.5
Diced: 1 cup, 4½ oz	530	40	2
Grated: 1 Tbsp, ¼ oz	30	2.5	0
Shredded: Cheddar, ¼ cup, 1 oz	115	9	0.5
1 cup, 4 oz	455	37	1.5
Cheddar, Red.-Fat, ¼ cup, 1 oz	80	6	1
Mozzarella: ¼ cup, 1 oz	85	6.5	0.5
Part-Skim, ¼ cup, 1 oz	70	5	1
Sliced: 1 thin (3½" sq.), ¾ oz	85	7	0.5
Rectangular (7"x 4"x ⅛"), 1½ oz	170	14	0.5
Round (3¼" diam. x ⅛ "), ¾ oz	85	7	0.5
Semi-circular, 1¼ oz			
(5½" long, 3½" radius, ⅛" thick)	140	12	0.5
Fat-Free: Average all brands, 1 oz	40	0	2
Low-Fat: Average all brands, 1 oz	50	2	0.5
Reduced Fat: Avg. all brands, 1 oz	80	5	0.5

Cheese   C F Cb

Per 1 oz Unless Indicated

American:

	C	F	Cb
Regular: 1 slice, 1 oz	105	9	0.5
Alpine Lace, 1 oz	90	7	2
Kraft, 0.7 oz slice	70	5	2
Shredded, ¼ cup, 1 oz	115	9	0.5
Land O'Lakes, 0.7 oz slice	80	5	2
Light: Kraft (2% Milk), 0.7 oz slice	50	3	1
Fat-Free: Kraft, 0.7 oz slice	30	0	2
Borden, Singles, 0.7 pce	80	0	2
Babybel (Laughing Cow), 21g	70	6	0
Light Original, 21g pce	50	3	0
Bonbel (Laughing Cow), 1 pce	70	6	0
Brick (Land O'Lakes), 1" cube, 1 oz	110	8	1
Brie, 1 oz	95	8	0
Camembert, 1 oz	85	7	0
Caraway, 1 oz	105	8	1
Castello (Wegman's), avg., 1 oz	120	12	0

Cheddar: (Also see 'Quick Guide')

	C	F	Cb
Regular: 1 oz	115	9	0.5
Alpine Lace, 1 oz	90	7	0
Reduced-Fat/Low-Fat:			
Borden, Shredded, ¼ cup, 1 oz	80	6	1
Cabot Vermont, 50% Light, 1 oz	70	4.5	0.5
Lifetime, 1oz	45	1.5	3
Fat-Free, Kraft, 0.7 oz slice	30	0	2
Cheese Balls (Kaukauna), 1 oz, avg.	100	7	0.5
Cheese Nut, average, 1 oz	100	7	2
Cheese Logs (Kaukauna), avg., 1 oz	100	7	0.5
Cheshire, 1 oz	110	9	1.5
Colby: Regular, 1 oz	110	9	0.5
Reduced-Fat (Kraft), 1 oz	80	6	0
Colby-Jack, regular, 1 oz	110	9	1

Cottage Cheese: *Average All Brands*

	C	F	Cb
Creamed (4% milk fat): 2 Tbsp, 1 oz	30	1	1.5
½ cup, 4 oz	120	5	6
w. fruit, ½ cup, 4 oz	130	4	15
Reduced-Fat (2%): 2 T., 1 oz	25	0.5	1
½ cup, 4 oz	100	2	4
Low-Fat (1%): 2 Tbsp, 1 oz	20	.5	1
½ cup, 4 oz	80	1	3
Fat-Free/Non-Fat: 2 Tbsp, 1 oz	20	0	1
(Jewel), ½ cup, 4 oz	80	0	5
Friendship: Low-Fat P'apple, 4 oz	120	1	16
Non-Fat w. Peach, ½ c., 4 oz	110	0	15
Pot Style, ½ cup, 4 oz	90	2.5	3
Hood w. Chive/Onion, 4 oz	90	1	5
Knudsen:			
Free: Non-Fat, ½ cup, 4.oz	80	0	7
2% Milk Fat, ½ cup, 4 oz	100	2.5	6
Cottage Doubles, avg, 5.5 oz ctn	150	2.5	18
On the Go! Free, 4 oz ctn	70	0	7
Low-Fat, 4 oz ctn	90	2.5	6
Lactaid: Low-Fat, ½ cup, 4 oz	80	1	7
Light N' Lively: Fat-Free, 4.4 oz	80	0	8
Low-Fat, ½ cup, 4.4 oz	80	1.5	6
Cream Cheese: *See Page 45*			
Edam, Regular, 1 oz	100	8	0.5
Farmer (Friendship), 2 Tbsp, 1 oz	50	2.5	0
Feta: Regular, 1 oz	75	6	1
Crumbled, ½ cup, 2½ oz	190	15	3
Reduced-Fat (Athenos), 1 oz	60	4	1
Fontina, 1 oz	110	9	0.5
Gjetost (Goat's Milk, fresh), 1 oz	130	8	12
Wegman's, 1 oz	130	9	11

Goat's Milk Cheese:	C	F	Cb
Chevre, Soft, 1 oz	80	6	1
Chavril: 3 Tbsp, 1 oz	60	4.5	0.5
Semi-Soft, 1 oz	100	8.5	1
Hard, 1 oz	130	10	0.5
Gorgonzola, 1 oz	100	8	0.5
Galbani Dolcelatte, 1 oz	95	8	1
Gouda, 1 oz	100	8	0.5
Gruyere, 1 oz	115	9	1
Havarti (Land O'Lakes), 1 oz	110	8	1
Italian Blend (Sargento), 1 oz	90	7	1
Jarlsberg (Wegman's), 1 oz	100	8	0
Jarlsberg Red. Fat, shredded, 1 oz	70	4	0
Kefir (Alta Dena), 2 Tbsp, 1 oz	70	6	2
Labneh (Lebanese cream chse), 1.8 oz	70	4	1
Lactose Free Cheese (Lifetime), 1 oz	40	0	1
Limburger, 1 oz	95	8	0
LiveActive (Kraft) ~ See Page 44			
Mascarpone (Wegman's), 1 oz	130	13	1
Mexican:			
Cacique: Cotija, 1 oz	110	9	0
Queso Fresco, 1 oz	80	6	0
Queso Quesadilla, 1 oz	70	5	2
Ranchero, 1 oz	80	6	0
Chi-Chi's: Con Quéso, 2 Tbsp	90	7	4
Hot/Medium/Mild/Acante, 2 T.	10	0	2
Kraft, Taco, shredded, 1 oz	100	8	2
Sargento, Shredded, ¼ cup	110	9	0.5
Supremo Chihuahua: Quéso Bianco	100	8	0
Quéso Fresco; Rancherito	80	6	0
Monterey, 1 oz	105	8.5	0
Monterey Jack: Regular, 1 oz	110	9	0
Kraft 2% Milk Red. Fat, 1 oz	80	6	1
Alpine Lace, Co-Jack, 1 oz	90	7	0
Weight Watchers, 1 oz	90	6	1
Mozzarella:			
Regular: 1 oz	85	6.5	0.5
Land O'Lakes/Polly-O, 1 oz, avg.	90	6	1
Shredded, ¼ cup, 1 oz	90	7	1
Light: Polly-O Lite, Shred., 1 oz	60	2.5	1
Kraft 2% Milk Fat, Red. Fat, 1 oz	70	4	1
Sargento Reduced Fat, ¼ c, 1 oz	80	4.5	1
Part Skim: Alpine Lace, 1 oz	70	5	1
Borden/Kraft, Shred., ¼ c, 1 oz	80	5	1
Polly-O, 1 oz	70	5	1
Fat-Free: Polly-O, 1 oz	35	0	1
Kraft, shredded, ¼ cup, 1 oz	45	0	2
Muenster: Regular, 1 oz	105	9	0.5
Low-Fat, 1 oz	85	5	1
Myzithra, 4 Tbsp, 1 oz	80	4	1
Neufchatel: 1 oz	75	6	1
Philadelphia, 1 oz	70	6	1
Flavored: Fruit/Herbs	80	7	1
Chocolate (Hickory Farms), 1 oz	110	8	

Parmesan: Fresh/Block, 1 oz	C	F	Cb
Parmesan: Fresh/Block, 1 oz	110	7.5	1
Grated (Packaged): 1 tbsp	20	1.5	0
1 oz quantity	120	8	1
½ cup, 1¾ oz	215	14	2
w. Romano (Frigo), grated, 1 oz	110	7	0
Kraft Reduced-Fat Topping, 1 T.	20	1	2
Pizza Cheese, shredded:			
Regular (Kraft) ¼ cup, 1 oz	90	7	1
Port de Salut, 1 oz	100	8	0
Port Wine (Kaukauna), 1 oz	90	6	4
Pot (Sargento), 1 oz	25	0	1
Provolone: Regular, 1 oz	100	7.5	0.5
Reduced-Fat: Alpine Lace, 1 oz	80	5	1
Sargento, 1 slice, ⅔ oz	50	3.5	0
Pub (Rondele), 1 oz, avg.	95	7	1
Quark: 40% fat, 1 oz	47	3	1
20% fat, 1 oz	32	1.5	1
Skim/Non-Fat, 1 oz	22	0	1.5
Queso: Anejo/Asadero/Blanco, 1 oz	105	9	1
Chichuahua/De Papa, 1 oz	110	9	2
Ricotta Cheese:			
Whole Milk, 2 Tbsp, 1 oz	50	3.5	1
½ cup, 4½ oz	215	16	4
Part Skim, 2 Tbsp, 1 oz	40	2	1.5
½ cup, 4½ oz	170	10	6
Light/Low-Fat, 2 Tbsp, 1 oz	25	1	1.5
½ cup, 4½ oz	125	5	6
Fat-Free, ½ cup, 4½ oz	100	0	10
Baked Ricotta, 2 oz portion	130	9	3
Romano: Block/Loaf, 1 oz	110	8	1
Grated (Pkg): 1 oz	120	9	1
1 Tbsp, 5g	20	1.5	0
Roquefort, 1 oz	105	9	0.5
Sheep's Milk, 1 oz	45	3	1
Smoked: Wegman's, 1 oz	100	8	0
Tillamook, Smoked Cheddar, 1 oz	110	9	0
Stilton (Wegman's), 1 oz	110	10	1
String (Frigo/Kraft/Sargento), 1 oz	80	6	0.5
Light String-Ums (Kraft), 1 oz	80	4.5	1
String Lite (Frigo), 1 oz	60	2.5	1
Light (Sargento) 1 stick, 0.7 oz	50	2.5	0.5
Swiss: Regular, 1 oz	110	8	1.5
Reduced-Fat: Alpine Lace, 1.2 oz	110	7	1
Kraft, 2% Milk, 0.7 oz slice	50	2.5	2
Taco Cheese (Kraft) shredded, ¼ cup	120	10	1
Tilsit, 1 oz	100	7.5	0.5
Tybo, 1 oz	100	7	0.5
Vermont (Cabot), 1 oz	110	9	0
Wensleydale, 1 oz	100	8	0.5
Whey Cheese, 1 oz	125	8	9

Cheese (Cont)

Cheese Products

	C	F	Cb
Cheese Food:			
Average all flavors: ¾ oz slice	70	5	2
1 oz slice	95	7	2.5
Alouette: Sundr. Tomato, 2 T., 0.8oz	80	7	1
Light Garlic, 2 Tbsp, 0.8 oz	50	4	2
Peppercorn Cajun, 2 T., 0.8 oz	80	8	1
Savory Vegetable, 2 T., 0.8 oz	70	6	1
Cabot, Jalapeno, 1 oz	70	4.5	0
Cracker Barrel, Cheddar, 1 oz	120	10	0
Handi-Snacks: *(Kraft)*			
Breadsticks 'n Cheez, 1.1 oz pkg	110	4.5	14
Pretzels 'n Cheez, 1 oz pkg	90	3.5	12
Ritz Crackers 'n Cheez, 1 oz pkg	100	5	10
Mozzarella Stringchse Stick, each	80	6	0.5
Kraft: American shredded, 1Tbsp.	25	2	0.5
Singles, 1 slice, ¾ oz	70	5	2
Free Singles, 1 slice, 0.7 oz	30	0	2
Pimento Spread, 2 Tbsp, 1.1 oz	80	6	3
Light String-Ums, 1 stick, 1 oz	80	4.5	1
LiveActive:			
Cheese Sticks: Cheddar,(1), 1 oz	120	10	0
Mozzarella, 1 stick, 1 oz	80	5	0
Colby Jack, Reduced Fat (1), 1 oz	90	6	0
Cheese Cubes:			
Colby Jack, 7 cubes, 1 oz	110	9	0
Cheddar (Red. Fat), 7 cubes 1 oz	90	6	0
Lifetime Cholesterol Reducing,			
Slices, 1 Slice, 19g	30	1	2
Block, 1" cube, 1 oz	55	2.5	1
Lifeway Farmers Kefir, 2 Tbsp, 1 oz	25	1.5	1
Precious String Chse Stuffers, 1 oz	70	3	1
Rondele: Soft Spread., 2 T., 1 oz	100	9	1
Light, 2 Tbsp, 1 oz	60	5	2
Velveeta: Regular, ⅜" slice, 1 oz	80	6	3
Light, ¾" slice, 1 oz	60	3	4
Shredded, ¼ cup, 1.3 oz	130	9	3
WisPride: Port Wine,			
Ball/Cup, 2 Tbsp, 1.1 oz	90	5	5.5
Light, 2 Tbsp, 1.1 oz	80	3	5

Cheese Whiz (Sauce)

	C	F	Cb
Original, 2 Tbsp, 33g	90	7	2
Light, 2 Tbsp, 33g	80	3	6
Salsa Con Queso, 2 Tbsp, 33g	90	7	4

Cheese Substitutes

	C	F	Cb
Per 1 oz Unless Indicated			
Galaxy:			
Veggie Yellow American, 1 sl., ½ oz	35	2	1
Veggy Mozz. Singles, 1 sl., ½ oz	40	2	1
Lifetime Rice Cheese, 1" cube, 1 oz	60	3	5
Mori Nu Tofu: Mozzarella, 1 oz	70	4	2
Fat-Free Mozz./Ched./Jack, 1 oz	40	0	2
Sargento Chef Style,			
Cheddar, shredded, ¼ cup, 1 oz	110	9	1
Mozzarella, shrd, ¼ cup	80	6	0.5
Smart Beat, Fat-Free, 0.6 oz sl.	25	0	3
Soya Kaas: Regular, 1 oz	70	5	1
Fat-Free, all varieties, 1 oz	40	2	1
Soyco: Almond/Oat/Rice Slices,			
1 slice, 0.7 oz	40	2	1
Veggy Singles, 1 slice, 0.7 oz	40	2	1
Grated Parmesan, 2 tsp, 5g	15	0.5	1
Soy-Sation: Shredded Cheese, 1 oz	70	4	2
Tofu Rella, avg. all varieties, 1 oz	60	4	0
Tofutti Better Than Cream Chse, 1 oz	80	8	1
Trader Joe's:			
Soy Cheese: Cheddar Flavor, 1 sl.	45	2	3
Mozzarella Flavor, 1 oz	70	4	3
Sliced Yogurt Cheese, 1 oz	100	8	0
Yves, Good Slice, ¾ oz slice, avg.	35	2	1

NOTICE
THIS IS AN
EQUAL
OPPORTUNITY
KITCHEN

Snack & Cheese Dips, Spreads

PHILADELPHIA

Cream Cheese C F Cb

Regular/Soft, average all brands:
2 Tbsp, 1 oz	90	9	2
8 oz pkg	720	72	13
w. Chives/Herbs/Pimento, 1 oz	75	2.5	10
w. Fruit/Strawb./P'apple, 1 oz	90	8	4
Lox, 1 oz	80	7	1

Philadelphia *(Kraft):* Per 2 Tbsp
Original, 2 Tbsp, 1 oz	100	10	0.5
3 oz package	300	30	2
Regular, 2 Tbsp, 1.1 oz	90	9	2
Neufchatel ⅓ Less Fat, 1 oz	70	6	1
Light: Plain, 2 Tbsp, 1.1 oz	60	4.5	2
Flavors, avg., 0.7 oz	70	4	6
Fat-Free Varieties, 1 oz	25	0	1
Flavored: Blueb./Raspberry, 1 oz	80	6	4.5
Honey Nut; Strawberry, 1 oz	80	7	4.5
Garden Vegetable, 1 oz	80	7.5	2
Jammin' Swirls, 2 Tbsp, 1.1 oz	80	6	7
Whipped: Regular, 2 Tbsp, 0.7 oz	60	6	1
Mixed Berry, 2 Tbsp, 0.7 oz	70	5	3
Snacks: Bars (1), 1½ oz	180	11	20
Snack Bites (1) 1 oz	130	7	15
Bagel & Crm Chse To Go, 3.2 oz	240	9	36

Dips/Spreads

Per 2 Tbsp (1 oz), Unless Indicated
Average All Brands
Avocado/Guacamole, 2 Tbsp, 1 oz	45	4	2
Baba Ghannoush *(Eggplant/Sesame)*	70	6	2
Cheese Fondue, ½ cup, 4 oz	260	15	4
French Onion Dip, 2 Tbsp	60	4.5	3
Hummus: 2 Tbsp, 1 oz	50	1	5
½ cup, 4.5 oz	220	4.5	23
Tzatziki *(Cucumber/Yogurt)* 2 T.	30	2.5	2
Clearman's: Original Spread, 1 oz	150	15	2
Frito Lay: Chili Cheese; Jalapeno	50	3	4
French Onion	60	5	4
Bean/Jalapeno Bean	40	1	6
Guiltless Gourmet: Hummus, 2 T.	35	1.5	4
Other varieties	30	0	5
Heluva Good Cheese: Chse 'N Salsa	80	3	3
French Onion; Jalapeno Cheddar	80	4	6
Bacon/Homestyle/Ranch	60	5	2
De La Casa, 5 Layer Party Dip, 2 T.	40	2.5	4
Frito Lay, French Onion, 2 Tbsp	60	5	4
Kaukauna: Nacho Cheese	90	7	4
Veggie Ranch	50	3	3

Dips/Spreads (Cont) C F Cb

Per 2 Tbsp (1 oz)
Knudsen: Nacho Cheese	60	4	3
Sour Cream Bacon & Onion	60	5	2
Sour Cream French Onion	50	4	2
Kroger, The Big Dipper; all flavors	60	5	2
Kraft: Average all flavors, 2 Tbsp	60	5	4
Cheez Whiz Dip: Orig., 2 Tbsp	90	7	4.5
Light, 2 Tbsp	80	3.5	6
Lay's Dip Mix, prepared, 2 Tbsp	60	6	3
Marie's Dips, average all varieties	90	9	2
Nalley's, all flavors, average	120	12	3
Naturally Fresh: Chocolate Dip	100	0	23
Cream Cheese Dip, 2 Tbsp	90	3.5	14
Fruit Dip, 2 Tbsp	80	4.5	10
Old Dutch French Onion, 2 Tbsp	50	5	2
Old El Paso: Black Bean, 2 Tbsp	25	0	5
Cheese 'n Salsa: Mild; Medium	40	3	3
Low-Fat, medium	30	1.5	4
Chunky Salsa varieties, avg.	15	0	3
Olys Bagel Spread: Berry	100	8	3
Garden Veg; Garlic & Herb	90	9	1
Prices: Pimiento Cheese Spread	80	7	2
Light Pimiento, 1 oz	55	3	3
Ruffles, French Onion; Ranch	60	5	3
Snyder's Mustard Pretzel	70	1	15
Stop & Shop: Veggie Dip, 2 Tbsp	110	10	3
Sour Crm French Onion, 2 T.	60	5	2
TGI Fridays: Spinach,Chse,Artichoke	45	3.5	3
Spinach Dip, 2 Tbsp	50	3.5	4
T. Marzetti: Choc Fruit, 2 Tbsp	110	2	23
Guacamole	130	13	2
Veggie: Ranch	120	12	2
Light Ranch	60	6	2
Fat-Free Ranch	30	0	6
Toby's: Tofu Pate, 2 Tbsp	80	7	2
Other Spreads, average, 2 Tbsp	40	2.5	2
Tostitos Dip: Con Queso variety	40	2.5	5
Reduced-Fat Zesty Cheese, 2 T.	40	2	4
Wise: French Onion, 2 Tbsp	60	5	3
Nacho Cheese	50	4.5	3
Salsa: *See Page 85*			

45

Egg & Egg Dishes

Chicken Eggs

Fresh Eggs

	C	F	Cb
Raw (weight with shell):			
Small, 40g	65	4	0
Medium, 44g	70	4	0
Large, 50g	75	4.5	0
Extra Large, 56g	80	5	0
Jumbo, 63g	90	5.5	0
Egg Yolk, 1 extra large	63	5	0
Egg White, 1 extra large	16	0	0
Dried Egg Powder			
Whole Egg: ¼ cup, 1 oz	170	12	0
1 Tbsp	30	2	0
Egg White, ¼ cup, 1 oz	105	0	0
Egg Yolk, ¼ cup, 1 oz	195	18	0

Egg Substitutes

¼ Cup (Equivalent to 1 Egg) ~ Zero Cholesterol.

	C	F	Cb
Better 'n Eggs *(Papetti)*, ¼ cup, 2 oz	30	0	1
EggBeaters *(Fleischmann's)* Frozen/Liquid Regular/Flavors, ¼ cup, 2.2 oz	30	0	1
Egg Watchers *(Tofutti)*, ¼ c., 2 oz	30	0	1
Ener-G, Egg Replacer, 1½ tsp, 4 g	15	0	4
Egg Substitute *(Jewel)*, ¼ cup	30	0	1
Nature Egg, Simply Egg White, ¼ c., 2 oz	25	0	0
Scramblers *(Morning Star)*, ¼ cup	35	0	1
Second Nature, Fat-Free, ¼ c., 2 fl.oz	35	0	1

Other Eggs

	C	F	Cb
Duck, 1 large, 2½ oz	130	9.5	0
Goose, 1 large, 5 oz	280	19	0
Quail, 3 eggs, 2 oz	42	3	0
Turkey, 1 large, 3 oz	135	9.5	0
Turtle, 1 egg, 1¾ oz	75	5	0

Omega-3 Fat Enriched

	C	F	Cb
Eggland's Best, 1 large	70	4	0
Eggs Plus *(Pilgrim's Pride)*, 1 large	70	4.5	1

Note: Cholesterol content same as regular eggs, but Omega-3 fats inhibit blood cholesterol increase. (Extra Notes ~ See Page 271)

Cooked Eggs

	C	F	Cb
Boiled Egg: Same as raw egg			
Hard-Cooked *(Egg·Lands)*, Peeled	60	3.5	0
Fried Egg:			
With fat: 1 large egg	105	9	0.5
2 small eggs	175	13	1
No fat/nonstick pan, 1 large	75	5	0.5
Deviled Egg, 2 halves	145	13	0.5
Eggs Benedict (2) on toast or English muffin	860	56	25
Eggs Florentine (2) on toast or English muffin	890	59	25
Pickled Egg, 1 large	80	5.5	0
Poached Egg, 1 large	65	4	0
Quiche (Home-Made):			
Egg & Bacon, 1 slice, 5.3 oz	580	43	27
Ham & Cheese, 1 slice, 5.3 oz	475	33	29
Scotch Egg, 1 egg	300	21	16
Scrambled Eggs: 1 large egg:			
w. 1 Tbsp milk + 1 tsp fat	120	9	1
w. 1 Tbsp skim milk/no fat	85	5.5	1
2 large eggs:			
w. 2 Tbsp milk + 2 tsp fat	260	20	2
w. 2 Tbsp skim milk/no fat	180	11	2

Omelets

	C	F	Cb
1 Egg: Plain (w. 1 tsp fat)	125	10	0.5
with ½ oz cheese	175	15	0.5
w. ½ oz cheese + ½ oz ham	200	16	0.5
2 Eggs: Plain (w. 2 tsp fat)	250	20	1
with 1 oz cheese	360	29	1
w. 1 oz cheese + 1 oz ham	410	32	1
3 Eggs: Plain (w. 1 Tbsp fat)	360	29	1.5
w. 2 oz cheese	580	47	2.5
w. 2 oz cheese + 2 oz ham	680	53	2.5
Extras: Tomato/Onion/Veges	20	0	4.5
Egg Substitute *(EggBeaters)*:			
2 eggs (½ cup) + 1 tsp fat	100	4	2
3 eggs (¾ cup) + 2 tsp fat	160	8	3
Extras: 1 oz cheese	110	9	1
1 oz ham	50	3	1
Tom./Onion/Veges	20	0	4.5

Egg Nog ~ *Per ½ Cup (4 fl.oz)*

	C	F	Cb
Average all Brands, ½ cup	170	9.5	17
Regular: *Borden*	160	9	17
Hood (Golden)	180	9	22
Light/Low-Fat: *Horizon; Hood*	140	4	22
Fat-Free: *Hood*	55	0	9

Egg & Egg Dishes (Cont)

Breakfast Sides

	C	F	Cb
Toast: Plain, 1 thick slice	85	1	13
with 2 tsp butter/marg.	155	9	13
with 3 tsp/1 Tbsp fat	190	13	13
English Muffin: Plain, 2 oz	130	1	26
with 3 tsp fat	230	12	26
Bacon, 2 strips	70	5	0
Ham, Lean, 2 oz	100	3	0
Hash Browns: ½ cup	125	6.5	14
1 cup serving	250	13	28
Sausages, 2 links (1 oz ea.)	180	16	1.5

Frozen Egg Breakfasts

Aunt Jemima Great Starts: *Per Package*

	C	F	Cb
French Toast & Sausage Bkfst	440	27	35
Griddle Cake w. Ham, Egg, Cheese	240	8	33
Pancakes & Sausage Breakfast	470	25	50
Sausage, Egg & Chse Biscuit	340	21	27
Sausage, Egg & Chse Croissant	350	23	22
Scrambled Eggs & Saus. Bkfst	370	27	18

Jimmy Dean

Bacon, Egg, Cheese Muffin (1)	230	9	27
Croissant: Egg & Cheese (1)	310	20	23
Egg, Sausage, Cheese (1)	450	33	24
Egg, Sausage, Cheese Biscuit (1)	430	30	28
Omelet: 3 Cheese (1)	290	23	5
Ham & Cheese (1)	280	17	5

Pillsbury: Toaster Scrambles,

Cheese, Egg & Bacon	180	12	15
Cheese, Egg & Sausage	180	11	15

Red Baron

Scrambles: Ham (1), 5 oz	330	15	33
Bacon (1), 5 oz	400	22	35
Minis, 4 pieces, 5½ oz	390	17	45

Swanson Great Starts

Hungryman Hearty Breakfast	1170	61	125
Weight Watchers: Omelet	220	5	30

Frozen Pancake/Waffles: *See Page 122*

Frozen Egg Rolls

Chun King/La Choy: *Average All Brands*

	C	F	Cb
Chicken Egg Rolls: Mini, 6 rolls	210	9	25
Restaurant Style, 1 roll, 3 oz	210	9	25
Pork & Shrimp Egg Rolls:			
Mini, 6 rolls, 3 oz	210	9	27
Shrimp Egg Rolls: Mini, 6 rolls	190	6	28
Restaurant Style, 1 roll, 3 oz	180	7	25
Lotus: Pork, 3 oz	180	7	18
Vegetable, 3 oz	70	1.5	13
Kahiki: Pork, 3 oz	140	3.5	20
Chicken, 3 oz	160	6	19
Vegetarian, 3 oz	130	3.5	21

Fast Food/Restaurants

	C	F	Cb
Au Bon Pain: Egg on a Bagel	400	4	63
w. Bacon & Cheese	560	18	63
Bob Evans: Eggs Benedict	420	20	35
Three Cheese Omelette	770	67	4
Bojangles: Egg Biscuit	400	30	26
Bacon, Egg & Cheese Biscuit	550	42	27
Bruegger's Bagels: Breakfast Sandwiches,			
Egg & Cheese	420	18	71
Egg & Cheese & Sausage	640	38	72
Burger King: Ham, Egg & Chse Bisc.	390	22	31
Egg & Cheese Croissan'wich	300	17	26
Saus., Egg & Chse Croissan'wich	470	32	26
Carl's Jr: Steak & Egg Burrito	600	32	44
Chick-Fil-A			
Chicken, Egg & Cheese Bagel	500	20	49
Denny's: Two Eggs & More B'Fast	630	46	21
All American Slam, no toast	950	75	21
Heartland Scramble, no syrup/marg.	1190	59	118
Eat 'N Park: Cheese Omelette	390	30	2.5
Hardee's: Bacon Platter	980	56	90
Steak N Egg Burrito	470	22	38
IHOP: T-Bone Steak & Eggs	1325	86	63
Country Fried Steak/Eggs	1535	105	73
McDonald's: Egg McMuffin	300	12	30
Bacon, Egg & Cheese Bisc., Reg.	440	25	36
Scrambled Eggs (2)	170	11	1
Whataburger			
Breakfast Platter w. Bacon (2 sl.)	740	45	53

"He misses the way you used to bend over and pat him."

Note: Cooking reduces weight of meat by 20-45% due to water and fat losses. Average weight loss is 30%. Actual loss depends on cooking method and cooking time. Examples:
4 oz raw wt. = approx. 3 oz cooked wt.
4 oz cooked wt. = approx. 5½ oz raw.

What 3 oz Cooked Meat Looks Like
• Half the size of this book (4¼" x 3" x ⅜ " thick)
• Rectangular piece (4" x 2½" x ½" thick)
• Deck of cards (3½" x 2½" x ⅝ " thick)

Quick Guide

Steak
Sirloin (Choice Grade)
External fat trimmed to ¼"
Broiled, Edible Portion (no bone)

	C	F	Cb
Small Serving, 3 oz (cooked)			
(3 oz cooked, from 4-4½ oz raw)			
Lean + fat (¼"), 3 oz	225	13	0
Lean + marbling, 3 oz	195	10	0
Lean only, 3 oz	160	6	0
(No external fat or marbling)			
Medium/Regular Serving, 5 oz (cooked wt)			
(from approx. 7 oz raw)			
Lean + fat (¼"), 5 oz	350	21	0
Lean + marbling, 5 oz	325	17	0
Lean only, 5 oz	265	10	0
Large Serving, 8 oz (cooked wt)			
(from 11-12 oz raw)			
Lean + fat (¼"), 8 oz	600	36	0
Lean + marbling, 8 oz	520	27	0
Lean only, 8 oz	425	15	0
Extra Large Serving, 12 oz (cooked wt)			
(from approx. 16-17 oz raw)			
Lean + fat (¼"), 12 oz	900	52	0
Lean + marbling, 12 oz	740	40	0
Lean only, 12 oz	640	23	0
Pan Fried			
Sirloin (choice), medium serving:			
Lean + fat (¼"), 5 oz	460	32	0
Lean only, 5 oz	340	16	0

Other Steaks

	C	F	Cb
Filet Mignon (Tenderloin):			
1 Medium steak, 6 oz raw wt.			
Broiled, with ¼" fat trim			
Lean + fat (¼"), 4 oz	380	28	0
Lean only, 3½ oz	230	12	0
New York/Club Steak:			
Top Loin/Short Loin			
1 steak, regular (9¼ oz raw, ¼" fat)			
Broiled: Lean + fat (¼"), 6¼ oz	580	43	0
Lean + marbling, 5½ oz	400	25	0
Lean only, 5¼ oz	360	20	0
Porterhouse Steak:			
1 Medium, (6 oz raw wt. no bone), broiled			
Lean + fat (¼"), 4¼ oz	410	33	0
Lean only, 3½ oz	210	11	0
1 Large (12 oz raw wt. no bone), broiled			
Lean + fat (¼"), 8½ oz cooked	820	66	0
Lean only, 7 oz cooked	420	22	0
With Bone: See T-Bone Steak			
T-Bone Steak (Broiled/Grilled): wts. include bone			
Medium, 8 oz raw wt. (with bone)			
Lean + fat (¼")	410	32	0
Lean only, 4 oz raw	230	12	0
Large, (12 oz raw wt.) ¼" fat	620	48	0
Supersize, (20 oz raw wt.) ¼" fat	1025	88	0

Also See Fast-Foods & Restaurants Section ~
LoneStar Steakhouse, Outback Steakhouse, Western Sizzlin

Beef - Average All Cuts

Average All Retail Cuts
Edible weight (no bone)

Raw	C	F	Cb
(1 lb raw yields approx. 11-12 oz cooked)			
Lean + fat (¼" trim), 1 oz	70	6	0
½ Pound, 8 oz	560	44	0
Lean only, 1 oz	40	2	0
½ Pound, 8 oz	320	17	0
Fat only, 1 oz	190	20	0
Cooked (No Added Fat)			
Lean + fat (¼"), 1 oz	86	6	0
Small serving, 3 oz	260	18	0
Lean + marbling, (no ext. fat) 1 oz	78	5	0
Small serving, 3 oz	235	15	0
Lean only, 1 oz	60	3	0
Small serving, 3 oz	180	9	0
Fat only, 1 oz	255	28	0

Beef - Individual Cuts

Average All Grades Edible Weight (no bone)	**C**	**F**	**Cb**
Brisket, whole, braised:			
Lean + fat ¼", 3 oz	330	27	0
Lean + marbling, 3 oz	280	21	0
Lean only, 3 oz	250	17	0
Chuck, blade, braised:			
Lean + fat (¼"), 3 oz	295	22	0
Lean + marbling, 3 oz	290	21	0
Lean only, 3 oz	245	21	0
Flank: Raw, 4 oz	175	8	0
Braised, 3 oz	225	14	0
Broiled, 3 oz	155	6	0
Ribs, whole (ribs 6-12): Roasted			
(1 lb raw yields 10¼ oz roasted)			
Lean + fat (¼")			
(3.6 oz w. bone, 3 oz no bone)	305	25	0
Lean only 3 oz (no bone)	280	22	0
Round, bottom, braised:			
Lean + fat (¼"), 3 oz	190	7.5	0
Lean only, 3 oz	185	6.5	0
Round, eye/tip, roasted:			
Lean + fat (¼"), 3 oz	205	11	0
Lean, 3 oz	145	4	0
Round, top: Per 3 oz (cooked wt)			
Braised, Lean + fat	210	10	0
Lean only	175	5	0
Broiled, Lean + fat	180	8	0
Lean only	155	5	0
Pan-fried, Lean + fat	235	13	0
Lean only	190	7	0

Ground Beef

Ground Beef, Raw: Per 4 oz	**C**	**F**	**Cb**
73% lean (27% fat)	380	34	0
80% lean (20% fat)	290	22	0
85% lean (15% fat)	240	17	0
90% lean (10% fat)	200	11	0
93% lean (7% fat)	170	8	0
96% lean (4% fat)	150	4.5	0
Baked/Broiled: Reg., 3 oz	230	16	0
Lean (80%), 3 oz	230	15	0
Extra lean (90%), 3 oz	185	10	0
Pan-fried: Regular, 3 oz	230	15	0
Lean, 3 oz	230	15	0
Extra lean, 3 oz	195	10	0
Ground Beef Patties: Average (23% Fat)			
Frozen, raw, 4 oz	320	26	0
Broiled, 3 oz (from 4 oz raw)	240	17	0

Quick Guide

Roast Beef	**C**	**F**	**Cb**
Round (Eye/Tip, average) Average All Cuts			
Small Serving, 3 oz			
(2 thin slices/1 thick slice)			
Lean + fat (¼"), 3 oz	200	11	0
Lean only, 3 oz	150	5	0
Medium Serving, 5 oz (3-4 thin slices)			
Lean + fat, 5 oz	330	19	0
Lean only, 5 oz	245	9	0
Large Serving, 8 oz (3 thick slices)			
Lean + fat, 8 oz	525	30	0
Lean only, 8 oz	390	14	0

Roast Dinner Extras

	C	**F**	**Cb**
Gravy: Thin, 2 Tbsp	20	0.5	3.5
Thick, 2 Tbsp	50	2	0.5
1 Ladle/4 Tbsp	100	4	1
Veges: Beans, green, ½ cup	20	0	5
Cauliflower w. cheese sce, 4 oz	135	9	15
Corn, kernels, ¼ cup	35	0	9
Carrots, ¼ cup	20	0	3
Peas, ¼ cup	35	0	6
Pumpkin baked: w. fat, 4 oz	90	7	6
No added fat, 4 oz	25	0	5
Potato: Roasted w. fat, 1 small	155	8	30
Baked in Jacket, 1 large	280	0	63
with 1 Tbsp whipped butter	350	8	63
with Sour Cream, 2 Tbsp	270	5	64
Sweet Potato/Yam, 1 medium	105	1	24
Beef Kabobs: Beef & Veggies, 2 oz	160	10	4
If very lean meat	100	4	4

"347 ~ 348 ~ 349..."

Lamb

	C	F	Cb
Choice Grade			
Leg (Whole), roasted:			
Lean + fat, 3 oz	250	18	0
Lean only, 3 oz	155	6	0
Leg (Sirloin Half), roasted:			
Lean + fat, 3 oz	250	18	0
Lean only, 3 oz	175	8	0
Leg (Shank Half), roasted:			
Lean + fat, 3 oz	190	11	0
Lean only, 3 oz	155	6	0
Loin Chop, broiled:			
1 chop (raw wt., 4¼ oz):	250	17	0
Lean + fat (2¼ oz edible)	180	12	0
Lean only (1.6 oz edible)	85	3.5	0
Rib Chop, broiled/roasted:			
1 chop (raw wt., 3½ oz)			
Lean + fat (2½ oz edible)	255	21	0
Lean only (1¾ oz edible)	105	6	0
Shoulder (Arm/Blade):			
Braised: Lean + fat, 3 oz	290	21	0
Lean only, 3 oz	240	12	0
Broiled: Lean + fat, 3 oz	240	16	0
Lean only, 3 oz	170	8	0
Roasted: Similar to Broiled			
Cubed Lamb (Leg/Shoulder):			
For stew or kabob			
Raw, lean only, 8 oz	305	12	0
Braised, lean only, 3 oz	190	8	0
Broiled, lean only, 3 oz	160	6	0
New Zealand Lamb (Imported):			
Similar calories and fat to domestic.			

Veal

	C	F	Cb
Edible Weights			
Leg (Top Round):			
Braised: Lean + fat, 3 oz	180	6	0
Lean only, 3 oz	170	5	0
Pan-fried, breaded:			
Lean + fat, 3 oz	195	8	9
Lean only, 3 oz	175	6	9
Pan-fried, not breaded:			
Lean + fat, 3 oz	180	7	0
Lean only, 3 oz	155	4	0
Roasted: Lean + fat, 3 oz	135	4	0
Lean only, 3 oz	130	3	0

Veal (Cont)

	C	F	Cb
Loin Chop: 1 chop, 7 oz raw wt.			
Braised: Lean + fat, 3 oz	240	14	0
Lean only, 3 oz	190	8	0
Roasted: Lean + fat, 3 oz	185	10	0
Lean only, 3 oz	150	6	0
Rib, roasted: Lean + fat, 3 oz	195	12	0
Lean only, 3 oz	150	7	0
Shoulder, Arm/Blade, roasted:			
Lean + fat, 3 oz	155	7	0
Lean only, 3 oz	145	6	0
Sirloin, roasted:			
Lean + fat, 3 oz	170	9	0
Lean only, 3 oz	145	6	0
Cubed for Stew: braised			
Leg/Shoulder, lean only, 3 oz	160	4	0
(1 lb raw yields approx. 9¼ oz cooked)			

Pork

	C	F	Cb
Figures based on NLMB data (1990)			
Fresh Pork (Cooked Wt., no bone)			
(4 oz raw wt. = approx. 3 oz cooked wt.)			
Blade Steak, broiled:			
Lean + fat, 3 oz	220	15	0
Lean only, 3 oz	190	11	0
Country Style Ribs, broiled:			
Lean + fat, 3 oz	280	22	0
Lean only, 3 oz	210	13	0
Spareribs, braised: lean & fat, 6 oz	675	51	0
(from 1 lb raw wt)			
Leg (Ham), roasted:			
Lean + fat, 3 oz	230	15	0
Lean only, 3 oz	180	8	0
(Ham, cured -- See Cold Meats)			
Loin Chops, broiled: Average			
(From 1 chop: 5 oz raw wt. w. bone			
or 4 oz raw wt., no bone)			
Lean + fat, 3 oz	200	11	0
Lean only, 3 oz	165	7	0
Rib Chops, broiled:			
Lean + fat, 3 oz	220	14	0
Lean only, 3 oz	185	9	0
Rib Roast, roasted:			
Lean + fat, 3 oz	215	13	0
Lean only, 3 oz	180	9	0
Loin Roast, roasted:			
Lean + fat, 3 oz	190	10	0
Lean only, 3 oz	160	7	0

Pork (Cont)

	C	F	Cb
Sirloin Chop, broiled:			
Lean + fat, 3 oz	175	8	0
Lean only, 3 oz	165	6	0
Sirloin Roast, roasted:			
Lean + fat, 3 oz	175	8	0
Lean only, 3 oz	170	7	0
Tenderloin, roasted:			
Lean + fat, 3 oz	147	5	0
Lean only, 3 oz	140	4	0
Ground Pork			
Raw: Average, ¼ lb, 4 oz	300	24	0
Broiled, 3 oz	250	18	0
Pan-fried, drained, 3 oz	260	19	0

Bacon

	C	F	Cb
Raw: 1 med. slice (20 lb), ¾ oz	95	9	0
1 thick slice (12 lb), 1⅓ oz	175	17	0
(1 lb raw yields approx. 5 oz cooked)			
Broiled/Pan-Fried: 1 med. sl., 8 g	40	3	0
3 medium slices, 24g	125	10	0
2 thin slices, ½ oz	75	6	0
1 thick slice, 12g	65	5	0
Canadian-style: Cooked, 1 slice	35	1.5	0.5
As purchased, 1 slice, 1 oz	35	1.5	0.5
Bacon Bits, 1 Tbsp, ¼ oz	35	2.5	0
Breakfast Strips, Broil., 1 sl., 12 g	50	4	0

Ham

	C	F	Cb
Boneless Ham, cooked:			
Regular, (approx. 11% fat):			
Unheated (as purch.), 1 oz	50	2.5	0
Roasted, 3 oz	150	8	0
Extra Lean (5% fat):			
Unheated, 1 oz	45	2.5	0
Roasted, 3 oz	125	5	0
Whole Ham, cooked:			
Lean + fat (as purchased)			
Unheated, 1 oz	70	5	0
Roasted, 3 oz	210	15	0
Lean only, unheated, 1 oz	40	2	0
Roasted, 3 oz	135	5	0
Canned Ham: Similar to boneless ham			
Chopped, canned, 3 oz	200	16	0
Ham Patties, ckd, 1 pty, 21/4 oz	215	20	1
Ham Steak, extra lean, 2 oz	70	2.5	0
Luncheon Slices: See Deli Meats, Page 53			

Game & Other Meats

	C	F	Cb
Bison Steak,			
lean, 6 oz (raw)	205	4	0
Boar (wild), roasted, 3 oz	140	4	0
Buffalo Steak: *New West Foods,* 4 oz	70	3	0
Trader Joes, 1 patty	430	30	1
Caribou, roasted, 3 oz	140	4	0
Deer/Venison, roasted 3 oz	135	3	0
Goat (Capretto): Raw, 3 oz	95	2	0
Roasted, 3 oz	120	2.5	0
Ostrich: *Blackwing Ostrich Meats,*			
Sport Jerky, ½ oz pce	25	0	0
Sausage Patties (2) 2 oz	60	0.5	0
New West Foods:			
Ground Ostrich, 4 oz	165	7	0
Ostrich Steak, 4 oz steak	130	2.5	0
Rabbit: Roasted, 3 oz	165	7	0
Stewed, 1 cup, diced, 5 oz	290	12	0

Variety & Organ Meats

	C	F	Cb
Brains: Braised, 3 oz	130	9	0
Pan fried, 3 oz	200	14	0
Chitterlings, pork, simmered, 3 oz	200	17	0
Ears, pork, simmered, 1 ear	185	12	0
Feet, pork: Simmered, 3 oz	200	14	0
Cured, pickled, 3 oz	170	14	0
Hormel, 2 oz	80	6	0
Head Cheese (Pork Snouts/Ears/Vinegar/Spices):			
1 oz slice	50	4	0
Heart: Average, braised, 3 oz	125	5	0
Jowl, pork, raw, 4 oz	750	80	0
Kidneys, simmered, 3 oz	135	4	0
Liver (beef): Raw, 4 oz	150	4	4
Braised, 3 oz	145	4	4
Pan-fried, 3 oz	160	4.5	4
Pancreas, pork, braised, 3 oz	185	8	0
Pork Cracklins, 0.5 oz	80	6	0
Pork Hocks, 1 piece, 6 oz	340	23	0
Scrapple, 2 oz	120	8	8
Spleen, pork, braised, 3 oz	130	3	0
Stomach, pork, raw, 4 oz	185	12	0
Sweetbreads: Beef, ckd., 3 oz	125	9	0
Lamb, cooked, 3 oz	125	9	0
Tail, pork, simmered, 3 oz	340	31	0
Tongue, braised, 3 oz: Veal	170	9	0
Beef/Lamb/Pork, average, 3 oz	235	17	0
Tripe, beef, raw, 4 oz	95	4	0
Lean + fat, 3 oz	80	3.5	1.5

Sausages, Franks

Quick Guide

Franks & Weiners
Average All Brands   **C** **F** **Cb**

Regular/Smoked: *Per Frank*

	C	F	Cb
Regular, 1.5oz (10/16 oz pkg)	140	13	1
Jumbo, 2 oz (8/16 oz pkg)	170	16	0
Bun Length, 2 oz	180	17	2
Extra Long, 2.75 oz	240	21	2
Small/Cocktail (50/lb) each	30	3	0.5

Beef Franks: *Per Frank*

Regular, 1.6 oz (10/16 oz pkg)	140	13	2
Jumbo, 2 oz (8/16 oz pkg)	170	15	2
Bun Length, 2 oz	180	16	2
¼ lb Dog, 4 oz	300	24	4

Brands

Ball Park

Reg./Smoked, Fat-Free (1), 1.76 oz	40	0	4
Beef: Fat-Free, 1.76 oz link	45	0	5
Reduced-Fa, 2 oz link	100	7	3
Turkey Frank, 1.76 oz link	45	0	5

Beef Kosher

Beef: 2 oz link	180	14	4
2.6 oz link (6/16 oz)	230	19	6

Foster Farms

Chicken Franks, 2 oz (8/16 oz)	140	12	1

Healthy Choice

Turkey Franks, 1.76 oz link	70	2.5	6

Hebrew National

Beef: 1.72 oz link	150	14	1
14 lb link, 4 oz	340	32	1
97% Fat-Free, 1.72 oz link	50	1.5	2

Jennie-O

Turkey Franks: 1 oz link	70	5	1
2 oz link	120	10	2

Oscar Mayer

Reg./Smoked, Fat-Free, 1.76 oz link	40	0	3
Beef, Reduced-Fat, 2 oz link	110	8	2
Cheese Frank, 1.6 oz link	140	13	1
Turkey Franks, 1.6 oz link	100	8	2
2 oz link	120	10	3

Shelton's

Chicken Franks, 1.2 oz link	70	6	0
Turkey Franks, 1.2 oz link	60	4.5	1

Zacky Farms

Chicken Frank, 2 oz link	160	12	1

Vegetarian Sausages

See Frozen/Canned & Packaged Meals

Quick Guide

Fresh Sausages
Pork/Beef: *Average All Types*   **C** **F** **Cb**

	C	F	Cb
Small: Raw, 4" link, 1 oz	85	7.5	0
Broiled/Pan-fried	80	7	0
Medium: Raw, 2 oz	170	15	0
Broiled/Pan-fried	165	14	0
Large: Raw, 3 oz	255	22	0
Broiled/Pan-fried	245	21	0
Italian: Raw, 3.2 oz	315	28	0.5
Cooked, 2.4 oz	230	18	3
Chorizo: Beef Chorizo, 2.5 oz pce	250	23	5
Pork Chorizo, 2 oz piece	250	23	5

Note: Fat is lost in broiling/pan frying.
(Cooked wt. = approx. 60-70% raw wt.)

Smoked Sausage

	C	F	Cb
Average All Brands: 2 oz link	170	15	0
3 oz link	255	22	0
Ball Park, Bun Size, 2 oz	180	17	2
Butterball (w. Turkey), 2 oz	100	6	4
Eckrich, 2 oz	180	16	2
Healthy Choice, Beef/Polska, 2 oz	80	2.5	6

Breakfast Sausages/Patties

Armour Brown 'n Serve

Pork/Turkey, 3 links, 2.1 oz	210	19	2
Lite Original, 3 links	120	8	3
Beef Sausage, 3 links, 2 oz	230	22	1

Butterball: Turkey Brkfast Pats (2)	120	7	2
Turkey Breakfast Links (3)	120	8	2
Healthy Choice, Patties/Links (3), 2 oz	70	3	3
Jennie-O, Italian Turkey Saus. (2)	160	10	0
Jimmy Dean: Pork Saus. Patties (2)	260	24	0
Pork Sausage Links: Original (3)	290	28	0
Country Maple (3)	230	20	3
Breakfast Sandwiches: *See Page 47*			
Jones/Golden Brown:			
Pork Sausage Patties: Original (1)	75	7	0.5
All Natural (1)	95	9	0
Sandwich Patties (1)	170	16	1
Pork Sausage Links: 2 links	180	18	2
Light, 2 links	110	8	1

Swanson 'Great Starts': *See Page 47*

Vegetarian Patties:
Boca: *See Page 61*
Garden Burger: *See Page 62*

Bagel, Corn & Hot Dogs

Hot Dogs, Ready-To-Go

	C	**F**	**Cb**
(Includes Ketchup/Relish; no Mayo)			
Regular (1.5 oz frank, 1.5 oz bun)	260	15	22
Bun Length (2 oz frank, 1.5 oz bun)	290	18	21
Jumbo Dog (2 oz frank, 2 oz bun)	360	20	36
¼ lb Beef Dog (¼ lb frank, 2 oz bun)	480	15	36
Mile Long Dog (2.6 oz dog, 1.5 oz bun)	360	24	23

Weinerschnitzel: See Fast-Foods

Corn Dogs

Beef/Pork Frank: Average, 2.6 oz	170	10	16
Foster Farms Chicken Franks:			
1 dog, 2.6 oz (75g)	180	10	15
Chili Cheese, 1 dog, 2.6 oz (75g)	200	9	24
Mini Corn Dogs (4), 2.68 oz	210	12	18
Oscar Mayer Turkey & Pork, 3.2 oz	260	15	25
State Fair w. Ball Park Franks,			
Corn Dogs, 1 dog, 2.7 oz (76g)	210	12	23
Mini Corn Dogs (4)	230	13	22

Bagel Dogs

Best's Kosher: 1 dog, 1 oz	320	11	43
Mini, 1 piece, 0.8 oz	60	2	8
Vienna Beef: 1 piece, 1 oz	85	3.5	7

Hot Dog Toppings/Extras:

American Chse, 1 slice, 1 oz	110	9	1
Catsup, 1 Tbsp	16	0	4
Chili (w. Beans), ¼ cup	70	3.5	9
Mustard, 1 Tbsp	20	0	1
Pickle Relish, 1 Tbsp	20	0	5
Sauerkraut, ½ cup	20	0	5

WILL-POWER TONIC
~ RECIPE ~

- 1 Cup of Desire
- 1 Quart of Determination
- 1 Tbsp of Common Sense
- 1 Tbsp of Stick-to-itiveness
- 1 Tbsp of Foresight
- 1 Cup of Energy

Deli & Luncheon Meats

	C	**F**	**Cb**
Beef Jerky:			
Bridgeford Beef Jerky, 1 oz	100	0.5	5
Beef Stick (5.5 oz stick), 1 oz	150	13	2
Beef Steak, 1 oz	70	0.5	2
Beef & Cheese (Giant Size),			
½ pkg, 1.5 oz	170	14	1
Pepperoni Sticks (2), 1 oz	160	13	2
Pepperoni (1" diam.), 1 oz	130	12	0
Teriyaki, 1 oz pkg	80	0.5	4
Original; Hot 'n Spicy	70	1	5
Berliner (pork/beef), 1 oz	65	5	1
Beerwurst (Beef):			
Small (2.75"diam), ¹⁄₁₆" slice	20	2	0
Large (4"diam), ⅛" slice	75	7	0.5
Beerwurst (Pork):			
Small (2.75"diam), ¹⁄₁₆" slice	15	1	0
Large (4"diam), ⅛" Slice	55	4	0.5
Bologna: 1 Slice, 1 oz	65	6	1
Fat-Free, 1 slice, 1 oz	20	0	2
Beef Bologna: 1 slice, 1 oz	90	8	1
Light, 1 slice, 1 oz	60	4	2
Light *(Oscar Mayer),* 1 sl., 1 oz	60	4	2
Red. Fat *(Hebrew Nat.),* 2 sl.,1 oz	40	2.5	0.5
Fat Free *(Osc. M.),* 2 sl., 1.6 oz	40	0	1
Healthy Choice, 1 oz	35	1	3
Weight Watchers, 2 sl., ¾ oz	35	2	0
Beef *(Tyson),* 1 slice	80	7	1
Ring *(Boar's Head),* 2 oz	145	13	0
Turkey, average, 1 oz	60	5	0.5
Blood Sausage, 1 oz	100	9	0.5
Bratwurst: Average, 1 oz	80	7	1
Boar's Head, cook., 1 wurst, 4 oz	300	25	0
Bob Evan's, Beer, 2.6 oz link	270	21	0
Braunschweiger (Pork/Liver/Sausage),			
Oscar Mayer, 1 oz	110	10	1
Chicken, *Average All Brands*			
1 thick or 2 thin slices, 1 oz	30	1	1
Chicken Roll, 1 slice, 2 oz	90	4	1.5
Corned Beef: Average, full fat, 1 oz	60	5	0.5
Healthy Choice, Hillshire Farm, 1oz	30	1	0
Hebrew National, 4 slices, 2 oz	90	4.5	0
Loaf, jellied, 1 oz	45	2	0
Hash, canned, average, 1 oz	50	3	3
Dutch Brand Loaf, average, 1 oz	70	5	1.5

Continued Next Page

Deli & Luncheon Meats

Ham, Luncheon:	C	F	Cb
Baked/Boiled, sliced, 1 oz	30	1	0.5
Chopped: *Eckrich (97% FF)*, 1 oz	25	1	1
Armour: Canned, 1 oz	35	1.5	0.5
97% Fat Free, 1 oz	25	1	1.5
Healthy Choice, 2 sl., 2 oz	60	1.5	1
Hormel (Black Label), 1 oz	70	6	0
Oscar Mayer, 1 oz slice	60	2	0.5
Honey/Brown Sugar: Avg., 1 oz	30	1	1
Healthy Choice Deli Traditions:			
2 slices, 2 oz	60	1.5	2
Prosciutto, average, 1 oz	70	5	0
Ham & Cheese Loaf, avg., 1 oz	70	5	1
Head Cheese *(Osc. Mayer),* 1 oz sl.	50	4	0
Honey Loaf *(Osc. Mayer),* 1 oz sl.	35	1	2
Italian Sausage, 2.6 oz	250	20	3
Kielbasa (Polish Sausage), 1 oz	65	5	1
Scott Petersen, 3.4 oz link	320	27	4
Beef, 2 oz link	190	17	1
Boar's Head, 1 oz	60	5	0
Kippered Beefsteak:			
Hickory Farms, 3 slices, 0.75 oz	50	1	1
Knockwurst, 1 oz	90	8	0.5
Linguica *(Gaspar's),* 2 oz	180	8	1
Liverwurst, 1 oz	65	5	2
Liver Pate, fresh, average, 1 oz	90	8	1
Luncheon Loaf *(Foods Co),* 1 oz	65	5	2
Mortadella, 1 oz	105	9	0
Olive Loaf: Average, 1 oz	70	5	3
Oscar Mayer, 1 oz	75	6	2
Pastrami (Beef): Average, 1 oz	45	3	0.5
Healthy Deli, 1 oz	34	1	0.5
Hillshire (DeliSelect), 6 sl., 2 oz	60	1	0
Boar's Head, 2 oz	70	4	2
Peppered Beef, 1 oz slice	40	2	1
Pepperoni, 5 slices, 1 oz	140	13	0
Pickle Loaf, average, 1 oz	70	5	5
Pickle & Pimento Loaf			
Oscar Mayer, 1 oz	75	6	3
Polish Sausage: *See Kielbasa*			
Proscuitto/Proscuitti: Avg., 1 oz	70	5	1
Hormel, 1 oz	90	7	1
Roast Beef: Lean, 1 oz	40	2	0
Healthy Choice, all types, 2 oz	60	1.5	1
Salami: Beef, average, 1 oz	80	7	1
Beer Salami, average, 1 oz	50	4	0.5
Cotto: *Oscar Mayer,* 1 slice, 1 oz	70	6	1
Dry: Hard, avg., 4 slices, 1 oz	110	10	3
Oscar Mayer, 2 slices, 1.6 oz	100	8	1

Salami (Cont):	C	F	Cb
Genoa: Average, 1 oz	120	9	1
Stick *(Best's Kosher),* 2, 1.75 oz	180	15	2
Italian *(Bridgeford),* 1 oz	120	11	0
Turkey, average, 1 oz	55	4	1
Spam *(Hormel):*			
Regular: ¼" slice, 1 oz	90	8	1
½" slice, 2 oz	180	16	2
Lite: ¼" slice, 1 oz	55	4	0
½" slice, 2 oz	110	8	1
Turkey: ¼" slice, 1 oz	40	2	1
½" slice, 2 oz	80	4	2
Singles: Classic, 3 oz pkg	210	16	2
Turkey, 3 oz pkg	110	4	3
Summer Sausage:			
Bridgeford, 1 oz	100	9	1
Oscar Mayer, 1 slice, 0.8 oz	70	7	0.5
Treet *(Armour),* canned, 1 oz	100	9	1.5
Turkey: Average, 1 oz slice	30	1	0.5
¾ oz slice	22	0.5	0.5
Turkey Breast:			
Butterball Fat Free, 3 sl., 2 oz	60	0	4
Deli Thin Smoked, 2 sl., 1 oz	50	0.5	2
Hillshire Deli Select, 6 sl., 2 oz	50	0.5	2
Louis Rich Carvery Board,			
2 slices, 1.8 oz (52g)	50	0	2
Free, 2 slices, 2 oz	50	0	2
Healthy Choice: Deli Thin: Per 4 Slices, 52g (1.8 oz)			
Oven-Roasted	60	1.5	2
Smoked/Rotisserie Seasoned	60	1.5	3
Honey Roasted & Smoked	60	1.5	4
Hearty Deli Sliced:			
Oven Rstd Turkey Brst. 1 sl., 1 oz	30	1	1
Turkey Ham, 1 slice, 1 oz	35	1.5	0.5
Turkey Pastrami, 1 oz	35	1.5	1
Turkey Roll, 1 oz	40	2	0.5
Turkey Loaf, 1 oz	35	1	0.5
Vegetarian Deli *(Worthington, Yves):* See Page 76			

Meat Spreads

	C	F	Cb
Average All Brands: *Per ¼ Cup (2 oz)*			
Chicken	90	10	2
Ham, deviled	140	11	0
Liverwurst	190	16	2
Roast Beef	130	10	2
Sandwich Spread	140	10	9
Turkey	110	7	2

Paté

C **F** **Cb**

	C	F	Cb
Canned: *Average All Brands*			
Chicken Liver, 2 Tbsp, 1 oz	60	4	2
Paté de Foie Gras, goose liver, 1 oz	130	12	2
Fresh (Refrigerated):			
Average all types, 1 oz	110	10	1
Boar's Head Liverwurst Pate, 2 oz	145	12	0
Marcel Henri			
Pate de Champagne	210	18	2
Chicken Liver w. Port Wine, 2 oz	210	18	2
Duck Truffle w. Port Wine, 2 oz	240	24	2
Old Wisconsin Pate			
All types, 1 oz	105	9	1.5
Vegetable Pate; Spin/Mushr., 2 oz	105	7	10
Trois Petit Cochons			
Mediterranean, 2 oz	130	11	3
Smoked Salmon, 2 oz	115	9	2
Wegmans			
Alexian Wild, 2 oz	270	27	1
Cognac; Black Peppercorn, 2 oz	160	17	4

Lunch Packs

C **F** **Cb**

	C	F	Cb
Lunchables *(Oscar Mayer): Per Package*			
Cracker Stackers Ham & Cheddar	420	23	37
Nachos Cheese & Salsa, 4.4 oz	380	21	39
Pizza varieties, avg., 4.5 oz	300	13	28
Taco Bell Beef Tacos, 5.35 oz	310	11	34
Fun Fuel: Ham Bagels, 5.6 oz	410	10	64
Chicken/Ham Wraps, 5.5 oz	435	13	64
Peanut Butter Soft White Bread	600	19	85
Turkey Bagels, 5.6 oz	420	10	64
Pizza Dunks Soft Breadsticks	500	13	84
Beef Taco, 5.7 oz	495	15	69
Waffles & Sausage, 4.8 oz	460	16	66
Fun Snacks: Chips Ahoy!, 3.1 oz	200	9	30
Fudge Brownie, 4.3 oz	260	9	42
Oreo Cookies 'N Frosting, 3.7 oz	230	9	37
S'Mores, 3.4 oz	200	6	35
Star Cookies 'N Frosting, 3.6 oz	230	10	34
Mega Pack: Combo Ham & Ched.	765	32	101
Combo Turkey & Cheddar, 5.4 oz	750	31	101
Pizza: Pepperoni, 6.85 oz	760	28	105
Extra Cheesy, 6.8 oz	700	25	104
Pizza Stix, 7.15 oz	680	16	118
Ultimate Nachos Cheese & Salsa	780	32	113
Lunch Bucket *(Armour)*			
Beans 'n Weiners, 7.5 oz	290	10	37
Chili w. Beans, 7.5 oz	235	9	25
Hearty Beef Stew, 7.5 oz	155	8	15
Rings 'n Franks, 7.5 oz	225	9	30
Lunchmakers *(Armour)*			
Loco Nachos	370	13	59
Cheese Pizza	310	13	36
Smuckers			
Snackers, 3.3 oz package	410	20	47
Uncrustables Sandwiches:			
Grilled Cheese Sandwich, 1.76 oz	150	6	17
Peanut Butter Sandwich, 1.72 oz	200	11	18
Peanut Butter & Honey, 1.76 oz	210	9	26
Peanut Butter & Grape Jelly: 1.76 oz	210	9	25
Large, 80g	320	16	33
Peanut Butter & Strawb. Jam: 1.76 oz	210	9	25
Large, 80g	320	16	33
South Beach Diet *(Kraft)*			
Wraps: *Per Package*			
Deli Ham & Turkey, 1 pkg	220	10	24
Grilled Chicken Caesar, 1 pkg	230	10	24
Southwestern Style Chicken	240	10	26
Turkey & Bacon Club, 1 pkg	250	12	25

STOP!
ARE YOU REALLY HUNGRY?
Or Simply Eating Out Of Habit, Or To Relieve
Boredom, Stress Or Feeling Low?!

INSTEAD, TRY ONE OF THESE:

Drink Some Water or Diet Soda · Take A Walk · Take A Bike Ride!
Phone A Friend · Relax In A Hot Tub · Have A Cuddle
Read A Book · Meditate · Relax To Music
Go Dig In The Garden · Play With The Kids

COPYRIGHT © 1998 ALLAN BORUSHEK
SALES: PH (714) 642 0500 FAX (714) 642 0900

Do you snack compulsively
when you are bored,
stressed or irritable?

If so, place this magnetic
STOP! poster on your fridge.

To Order, See Page 303

Chicken

Quick Guide

	C	F	Cb
Chicken			
From 3lb ready-to-cook chicken			
Breast/Wing Quarter			
Roasted: With skin	300	15	0
Without skin	185	5	0
Fried, batter dipped	530	30	17
Leg Quarter: Thigh & Drumstick			
Roasted: With skin	270	16	0
Without skin	185	8	0
Fried, batter dipped	435	25	15
KFC: *See Fast-Foods Section*			

Average - All Meats

	C	F	Cb
Average of Light Meat: *Per 4 oz (no bone)*			
Roasted: with skin	250	12	0
without skin	190	5	0
Stewed: with skin	225	12	0
without skin	180	4.5	0
Fried: Batter-dipped, 4 oz	310	17	12
Flour coated, 4 oz	275	14	2
Average of Dark Meat: *Per 4 oz (no bone)*			
Roasted: with skin	285	18	0
without skin	230	12	0
Stewed: with skin	260	16	0
without skin	215	10	0
Fried: Batter-dipped, 4 oz	330	21	12
Flour coated, 4 oz	320	20	5

Chicken Parts

	C	F	Cb
Broilers or Fryers: Edible Weights (no bone)			
Breast: *Per ½ Breast*			
Raw: With skin, 5 oz	240	13	0
Without skin, 4¼ oz	130	1.5	0
Roasted: With skin, 3½ oz	195	8	0
Without skin, 3 oz	140	3	0
Stewed: With skin, 4 oz	210	8	0
Without skin, 3¼ oz	145	3	0
Fried: Batter-dipped, 5 oz	365	19	12
Flour coated, w. skin, 3½ oz	220	9	7
Drumstick: *Per Drumstick*			
Roasted: With skin, 2 oz	115	6	0
Without skin, 1½ oz	75	2.5	0
Fried: Batter-dipped, 2½ oz	195	11	7
Flour coated, 1¾ oz	120	7	1
Stewed: With skin, 2 oz	115	6	0
Without skin, 1½ oz	80	3	0

	C	F	Cb
Thigh Portion: Edible Wt. (no bone)			
Raw: With skin, 3.3 oz	200	14	0
(4¼ oz with bone)			
Without skin, 2.4 oz	80	3	0
Roasted: With skin, 2¼ oz	155	10	0
Without skin, 2 oz	110	6	0
Stewed: With skin, 2½ oz	160	10	0
Without skin, 2 oz	105	5	0
Fried: Batter-dipped, 3 oz	240	14	8
Flour coated, 2¼ oz	165	9	2
Wing: *Per Wing*			
Raw Weight 3.2 oz (with bone)			
Raw: With skin	110	8	0
Without skin	35	1	0
Roasted: With skin	100	7	0
Without skin	45	2	0
Fried: Batter-dipped	160	11	5
Flour coated	105	7	1
Stewed: With skin, 4 oz	100	7	0
Buffalo Wings: *See Fast-Foods Section*			
Neck: Simmered, with skin	95	7	0
Without skin	30	2	0
Skin Only: *Skin from ½ Chicken*			
Raw skin, 2¾ oz	275	26	0
Roasted skin, 2 oz	255	23	0
Stewed skin, 2½ oz	260	24	0
Fried, Flour coated, 2 oz	280	24	5
Fried, Batter-dipped, 6¾ oz	750	55	45
Roasters			
Average of Light & Dark Meat:			
Roasted: With skin, 4 oz	250	15	0
Without skin, 4 oz	190	8	0
Light Meat: Without skin, roasted	175	5	0
Dark Meat: Without skin, roasted	200	10	0
Stewing Chicken			
Average of Light & Dark Meat: *Per 4 oz Stewed*			
With skin	320	21	0
Without skin	265	14	0
Light Meat: Without skin	240	9	0
Dark Meat: Without skin	290	17	0
Capon Chicken			
Roasted: With skin, 4 oz	260	13	0
½ Chicken, with skin	1460	74	0
Chicken Offal & Stuffing			
Giblets: Simmered, 1 cup	230	7	0.5
Fried, flour-coated, 1 cup	400	20	6
Gizzard, simmered, 1 cup	225	4	0
Heart, simmered, 1 cup	270	12	0.2
Liver: Raw, 4 oz	135	5.5	1
Simmered, 1 cup	215	8.5	1
Liver Pate Fresh, 1 Tbsp, ½ oz	30	2	1
Stuffing: Average, ½ cup	180	9	22

Chicken Products | **C** | **F** | **Cb** |

Shop Stop

Item	C	F	Cb
Blazing Chicken Wings, 3 oz	200	12	1
Breaded Tenderloins (3), 4 oz	240	12	15
Boneless Skinless Breasts (1), 8 oz	210	5	3

Stove Top

Item	C	F	Cb
Chicken Stuffing Mix: 1 oz	110	1	20
½ cup prepared	170	9	20
Tyson: Breaded Nuggets (5)	280	18	16
Breast Nuggets (5)	280	16	21
Southern Fried Nuggets (6)	270	21	11
Breast Patties: Regular, 2.6 oz	180	11	12
Southern Fried (1), 2.6 oz	240	18	10
Wings: Flavored, average (3)	220	15	1
BBQ Style (3), 3½ oz	250	15	13
Stir Fry Kit: Chicken, 2¾ c. froz.	430	4.5	73

Duck, Goose, Quail

Item	C	F	Cb
Duck: Roasted, with skin, 3 oz	285	24	0
Without skin, 3 oz	170	10	0
½ whole duck, with skin	1290	108	0
Goose: Roast, with skin, 3 oz	260	19	0
Without skin, 3 oz	200	11	0
Pheasant: ½ bird, raw	725	37	0
Quail: 1 whole, raw	210	13	0

Turkey

Fryer-Roasters: *Per 3 oz Serving*

Item	C	F	Cb
Roasted: Light Meat, with skin	140	4	0
without skin	120	1	0
Dark Meat: with skin	155	6	0
without skin	140	4	0

½ of Whole Turkey: (Approx. 3¼ lbs raw wt. w/out neck and giblets; 1.8 lbs cooked wt.)

Item	C	F	Cb
Roasted: With skin	1400	46	0
Without skin	1030	18	0

Ground Turkey, Raw: (4 oz raw wt. = 3 oz ckd wt.)

Item	C	F	Cb
Regular (85% lean), 4 oz	170	10	0
Lean (90% lean), 4 oz	160	8	0
Foster Farms (94% lean), 4 oz	150	7	0
Jennie-O (93% lean), 4 oz	160	8	0
Breast, no skin, 4 oz	115	1	0
Patties: Small, 3 oz	110	6.5	0
Medium, 4 oz	160	9	0
Large, 5.3 oz	175	10	0

Turkey Parts | **C** | **F** | **Cb** |

Roasted, Edible Weights (no bone)

Breast (½): (from 17¼ oz raw wt. w/bone)

Item	C	F	Cb
With skin, 12 oz (no bone)	525	11	0
Without skin, 10¾ oz	415	2	0

Back (½): With skin, 4½ oz

Item	C	F	Cb
With skin, 4½ oz	305	18	0
Without skin, 3½ oz	165	6	0

Leg (Thigh & Drumstick): (from 1 lb raw wt. w/bone)

Item	C	F	Cb
With skin, 8½ oz (no bone)	345	16	0
Without skin, 7¾ oz	235	5	0

Wing: (from 7¼ oz raw wt. w/bone)

Item	C	F	Cb
With skin, 3 oz (no bone)	185	9	0
Without skin, 2 oz	100	2	0
Neck: Simmered, 1 neck, (9 oz w. bone)	275	11	0
Giblets, simm., 1 cup, 5 oz	240	7	3

Young Hens (Roasted)

Item	C	F	Cb
Light Meat: With skin, 3 oz	175	8	0
Without skin, 3 oz	135	3	0
Dark Meat: With skin, 3 oz	200	11	0
Without skin, 3 oz	165	7	0

Young Toms – Similar to Young Hens

Turkey Products

Banquet: *See Frozen Meals, Page 61*

Item	C	F	Cb
Circle L: Boneless Bacon, 3 oz	120	9	1

Hormel: Turkey Ham & Chunks (canned), ckd:

Item	C	F	Cb
Breast & White Turkey, 2 oz	60	1	2
Turkey Ham/Pastrami, 2 oz	70	3	1
Turkey Salami, 2 oz	100	8	0
Jennie-O: Turkey Bacon, 2 slice	35	3	0
Turkey in BBQ Sauce, 5 oz	200	2	17

Louis Rich: 98% Fat Free Breast of Turkey

Item	C	F	Cb
Rotiss'd/Smoked/Rstd, 2 oz, 3 sl.	60	1	0
Franks: Medium, 1½ oz	100	8	2
Large, 2 oz	125	10	3.5
Smoked Sausage/Kielbasa, 1 oz	45	2.5	1
Turkey Bacon, 1 oz	70	5	0
Turkey Nuggets/Sticks, ckd, ea.	75	5	4.5

Luncheon Slices: *See Deli Meats, Page 54*
Swanson: *Frozen Meals, Page 67*
Turkey Store (Jennie-O)

Item	C	F	Cb
Gobble Stix (1)	25	0	1

Fish ~ Fresh & Canned

Quick Guide

Fresh Fish

C **F** **Cb**

Low Oil (Less than 2.5% fat)
White/pale colored flesh. Examples:
Cod, Flounder, Haddock, Halibut, Mahi Mahi
Perch, Pike, Pollock, Snapper, Sole, Whiting.

Per 4 oz Edible Portion

	C	F	Cb
Raw, 4 oz (no bones)	90	1	0
Steamed, Broiled, Baked	130	1	0
Fried: Lightly Floured	210	8	3.5
Breaded	260	12	8
In Batter	320	16	27

Medium Oil (2.5-5% fat)
Pale colored flesh. Examples: **C** **F** **Cb**
Bluefin Tuna, Catfish, Kingfish, Orange Roughy,
Salmon (Pink), Swordfish, Rainbow Trout, Yellowtail.

	C	F	Cb
Raw, 4 oz (no bones)	140	5	0
Baked, Broiled, 4 oz	175	6	0
Fried, 4 oz	230	11	8

High Oil (Over 5% fat) **C** **F** **Cb**
Darker colored flesh. Examples:
Albacore Tuna, Bluefish, Herring, Mackerel,
Salmon (Atl./Chinook/Sockeye), Sardines, Trout,
Whitefish.

	C	F	Cb
Raw, 4 oz (no bones)	230	16	0
Baked, Broiled, 4 oz	275	17	0
Fried, 4 oz	340	23	12

Cooking Yields (Fin Fish):
4 oz Raw wt. = 3½ oz Cooked wt.
4 oz Cooked wt. = 5 oz Raw wt.

Calorie & Fat Variations
The amount of fat/oil in fish varies with the species,
season and locality. Within the same fish, fat/oil content
is generally higher towards the head.

Fish & Shellfish

C **F** **Cb**

Edible Weights: (no bones/shell)

	C	F	Cb
Abalone, Raw, 3 oz	90	0.5	5
Ahi Tuna, grilled, 6 oz fillet (no fat)	220	2	0
Anchovy: Paste, 1 Tbsp, ¼ oz	15	1	0.5
Cnd. in oil, drnd., 5 only, ¾ oz	40	2	0
Pickled, 1 oz	50	3	0
Barracuda (Pacific), raw, 4 oz	130	3	0
Bass: Sea, raw, 4.6 oz fillet	125	2.5	0
Striped: Raw, 1 fillet, 5½ oz	150	3.5	0
Baked, 3 oz	105	3	0
Blue Fish: Raw, 1 fillet, 5¼ oz	185	6.5	0
Baked, 3 oz	130	5	0
Butterfish, raw, 3 oz	125	7	0
Cajun & Creole Dishes: *See Page 176*			
Calamari, breaded/fried, 1 serve	360	21	10
Carp, raw, 3 oz	110	5	0
Catfish: Raw, 4 oz	115	6.5	0
Fried, breaded, 1 fillet, 3 oz	200	12	7
Baked, 3 oz	130	7	0
Caviar, black/red, 1 Tbsp, 16g	40	3	0.5
Clams: Raw, 3 oz (4 lge/9 small)	65	1	2
Fried, breaded, 6.6 oz (20 small)	380	21	20
Canned, drained, ½ cup, 2½ oz	105	1.5	3.5
Minced, ¼ cup, 2 oz	25	0	2
Clam Juice: (*Snow's*) 1 Tbsp	0	0	0
Cod, Atlantic/Pacific: Raw, 4 oz	95	1	0
Baked/Broiled, 1 fillet, 6¼ oz	190	2	0
Canned, 3 oz	90	1	0
Minced, ¼ cup, 2 oz	25	0	0
Smoked/Dry Heat, 3 oz	95	1	0
Crab: Alaska King, raw, 1 leg, 6 oz	145	1	0
1 leg, cooked, 4¾ oz	130	2	0
Blue: Raw, 1 crab			
(⅓ lb whole crab, ¾ oz flesh)	20	0.2	0
Steamed, 3 oz	85	1	0
Canned, drained, ½ cup, 2½ oz	65	1	0
Dungeness, 1 crab, 5¾ oz edible			
(from 1½ lb whole crab)	180	2	0
Imitation Crab Legs/Stix, 3oz	85	1	8.5
Crab Cakes (Low-fat), (1), 2 oz	95	4.5	0.5
Regular (1), 3 oz	130	6.5	0
Crab Legs, restaurant (*Red Lobster*)	260	4.5	0
Crayfish, raw, 4 oz (edible)	100	1	0
Croaker, raw, 3 oz	90	3	0
Cuttlefish, raw, 3 oz	70	1	0
Dolphinfish, raw, 1 fillet, 7 oz	175	1.5	0
Eel: Raw, 3 oz	155	10	0
Smoked/Dry Heat, 3 oz	200	13	0
Fish & Chips: *Arthur Treacher*	1540	101	132
Denny's, no condiments	960	54	83
Fish S'wich w. Tartar Sce, 5½ oz	430	23	41
Fish Sticks (1), frozen, breaded, 1 oz	70	3.5	6

Fish & Shellfish (Cont)

Edible Weights: (no bones/shell)

	C	F	Cb
Fish Oil, 1 Tbsp, ½ oz	125	14	0
Flounder/Sole: Raw, 4 oz	105	1.5	0
Baked, 1 fillet, 4½ oz	150	2	0
Frozen Fish & Entrees: *See Page 60*			
Gefilte Fish: *See Kosher/Deli Foods, Page 179*			
Grouper, raw, 4 oz	105	1	0
Haddock: Raw, 4 oz	100	1	0
Broiled, 1 fillet, 5¼ oz	170	1.5	0
Smoked, 3 oz	100	1	0
Baked, 3 oz	90	1	0
Halibut: Raw, 4 oz	125	3	0
Baked, ½ fillet, 2¾ oz	225	5	0
Herring: Atlantic, raw, 4 oz	180	10	0
Pickled, 2 pieces, 1 oz	80	5	3
In Sour Cream, 1 oz	55	3	5
Party Snacks, ¼ cup, dr., 2 oz	120	5	0
Rollmops, 1½ oz	110	8	6
Canned: Plain, drained, 3 oz	130	8	0
in Tomato Sauce, 3.5 oz	140	8	2
Smoked, kippered, 4 oz	245	14	0
Jellyfish: Raw, 4 oz	30	0	0
Dried, Salted, 1 cup, 2 oz	20	1	0
King Fish, raw, 4 oz	120	2.5	0
Ling, raw, 4 oz	100	0.5	0
Lobster, Northern: Raw, 4 oz	105	1	0.5
1 Lobster, 6¼ oz			
(from 1½ lb whole lobster)	160	1.5	1
Cooked, 1 cup, 5 oz	140	1	2
Lobster Newberg, ¾ cup	360	20	9
Lobster Thermidor, 1 serving	370	22	15
Lobster Salads, ½ cup	220	13	5
Lobster Tail, restaurant *(Red Lobster)*	260	3	0
Lomi Salmon, ¼ cup, 4 oz	20	1	3
Lox, Regular/Nova, 2 oz	65	2.5	0
Mackerel: Atlantic, raw, 4 oz	230	16	0
Broiled, 3 oz fillet	230	16	0
Jack, canned, ½ c., 3⅓ oz	150	6	0
King, raw, 4 oz	120	2	0
Pacific/Jack: Raw, 4 oz	180	9	0
Broiled, 3 oz	170	9	0
Spanish, raw, 4 oz	160	7	0
Mahi-Mahi, raw, 4 oz	125	1	0
Milkfish, raw, 4 oz	170	7.5	0
Monkfish: Raw, 4 oz	85	1.5	0
Baked, 3 oz	80	2	0
Mullet, striped, raw, 4 oz	135	4.5	0
Mussels: Raw, 4 oz (edible wt.)	100	2.5	4
1 cup, 5¼ oz (edible wt.)	130	3.5	5
Cooked, moist heat, 3 oz	150	4	6

	C	F	Cb
Ocean Perch: Raw, 4 oz	105	1	0
Baked, 3 oz	100	1	0
Octopus, common, raw, 4 oz	95	1	2.5
Orange Roughy, raw, 4 oz	85	1	0
Oysters: Common, raw, 3 oz	70	2	0
Eastern raw: 6 medium, 3 oz	50	1.5	4.5
1 cup, 8¾ oz	150	4	14
Fried/breaded, 6 med., 3 oz	170	11	10
Pacific, raw, 1 med., 1¾ oz	40	1	2
Oysters Rockerfeller, 3 oysters	220	13	12
Perch, average, raw, 4 oz	105	1	0
Pike: Northern, raw, 4 oz	100	1	0
Walleye, raw, 4 oz	105	1.5	0
Pollock, raw, 4 oz	105	1	0
Pout (Ocean), raw, 4 oz	90	1	0
Pompano, Florida, raw, 4 oz	190	10	0
Porgy/Scup, raw, 4 oz	150	4	0
Quahogs ~ See Clams			
Red-Snapper, raw, 4 oz	115	1.5	0
Rockfish, Pacific, raw, 4 oz	110	2	0
Roe, raw, 2 Tbsp, 1 oz	40	2	0.5
Sablefish, raw, 4 oz	220	17	0
Smoked, 3 oz	220	17	0
Salmon:			
Raw: Chinook, 4 oz	205	12	0
Atlantic; Coho/Silver, 4 oz	210	12	0
Chum; Pink, 4 oz	135	4	0
Red/Sockeye, 4 oz	190	10	0
Baked: Atlantic/Coho, 3 oz	150	7	0
Smoked Salmon: Chinook, 3 oz	100	4	0
Pacific Supreme, 2 oz	100	4	0
Wild Oats, Pastrami Style, 2 oz	130	9	0
Canned Salmon: *Average All Brands*			
Pink: 1 oz	40	2	0
¼ cup, 63g (2.2 oz)	90	5	0
3¾ oz can, whole	155	8.5	0
7½ oz can, whole	300	17	0
Skinless/boneless, ¼ c., 2 oz	70	2	0
Red Sockeye: 1 oz	50	3	0
¼ cup, 63g (2.2 oz)	110	7	0
3¾ oz can, whole	190	12	0
Atlantic, ½ cup, 3½ oz	230	14	0
Chinook/King, ½ cup	210	14	0
Chum, ½ cup, 3½ oz	140	5	0
Coho/Silver, ½ cup	155	5	0
Atlantic Steaks: Small, 8 oz	320	14	0
Medium, 12 oz	480	21	0
Large, 16 oz	640	28	0
Salmon Cake, take-out, 3 oz	240	15	6

Fish ~ Fresh & Canned (Cont)

Fish (Cont)

	C	F	Cb
Sardines (Canned): *Average All Brands*			
In Oil, undrained, 1 oz	85	7	0
Drained of oil, 1 oz	60	3	0
3¾ oz can, drained, (3¼ oz)	190	11	0
1 lge/2 med. ⅗" small, 0.8 oz	50	3	0
In Tom./ Mustard Sce, 1 oz	45	3	0
3¾ oz can (3 sardines)	210	12	1
Sashimi: *See Japanese Foods, Page 178*			
Scallop: Raw, 6 lge/15 small, 3 oz	80	0.5	2
Breaded/fried, 6 pces, 3½ oz	200	10	10
Sea Bass, raw, 4 oz	110	2	0
Seafood Salad, 1/2 cup	190	16	7
Shark: Raw, 4 oz	150	5	0
Batter-dipped, fried, 4 oz	260	16	0
Baked, 4 oz	185	7	0
Shark Fin, dried, 1 oz	30	0	0
Shrimp: Raw, in shell, ½ lb	140	2	1.5
Raw, shelled, 3 oz (12 lge)	90	1.5	0.5
Breaded/fried, 3 oz (11 lge)	210	11	10
Canned, 1 oz (10 shrimp)	65	1	0
Tiger, cooked, 1 shrimp, ½ oz	15	0.5	0
Battered, fried, 1 shrimp	60	4	3
Shrimp Cocktail, restaurant-style	140	2	1
Smelt, Rainbow, raw, 4 oz	110	3	0
Snapper: Raw, 3 oz	85	1	0
Cooked, 1 fillet, 6 oz	215	3	0
Sole, raw, 4 oz	105	1.5	0
Squid: Raw, 4 oz	105	1.5	3.5
Fried, 3 oz	150	6	7
Surimi (Imitation Crab), 4 oz	115	1.5	11
Sweet & Sour Fish, ½ dish, 10 oz	580	29	53
Swordfish raw:			
Small Steak, 4 oz	135	4.5	0
Medium Steak, 6 oz	205	7	0
Tilapia, Rain Forest Fillets, 4 oz	110	2	0
Trout, Rainbow: Raw, 4 oz	135	4	0
Broiled, 3 oz	125	5	0
Smoked, 2 oz	110	6	0
Tuna: *Average All Brands*			
Raw: Albacore, 4 oz	190	8	0
Bluefin, 4 oz	165	5.5	0
Skipjack, Yellowfin, 4 oz	125	1	0
Broiled, 3 oz	115	1	0
Canned:			
In Water, drained:			
Chunk/Solid: 2 oz can	75	1.5	0
3 oz can	110	2.5	0
6 oz can	220	5	0
In Oil, drained:			
Chunk Light: 2 oz	110	5	0
6 oz can, drained	340	14	0

Tuna (Cont)

	C	F	Cb
Solid White, 2 oz	105	4.5	0
6.3 oz can, drained	330	14	0
Tuna Salad: Deli Style, ½ c., 4oz	300	24	15
Lower fat, 4 oz	210	10	11
Whitefish: Raw, 4 oz	150	6.5	0
Baked, 3 oz	145	6.5	0
Smoked, 3 oz	90	1	0
Whiting: Raw, 4 oz	100	1.5	0
Baked, 3 oz	85	1	0
Yellowtail: Raw, 4 oz	165	6	0
Grilled, 3 oz (from 4 oz raw)	160	6	0

Other Canned/Packaged Fish

	C	F	Cb
Bumble Bee: *Incl. Mayo & Crackers*			
Tuna Salad Kit: Original	280	20	18
Fat-Free Kit	150	1.5	24
w. Mayonnaise Kit	420	22	24
Seafood Salad w. Crab Kit	180	5.5	27
Sensations: Spring Thai Chili Kit	250	12	20
Other varieties, average	200	8.5	13
Lunch on the Run, Tuna Salad Kit	320	14	19
Chicken of the Sea			
Albacore Tuna, 3 oz pouch	100	1.5	0
Light Tuna, 3 oz pouch	90	1	0
Shrimp, 2.5 oz pouch	55	0.5	1
Smoked Pacific Salmon, 3 oz pouch	120	3.5	0
Starkist			
Pouch: *Per 3 oz Pouch (Drained)*			
Tuna Chunk Light, in water, 2 oz	90	1	0
Albacore Tuna, in water, 2 oz	105	1.5	0
Lunch-To-Go Kit: Chunk Light Tuna			
w. Mayo/Crackers, 4.5 oz	210	9	27
Tuna Creations, all varieties, 2 oz	60	0	0

Frozen Fish Products

Gorton's: *See Page 63*
Kroger: *See Page 64*
SeaPak: *See Page 66*
Van De Kamp's: *See Page 68*
Fast-Foods & Restaurant Chains: *See Page 183*
Captain D's Seafood: *See Fast-Food Section*
Long John Silvers: *See Fast-Food Section*
Shoney's: *See Fast-Food Section*

Amy's (Vegetarian)

	C	F	Cb
Per Serving			
Bowls: Brown Rice & Vegs, 10 oz	260	9	36
Santa Fe Enchilada, 10 oz	350	11	47
(Other Varieties ~ *www.CalorieKing.com*)			
Asian Meals: Thai Stir Fry, 9.5 oz	310	11	45
Asian Noodle Stir Fry, 10 oz	290	7	50
Entrees: Chse Enchilada, 4.7 oz	240	14	18
Cheese Lasagna, 10.3 oz	380	14	44
Macaroni & Cheese, 9 oz	410	16	47
Macaroni & Soy Cheeze, 9 oz	370	15	42
Whole Meals: Chse Enchilada, 9 oz	350	15	38
Black Bean Enchilada, 10 oz	330	8	53
Veggie Loaf, 10 oz	280	7	47
Pot Pies: Country Vege, 7½ oz	370	16	47
Mex. Tamale; Shepherd's Pie, avg.	160	4	27
Vegetable (Non Dairy), 7½ oz	360	13	50
Burgers: Californian (1), 2½ oz	140	5	19
Other varieties (1), avg., 2½ oz	120	2.5	14
Burritos: Bean & Rice, 6 oz	280	6	48
Bean & Cheese, 6 oz	280	8	43
Breakfast Burrito, 6 oz	250	7	38
Snacks: Nacho, 5-6 pieces, 3 oz	210	8	26
Cheese Pizza, 5-6 pieces, 3 oz	190	7	22
Extra Product Listings ~ www.CalorieKing.com			

Banquet

	C	F	Cb
Pot Pies: Beef, 7 oz	450	27	36
Chicken/Turkey, average, 7 oz	380	21	36
Chicken: Breast Patties (1)	260	19	13
Chicken Brst Tenders/ Nuggets (5)	220	13	14
Crispy Chicken, Skinless, 4.2 oz	330	19	16
Popcorn Chicken, 11 pieces	180	9	18
Wings: Hot & Spicy, 3 oz	260	17	8
Honey Barbecue, 3 oz	270	17	12
Crock Pot Classics: *Per Cup*			
Beef Stew	210	5	23
Chicken & Dumplings	310	14	27
Chicken & Red Potatoes	240	11	21
Creamy Chicken & Pasta	430	20	39
Herb Chicken & Rice, 1 cup	310	3.5	51
Homestyle Pork	200	4	24
Stroganoff Beef & Noodles	350	12	38
Hearty One Dinners: Turkey, 16 oz	520	22	48
Boneless Pork Rib, 16 oz	650	34	55
Chicken Fried Beef Steak, 16 oz	730	40	65
Fried Chicken, 16 oz	820	40	70
Salisbury, 16 oz	600	30	50

Banquet (Cont)

	C	F	Cb
Meals: BBQ Chicken	280	8	35
Boneless Pork Rib, 10 oz	370	18	37
Cheese Enchilada Meal, 11 oz	410	12	64
Chicken Fingers, 7 oz	550	26	60
Chicken Fried Beef Steak, 10 oz	380	18	41
Corn Dog Meal, 7.5 oz	490	18	68
Fettuccine Alfredo	420	18	50
Fried Chicken, 9 oz	450	20	35
Fried Rice w. Chicken & Egg Roll	320	7	46
Homestyle Noodles & Chicken	450	20	46
Lasagna w. Meat Sauce, 11 oz	340	9	50
Mac & Cheese, 6.5 oz	400	11	59
Macaroni & Beef, 11 oz	320	6	50
Meatloaf Meal, 9.5 oz	280	14	25
Mexican Style Enchilada Combo	400	15	60
Our Original Fried Chicken	470	27	35
Pepperoni Pizza, 6.75	400	13	61
Salisbury Steak Meal, 9.5 oz	300	15	27
Spaghetti & Meatballs, 10.5 oz	400	17	40
Swedish Meatballs, 10.25 oz	400	19	33
Sweet & Sour Chicken, 10 oz	430	16	60
Turkey Mostly White Meat	230	6	30

Bertolli

	C	F	Cb
Per ½ Package			
Chicken alla Vodka & Farfalle	500	24	40
Chicken Florentine & Farfalle	560	31	40
Chicken Parmesan & Penne	530	25	52
Grilled Chicken Alfredo	710	42	54
Meatballs Pomodoro & Penne	600	31	54
Roasted Chicken & Linguini	420	17	41
Shrimp Asparagus & Penne	480	21	50
Shrimp Scampi & Linguini	500	25	53
Spicy Shrimp Fra Diavolo & Penne	410	19	41
Spinach & Ricotta Cheese Ravioli	500	28	46

Birds Eye – Voila!

	C	F	Cb
Per Cup, Cooked (2 Cups Frozen)			
Chicken Voila!: Garlic Chicken	240	8	21
Other varieties, average	220	7	28
Steak Voila! Beef Sirloin/Potato	190	7	22
Reduced Carb Voila: *Per 1 cup Cooked*			
Chicken & Sausage Tuscano	170	8	10
Chicken Teriaki & Vegetables	160	4	15
Down Home Chicken and Vegetables	180	5	17
Roasted Garlic Chicken & Vege.	120	2.5	13
Teriaki Chicken & Vegetables	150	2.5	15

Frozen Entrees & Meals (Cont)

Boca (Vegetarian)

	C	F	Cb
Burger: Cheeseburger, 1 patty	100	5	5
All American Flame Grilled (1)	90	3	5
Vegan, Original, 1 patty	70	0.5	9
Organic Burgers: Vegan, Orig. (1)	100	2.5	9
Roasted Garlic/Onion, 1 patty	70	1.5	6
Chik'n: Nuggets (4), 3 oz	180	7	17
Hot & Spicy Buffalo Wings (4)	160	7	14
Patties (1), 2.5 oz	160	6	15
Sausages: Bratwurst (1), 2.5 oz	140	7	6
Italian, 2.5 oz	130	6	6
Organic Pizza, ⅓ Pizza	260	8	36

Boston Market

	C	F	Cb
Meals: *Per Serving*			
Beef Sirloin & Noodles	470	12	59
Chicken Pot Pie, 1 cup (½ box)	560	36	43
Meatloaf	670	39	50
Salisbury Steak	720	28	61
Swedish Meatballs	860	49	70

Budget Gourmet (Michelina's)

	C	F	Cb
Classics: *Per Container (8 oz)*			
Escalloped Noodles & White Turkey	300	10	44
Fettuccini Alfredo w. 4 Cheeses	300	9	43
Pizza Snacks, 5 oz	410	21	41
Spicy Szechwan Vege w. Chicken	310	6	51
Stir Fry Rice & Vegetables	450	20	60
Other varieties, average	290	12	37
Premium: Beef Stroganoff, 8 oz	290	7	38
Beef Pepper Steak w. Rice, 8 oz	260	4.5	43
Cheese Manicotti	300	13	31
Chicken and Pasta, 8.5 oz	380	15	43
Lasagne w. Meat Sauce	320	8	47
Stuffed Pepper Casserole	260	10	32
Swedish Meatballs, 10 oz	470	22	50
Lean Gourmet: Shrimp Scampi	220	2.5	44
Salisbury Steak w. Pot. & Gravy	210	7	26
Santa Fe Style Rice & Beans	350	9	59
Shrimp w. Pasta & Veges, 8 oz	260	6	37
Swedish Meatballs, 9 oz	310	9	41

Cedarlane (Vegetarian)

	C	F	Cb
Burrito, Beans, Rice, Chse (1), 6 oz	260	1	48
Eggplant Parmesan, ½ pkg, 5 oz	480	8	16
Dr Sears Zone: Chse Omelet, 1 ctn	350	13	37
Spinach & Cheese Pizza (1)	370	14	40
Vegetable Lasagne, 1 pkg	310	12	33
Enchilada: Garden Vege (1), 4.8 oz	140	3	20
Three-Layer Pie, ½ pkg, 5.5 oz	215	7	27
Lasagne: Cheese, ½ ctn, 5 oz	190	6	22
Garden Vege, ½ ctn, 5 oz	180	3	26

Claim Jumper

	C	F	Cb
Meals: Baby Back Pork Ribs (3)	210	14	2
Beef Pot Pie	580	41	39
Beef Pot Roast	500	20	48
Buffalo Wings (2)	160	9	5
Chicken Fried Beef Steak	660	36	68
Chicken Pot Pie, ½ pie, 8 oz	550	37	39
Chicken Tenderloins, 2 pieces	160	6	12
Country Fried Chicken, 19 oz	610	26	72
Lasagna w. Meat Sauce, 8 oz	280	13	26
Meatloaf Dinner	570	36	38
Rst Turkey Brst w. Gravy & Dressing	520	24	53
Salisbury Steak	630	36	43
Spicy Chicken Tenderloins, 3 oz	210	8	20
Turkey Pot Pie, ½ pie, 8 oz	540	39	37
Sauce: Hot Sauce, ½ Tbsp	0	0	0
Original Barbecue, 4 Tbsp	70	0.5	17

Contessa

	C	F	Cb
Meals: *Per Serving*			
Beef Goulash, 8 oz	210	5	32
Burgandy Beef Stew, 8 oz	210	11	22
Chicken Cacciatori, 8 oz	230	7	24
Chicken Chow Mein, 8 oz	320	2.5	55
Chicken Tandoori, 1⅓ cups, 8 oz	200	3.5	27
Kung Pao Shrimp, 8 oz	200	3.5	30
Shrimp Mediteranean, 1¾ cups	180	3	27
Shrimp Primavera, 1½ cups	350	21	30
Shrimp Stir Fry, 1¾ cups	120	2.5	16
Sweet n Sour Shrimp, 1½ cups	180	0	40

Croissant Pockets

	C	F	Cb
Egg, Sausage & Cheese	360	20	37
Five Cheese Pizza (1)	390	20	40
Ham & Cheddar	340	16	39
Pepperoni Pizza	390	20	42
Philly Steak & Cheese	360	19	36
Other varieties, average	320	15	35

El Monterey

	C	F	Cb
Shredded Beef Tamales (1)	310	19	27
Soft Taco: Beef & Cheese (1)	440	22	42
Spicy Beef & Cheese (1)	420	22	40
Spicy Chicken & Cheese (1)	340	11	44
Quesadilla: Gr. Chkn & 3 Chse (1)	260	14	20
Char Broiled Chicken & Chse (1)	230	10	20
Taquitos: Fiesta Appetizers Pack	370	23	29

Essensia (Albertson's)

	C	F	Cb
Entrees: Corn Souffle, 1 cup	300	19	17
Eggplant Parmesan, 1 cup	310	18	26
Herbed Chicken, 1/3 pkg	180	4.5	1
Jambalaya, 1 cup	220	5	26
Mac & Cheese, 1 cup	300	10	36
2 Meat Lasagna, 1 cup	360	20	31
Pork & Vege Spring Roll (1)	210	10	23
Roast Garlic Mash Potatoes, 5 oz	190	9	26
6 Cheese Cannelloni (1)	180	7	18
7 Cheese Lasagna, 5 oz	310	13	33
Striped Ravioli, 1 cup	360	20	31
Vegetable Lasagna, 1 cup	230	6	32

GardenBurger (Vegetarian)

	C	F	Cb
Meals: Chicken n Grill, 1 patty	100	2.5	5
Herb Crusted Chicken Cutlet (1)	150	9	10
Mamma Mia Meatballs (6)	110	4.5	7
Riblets, 1 riblet + sauce	230	4.5	27
Burgers: Per 2½ oz Patty			
Original Burger; Black Bean, avg	90	3	13
Flame Grilled, Homestyle Classic, avg.	120	4	7
Garden Vegan	100	1	12
Other varieties, average	100	3	1
Wraps: Margherita Pizza	240	8	34
Black Bean Chipotle (1)	240	8	32

Gorton's

	C	F	Cb
Fish Fillets: Beer Batter (1)	115	7	9
Crispy Battered (1)	130	8.5	8.5
Crunchy Golden (1)	120	6	12
Grilled, average all flavors (1)	100	3	1
Grilled Salmon, average (1)	100	3.5	1
Fish Sticks, Breaded (6), 3.7 oz	250	14	20
Grilled Fillet Meal: Alfredo	160	3	19
Lemon & Herb Butter	240	3.5	34
Popcorn Shrimp (11), 4 oz	280	17	22
Shrimp Bowl: Alfredo, 1 bowl	250	5	49
Fried Rice, 1 bowl	350	2.5	68
Garlic Butter, 1 bowl	260	6	38
Primavera, 1 bowl	270	6	41
Teriyaki, 1 bowl	320	6	57
Tenders: Extra Crunchy, 3½ pieces	260	12	29
Original, 3½ pieces, 4 oz	270	15	25

Green Giant

Create A Meal: Prepared with Meat & Oil
(Prepared Wt. ~ Approx 10 oz)

	C	F	Cb
Oven Rstd: Garlic Herb, 1¾ cup	350	9	35
Parmesan Herb Chicken, 1¾ c.	340	11	29
Stir Fry: Lo Mein, 1 cup	270	7	28
Szechuan; Teriyaki, avg., 1 cup	190	9	10

Green Giant (Cont)

	C	F	Cb
Complete Skillet: Per 1¼ Cup (Prep.)			
Beef Stew	180	3.5	27
Chkn Alfredo/& Cheesy Pasta, avg.	270	6	40
Chicken Lo Mein	190	2	31
Chicken Noodle, 1¼ cups	320	6	45
Chicken Teriyaki, 1½ cups	240	1	36
Garlic Chicken & Pasta, 1 cup	230	6	33
Steak Teriyaki, 1½ cup	300	3.5	53
Pasta Accents: Per Cup (Cooked)			
Alfredo Pasta	210	4	34
Primavera Pasta	250	11	33
Roasted Garlic Pasta	240	10	31

Healthy Choice

Entrees/Familiar Favorites: Per Meal

	C	F	Cb
Cheesy Rice & Chicken	230	4	33
Chicken Enchilada	360	7	59
Lasagna Bake	270	7	36
Macaroni & Cheese	270	6	40
Roast Turkey Breast	230	6	25
Dinners: Beef Pot Roast	320	9	39
Beef Tips Portabello	280	8	28
Chicken Enchilada	310	7	46
Chicken Parmigiana	320	9	40
Chicken Teriyaki w. Rice	270	6	37
Lemon Pepper Fish	280	5	49
Roasted Chicken Breast	280	8	32
Salisbury Steak	360	9	45
Sweet & Sour Chicken	340	7	54
Flavor Adventures: Beef Merlot	240	8	26
Chicken Tuscany	330	9	42
Grilled Chicken Baja	270	5	33
Oriental Style Beef	300	9	27

Home Bistro

Meals: Per Package

	C	F	Cb
Blackened Chkn in Champagne Sce	560	32	8
Chicken Stir Fry	310	7	15
French Toast Breakfast	720	59	28
Grilled Chkn Brst in Carmen Parmesan	480	31	7
Poached Salmon Fillet in Sauce	580	44	10
Roasted Turkey Breast w. Stuffing	440	20	19
Sea Scallops in Chili Hollandaise Sce	590	31	51
Shrimp Scampi	710	44	9
Low Carb: Beef Stir Fry	400	17	15
Filet Mignon w. Bearnaise Sce	870	73	14
Grilled Chicken Satay	640	40	20
Roasted Crab Cakes w. Sauce	540	43	10
Roasted Rack of Lamb w. Sauce	700	41	16
Szechuan Beef	390	21	10
Western Omelette w. Sausage	660	57	9

Hot Pockets

	C	F	Cb
Breakfast Pastries: Ham, Egg & Chse	150	7	17
Sausage, Egg & Cheese	170	9	18
Fruit Pastries: Apple/Strawb., avg.	240	9	39
Cream Cheese & Strawb. w. Icing	240	10	34
Pizza Mini's, avg. 5 pces, 3 oz	240	12	29
Sandwiches: Pepperoni Pizza	360	17	44
Barbecue Sce w. Beef; Italian	340	12	50
Chicken Melt with Bacon, 4½ oz	350	17	39
Four Cheese Pizza (no meat), 4½ oz	390	20	44
Steak Fajita, 4½ oz	260	7	39
Other varieties, average, 4½ oz	310	13	36
Subs: Ham & Cheese, 5.6 oz	360	10	49
Meatballs & Mozzarella, 5.6 oz	360	14	44
Other varieties, average, 5.6 oz	390	16	44
Pot Pie Express: Turkey, 1 pce	340	18	35
Other varieties, average, 1 pce	350	17	40

Impromptu Gourmet (Schwan's)

	C	F	Cb
Entrees: Choice Beef Filet Mignon	620	50	0
Choice Bison Rib Eye Steak, 10 oz	410	16	0
French Cut Rack of Pork, 4 oz	150	5	1
Fully Cooked Cajun Turkey, 3 oz	140	8	2
Gourmet Chkn Wellington, 8 oz	420	19	13
New York Strip, 10 oz	660	48	0
Orange Ginger Mahi Mahi, 7 oz	240	6	9
Prime Rib Roast, 12 oz	840	67	2
Spiral Sliced Ham, 3 oz	150	7	7
Stuffed Chkn Breast Saltimbocca	330	14	3
T-Bone Steak, 16 oz	250	18	0

José Olé

	C	F	Cb
Breakfast Burrito			
Egg, Sausage & Cheese, 4 oz	270	11	34
Egg, Ham & Cheese, 4 oz	260	9	34
Taquitos, average, 3 pieces	180	8	22
Mexi-Minis: Beef & Chse Tacos (4)	200	11	19
Chimichangas, 3 pces	240	12	25
Taquitos, 4 pces	180	8	21
Quesadillas, 3 pces	220	8	28
Burrito: Beef & Cheese (1)	300	10	39
Chicken Monterey (1)	270	6	40
Chimichanga: Beef, 1 pce	350	15	39
Chicken , 1 pce	330	12	44

Kid Cuisine

	C	F	Cb
Meals: Cheese Pizza Painter	400	8	68
Chicken Nuggets	440	17	53
Dip & Dunk Cheese Pizza Strips	470	13	65
Fiesta Beef Taco Dippers	390	18	44
Macaroni & Cheese	400	11	61
Pepperoni Pizza	390	7	69
Popstar Popcorn Chicken	420	13	61

Kroger

	C	F	Cb
Stir Fry: Beef Stir Fry, 1¾ cup	180	4	26
Calamari Rings (15)	200	11	19
Chicken Stir Fry, 1½ cup	200	2	30
Chicken Alfredo, 1¾ cup	270	9	30
Coconut Shrimps (5) w. Sauce	360	22	30
Grilled Fillet varieties, avg., 1 pce	100	3	1
Popcorn Shrimp (19)	200	11	14
Shrimp Fried Rice, 1 cup	190	0.5	36
Shrimp Linguini, 1¾ cups	340	8	51
Swedish Style Meatballs (6)	250	18	7

Lean Cuisine

	C	F	Cb
Cafe Classics Entrees: *Per Meal*			
Beef Portabello	210	5	25
Bow Tie Pasta & Chicken	240	4.5	33
Garlic Beef & Broccoli	170	6	13
Sweet & Sour Chicken	300	3	51
Thai Style Chicken	220	4	30
Cafe Classics Bowls: *Per Bowl*			
Chicken Teriyaki	250	2	44
Grilled Chicken Caesar	230	6	24
Three Cheese Stuffed Rigatoni	240	6	35
Comfort Classics Entrees: *Per Meal*			
Baked Chicken	240	4.5	34
Cheese Lasagna w. Chicken	290	8	35
Honey Roasted Pork	180	6	14
Meatloaf & Whipped Potato	250	7	27
Roasted Turkey Breast	260	2.5	46
Salisbury Steak	270	8	27
Dinnertime Selects: *Per Meal*			
Beef Steak Tips Dijon	320	8	44
Grilled Chicken & Penne Pasta	330	4.5	52
Salisbury Steak	310	8	34
One Dish Favorites: Rstd Chicken	240	6	30
Angel Hair Pasta	260	4	48
Chicken Enchilada	270	4.5	47
Lasagna w. Meat Sauce	320	7	44
Macaroni & Cheese	290	7	41
Santa Fe Rice & Beans	290	6	49
Stuffed Cabbage	200	6	25
Swedish Meatballs	280	7	32
Teriyaki Stir-Fry	300	4.5	49

Lean Cuisine (Cont)

	C	F	Cb
Skillets: Chkn Alfredo	190	4.5	25
Chicken Primavera	180	2.5	28
Garlic Chicken	240	4	40
Herb Chicken & Roasted Potatoes	160	3.5	22
Spa Cuisine: Chicken Pecan	260	6	32
Pork w. Cherry Sauce	260	4	41
Salmon w. Basil	230	6	25

Lean Pockets

Per Piece

	C	F	Cb
BBQ Sauce w. Beef	290	7	48
Ham/Philly Steak & Cheese, 1 pce	280	7	41
Meatballs & Mozzarella	290	7	45
Steak Fajita	260	7	40
Three Cheese & Chicken Quesadilla	280	7	42
Turkey/Broccoli/Cheese	270	7	40
Other varieties, avg.	280	7	43
Lean Pockets Subs, average	310	7	44
Lean Pockets Ultra, 4 oz	200	6	19

Lightlife (Vegetarian)

	C	F	Cb
Smart Menu: Breakfast Patties (1)	45	1.5	3
Burgers (1)	100	1	9
Chick'n Nuggets (4)	220	11	16
Chick'n Patties (1)	160	7	14
Meatless Meatballs (5)	160	7	6
Gimme Lean! Meals, avg., 2 oz	50	0	4
Grab'n Go: Smart Pretzel Dog (1) 5 oz	350	8	50
Smart Tortilla Wrap Burrito:			
Breakfast Scramble (1)6 oz	320	1	41
Chick'n Ranchero (1) 6 oz	300	6	48
Mexican Beef Style (1) 6 oz	340	7	54
Hot Dogs, Tofu Pups, 1 link, 1.5 oz	60	2.5	2
On The Go: Smart BBQ, ¼ cup, 2 oz	70	0	13
Smart Chili, 1 cup, 8.3 oz	210	0	34
Smart Garlic Teriyaki Chick'n	290	4	50
Smart Orange Sesame Chick'n	270	5	46
Smart Veggie Bolognese	220	1	37
Smart Tex Mex, ¼ cup, 2 oz	50	0	6
Smart Dogs!, Jumbo, Fat-Free (1)	80	0	3
Original, Fat-Free (1)	45	0	2
Smart Franks Deli Style Dogs (1) 2 oz	110	4.5	5
Smart Ground: Original, ⅓ cup, 55g	70	0	5
Taco & Burrito, ⅓ cup, 55g	70	0	7
Smart Links: Brats, German Style (1)	120	5	5
Country Breakfast Style (2) 2 oz	100	3.5	8
Old World Italian Style (1) 2 oz	110	4.5	5
Smart Menu Strips: Chick'n, 3 oz	80	0	5
Steak-Style, 3 oz	80	0	5

Marie Callender's (Cont)

	C	F	Cb
Complete Dinners: *Per Serving*			
Beef Pot Roast	330	10	32
Beef Stroganoff	420	18	40
Beef Tips in Mushroom Sce, 13.6 oz	360	12	35
Chicken Fried Beef Steak	540	28	51
Chicken Parmigiana, 1 dinner	650	29	66
Country Fried Chick. & Gvy, 1 din.	670	37	58
Fish w. Mac & Cheese	450	16	53
Golden Battered Fish Fillet	450	16	53
Grilled Chkn & Mashed Pot., 15 oz	450	17	39
Herb Rstd Chicken & Mashed Pot.	530	35	20
Homestyle BBQ Chicken, 14¾ oz	590	28	44
Meatloaf & Gravy w. Mashed Pot.	560	31	39
Pork Chop, 1 dinner	590	33	50
Salisbury Steak & Gravy, 14 oz	400	16	38
Sweet & Sour Chicken, 1 dinner	620	20	90
Pot Pies: Beef	530	32	43
Chicken (10 oz); Turkey, 1 cup	670	41	56
One Dish Classics:			
Cheesy Chicken Breast & Rice	470	19	44
Country Beef Stew w. Cornbread	440	16	52
Fettucini Alfredo, 14 oz	870	51	76
Fettuccini w. Chicken/Broc., 13 oz	630	37	43
Macaroni & Cheese, 8 oz	350	15	36
Meat Lasagna, 8 oz	240	9	24
Crockpot Meals: Turkey & Veges	170	6	21
Chunky Chicken & Noodles	220	10	18
Hearty Beef Vege Soup	130	3	16
Homestyle Chicken Noodle Soup	120	3.5	13
Old Fashioned Beef & Veges	150	4.5	14

Michael Angelo's

	C	F	Cb
Entrees: Chicken Parmesan	260	10	25
Eggplant Parmesan, 6 oz	285	19	23
Fettuccine Alfredo	280	8	40
Manicotti w. Sauce	230	12	11
Sausage & Pepper & Onion	230	7	31
Spaghetti & Meatballs, 15.25 oz	230	9	26
Bowls: Angel Hair & Shrimp, 6 oz	200	6	28
Angel Hair Pasta Pomodoro, 7 oz	200	5	34
Chicken Milano Pasta, 6 oz	290	11	30
Chkn Rosemary Pasta; Saus., 6 oz	250	8	30
Lasagna: Chicken, 8 oz	290	7	37
Four Cheese, 8 oz	400	22	28
Meat Lasagna, 8 oz	290	10	26
Vegetable, 8 oz	230	7	23
Snacks: Four Chse Calzone (1)	360	13	50
Meatball Calzone (1), 5 oz	390	15	45
Mini Calzone (1), avg. 0.7 oz	60	2.5	8

Frozen Entrees & Meals (Cont)

Morningstar Farms

	C	F	Cb
Breakfast Pattie, 1 patty	80	3	3
Burgers: *Made with Organic Soy*			
Classic Burger	150	7	10
Tex Mex Burger	120	1.5	17
Vegan Burger; Veggie Medley, avg.	100	2	8
Zesty Tomato Basil Burger	120	6	7
Thai Burger	100	3.5	9
Grillers: Veggie Burger	130	6	5
Prime Veggie Burger	170	9	4
Vegan	100	2.5	7
Patties: Parmesan Ranch	170	7	17
Breaded Veggie Patties	150	6	16
Poultry: *Made with Organic Soy*			
Buffalo Wings (5)	200	9	18
Chik'n Nuggets (4)	190	7	18
Okara Pattie	120	5	6
Roasted Herb Chicken	150	4	22
Veggie Corn Dogs (1)	170	6	22
Entrees: Lentil Rice Loaf, 1" slice	160	7	16
Nine Bean Loaf, 1" slice	150	7	15
Recipe Crumbles: Grillers, ⅔ cup	90	2.5	5
Sausage Style, ⅔ cup	80	2.5	5

Ore-Ida

	C	F	Cb
Bagel Bites: *Per 4 Pieces (3 oz)*			
Three Cheese, 4 pieces	200	6	28
Cheese, Sausage, Pepperoni	200	6	29
Spicy Nacho; Nacho Cheese	240	10	26

Quorn (Vegetarian)

	C	F	Cb
Garlic & Herb Ckn-Style Cutlets (1)	190	8	20
Gruyer Cutlet	260	15	23
Meat-free Dogs (1), 1.5 oz	80	4	8
Meat-free Links (2), 1.6 oz	90	2	9
Meat-free Meatballs (4), 2.4 oz	110	3	7
Naked Cutlets (1), 2.4 oz	80	2.5	5
Nuggets (1), 3-4 pieces, 3 oz	190	10	17
Patties (1), 2.6 oz	140	7	13
Tenders, 1 cup, 3 oz	90	2	8
Turkey Style Roast, 3 oz	90	1.5	9

Rosina/Celentano

	C	F	Cb
Entree: *Per Serving*			
Cheese Ravioli, 4 pieces	230	3.5	36
Eggplant Parmigiana, 10 oz	460	29	38
Manicotti, 7 oz	420	14	53
Ravioli Stuffed Cheese, Mini, 4 oz	220	2.5	36
Stuffed Shell: 6.5 oz	320	12	36
Light Broccoli, 10 oz	330	5	54

Safeway Select

	C	F	Cb
Gourmet Club Meals: *Per Serving*			
Cha Siu Bao, 1 bau, 3 oz	210	4.5	34
Enchiladas	210	8	25
Low Fat Turkey Lasagna, 1 cup	230	3	36
Macaroni & Cheese	350	19	32
Meat Lasagna, 1 cup	270	7	34
Tamale Bake, 1 cup	290	16	25
6 Vegetable Lasagna, 1 cup	310	17	27
St. Louis Ribs (2), 125g	370	23	17
Stir Fry: Chicken Fajita	130	3	14
Shrimp & Vegetable	120	0	20
Teriyaki Beef	170	4	24
Gourmet Club Eating Right: *Per ½ Package*			
Burgundy Beef Stew	250	9	38
Cashew Chicken, 16 oz	330	5	53
Chicken Lettuce Wraps, 2 oz	80	3.5	8
Chicken Penne Pasta	280	8	34
Chicken Tamales Verde	220	9	25
Creamy Broccoli Beef	290	7	40
Ginger Chicken	350	6	49
Meatloaf Dinner	230	6	31
Orange Glazed Chicken	350	5	56
Shrimp Lo Mein, 10 oz	290	6	41

SeaPak

	C	F	Cb
Coconut Shrimp, 4 pces	270	17	19
Jumbo Butterfly Shrimp, 4 pces	210	10	20
Popcorn Shrimp, 15 pces, 3 oz	210	10	20
Shrimp Scampi, 8 pces	330	29	2
Shrimp Tempura, 4 pieces	240	8	35

Seeds of Change

Per Bowl (11 oz)	C	F	Cb
Creamy Spinach Lasagna	340	10	40
Ginger Stir Fry	260	3	47
Penne Marinara	300	8	40
Seven Grain Pilaf	310	9	46
Spicy Peanut Noodles	350	9	51
Spicy Yucatan Frijoles	340	5	54
Teriyaki Stir-Fried Rice	310	2	49
Vegetarian Chicken Teriyaki	300	3.5	47

Stouffer's

	C	F	Cb
Homestyle Dinners: *Per Serving*			
Chicken Fettucini, 16.75 oz	610	33	55
Country Fried Beef Steak, 16 oz	520	33	52
Grilled Lime Chicken, 14 oz	490	14	66
Meatloaf, 17 oz	590	32	43
Monterey Chicken, 14.25 oz	500	17	58
Roast Turkey Breast, 16 oz	390	13	48
Slow Roasted Beef, 14 oz	320	15	27

Frozen Entrees & Meals (Cont)

Stouffer's (Cont)

Entrees:	C	F	Cb
Stroganoff, 9.75 oz	380	17	34
Breaded Boneless Pork Cutlet	370	21	31
Creamed Chipped Beef	140	8	9
Grilled Teriyaki Chicken	300	3.5	45
Chicken a la King	410	14	53
Fish Fillet w. Mac Cheese, 9 oz	420	18	45
Lasagna w. Meat Sce, 10½ oz	350	11	38
Macaroni & Beef w. Tomatoes	330	11	38
Macaroni & Cheese, 1 cup, 8 oz	350	17	34
Salisbury Steak, 16 oz	470	24	34
Spaghetti w. Meat Sauce	360	12	45
Stuffed Pepper, 10 oz	220	10	22
Swedish Meatballs w. Pasta	500	25	40
Tuna Noodle Casserole	370	17	35
Turkey Tetrazzini	380	20	32
Family Style Recipes: *Per Serving*			
Grandma's Chkn & Vege Bake	360	15	36
Lasagna w. Meat Sce, 1 cup	270	10	30
Macaroni & Cheese, 1 cup	350	17	34
Italian Style: Chkn Ravioli, 8.2 oz	360	14	40
Cheese Stuffed Rigatoni, 8.2 oz	460	20	52
Italian Sausage Stuffed Rigatoni	390	15	44
Skillets: *Per Bowl*			
Broccoli & Beef; Garlic Chkn, avg.	330	6	46
Chicken Alfredo	410	11	49
Chicken & Pasta	340	7	42
Chicken & Veges	360	9	43
Homestyle Beef	300	11	32
Teriyaki Chicken, 12.5 oz	310	4.5	44
Steak Teriyaki	310	5	49
Yankee Pot Roast	300	8	39
Corner Bistro: Paninis, average	355	17	31
Chicken Carbonara, 12 oz	530	22	50
Garlic/Rosemary Chicken, 12 oz	420	17	42
Monterey Chicken, 12 oz	500	23	46
Seafood Scampi, 14 oz	410	11	57
Sesame Chicken, 12½ oz	510	15	72

Swanson

Hungry Man Dinners: Meatloaf	680	37	61
Boneless Pork Rib	920	35	71
Boneless White Meat Fried Chkn	710	29	86
Buffalo Chicken Strips	920	35	71
Classic Fried Chicken	960	45	91
Hearty Breakfast	450	27	35
Mexican Style Fiesta	870	38	113
Rotisserie Chicken	690	35	48
Salisbury Steak	490	18	55
Turkey Breast	660	27	81
Hungry Man XXL: Backyard BBQ	860	48	62
Roasted Carved Turkey Dinner	820	36	84
Southern Fried Boneless Chicken	760	16	84

Swanson (Cont)

Pot Pies:	C	F	Cb
Flaky Crust Chicken/Turkey	320	17	31
American Recipe: Salisbury Steak	500	26	48
Boneless White Meat Fried Chkn	520	22	75
Breaded Fish Fillet, 10 oz	510	23	57
Chicken Strips w. Fries	640	30	80
Classic Fried Chicken, 11½ oz	770	37	72
Turkey Breast w. Stuffing & Gravy	380	17	40

TGI Friday's

Buffalo Wings (3)	150	10	2
Honey BBQ Wings (3)	150	9	6
Mozzarella Sticks & Sce, 1 Serve	110	6	10
Popcorn Chicken, 3 pces, 2.6 oz	250	8	29
Potato Skins, Ched. & Bacon, 3 pces	210	12	20
Quesadilla Rolls: Chicken (2)	250	12	26
Steak (2)	230	10	26
Sides: Spinach Dip, 2 Tbsp, 1 oz	45	3.5	2

Trader Joe's

Meals: *Per Serving*			
Asian Style Chkn Stir Fry w. Sce, 8 oz	90	1	30
BBQ Chicken Teriyaki, 1 cup	150	3.5	11
Chicken Chow Mein, ⅓ pkg, 6.75 oz	240	2	45
Chicken Fried Rice, 1 cup, 5 oz	200	3.5	33
Chicken Marsala, 1 pkg, 11 oz	320	6	34
Citrus Glazed Chicken, 8 oz	270	5	40
Mandarin Orange Chicken, 1 cup	270	10	23
Rice Bowls, average, 11 oz bowl	350	2	62
Shrimp Stir Fry, 6.4 oz	70	0.5	6
Swt & Sr Shrimp w. Rice, ⅓ pkg 7.4 oz	190	0	39
Turkey Saus. Stromboli, ¼ loaf, 4.5 oz	250	7	31
Pies: Shepherds Pie, ½ pie, 8 oz	190	3.5	23
Spinach Pie, ¼ pie, 6 oz	240	4	37
Quiche: Broccoli & Cheddar, 6 oz	460	30	32
Mexicaine, 6 oz	500	34	31
Spinach & Mushroom, 6 oz	460	26	38

For Complete Nutritional Data ~ see CalorieKing.com

Tyson

Meal Kits: Beef Fajita (1)	140	4	17
Chicken Fajita (1)	130	3.5	17
Chicken Fried Rice, 2½ cups	440	6	69
Chicken Quesadilla (1)	250	10	26
Chicken Stir Fry, 2¾ cups	430	4.5	73
Meals: Buffalo Hot Wings, 4 pieces	220	15	1
Chicken Bites, 13 pieces	270	18	15
Chicken Brst Fillets, breaded (1)	240	9	20

Frozen Entrees & Meals (Cont)

Tyson (Cont)

	C	F	Cb
Meals: Chkn Brst Nuggets, 5 pces	280	16	21
Chicken Breast Strips, 3 oz	120	3.5	1
Chicken Breast Tenderloins, 1 pce	150	7	12
Country Fried Steak, 1 piece	310	23	15
Crispy Chicken Strips, 2 pces	200	10	13
Fajita Style Chicken Strips, 3 oz	110	4	1
Fun Nuggets, 5 pieces	280	18	16
Honey Barbecue Wings, 3 pces	250	15	13
Honey Chicken Brst Tenders, 5 pce	220	13	13
Popcorn Chicken, 9 pces	200	8	17
Southern Style Chkn Brst Patties (1)	240	18	10
Steak Fingers, 2 pces	250	18	14

Van De Kamp's

	C	F	Cb
Butterfly Shrimp, 7 pces, 4 oz	270	13	26
Crispy Battered Halibut, 3 fillets	240	12	22
Crispy Fish Tenders, 4 pces, 4 oz	210	10	22
Crispy Fish Portions, 1 pce	150	8	14
Popcorn Shrimp, 20 pces, 4 oz	260	11	30
Fish Sticks, Breaded, 6 stix, 4 oz	260	13	23
Battered Fillets, 2.6 oz fillet	130	6	11
Crunchy Fish Fillets, 1 pce, 2.6 oz	230	13	18
Crisp & Healthy, Breaded (2), 1.8 oz	170	2.5	25

Weight Watchers

	C	F	Cb
Smart Ones Bistro Selections: *Per Meal*			
Chicken Fettucini	340	8	42
Chicken Parmesan	290	5	35
Chkn Tenderloins w. Barbecue Sce	240	4.5	34
Fajita Chicken Supreme	260	7	32
Glazed Chicken	260	2.5	45
Golden Baked Garlic Chicken	270	5	42
Grilled Mandarin Chicken	280	4.5	42
Meatloaf w. Mashed Potatoes	260	8	22
Oven Roasted Chicken	260	6	37
Roasted Chicken w. Sour Cream	180	4	20
Southwest Style Adobo Chicken	310	10	36
Stuffed Turkey Breast	290	6	42
Thai Style Chicken & Rice Noodles	260	4	43
Smart Ones Entrees: *Per Meal*			
Angel Hair Marinara	230	1.5	41
Broccoli & Cheddar Roasted Pot.	220	6	34
Chicken Enchiladas Suiza	310	8	45
Honey Dijon Chicken	220	3.5	38
Lasagna Bolognese	270	4	43
Lemon Herb Chicken Piccata	250	5	36
Macaroni & Cheese	270	2	52
Radiatore Romano	290	7	43
Roast Turkey Medallions	220	1.5	38

Weight Watchers (Cont)

	C	F	Cb
Smart Ones Entrees (Cont):			
Salisbury Steak	260	7	26
Santa Fe Style Rice & Beans	310	7	51
Spaghetti Bolognese; 3 Chse Mac	310	6	48
Spaghetti Marinara	300	4.5	54
Spicy Szechuan Style Vege & Chkn	240	5	36
Traditional Lasagna w. Meat Sce	300	6	43
Tuna Noodle Gratin	250	4.5	37
High Protein, avg. all varieties	210	8	12
Smart Ones Bowls: *Per Bowl*			
Southwestern Style Chicken	230	3.5	33
Teriyaki Chicken & Vegetable	270	3	46
Smartwiches, avg. all, 127g	270	6	40
For Complete Nutritional Data ~ see CalorieKing.com			

White Castle

	C	F	Cb
Cheese Burger, Microwaveable, 1 pkg, 3.7 oz	320	18	26
Hamburgers, 1 pkg (2 sandwiches)	280	14	26

Worthington/Loma Linda

	C	F	Cb
Bolono, 3 slices, 2 oz	80	3	3
Chik-Nuggets, 5 pieces	250	15	14
Chicken Roll, ⅜ slice, 1.9 oz	90	4.5	2
Chicken Slices, 3 slices, 2 oz	90	4.5	2
ChikSticks, 1 pce, 1.6 oz	100	6	4
Corn Dogs (1)	150	4	22
Corned Beef Slices, 3 slices, 2 oz	140	9	5
Dinner Roast, ¾" slice	180	11	6
Fillets, 2 pieces, 2.9 oz	180	9	8
Fried Chik'n w. Gravy, 2 pieces	150	10	5
FriPats, 1 pattie, 2¼ oz	130	6	5
Golden Croquettes, 4 pieces, 2.9 oz	210	11	14
Leanies, 1 link, 1.4 oz	100	7	2
Meatless Smoked Beef, 3 slices	130	7	7
Prosage: Links, 2 links, 1.6 oz	80	3	3
Patties, 1.3 oz Pattie	80	3	3
Salami, 3 slices, 2 oz	120	7	3
Smkd Turkey Slices, 3 slices	140	9	4
Stakelets, 2.5 oz piece	150	7	7
Stripples, 2 slices	60	4.5	2
Swiss Steak, 1 piece	130	6	9
Tuno (tuna substitute), ½ cup	90	6	3
Wham Vege Slices, 2 slices	110	7	3

Zatarain's

	C	F	Cb
Blackened Chicken Alfredo, 10.5 oz	535	30	44
Jambalaya seasoned w. Chicken w. Sausage	360	8	53
	390	12	58
Red Beans & Rice w. Sausage	565	19	76

Frozen Pizzas	C	F	Cb
Amy's: *Per 1/3 Pizza*			
Cheese; Spinach; Pesto, avg.	310	12	38
Cheese Pesto (Whole Wheat Crust)	360	18	37
Cheese Pizza (Rice Crust), 1/3 pizza	300	14	31
Mushroom & Olive	250	9	33
Roasted Vegetable	270	9	42
California Pizza Kitchen			
Large: Five Cheese & Tomato, 1/6	320	15	29
BBQ Chicken, 1/6 pizza	290	9	33
Small: BBQ/Thai Chkn, average, 1/3	290	10	33
Five Cheese & Tomato, 1/3	320	15	29
Crispy Thin Crust: Sicilian, 1/3 pizza	310	14	30
Margherita, 1/3 pizza	300	13	31
Other varieties, avg., 1/3 pizza	290	12	30
Celeste			
Pizza For One: Cheese, 1 pizza	360	14	42
Deluxe; Pepperoni; Chseburger	410	21	42
Original/Zesty Four Cheese, avg.	400	18	41
Sausage & Pepperoni; Suprema	470	26	44
Zesty Chicken Supreme	340	15	39
Di Giorno			
Rising Crust (Large): *Per 1/6 Pizza*			
Four Cheese	310	11	40
Other varieties, average	355	16	40
Rising Crust (Small): Supreme, 1/3	320	14	35
Four Cheese	350	14	41
Pepperoni/Supreme	370	16	40
Deep Dish: Three Meat, 1/6 pizza	310	15	32
Supreme, 1/6 pizza	320	15	33
Pepperoni, 1/6 pizza	340	18	32
Cheese Stuffed Crust: Supreme, 1/6	350	16	35
Four Cheese, 1/3 pizza	360	14	41
Pepperoni, 1/3 pizza	370	16	40
Three Meat Pizza, 1/2 pizza	340	16	34
Half & Half: *Per 1/6 Large Pizza*			
Pepperoni/Cheese: Pepperoni	390	18	40
Cheese	310	11	40
Microwave: 3 Meat, 1/2 pizza	420	19	44
4 Cheese, 1/2 pizza	370	15	44
Pepperoni/Supreme, avg., 1/2	390	18	44
Thin Crispy Crust:			
Four Meat, 1/5 large	320	13	37
Grilled Chicken/Tom./Spinach, 1/6	260	8	33
Other varieties, average, 1/6	305	12	34
Ellio's Pizza (McCain)			
9 Slice Pizza: All Cheezy, 1 slice	160	5	23
Cheese; Pepperoni, avg., 1 slice	160	5	20
27 Slice Pizza: Cheese, 1 slice	150	3	21
Pepperoni, 1 slice	160	5	20

	C	F	Cb
Essensia *(Albertson's)*			
5 Cheese, 1/6 pizza	320	11	42
3 Meat, 1/6 pizza	360	15	41
Supreme, 1/8 pizza	270	11	31
Freschetta			
Hand Tossed (Large): 4 Chse, 1/5	390	14	47
4 Meat, 1/6 pizza	350	15	40
Pepperoni, 1/6 pizza	340	14	40
Canadian Bacon Pineapple, 1/5	340	9	49
Supreme, 1/6 pizza	350	15	38
Vegetable Primavera, 1/6 pizza	310	11	40
Brick Oven 8": BBQ Chicken, 1/3 pizza	280	11	39
Ham & Mushroom, 1/2 pizza	325	11	39
Potato, Bacon & Cheese, 1/2 pizza	395	17	43
Thai Chicken, 1/3 pizza	300	14	27
Italian Style Pepperoni, 1/4 pizza	410	21	38
Sauce Stuffed Crust: 4 Chse, 1/5	340	12	43
Sausage & Pepperoni, 1/5 pizza	370	16	43
Pepperoni, 1/5 pizza	360	15	43
8" Hand Tossed, Pepperoni, 1/5	460	19	51
12" Ultra Thin: Supreme, 3 slices	350	19	27
5 Cheese, 3 slices	330	17	25
Healthy Choice: *Per Pizza (6 oz)*			
French Bread Pizza: Pepperoni	360	5	56
Supreme; Vegetable, avg.	325	5	50
Cafe Selections Pizza: Four Chse	370	3	58
Gourmet Supreme	360	4	56
Italian Style Pepperoni	370	4.5	58
Jeno's: *Per Pizza (7 oz)*			
Crispy & Tasty: Cheese	440	21	47
Pepperoni; Supreme; Comb., avg.	490	25	50
Three Meat; Sausage, average	480	24	49
Heaven's Bistro: *Per 1/3 Pizza*			
Chicken w. BBQ Sauce	270	2	48
Grilled Vegetable	230	1	42
Pepperoni; Sausage, average	250	3	42
Lean Cuisine			
French Bread Pizza: Cheese, 6 oz	370	7	50
Deluxe, 6 oz	310	9	44
Pepperoni, 5.25 oz	300	7	44
Casual Eating: Deluxe, 6 oz	370	9	55
BBQ Chkn; Margherita, avg., 6 oz	320	9	46
Four Cheese, 6 oz	400	9	59
Rstd Garlic; Mushroom, avg., 6 oz	285	7	39
Roasted Vegetable, 6 oz	330	5	58
Pizza Fit 'n Free			
7" Pizza, 7 oz	250	0	43

Frozen Pizzas (Cont)

	C	F	Cb
Ralph's			
Pizza Pals: *Per Pizza*			
Cheese; Hamburger, average	410	12	57
Taco Supreme	380	12	47
Other varieties, average	455	17	58
Self Rising Crust: 4 Cheese, ⅙	300	8	43
Pepperoni, ⅙ pizza	390	16	45
Other varieties, avg., ⅙ pizza	355	14	45
Red Baron			
Classic (Large): 4 Cheese, ¼ pizza	410	19	40
Pepperoni, ⅕ pizza	330	16	32
Other varieties, average, ⅕ pizza	350	18	33
Deep Dish Pan Style:			
4 Cheese, ⅓ pizza	380	17	41
Pepperoni; Meat Trio, avg., ⅓ pizza	400	20	41
Supreme, ⅓ pizza	420	20	43
Deep Dish Singles: 4 Cheese, 1	430	30	44
Pepperoni, 1 pizza	450	22	45
Other varieties, average, 1 pizza	420	21	43
French Bread Pizzas: Supreme (1)	360	15	42
5 Cheese & Garlic (1)	410	22	39
Pepperoni; 3 Meat, average	360	15	42
Microwaveable Classic: 4 Chse (1)	740	39	62
Supreme, 1 pizza	760	42	64
Other varieties, avg. (1)	795	46	62
Pizzeria Style: *Per ⅙ Pizza*			
4 Cheese; Pepperoni, avg.	350	14	40
Special Deluxe; Supreme, avg.	370	16	41
Thin Crust: *Per ¼ Pizza*			
Mozzarella Tomato Basil	270	13	27
Five Cheese; Meat Trio, average	310	16	27
Pepperoni varieties, average	360	20	27
Reggio's			
Individual Pizza: Cheese (1)	250	8	33
Pepperoni, 1 pizza	290	13	33
Sausage & Mushroom (1)	280	10	34
Dinner Size: Cheese, ¼ pizza	330	12	41
Pepperoni & Sausage, ¼ pizza	400	18	41
Sausage; Supreme, ¼, avg.	380	16	41
Stop & Shop			
Single Serving, Cheese, 1	390	19	42
9 Slices, Cheese, 2 slices	350	10	49
Stouffer's			
French Bread Pizzas: Deluxe, 1 pce	430	21	44
Cheese, 1 piece (½ pkg)	360	15	43
Extra Cheese, 1 piece	400	18	44
Pepperoni, 1 piece	410	20	43
Tombstone			
Original Pizza, 12 inch: *Per Serving*			
Extra Cheese, ¼ pizza	340	15	37
Pepperoni, ¼ pizza	380	20	37
Sausage & Pepperoni, ¼ pizza	370	17	37
Supreme, ⅕ pizza	300	14	31
Light Pizza, Vegetable, ⅕ pizza	230	6	31
Half & Half Pepperoni & Cheese:			
Pepperoni, ⅕ pizza	410	21	37
Cheese, ¼ pizza	330	16	31
Deep Dish Individual: Cheese (1)	420	17	50
Pepperoni (1)	460	22	50
Supreme (1)	440	20	51
Thin Crust: 3 Cheese, ¼ pizza	330	18	30
Harvest Wheat Supreme, ¼	260	10	29
Brick Oven Style: Cheese, ¼ pizza	350	15	38
Other varieties, average, ¼	310	16	29
Tony's			
Original: Cheese, ⅓ pizza	370	15	42
Pepperoni, ⅓ pizza	400	19	42
Sausage & Pepperoni, ⅓ pizza	430	21	42
Supreme, ⅓ pizza	420	20	43
Thin Crust: Cheese, ⅓ pizza	340	15	36
Sausage &/Pepperoni, ⅓ pizza	390	19	32
Supreme, ⅓ pizza	360	19	34
Deep Dish (Individual): Cheese (1)	390	16	47
Pepperoni (1)	480	24	48
Totino's			
Crisp Crust Party Pizza: *Per ½ Pizza*			
Cheese	320	15	34
Pepperoni; Supreme	380	22	34
Trader Joe's: *Per ⅓ Pizza*			
4 Cheese	350	14	42
Formaggio di Capra	360	17	37
Pizza Mascarpone	340	15	45
Vegetarian	300	11	43
Verdi (Safeway Select)			
Self-Rising Crust (Large): *Per ⅙ Pizza*			
Meat Magnifico	350	15	41
4 Cheese	310	11	41
Other varieties, average	365	16	41
Thin Crispy Crust: Supreme, ⅓	360	16	38
Four Cheese, ⅓ pizza	310	11	37
Pepperoni, ⅓ pizza	315	16	37
Weight Watchers (Smart Ones): *Per Pizza*			
Deluxe	360	9	52
Four Cheese	390	10	56
Pepperoni	390	11	50
Veggie Ultimate	330	6	54

Canned & Packaged Meals

	C	**F**	**Cb**
Annies Homegrown: *Per Cup (Prepared)*			
Arthur Mac & Cheese	370	14	50
Beef Stroganoff	320	13	24
Cheeseburger Macaroni	350	13	27
Cheesy Lasagna	280	9	26
Penne Pasta w. Alfredo Sauce	360	13	47
Shells & Cheddar	280	4.5	48
B & M: *Per ½ Cup (4½ oz)*			
Baked Beans: Original	170	2	31
Barbeque	190	0.5	39
Vegetarian	160	1	28
Brown Raisin Bread, ½" slice, 2 oz	130	0.5	29
Banquet			
Homestyle Bakes: *Per Serving (Prepared)*			
Asian Style Fried Rice	250	1.5	49
Beef Stew & Biscuits, ⅔ cup	300	8	43
Chicken & Dumplings, 7.8 oz	230	4.5	33
Creamy Cheesy Chicken Alfredo	400	22	36
Country Chicken, Potato, Biscuits	250	11	31
Creamy Chicken & Biscuits, 7.4 oz	350	18	39
Lasagne	290	11	36
Pasta & Meatballs	310	10	41
Betty Crocker			
Complete Meals: *Per Serving (⅓ Pkg)*			
Cheesy Beef Taco	250	5	43
Chicken & Buttermilk Biscuits	280	11	37
Chicken Fettuccini Alfredo	240	9	31
Stroganoff	200	4.5	30
Three Cheese Chicken	260	10	33
Hamburger Helper: *Per Cup (Prep. as Directed)*			
Bacon Cheeseburger	380	15	38
Beef Pasta	270	11	24
Cheeseburger Macaroni	300	13	27
Cheesy Enchilada; Quesadilla	350	13	40
Cheesy Hashbrown	400	19	39
Cheesy Italian Shells	350	13	37
Chili Macaroni	290	11	29
Crunchy Taco	300	14	27
Salisbury	280	11	26
Tuna Helper: *Per Serving (Prep. as Directed)*			
Creamy Parmesan	290	9	37
Other varieties, average	310	12	37
Chicken Helper: *Per Cup (Prep. as Directed)*			
Cheesy Chicken Enchilada	320	7	40
Chicken Fried Rice	260	9	25
Fettuccini Alfredo	300	9	37
Banquet Style Bakes: *Per Serving (¼ Pkg)*			
Asian Style Fried Rice	250	1.5	49
Lasagne	290	11	36
Pasta & Meatballs	310	10	41

	C	**F**	**Cb**
Betty Crocker (Cont)			
Mashed Potatoes: *Per Serving (Prepared)*			
Potato Buds, ⅓ cup	160	8	19
Other varieties, average, ½ cup	170	7	22
Side Dishes/Casseroles: *Per Serving (Prepared)*			
Au Gratin; Cheesy Scalloped, ½ cup	150	5	22
Cheddar & Bacon; Cheesy Scallops	120	3	22
Roasted Garlic	120	4	20
Scalloped Potatoes, ⅔ cup	130	4	22
Other varieties, ⅔ cup	120	3.5	22
Deluxe Potatoes: *Per ½ Cup (Prepared)*			
Cheesy Cheddar Au Gratin	170	8	23
Loaded Au Gratin	140	4	23
Three Cheese Mashed Pot. Bake	190	9	24
Microwaveable Mashed Potato:			
Creamy Butter; Rstd Garlic, ⅔ cup	90	1	18
Seasoned Skillets:			
Hash Brown, ½ cup	120	4	19
Roasted Garlic & Herb, ⅔ cup	170	9	22
Traditional, ½ cup	180	9	22
Suddenly Salad: *Prepared As Directed*			
Caesar, ½ cup	250	10	34
Classic, 1 cup	240	8	37
Ranch & Bacon, ¾ cup	330	20	31
Bowl Appetit: *Per Bowl*			
Pasta Alfredo	360	11	53
Three Cheese Rotini	360	10	55
Bush's Best: *Per ½ Cup*			
Chili Beans	120	1	20
Dark Red Kidney Beans, ½ cup	105	2	20
Frijoles Negras, ½ cup	110	0.5	23
Frijoles Pintos, ½ cup	80	0	18
Garbanzo Beans/Chick Peas, ½ c.	105	2	20
Refried Beans: Traditional	150	3	24
Fat Free	130	0	24
Baked Beans: Vegetarian	130	0	29
Other flavors, average	150	1	32
Campbell's: *Per Cup (8 fl.oz)*			
Chunky Chili: Roadhouse; Firehouse	230	8	25
Tantalizin Turkey	190	2.5	27
Pork & Beans in Tomato Sauce	140	1.5	25
Spaghetti O's Original	180	1	37
Spaghetti O's Meatballs	240	8	32
Sliced Franks	230	10	27
Supper Bakes: *Per ⅙ Box (Prepared as Directed)*			
Cheesy Chicken	170	4	27
Creamy Stroganoff	190	4	31
Garlic Chicken w. Pasta	230	1	44
Herb Chicken w. Rice	190	1	40
Lemon Chicken w. Rice	200	1	43
Savory Pork Chops	160	1	31
Southwestern Style Chicken	150	1	32
Trad. Roast Chicken w. Stuffing	160	3	29

Canned & Packaged Meals (Cont)

	C	F	Cb
Chef Boyardee			
Beefaroni, all types, 1 cup	260	9	32
Mini Bites (15 oz Can): Per Cup			
Mini Beef Ravioli w. Meatballs	280	13	31
Mini Pasta Shells w. Meatballs	260	10	32
Mini Spaghetti w. Meatballs	250	10	30
Jumbo (15 oz Can): Per Cup			
99% Fat Free: Beef Ravioli	170	1.5	33
Cheese Ravioli	240	2.5	45
Lasagna	270	10	36
Mini Ravioli	250	9	35
Spaghetti w. Jumbo Meatballs	270	12	28
Overstuffed Ital. Sausage Ravioli	240	4.5	40
Microwaveable Cups: Per Cup			
Beef Ravioli	190	5	29
Macaroni & Cheese	190	8	22
Mini Bites Spaghetti Rings	220	8	29
Spaghetti & Meatballs	200	8	23
Rice w. Chicken/Vegetables	230	9	30
Microwaveable Big Bowls: Per ½ Bowl			
Beefaroni	250	9	31
Mini Ravioli	240	8	33
Ravioli	220	7	32
Twistaroni: Cheesy Nacho, 1 cup	220	7	32
Chili Cheese Dog, 1 cup	220	6	32
Tomato & Beef, 1 cup	250	6	40
Dinner Kits: Per Serving			
Cheese Pizza	250	4	45
Lasagna	340	8	54
Spaghetti & Meatballs	300	8	45
Dennison's Chili (15 oz Can): Per Cup			
Chili Con Carne With Beans:			
Original; Hot, 1 cup, avg.	360	14	37
Chunky	300	10	32
99% Fat Free: Beef Chili w. Beans	210	2	29
Turkey Chili w. Beans	210	3	29
Dinty Moore (Hormel Foods)			
1½ lb Can: Beef Stew, 1 cup	180	8	17
7½ lb Can: Beef Stew, 1 cup	180	8	17
American Classics: Per Microwave Bowl			
Beef Stew, 10 oz	250	11	22
Noodles & Chicken, 7.5 oz	250	8	28
Microwave Cup: Beef Stew, 7.5 oz	150	6	15
Chicken & Dumplings, 7.5 oz	200	6	26
Other varieties, average	180	8	17
Dr. McDougall's: Per 10 oz			
Ramen Noodles	150	0.5	29
Rice Pilaf, average	260	2	52
Eden Soy (Vegetarian): Per ½ Cup (4½ oz)			
Baked Beans w. Sorghum, Mustard	150	0	27
Black Eyed Peas	90	1	16
Black Soybeans	120	6	8
Refried Black/Pinto/Kid. Beans, avg.	85	1	17
Other varieties, average	125	0	24

	C	F	Cb
Fantastic: Per Cup			
Bean Chili	160	2	33
Black Bean Chipotle	130	0.5	31
Sesame Miso, 1.8 oz	140	2	27
Spicy Thai	150	0.5	32
Tuscan Tomato & Shells	140	1	31
Farmhouse			
Pasta: Per ¾ Cup			
Chicken Pasta	370	15	49
Creamy Garlic	420	20	49
Herb & Butter	430	20	48
White Cheddar Pasta	380	14	50
Rice: Per ⅓ Cup (Prepared as Directed)			
Chicken Rice	230	5	41
Long Grain & Wild Herb Butter	220	4	41
Other varieties, average	230	5	41
French's Fried Onions			
Regular:			
2 Tbsp, ¼ oz	45	3.5	3
¼ cup, ½ oz	90	7	6
1 cup, 2 oz	360	28	24
Cheddar:			
2 Tbsp, ¼ oz	40	3	3
¼ cup, ½ oz	80	6	6
1 cup, 2 oz	320	24	24
Health Valley (Vegetarian)			
Fat Free Beans & Chili:			
Vegetarian/Chili, 1 cup	160	1	30
Turkey w. Chili Beans, 1 cup	220	3	34
Other varieties, ½ cup	80	0	15
Meal Cups, average all varieties	140	1	27
Heinz			
Vegetarian Beans, ½ cup	140	0.5	27
Hormel: Per Cup			
Completes: Per 10 oz Serving			
Beef & Beans in BBQ Sauce	390	11	43
Beef Pot Roast	230	3	27
Beef Steak Tips	280	9	29
Chicken & Dumplings	260	8	34
Chicken & Noodles	250	8	28
Chicken & Rice	260	10	30
Chicken Alfredo	360	20	28
Chicken Breast w. Mash Potatoes	210	3	24
Chicken Breast w. Dressing	280	5	35
Lasagne	280	7	42
Meatloaf	310	11	34
Roast Beef w. Mashed Potato	230	3	27
Salisbury Steak	280	11	30
Spaghetti & Meatballs	280	8	36
Teriyaki Chicken	270	1.5	57
Turkey & Hearty Vegetables	180	3.5	24
Turkey w. Dressing	280	8	31

Hormel (Cont): Per Cup	C	F	Cb
Kid's Kitchen: Beans & Wieners	320	13	37
Cheesy Mac 'N Cheese	280	16	24
Mini Beef Ravioli	250	6	38
Noodle Rings & Chicken	140	4	18
Chili (15 oz Can): Per ½ Can			
With Beans: Homestyle Chili	270	7	34
Reg./Hot/Chunky, average	270	7	34
Turkey (99% Fat Free)	200	3	26
Vegetarian (99% Fat Free)	200	1	38
Less Sodium Without Beans:			
Hot/Chili, 1 cup	210	9	17
Chunky No Beans	210	8	19
Turkey No Beans	190	3	17
Tamales (15 oz Can), 2 Tamales	140	7	15
Hungry Jack Potatoes			
Instant Potato Flakes, ⅓ cup	80	0	19
Hunt's			
Manwich Sloppy Joe, ¼ cup	30	0	7
Knorr Lipton			
Asian Sides: Per Cup (Prepared as Directed)			
Beef Lo Mein; Thai Sesame, avg.	280	9	42
Chicken Fried/Teriyaki Rice, avg.	280	7.5	48
Teriyaki Noodles	300	8	49
Cajun Sides: Per Cup (Prepared)			
Garlic Butter Rice	300	8	48
New Orleans Style Chicken	290	5.5	50
Dirty Rice	300	6.5	50
Red Beans & Rice	330	5.5	61
Fiesta Sides: Per Cup (Prepared as Directed)			
Taco Rice	290	7	51
Nacho Pasta	280	7.5	44
Pasta Sides: Per Cup (Prepared)			
Alfredo; Parmesan, avg.	320	12	43
Butter	290	11	46
Creamy Garlic Shells	350	12	50
Stroganoff	290	9	42
Rice Sides: Per Cup (Prepared)			
Cheddar Broccoli	260	5.5	47
Creamy Chicken	320	10	49
Herb & Butter	300	9	46
Other varieites, average	310	10	49
Sides Plus: Per Cup (Prepared)			
Alfredo Pasta Primavera	310	12	42
Roasted Chicken Rice	320	6.5	56
Southwestern Style Rice	310	7.5	51
Teriyaki Noodles	340	8	56
Whole Grain Sides: Per ⅔ Cup			
Alfredo	300	4	39
Sesame Chicken	300	4	51
Other varieties, avg.	270	7	45

Kraft	C	F	Cb
Minute White Rice, 1 cup	200	0	45
It's Pasta Anytime Meals: Per Package			
Fettuccine w. Classic Alfredo Sce	580	22	74
Bistro Deluxe: Sundried Tom. Parm	300	11	40
Other varieties, average	310	11	40
Dinners: Per Serving (Prepared as Directed)			
Macaroni & Cheese: Orig., ⅓ box	320	16	48
Scooby-Doo Spirals	410	19	47
Mac & Chse: Crazy Noodles, ½ box	410	18	48
Thick'n Creamy, ⅓ box	380	16	50
Easy Mac, avg. all varieties., 1 pch	230	4	42
Deluxe: Orig.; Sharp Chedd., ¼ box	320	10	45
Rotini White Cheese Sce, ½ box	390	15	48
Velveeta Shells & Cheese, ⅓ box	360	12	49
Velveeta Cheesy Potatoes: Per ½ Cup (Prepared)			
Au Gratin Potatoes	190	7	26
Bacon Scalloped Potatoes	200	8	26
Mashed Potatoes	200	12	21
La Choy			
Beef Chow Mein, 1 cup	90	2	11
Chicken Chow Mein, 1 cup	100	3	10
Beef Pepper Oriental, 1 cup	100	2.5	12
Chop Suey Vegetables, ½ cup	15	0	3
Chow Mein Noodles, ½ cup	130	5	19
Lightlife			
Tempeh: Flax; Soy, avg., 4 oz	225	9	16
Fakin' Bacon Strips, 3 sl., 2 oz	100	3	10
Garden Veggie, 4 oz	250	10	17
Three Grain; Wild Rice, avg., 4 oz	230	9	21
Smart Stuffers: Per 4 oz			
Chicken & Broccoli/Cordon Melts	210	8	16
Turkey w. Cranberry Stuffing	220	7	22
Light Burgers Patty (1) 3 oz	120	1.5	11
Smart Bacon, 2 slices, 22g	45	2	1
Smart Deli: Baked Ham	80	0	6
Country Ham Style, 4 slices	90	0	5
Old World Bologna Style, 4 sl., 2 oz	70	0	4
Pepperoni Slices, 13 slices, 1 oz	40	0	3
Roast Turkey Style, 4 slices, 2 oz	80	0	6
Maruchan			
Ramen Noodles: Beef/Chicken/Shrimp Flavors, ½ block, 1½ oz	190	7	26
Noodles: Instant Wanton,			
Hot & Sour, 1 pkg	200	12	20
Chicken, 1 pkg	210	13	18
Roast Beef Cup O Noodles	290	12	38
Morningstar Farms			
Kaffree Roma, 1 rounded tsp, 2g	10	0	2
Cheddar Burger, 4 pieces	150	7	10
Chick'n Nuggets, 4 pieces	190	7	18
Philly Cheesesteak	120	6	6

Canned & Packaged Meals (Cont)

Near East

Couscous: *Per Cup (Prepared)*

	C	F	Cb
Original Plain	230	2	46
Parmesan; Rst Garlic & Oil, avg.	220	5	59
Toasted Pine Nut	230	6	38
Other varieties, avg.	220	5	39

Whole Grain Blends: *Per Cup (Prepared)*

	C	F	Cb
Chicken & Herbs w. Brown Rice	280	6	52
Roasted Garlic w. Brown Rice	220	5	41
Roasted Pecan & Garlic w. Brown	250	9	38
Wheat Pilaf	200	4.5	40
Pasta, all types	240	6	41
Falafels, ¼ cup, (2½ patties)	220	14	18

Rice Pilaf: *Per Cup (Prepared)*

	C	F	Cb
Long Grain; Wild Rice; Garlic Herb	220	4	43
Spanish Mix	310	8	54
Tabouli Mix, Wheat Salad	120	3	23
Toasted Almond Mix	230	6	40
Other varieties, average	270	4.5	55

Nissin

	C	F	Cb
Cup Noodles, all types, avg.	300	13	38

Chow Mein: *Garlic Shrimp, ½ pkg*

	C	F	Cb
Garlic Shrimp, ½ pkg	280	14	32
Chicken Flavor, ½ pkg	240	9	34
Souper Meal, average, ½ pkg	270	11	39
Teriyaki Beef, ½ pkg	270	11	36

Noodle Chef

Delecta Bowl: *Per Bowl*

	C	F	Cb
Tomato Penne	380	4	74
Pizza Mac & Cheese	370	4	70

Nutritious Living: *Per Tray (8 oz)*

	C	F	Cb
Hi Low: Beef Stew	170	5	8
Chicken Vegetable Parmesan	160	4	14
Tuna Noodle Casserole	200	7	14
Turkey Chili w. Beans	180	6	13

Old El Paso

Dinner Kits: *Per Serving (Prepared)*

	C	F	Cb
Chicken Soft Taco (2)	310	10	32
Enchilada Bake, ¼ pkg	370	13	33
Fajita (2), 84g	320	12	34
Hard Taco (2)	290	16	18
Shells, Taco Sce, Seasoning (2)	160	6	23
Soft Taco, 82g	380	10	33
Taco Dinner (2)	260	14	18

Side Dishes: *Spanish Rice, ⅓ pkt*

	C	F	Cb
Spanish Rice, ⅓ pkt	280	4.5	55
Cheesy Mexican Rice, ⅓ pkt	290	6	55

Refried Beans: *Regular, ½ cup*

	C	F	Cb
Regular, ½ cup	100	0.5	17
w. Green Chilies, ½ cup	100	0.5	19
Vegetarian, ½ cup	100	1	17
Fat Free varieties, ½ cup	100	0	18

Pasta Roni: *Per Cup (Prepared)*

	C	F	Cb
Angel Hair Pasta varieties, avg.	310	14	39
Chicken & Broccoli	360	15	49
Chicken (flavor)	300	12	39
Chicken; Shells & White Cheddar	290	12	38
Fettuccine Alfredo	450	25	47
Four Cheese	370	16	49
Parmesan	310	14	39

Nature's Way: *Creamy Parmesano*

	C	F	Cb
Creamy Parmesano	280	9	41
Mushroom in Sauce	280	10	39
Olive Oil & Italian Herb	250	8	38

World Flavors: *Per Cup (Prepared)*

	C	F	Cb
Asian Garlic Chicken	280	11	39
Butter Herb Italiana	300	12	40
Chicken Quesadilla	310	13	40

Rice-A-Roni: *Per Cup (Prepared)*

	C	F	Cb
Beef; Herb & Butter; Rice Pilaf, avg.	310	9	51
Broccoli Au Gratin	360	17	46
Chicken	310	9	51
⅓ Less Salt	270	5	51
Chicken & Broccoli	230	5	40
Chicken & Garlic	260	8	41
Fried Rice	320	11	49
Spanish Rice	260	7	44

(Reduced Fat Recipe: If only 1 Tbsp fat is used instead of 2 Tbsp, deduct 35 calories and 4g fat.)

Express: *Per Cup (Prepared)*

	C	F	Cb
Asian Fried Rice	280	6	51
Golden Chicken	270	6	51
Other varieties, average	275	6	51

Nature's Way: *Parmesan & Romano*

	C	F	Cb
Parmesan & Romano	280	9	42
Italian Cheese & Herb	340	12	52
Long Grain & Wild Rice	250	7	43

Savory Whole Grains: *Per Cup (Prepared)*

	C	F	Cb
Chicken & Herb	260	8	41
Roasted Garlic Italiano	270	9	41
Spanish	250	8	42

Rosarita

Refried Beans: *Per ½ Cup*

	C	F	Cb
Traditional; Vegetarian; Spicy	120	2	19
Low-Fat Black Bean	110	0	19
Fat-Free varieties	100	0	19

Shedd's

Country Crock Side Dishes

	C	F	Cb
Mashed Potatoes: Homestyle, ⅔ cup	190	9	23
Garlic, ⅔ cup, 5 oz	170	7	23
Cheddar Mashed Potato, ⅔ cup	200	10	24
Chicken Rice w. Herbs, 1 cup	210	3.5	42
Deluxe, 1 cup	370	17	40
Elbow Macaroni & Cheese, 1 cup	380	17	40
Deluxe: Cheddar Broccoli Rice, 1 cup	270	11	35
Loaded Mashed Potatoes, ⅔ cup	200	11	23
Scalloped Potatoes, ⅔ cup	210	11	22

Simply Asia	C	F	Cb
Noodle & Sauce Meal Kits: *Per Cup (Prepared)*			
Chili Garlic	330	5	62
Roasted Peanut	385	14	55
Sesame Teriyaki	285	1	60
Other varieties, average	305	5	58
Noodle Bowls: *Per ½ Package (4 oz)*			
Roasted Peanut	340	6	60
Sesame Teriyaki	200	2	40
Soy Ginger; Spicy Kung Pao, avg.	330	5	51
Quick Noodles: *Per Tray*			
Pad Thai	660	9	133
Szechwan Garlic Chow Mein	650	12	121
Other varieties, average	630	8	126
Take Out Noodle Boxes: *Per ½ Box (5.3 oz)*			
Honey Teriyaki	380	3	73
Pad Thai	390	4	79
Sweet & Sour	370	2	75
Other varieties, average	390	5	71
Stagg Chili			
14.3 oz Box: *Per Cup (8.7 oz)*			
Chili w. Beans: Classic/Dynamite	335	17	29
Country/Laredo	320	16	29
Ranch House Chicken	240	8	26
Rio Blanco Chicken	260	12	20
No Beans: Steakhouse/Double	320	22	14
99% Fat Free: Veg. Gdn/4 Bean	200	1	37
Turkey Ranchers	240	3	31
Silverado	250	7	30
S & W: *Per ½ Cup*			
Baked Beans, avg. all types	140	0.5	28
Caribbean Black Beans	90	0	14
Kidney Beans	100	0.5	23
San Antonio; Santa Fe Beans, avg.	90	0.5	21
White Beans	80	0.5	19
Taco Bell			
Home Originals: *Per Serving*			
Dinner Kits: Fajita, ⅓ pkg	230	5	41
Cheesy Dbl Decker Taco, ⅙ pkg	350	14	30
Soft Taco, ⅓ pkg	370	13	40
Taco, ⅙ pkg	240	11	19
Ultimate Nachos, ¼ pkg	280	14	31
Refried Beans (16 oz Can): *Per ½ Cup Serving*			
Fat-Free (w. Green Chilies), 4.6 oz	100	0	18
Vege Blend, 4.6 oz	120	1	20
Bowlz (9 oz): Santa Fe Beef	360	7	49
Salsa Chicken; Fiesta Steak, average	270	6	43
Tasty Bite, Vegetarian Entrees: *Per ½ Package*			
Agra Peas & Greens	140	10	9
Bengal Lentils	160	8	16
Bombay Potatoes	105	4	13
Jaipur Vegetables	170	11	10
Jodhpur Lentils	105	4	12

Tasty Bite (Cont)	C	F	Cb
Vegetarian Entrees (Cont): *Per ½ Package*			
Kashmir Spinach	135	8	8
Madras Lentils	125	5	14
Punjab Eggplant	145	9	13
Ready Meals: *Per Package (w. Rice)*			
Peas Paneer	425	15	54
Spinach Dal	370	9	62
Vegetable Supreme	315	6	55
Thai Kitchen			
Bowls, avg. all types, 1.7 oz	120	2	24
Rice Noodles: *Per Serving*			
Curry Stir Fry, 1 cup	280	4	55
Lemongrass & Chili Stir Fry, 1 cup	270	2.5	55
Pad Thai varieties, 1 pkg, 4.5 oz	360	1	80
Savory Garlic, ½ package	230	2.5	47
Thai Peanut, 1 pkg, 2.25 oz	280	6	51
Thin/Stir Fry/Wide, 2 oz	180	0.5	40
Toasted Sesame Stir Fry, 1 cup	260	5	55
The Spice Hunter: *Per Cup Meal*			
Stuffed Potato: Creamy Butter	140	3.5	25
Broccoli & Cheddar	170	3	31
Sour Cream & Chives	160	2	31
Risotto: *Per Cup Meal*			
3 Cheese Wild Mushroom	260	3	47
Spinach & Garlic	240	1.5	47
Tofurky			
Deli Slices, average, 5 pces	100	3	6
Holiday: Dumplings (2), 4 oz	210	1	45
Tofurky Roast, 4 oz	190	5	10
Tofurky Wishstix, ½ piece	10	0	1
Jurky, 4 pieces	100	2	9
Sausages: Beer Brats (1), 3.5 oz	280	16	8
Kielbasa (1), 3.5 oz	240	12	12
Sweet Italian Sausages (1), 3.5 oz	280	13	12
Trader Joe's			
Bean Medley, ½ cup	150	1	26
Turkey Chili w. Beans, 1 cup	230	3	30
Black Bean Chili, 1 cup	230	1.5	37
Chicken Chili w. Beans, 1 cup	290	9	32
Pasta, Shells & White Cheddar, 1 cup	280	6	48
Refried Beans, avg., ½ cup	110	0	20
Organic Beans, avg., ½ cup	140	0	29
Black Beans: Regular, ½ cup	110	0	20
Cuban Style, ½ cup	120	2	20
Potatoes: Mashed Potatoes, ⅔ cup	120	4.5	20
Garlic Mashed Potatoes, ½ cup	150	7	19
Cheddar Cheese Au Gratin, ½ cup	140	5	21
Premium: Beef Stew, 1 cup	240	11	21
Chicken Stew, 1 cup	230	14	16
Tuna Helper: *See Betty Crocker, Page 71*			

Canned & Packaged Meals (Cont)

Uncle Ben's	C	F	Cb
Flavorful Rice: Per Cup (Prepared w. Margarine)			
Average all varieties	280	10	44
Country Inn: Per Cup (Prepared w/out Margarine)			
Broccoli Rice Au Gratin	200	2	43
Other varieties, avg.	200	1	43
Ready Rice: Per ½ Pouch (Prepared)			
Buttery Rice	190	4.5	47
Roasted Chicken	230	4	41
Teriyaki	260	3.5	51
Whole Grain Brown	220	4	41
Valley Fresh			
Chicken: Per 2 oz			
White & Dark Chunk	80	2	0
Premium Chunk White	70	1	0
Turkey, Premium Chunk White, ¼ can	80	1.5	0
Van Camps			
Pork & Beans, ½ cup	110	1.5	23
Original Baked Beans, ½ cup	160	1	30
Beanie Weanie Original, 7¾ oz	240	8	29
Baked Beans: w. Ground Beef, 1 c.	370	7	57
w. Chicken, 1 cup	360	2	62
Spanish Rice, 1 cup	180	3	37
White Wave (Vegetarian)			
Seitan: Chicken w. Broth, 5 oz	110	2	4
Traditional, 3 oz	90	1	3
Tofu Town: Per ½ Container			
Grilled Tenders: Havana Black Bean	210	8	18
Light Tamari, 5 oz	120	7	15
Mediterranean Tahini, 5 oz	240	13	16
Sesame Ginger Teriyaki, 5 oz	240	9	24
Soy Milks & Yogurts: See Pages 27, 30			
Tofu: See Page 77			
Worthington/Loma Linda (Vegetarian)			
Big Franks: 1 link, 1.8 oz	110	6	3
Low-fat, 1 link, 1.8 oz	80	2.5	3
Chili, 1 cup, 8 oz	280	10	25
Choplets, 2 slices, 3.2 oz	90	1	4
Diced Chik, 2 oz	50	0	1
Dinner Cuts, 2 slices, 3.2 oz	90	1	4
FriChik, 2 pces, 3.1 oz	140	8	3
Linketts, (1), 1¼ oz	70	4	1
Little Links, 2 links, 1.6 oz	90	5	8
Low-Fat Veja-Links (1), 1 oz	45	1.5	3
Multigrain Cutlets, 2 sl., 2¾ oz	100	1	5
Prime Stakes (1) 3.2 oz	120	6	7
Redi-Burger, ⅝" slice, 3 oz	120	2.5	7

Worthington/Loma Linda (Cont)	C	F	Cb
Saucettes, 4 pces, 3 oz	90	6	1
Super Links (1) 1.6 oz	110	8	2
Tender Bits, 6 pieces, 3 oz	120	4	7
Tender Rounds, 8 pieces, 2¾ oz	120	4.5	6
Turkee Slices, 3 sl., 3.3 oz	180	12	5
Vega-Links (1), 1 oz	50	3	1
Vege-Burger, ¼ cup, 2 oz	60	0.5	2
Vegetable Skallops, ½ cup, 3 oz	90	1	4
Vegetarian Burger, ¼ cup, 1.9 oz	70	1.5	3
Yves Veggie Cuisine (Vegetarian)			
Breakfast: Brkfast Links (2) 1.8 oz	70	2	3
Breakfast Patties (1) 2 oz	80	0.5	2
Canadian Veg. Bacon, 3 slices	80	0.5	1
Burgers: Meatless Beef Burger	110	4	8
Veggie Chick'n Burger (1) 2.6 oz	100	3	5
Deli: Roast Beef, 4 slices	110	2.5	4
Smoked Chicken, 4 slices	100	1.5	5
Dogs & Brats: Jumbo Dog (1) 2.6 oz	110	3	5
Brat Zesty Italian (1), 3.3 oz	150	5	9
Good Dog (1) 1.8 oz	70	3.5	2
Meatless Dog (1)	50	0.5	2
Tofu Dog, avg. (1), 1.3 oz	45	1	2
Veggie Brats Classic (1), 3.3 oz	160	5	9
Entree: Santa Fe Beef 10½ oz	360	9	57
Mac n Soy Cheese, 10½ oz	340	9	52
Skewers: BBQ Beef, 2.8 oz	100	0.5	10
Lemon Herb Chicken, 2.8 oz	100	1	5
Veggie Deli Slices: Bologna, 2 oz	80	2.5	2
Ham, 2 oz	100	2	5
Pizza Pepperoni, 1.7 oz	60	1	4
Salami, 2 oz	80	0	4
Veggie Turkey, 2 oz	100	1.5	5
Veggie Ground Round: Orig., ⅓ c.	60	0.5	4
Ground Turkey, ⅓ cup	60	1	4
Taco Stuffers, ⅓ cup, 1.93 oz	90	2.5	5
Veggie Entrees: Chili, 10.5 oz	240	1	37
Lasagne, 10.5 oz	300	3	51
Thai Lemongrass Veggie Chicken	330	9	49
Veggie Penne, 10.5 oz	210	1.5	36
Zatarain's: Pasta Dinner Mix (Prepared)			
Gumbo, 1 cup	120	0.5	23
Jumbalaya, 1 cup	130	0	29
Ready To Serve Complete Meals: Per Pkg			
Dirty Rice w. Pork, 8.8 oz	420	7	81
Jambalaya w. Sausage, 6.5 oz	350	12	48

Soybean Products	C	F	Cb
Cheeses (Soy): See Page 44			
Miso Paste, average, 1 Tbsp., ¼ oz	35	1	5
Miso Soup (dry mix), average			
1 Tbsp., dry mix	35	1	5
1 cup, prepared	35	1	5
Natto, ½ cup, 3 oz	160	7	14
Okara (Tofu fiber residue), ½ c., 2 oz	47	1	8
Tempeh: 1 piece, 3 oz	180	8	12
Fried, 3 oz	250	14	14
Seitan *(White Wave),* Trad., 3 oz	90	1	3
Soybean Protein (TVP), 1 oz	95	0	8
Soy Bean Paste, 1 tsp	10	0	2
Soy Beans: See Page 149			
Soy Drinks: See Page 27			
White Wave: See Page 76			

Tofu ~ Packaged	C	F	Cb
Tofu Stir Fried, average all, 4 oz	120	8	3
Azumaya Tofu: Soft (Silken), 3.2 oz	40	2	1
Soft, Light (Silken), 3.2 oz	40	1	3
Firm; Extra Firm, 2.8 oz	70	4	2
Light Extra Firm, 2.8 oz	60	2	3
Seasoned Tofu, 3 oz	90	5	3
House Foods			
Premium Tofu: Soft (Silken), 3 oz	50	2.5	2
Medium Firm (Regular), 3 oz	60	3	1
Firm, 3 oz	70	3.5	2
Extra Firm, 3 oz	80	4	1

Tofu ~ Packaged (Cont)	C	F	Cb
House Foods (Cont)			
Organic Tofu: Firm, 3 oz	60	3	0
Extra Firm, 3 oz	90	4.5	0
House Tofu: Tokusen Kinugoshi, 3 oz	90	4	3
Sukui/Soon (Extra Soft), 3 oz	45	2	2
Yaki Tofu: Yaki (Broiled), 3 oz	90	5	2
Tofu Steak: Original, 4.8 oz	80	9	0
Garlic & Pepper, 4.8 oz	80	9	1
Chili & Onion, 4.8 oz	70	8	4
Mori-Nu Tofu (Silken)			
Soft, 3 oz, 1" slice	45	2.5	2
Firm, 3 oz, 1" slice	50	2.5	2
Extra Firm, 3 oz, 1" slice	45	1.5	2
Organic, 3 oz, 1" slice	60	2.5	2
Lite: Firm, 3 oz, 1" slice	30	0.5	1
Extra Firm, 3 oz, 1" slice	35	0.5	1
Seasoned Tofu: *Per 3 oz*			
Japanese Miso	60	2.5	3
Chinese Spice	50	2	3
Nasoya Tofu: Soft, ⅕ pkg, 2.8 oz	60	3	1
Silken, 3.2 oz	45	2	1
Firm, ⅕ pkg, 3.2 oz	70	3	2
Extra Firm, ⅕ pkg, 2.8 oz	80	4	2
Super Firm, cubed, ⅕ pkg, 2.8 oz	100	5	3
Chinese 5 Spice, ¼ pkg, 3 oz	90	5	3
White Wave: Baked Tofu, 1 square	90	5	2
Soft/Firm Tofu, ⅕ block	110	6	3
Reduced Fat, ⅕ block	90	4	4
Firm, 3 oz	100	6	3

Soups

Homemade & Restaurant

Restaurant & Take-Out	C	F	Cb
Per 8 fl.oz			
Bean Medley	200	3	34
Beef Consomme	30	0	2
Borscht (w. Cream)	130	8	14
Bouillabaisse	400	15	10
Chicken & Corn	290	14	20
Chicken & Wild Rice	80	4	9
Chicken Consomme	50	0	2
Chicken Curry	180	8	18
Chicken Jambalaya	160	7	8
Chicken Noodle	80	2	12
w. Chicken	160	4	12
Chicken Soup	80	2	6
Chili with Beans	250	12	25
Clam Chowder	240	15	17
Corn & Crab	120	3	18
Corn Chowder	150	8	16
Cream of Broccoli	200	12	20
Cream of Potato	150	6.5	17
Cream of Mushroom	200	13	15
Creamy Pumpkin	210	10	26
Fish Chowder	220	15	6
French Onion	420	15	15
Gazpacho	50	0	5
Lentil Soup	250	9	28
Lobster Bisque	320	15	10
Matzo Ball (w. 1 large ball)	180	7	24
Minestrone	125	2.5	20
Mulligatawny	300	15	8
Pea & Ham	240	10	25
Potato & Bacon	170	7	19
Shark Fin Soup	100	4	8
Spicy Shrimp Soup, 1 bowl	160	7	10
Split Pea Soup	180	2.5	9
Vegetable (Fat Free)	75	0	18
Vegetable Beef	80	2	10
Vichyssoise	200	9	15
Watercress	90	4	13

Other Soups: See *International & Fast-Foods Sections (Arby's, Au Bon Pain, Boston Market, Dunkin' Donuts, Denny's, Schlotzsky's, Sizzler, Souplantation, Sweet Tomatoes, Zoup!)*

Homemade Soups: Calculate calories, fat and carbohydrates from ingredients.

Bouillon Cubes & Powders

	C	F	Cb
Bouillon Cubes: *Average all Types*			
Regular, 1 cube	5	0	1
Low Sodium (LiteLine)	12	0	1
Powders: Average, 1 tsp	10	0	1
Herb-Ox: Instant Broth & Seasoning,			
Beef, 1 envelope	5	0	1
Chicken; Vegetarian	5	0	1
Herbs, Spices: 1 tsp	5	0	1
Soup Oyster Crackers			
40 small/3 large, ½ oz	60	2	8

Amy's (Organic)

	C	F	Cb
Per Cup (½ Can)			
Alphabet (Fat-Free)	80	0	16
Black Bean Vegetable	130	1.5	25
Butternut Squash	100	2.5	20
Chunky Tomato Bisque	120	3.5	21
Chunky Vegetable	60	0	13
Corn Chowder	190	10	19
Cream of Mushroom, ¾ cup, (½ can)	140	9	13
Cream of Tomato	100	2	17
Lentil	150	4.5	19
Minestrone	90	1.5	17
No Chicken Noodle	90	3	12
Pasta & 3 Bean	130	5	19
Potato Leek	180	10	21
Split Pea (Fat-Free)	100	0	19
Vegetable Barley	70	1	13
Other varieties, average	150	4	23

'Light in Sodium' Range *(50% less sodium),*
(Calories/Fat/Carb ~ Same as Regular Range)

Andersen's ~ *Per Cup*

	C	F	Cb
Lentil	110	2	19
Split Pea	130	0	24
Split Pea w. Bacon	140	1	23
Tomato	130	3.5	22

Baxters

	C	F	Cb
Per Cup (Prepared as Directed)			
Cream of Asparagus	160	10	15
Cream of Scottish Smoked Salmon	150	8	16
French Onion	70	0	15
Stilton Cheese & White Port	210	15	14
Vichyssoise	210	15	16

Bean Cuisine

	C	F	Cb
Per Cup (Prepared as Directed)			
13 Bean Boullabaisse; Lentil, avg.	220	0	17
Island Black Bean	210	0	17
Santa Fe Corn Chowder	160	0	18
White Bean Provencal	250	1	32

Bear Creek — *Per Cup*

	C	F	Cb
Cheddar Potato	190	7	30
Chicken Noodle	120	1	23
Creamy Potato	160	4	28
Hot & Sour	90	0.5	18
Split Pea	110	1.5	20
Other varieties, average	145	5	28

Campbell's

	C	F	Cb
Classic Red & White: *Per ½ Cup*			
Bean w. Bacon; Fiesta Chili Beef, avg.	170	4	25
Beef Noodle	70	2	8
Beef w. Veges/Barley; Minestrone, avg.	90	1.5	16
Black Bean	110	1.5	18
Cheddar Cheese	110	5	12
Chicken & Dumplings	70	2.5	10
Chicken Won Ton	60	1	9
Cream of Asparagus	110	7	9
Cream of Broccoli	90	3.5	12
Cream of Chicken & Mushroom	80	6	7
Cream of Mushroom	100	6	9
Cream of Onion	100	6	10
Cream of Potato	90	2	15
Cream of Shrimp	90	5	8
Creamy Chicken Noodle	120	7	11
French Onion	45	1.5	6
Green Pea	180	3	28
Hearty Vegetable w. Pasta	90	0.5	19
Manhattan Clam Chowder	70	0.5	12
New England Clam Chowder	90	2.5	13
Old Fashioned Vegetable	80	1.5	14
Split Pea w. Ham & Bacon	180	3.5	27
Tomato	90	0	20
Tomato Bisque	130	3.5	23
Vegetable	100	0.5	20
Healthy Request: *Per ½ Cup*			
Chicken Rice	70	1.5	13
Vegetable Beef	90	1	15
Other varieties, average	80	2	15

Campbell's (Cont)

	C	F	Cb
98% Fat Free, prep., avg., ½ cup	70	2	10
Chunky: *Per Cup*			
Baked Potatoes w. Bacon Bits	180	8	23
Clam Chowder Manhattan	120	3.5	19
Classic Chicken Noodle	110	2.5	15
Grilled Chicken & Sausage Gumbo	140	2.5	21
Hearty Veges w. Pasta	120	2	23
Select: *Per Cup (8 fl.oz)*			
Beef w. Roasted Barley	130	1	22
Chicken & Pasta w. Roasted Garlic	100	1	18
Chicken Vegetable	110	0.5	19
Chicken w. Egg Noodles	110	1.5	14
Creamy Chicken Alfredo	180	7	18
Creamy Potato w. Roasted Garlic	180	10	20
Harvest Tomato w. Basil	80	0	18
Italian Saus. w. Pasta & Pepperoni	150	6	18
Italian Style Wedding	120	3	15
Mexican Style Chicken Tortilla	130	2.5	19
Minestrone; Tom. Garden; Vege	100	0.5	20
New England Clam Chowder	160	8	15
Potato Broccoli Cheese	120	4	18
Rosemary Chkn w. Rstd Potatoes	110	1	17
Savory Lentil	140	0.5	27
Savory White Bean w. Roasted Ham	170	1	30
Split Pea w. Ham	160	1	29
Other varieties, average	140	3	20
Soup at Hand: *Per Container*			
Chicken varieties, average	70	2	11
Cream of Broccoli	150	7	17
Creamy Mushroom	120	7	10
Creamy Tomato	190	4	34
Italian Style Wedding	90	4.5	10
New England Clam Chowder	120	6	13
Vegetable Beef	60	1	10
Velvety Potato	160	7	21

Soup is an excellent filler as part of a meal, or as a snack.

- *Add lots of veggies, and beans (for extra protein & fiber)*
- *Avoid Noodle Cups (high in fat)*
- *If using low-fat soup mixes, add extra microwaved veges, tofu or canned beans*

Soups (Cont)

Dr McDougall's   C   F   Cb

Per Serving (Mix)

	C	F	Cb
Split Pea w. Barley, 1.9 oz	190	1	35
Tortilla Soup w. Baked Chips. 1.8 oz	190	1.5	37
Vegetarian Vegetable, 1.5 oz	150	0.5	29
Big Cups: *Per Full Serving*			
Hot & Sour w. Noodles	170	1	35
Miso Soup w. Noodles	180	1	34
Pad Thai/Ramen, average	200	1	42
Black Bean & Lime	340	2	60
Minestrone & Pasta	200	1	40
Split Pea w. Barley	240	1	42
Tamale/Tortilla w. Baked Chips, avg.	200	2	34

Edward & Sons

Miso Cups: *Per Envelope (Dry Mix)*

	C	F	Cb
Golden Vegetable	30	1	3
Organic Traditional w. Tofu	35	1	4
Reduced Sodium	25	1	3
Savory w. Seaweed	30	1	3

Dixie Diners' Club

Per Cup (Prepared as Directed)
Carb Counters, Dine 'n Dash:

	C	F	Cb
Broccoli & Cheese	70	5	3
Chicken Cheese Enchilada	95	6	4
Chicken Noodle	40	1	3
Cream of Mushroom	50	4	2

Fantastic Cup Soups

Vegetarian Soup Cups: *Per Container (Prep'd as Directed)*

	C	F	Cb
Baja Black Bean, 1.6 oz	130	0.5	31
Buckeroo Bean Chili, 1.8 oz	160	2	33
Classic French Onion, 0.8 oz	90	2.5	15
Creamy Potato Leek, 1.2 oz	120	2.5	22
Great Lakes Cheddar Broccoli, 0.9 oz	100	3	15
Green Onion Miso w. Tofu, 1.4 oz	140	1.5	26
Hot & Sour, 1.6 oz	170	2	33
Mama's Minestrone, 1.7 oz	160	2.5	30
Sesame Miso, 1.4 oz	140	2	27
Southwest Tortilla Bean, 1.8 oz	170	3.5	34
Spicy Thai, 1.6 oz	150	0.5	32
Split Pea, 1.6 oz	140	0.5	28
Summer Vegetable Rice, 1.2 oz	110	0.5	25
Three Onion Noodle, 1.9 oz	180	2	36
Tuscan Tomato & Shells, 1.6 oz	140	1	31
Vegetarian Chicken Noodle, 1 oz	90	1	17

Health Valley   C   F   Cb

Per Cup

	C	F	Cb
Broths: Beef Flavored, Fat-Free	10	0	0
Chicken: Fat-Free	25	0	0
Low-Fat	35	1.5	0
Organic	15	1	1
Vegetable, Fat-Free	10	0	3
Fat-Free Soup: Split Pea & Carrots	110	0	24
Black Bean & Vegetable	120	0	24
Italian Minestrone	110	0	23
Other varieties, average	80	0	17
Organic Soup: Black Bean	130	1	26
Lentil	110	2	21
Minestrone	100	2	17
Mushroom Barley	90	2	15
Potato & Leek	80	2	15
Split Pea	110	0	23
Tomato	80	0	18
Vegetable	90	2	16
Soup Cup: *Per ½ Cup*			
Fat Free: Pasta Italiano	140	0	31
Zesty Black Bean w. Rice	100	0	22

Healthy Choice

Per Cup

	C	F	Cb
Bean & Ham	180	2	28
Chicken & Dumplingsf	140	2.5	21
Chicken w. Rice Soup	110	1.5	17
Chicken Tortilla Style	160	2	25
Country Vegetable	110	1	19
Fiesta Chicken	120	2	20
Garden Vegetable	120	0.5	24
Hearty Chicken	130	2	20
New England Clam Chowder	110	1	19
Old Fashioned Chicken Noodle	100	1.5	13
Split Pea and Ham	170	2	22
Vegetable Beef	130	1	22
Zesty Gumbo	100	2	16

Kikkoman

Dry Mix

	C	F	Cb
Chinese Style Egg Flower: 1⅓ tsp	40	1	7
w. Corn, 1 Tbsp, dry mix	50	6	11
Instant Miso:			
Shiro (White): 1 packet dry	35	1	4
w. Tofu, 1 packet dry	35	1	3

Campbell's BIG

Imagine	C	F	Cb
Per Cup			
No Chicken/Vegetable Broth	20	0	2
Free Range Chicken Broth	10	0	1
Organic Creamy: Broccoli	60	1.5	10
Butternut Squash	90	2	18
Chicken	70	1.5	12
Crab/Lobster Bisque, avg.	130	5	16
Portobello Mushroom	80	3	14
Potato Leek; Sweet Corn, avg.	115	3	19
Sweet Potato	110	1.5	23
Tomato	80	1	15
Tomato Basil	90	1.5	17

Knorr			
Recipe Classics: *Dry Mix*			
Cream of Spinach, 2 Tbsp	60	1.5	10
French Onion, 2 Tbsp	45	1	9
Leek Soup, 2 Tbsp	60	1	11
Spring Vegetable, 2 Tbsp, 0.3 oz	25	0	6
Tomato w. Basil, 3 Tbsp, 0.7 oz	70	1	15
Vegetable, 2 Tbsp, 0.5 oz	50	0.5	10
Bouillon Cubes: *Per ½ Cube (1 Cup, Prepared)*			
Beef; Chicken, average	20	1.5	0.5

Lipton			
Cup-a-Soup: *Per Envelope*			
Cream of Chicken	60	1	15
Chicken Noodle	80	1	17
Recipe Secrets: *Per Serving (Dry Mix)*			
Beefy Onion, 1 Tbsp	25	0.5	5
Onion, 1 Tbsp	20	0	4
Onion Mushroom, 1⅔ Tbsp	25	0	7
Soup Secrets: *Per Cup (Prepared)*			
Noodle Soup	60	1	10
Chicken Noodle	90	1	15

Manischewitz			
Condensed: *Per ½ Cup (Unprepared)*			
Chicken	15	0	2
Chicken w. Kreplach	40	1	6
Chicken w. Matzo Balls	80	3.5	9
Quart Jars: *Per 8 fl.oz (Prepared)*			
Borscht w. Beets	90	0	21
Borscht Low Calorie	25	0	6

Manischewitz (Cont)	C	F	Cb
Ready To Serve: Matzo Balls in Broth	220	9	27
Dry Mixes: *Per Cup*			
Matzo Ball & Soup Mix	40	0.5	9
Split Pea Cello	140	0	25
Vegetable Soup Cello	120	0	22

Maruchan			
Per Cup			
Instant Lunch, avg. all flavors	290	12	38
Ramen flavors, ½ pkt, 1½ oz	190	8	26

Miso Cup (Edward & Sons)			
Per Cup (Prepared as Directed)			
Original; Golden Seaweed	30	1	3
Traditional	35	1	4
Reduced Sodium	25	1	3

Nile Spice			
Per Cup			
Black Bean; Lentil	170	1.5	35
Chicken Flavored Vegetable	110	1.5	21
Country Mushroom	140	2.5	26
Minestrone	140	1	30
Split Pea, low-fat	200	1	35
Minestrone Couscous	180	1.5	34
Other varieties, average	190	2	36

Pacific Foods			
Per Cup			
Chicken Broth	10	0	1
Natural, Beef Broth	20	0	1
Organic: French Onion	35	0	6
Creamy Butternut Squash	90	2	17
Creamy Tomato	100	2	16
Roasted Red Pepper & Tomato	110	2	16
Vegetable Broth	15	0	3
Hearty Soups: Chicken Fajita	150	2.5	24
Other varieties, average	170	5	22

Pritikin			
Per Cup			
Fat Free Chicken Broth	5	0	0
Hearty Vegetable	90	0	15
Split Pea	180	5	32
Vegetarian Vegetable	80	0	15

Soups (Cont)

Progresso

	C	F	Cb
Vegetable Classic: *Per Cup*			
French Onion	50	1.5	8
Green Split Pea	170	1	28
Garden Vegetable	90	0	20
Hearty Tomato	110	1	23
Lentil; Tomato Basil, avg.	155	2.5	29
Minestrone	110	2	19
Tomato Rotini	140	1	29
Vegetable	80	0.5	16
Traditional: *Per Cup*			
Beef Barley	140	3.5	18
Chkn Herb Dumpling; Minestrone	100	2.5	14
Italian-Style Wedding; Chickarina, avg.	130	5	15
Manhattan Clam Chowder	100	2	17
New England Clam Chowder	190	10	20
Potato Broccoli & Cheese Chowder	180	10	18
Southwestern Style Chicken	120	2.5	19
Split Pea w/ Ham	150	1	25
Other varieties, average	100	2.5	14
Rich & Hearty: *Per Cup*			
Chicken & Homestyle Noodles	110	2	14
Chicken Pot Pie Style	170	6	21
Creamy Chicken Wild Rice	150	8	13
New England Clam Chowder	190	9	22
Savory Beef Barley Vegetable	130	1	22
Slow Cooked Vegetable Beef	120	1	19
Steak & Homestyle Noodles	110	2	16
Steak & Sauteed Mushrooms	110	2	18
Other varieties, average	125	2	21
Microwaveable Bowl: *Per Bowl*			
Chicken & Wild Rice/Noodle, avg.	100	1.5	17
Minestrone Soup	90	1.5	17
Vegetable Soup	80	0.5	17
Carb Monitor: *Per Cup*			
Chicken Cheese Enchilada	170	12	8
Chicken Vegetable	70	2	7
Tuscan Style Meatball	100	5	9

Safeway Select

	C	F	Cb
Signature Soups: *Per Cup (8.6 oz)*			
Baked Potato; Craving Crab, avg.	420	33	20
Broccoli & Cheesy Cheddar	280	21	14
Chkn Noodle; Harvest Vege Beef, avg.	130	3.5	13
Clam Chowder, all varieties	330	24	19
Fajita Chicken & Corn Chowder	350	23	25
Golden Split Pea	200	3	31
Savory Chicken & Wild Rice	170	6	20
Stompin' Steakhouse Chili	260	8	22
Tuscan Tomato & Basil Bisque	310	26	17

Shelton's

	C	F	Cb
All Natural: *Per Cup*			
Black Bean & Chicken	170	4	22
Chicken Noodle	80	2	9
Chicken Rice	90	1	14
Chicken Tortilla	110	1.5	16
Vegetable Chicken	150	2	28
Broths: Chicken	35	2.5	0
Organic Turkey	0	0	0

Simply Asia

	C	F	Cb
Noodle Bowls: *Per Bowl*			
Miso Tofu	420	3.5	82
Sesame Chicken	430	4.5	82
Soy Ginger	330	5	61
Spring Vegetable	270	3	56
Szechwan Garlic	650	12	121
Szechwan Hot & Sour	480	7	88

Spice Hunter

	C	F	Cb
Per Bowl (10 oz)			
Chicken Noodle	140	1.5	25
Creamy Thai Noodle	200	5	34
Split Pea	250	1.5	43

Swanson

	C	F	Cb
Per Cup			
99% Fat Free Chicken Broth	15	0.5	1
Beef Broth	15	0	1
Chicken Broth	10	0.5	1
Vegetable Broth	15	0	3

Tabatchnick

	C	F	Cb
Per Single Pouch			
Balsamic, Tomato & Rice	110	3.5	18
Barley Mushroom; Wild Rice, avg.	80	1	17
Black Bean	230	2.5	39
Broccoli & Cheese	200	12	15
Cabbage	90	1	21
Chicken w. Dumplings	150	6	19
Corn Chowder	130	4.5	21
Cream of Broccoli	130	5	18
Cream of Mushroom/Spinach, avg.	95	5	11
Creamed Spinach	40	1	7
Lentil	160	0	29
Macaroni & Cheese	250	8	34
Minestrone; Vegetable, avg.	100	1.5	18
New England Potato	110	5	17

Tabatchnick (Cont)

	C	F	Cb
New York Chicken	70	1	13
Old Fashioned Potato	100	1.5	21
Onion	60	1.5	11
Pea	140	0	34
Salmon Chowder	80	1.5	15
Seafood Chowder	130	6	15
Southwest Bean	220	5	35
Tomato Rice	110	3.5	18
Yankee Bean	180	1.5	33
Vegetarian Chili	180	3.5	28
Low Sodium: Mushroom	80	1	17
Pea	140	0	34
Vegetable	90	1.5	17

Thai Kitchen

Instant Rice Noodle: *Per Package (Prep. as Directed)*

Bangkok Curry; Thai Ginger	190	3.5	37
Garlic & Vege; Spring Onion	190	3	37
Lemongrass & Chili	190	3.5	37

Rice Noodle Soup Bowls: *Per ½ Bowl*

Hot & Sour	120	2.5	23
Lemongrass & Chili	110	1.5	23
Thai Ginger	120	2	23

Trader Joe's

Per Cup

Barley w. Vegetables	110	3	19
Black Bean	130	1.5	25
Chicken Broth	15	0	1
Chicken Noodle	90	1	14
Chunky Minestrone	110	2.5	19
Creamy Corn Chowder	170	6	28
Lentil w. Vegetables	140	3	21
Organic Lentil Vegetable	130	1.5	25
Rich Onion	90	3.5	12
Split Pea, Low Fat	100	0	19
Condensed: Clam Chowder	160	4	22

Vermont Country Soup

Per Cup

Chicken Noodle	180	8	16
Chicken Pomodoro	150	6	17
Country Vegetable	90	1	20
Cream of Potato	290	16	31
New England Clam Chowder	320	23	15
Tuscan Minestrone	120	1.5	22

Walnut Acres

Per Cup

Black Bean	150	0.5	29
Chicken and Wild Rice	80	2	11
Chicken Noodle	80	2	11
Classic Minestrone	120	2.5	22
Creamy Tomato	100	3	17
Portobello Mushroom	80	4	9
Split Pea	190	0.5	34
Tuscany White Bean	130	1.5	23

Westbrae Natural

Canned: *Per Cup (Unless Indicated)*

Alabama; Mediterranean Lentil, avg.	140	0	25
New York UnChicken Noodle	60	1	10
Old World Split Pea	150	0	28
Santa Fe Vegetable	160	0	31
Other varieties, average	125	0	25

Condensed: *Per ¾ Cup (Prepared as Directed)*

California UnChicken Broth	15	0.5	2
Monte Carlo Creamy Mushroom	70	3	10
Tuscany Tomato	70	0	16

Wolfgang Puck's

Per Cup

Original: Chicken & Egg Noodles	110	5	11
Minestroni Classic	160	4	25
Thick Hearty Vegetable	130	5	19
Organic Soup: Tortilla	160	3.5	27
Chicken w. Wild Rice	130	4	18
Creamy Broccoli/Tomato	210	16	41
Thick Hearty Lentil & Veggie	160	1	29
Thick Hearty Vegetable	90	3	14

Wylers

Dry Mix: Mrs Grass Onion, 10g	35	0.5	6
Homestyle Vegetable, 12g	35	0	7
Mrs Grass Hearty Soup Mix: *Per Cup*			
Chicken Noodle	70	1.5	11
Beef Vegetable	90	0.5	18

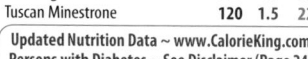

For Full Nutritional Data ~ See Author's Website www.CalorieKing.com

Herbs & Spices

Herbs & Spices | C | F | Cb

Per Teaspoon: Average all types — 5, 0, 1

	C	F	Cb
All Purpose, 1 tsp	0	0	0
Allspice, ground	5	0	1
Chili Powder	8	0	1
Cinnamon, ground	6	0	2
Curry Powder	6	0	1
Garlic Powder	9	0	2
Nutmeg, ground	12	0	1
Onion Powder	7	0	2
Parsley, dried	4	0	1
Pepper, black/red/white, avg.	6	0	1
Saffron	2	0	1
Salt Free Blends, 1 tsp	0	0	0
Tumeric, ground	8	0	1
Seeds: Fenugreek	12	1	2
Mustard, Poppyseed	15	1	1
Other types, average	7	0	1

Seasonings & Flavorings

	C	F	Cb
Accent Flavor Enhancer, 1 tsp	0	0	0
Angostura Bitters, 1 tsp	15	0	4
Bacon Bits, average, 1 Tbsp	35	2	2
Bacon Chips (Durkee), 1 Tbsp, 7 g	30	1	2
Bac-Os (Betty Crocker), 1½ Tbsp, 7g	20	1	1.5
Bragg Liquid Aminos, 1 tsp	5	0	0
Butter Buds, 1 tsp	5	0	2
Garlic Bread Sprinkle, 1 tsp	8	0.5	1
Garlic Salt, 1 tsp	2	0	0
Italian Seasoning, 1 tsp	4	0	1
Lemon Pepper Seasoning, 1 tsp	7	0	1
Meat Tenderizer, avg., 1 tsp	7	0	1
Molly McButter, 1 tsp	5	1	1
Mrs Dash Blends, 1 tsp	0	0	0
Salad Crunchies (*McCormick*), 1 tsp	10	0.5	2
Salt: Regular, Sea Salt, Lite Salt	0	0	0
Seasoning Mixes, avg., ¼ pkg	70	1	9
Taco Seasoning, avg., ¼ pkg	30	0.5	4
Old El Paso: Chili Season. Mix, 1 T.	8	0.5	1.5
Cheesy Taco Season. Mix, 1 Tbsp	10	0.5	2
Taco/Burrito Seasoning Mix, 2 tsp	15	0	4
Fajita Seasoning Mix, 1 tsp	5	0	1.5
Vegit Seasoning Mix, ¼ tsp	10	0	2

Condiments, Sauces | C | F | Cb

Average of Brands & Homemade

	C	F	Cb
Apple Sauce, *Also see Page 146*			
Sweetened, ¼ cup, 2½ oz	55	0	13
Unsweetened, ¼ cup, 2 oz	25	0	7
Barbecue Sauce, Avg., 2 Tbsp, 1 oz	40	0	10
Bull's Eye, Original, 1 Tbsp, ½ oz	30	0	7
Bearnaise Sauce, ¼ cup, 2½ oz	190	19	5
Buffalo Wing Sce: Honey Mustard, 1 T.	40	3	2
Average other varieties, 1 Tbsp	25	2	2
Catsup (Ketchup), regular, 1 Tbsp	15	0	4
Cheese, h/made, ¼ cup, 2½ oz	150	10	12
Chef-Mate, Hot Dog, ¼ cup	70	2.5	9
Chili Sauce: *Heinz,* 1 Tbsp, ½ oz	20	0	4.5
Del Monte, 1 Tbsp, ½ oz	20	0	5
Cocktail Sauce, ¼ cup	110	0	15
Fat-Free (*Walden Farms*) 1 Tbsp	0	0	0
Cranberry, all types, ¼ c., 2½ oz	110	0	27
Demi Glaze Gold, 2 tsp	30	0.5	3
Honey Mustard (*French's*) 1 tsp	5	0	1
Horseradish: 1 tsp	2	0	1
Kraft, 1 tsp	20	1.5	1
Ketchup: Regular, 1 Tbsp, ½ oz	15	0	4
Heinz One-Carb, 1 Tbsp	5	0	1
Mushroom Sauce, ½ cup, 2 oz	50	2	5
Mustard, average, 1 tsp	5	0	0.5
Pesto Sauce, ¼ cup, 2 oz	90	5	8
Pizza Sauce, cnd., ¼ cup, 2 oz	30	0	6
Seafood Cocktail Sce, ¼ cup	60	0	15
Soy Sauce: All types, avg., 1 Tbsp	10	0	1
Kikkoman Lite Soy, 1 Tbsp	10	0	1
Sour Cream Sce, ½ cup	250	15	22
Spaghetti Sce, ½ cup, 4½ oz	135	6	19
Steak Sauce: A1, 1 Tbsp, ½ oz	15	0	3
Lea & Perrins, 1 Tbsp, ½ oz	25	0	5
Carb Well (*A1*) 1 Tbsp, ½ oz	5	0	1
Str'berry Puree Sce: Unsweet., 2 T.	9	0	2
Sweet & Sour Sauce:			
Contadina, 1 Tbsp	40	1	8
Kraft, 1 Tbsp	60	0	13
La Choy, 2 Tbsp, 34g	60	0	14
Tabasco Sauce, 1 tsp	2	0	1
Taco Sauce, average, 2 Tbsp, 1 oz	10	0	1
Tartar Sauce: Heinz, 2 Tbsp, 1 oz	120	11	4
America's Choice, 2 Tbsp, 1 oz	160	17	1
Hellmann's, Regular, 2 Tbsp, 1 oz	80	7	4
McCormick, Fat-Free, 2 Tbsp, 1 oz	35	0	6
Teriyaki Sauce (*Kikkoman*) 1 T., ½ oz	15	0	3
Vinegar, White or Wine, 2 Tbsp	4	0	1
White Sauce, ½ cup, 5 oz	130	7	10
Worcestershire Sauce, 1 tsp	5	0	1

Pickles & Relish | C | F | Cb

Average All Brands

	C	F	Cb
Bread & Butter Pickles, 4 sl., 1 oz	25	0	6
Chutney, 2 Tbsp, 1¼ oz	50	0	11
Dill Pickle:			
Slices, 4 slices, 1 oz	4	0	1
1 large,			
(3¾"x 1¼" diam.), 2¼ oz	12	0	3
Extra lrg (4"x 1¾" diam.), 5 oz	30	0	6
Halves: Small, 1 oz	3	0	0.5
Large, 2½ oz	8	0	2
Sweet, small, ½ oz	22	0	6
Gherkins, sweet, 1 med., 1 oz	30	0	7
Green Chilies, chopped, 2 Tbsp	5	0	1
Horseradish, 1 Tbsp	10	0	2
Jalapenos, pickled, 2 whole, 2 oz	10	0.5	2
Jalapeno Relish, 1 Tbsp, ½ oz	5	0	1
Mustard, avg. all brands, 1 tsp	5	0	0.5
Peppers, Hot/Mild (1), 1.6 oz	20	0	4
Pickled: Beets, ½ cup, 4 oz	75	0	19
Onions, 1 medium, ¾ oz	10	0	2
Cocktail Onion, 1 onion	2	0	0
Red Cabbage, ½ cup, 3 oz	65	0	15
Pickles: Sweet, 2 Tbsp, 1 oz	35	0	0
Large (3"x ¾ diam.), 1¼ oz	40	0	10
Pickle in a Pouch, 1 large	12	0	3
Relishes: Sandwich Spread, 1 tsp	20	1	5
Cranberry-Orange, 1 Tbsp	30	0	7
Hot Dog *(Heinz)*, 1 Tbsp, ½ oz	17	0	3
Sweet Pickle, 1 Tbsp, ½ oz	20	0	5
Sauerkraut, ½ cup, 3½ oz	25	0	5
Sweet Cauliflower, 1 oz	35	0	8

Salsa

Average all Types: Per 2 Tablespoons

	C	F	Cb
Regular, no oil, 2 Tbsp	15	0	3.5
Homemade w. Oil, 2 Tbsp	40	3	8
Kaukauna, 2 Tbsp, 1 oz	15	0	3
La Victoria, 2 Tbsp, 1 oz	10	0	2
Old El Paso, 1 Tbsp, 1 oz	10	0	3
Wild Oats, 2 Tbsp, 1 oz	20	0	4

Gravy | C | F | Cb

	C	F	Cb
Homemade Gravy:			
Thin, little fat, 2 Tbsp, 1 oz	20	1	3
Thick, 2 Tbsp, 1¼ oz	50	2	9
¼ cup, 2½ oz	100	4	18
Franco-American (Canned)			
Beef; Turkey Gravy, 2 oz	25	0.5	3
Chicken Gravy, ¼ cup, 2 oz	40	4	4
Pillsbury (Gravy Mixes)			
Brown; Homestyle, ¼ cup, 2 oz	15	0	3
Chicken, as prep., ¼ cup, 2 oz	20	0	4

Gravy-In-Jars-Homestyle

	C	F	Cb
Boston Market, ¼ cup, 2 oz	40	2.5	3
Franco-American (In Jars):			
99% Fat Free, ¼ cup, 2 oz	20	0	3
Heinz, reg., all types, ¼ c., 2 oz	25	1	3
Fat Free Roast Turkey, ¼ c., 2 oz	10	0	2
Vons, all types, ¼ c., 2 oz	20	0.5	4

Tomato Products | C | F | Cb

Whole/Chopped/Crushed/Diced

	C	F	Cb
1 cup, 8½ oz	50	0	10
In Aspic, ½ cup	50	0	12
w. Green Chili, 1 cup, 8½ oz	60	0	16
Stewed, ½ cup, 1.7 oz	40	1.5	6.5
Wedges in Tom Juice, 1 cup	70	0.5	18
Salsa, average, 1 Tbsp	15	0	3.5
Tomato Ketchup:			
Regular, 1 Tbsp, ½ oz	15	0	4
One-Carb (Heinz), 1 Tbsp, ½ oz	5	0	1
Tomato Paste, 2 Tbsp, 1 oz	25	0	6
Regular, ¾ cup, 6 oz	140	1	32
Tomato Puree, ½ cup, 4½ oz	50	0	10
Tomato Sauce:			
Regular, ½ cup, 4.4 oz	50	0	11
Spanish Style, ½ cup, 4.3 oz	40	0	9
w. Mushrooms, ½ cup, 4.3 oz	45	0	10
w. Onions, ½ cup, 4.3 oz	50	0	12
Tomato Seasoning, 3 tsp	20	0	4
Sundried Tomatoes:			
Natural, 5-6 pces, 0.4 oz	22	0	5
In Oil, drained, 6 pces, ½ oz	40	2.5	4

Sauces ~ Pasta, Cooking

Brands	C	F	Cb

A-1

Steak & Marinades Sauce: *Per Tablespoon (½ oz)*

	C	F	Cb
Bold & Spicy; Teriyaki; New York	20	0	5
Carb Wel	5	0	1
Chicago	20	1	2
Jamaican Jerk	25	0.5	5
New Orleans Cajun	25	0	5
Steak Sauce	15	0	3

Barilla: *Per ½ Cup*

	C	F	Cb
Green & Black Olives; Garden Vege	90	4	12
Roasted Garlic & Onion	60	1.5	11
Other varieties, average	70	2.5	12

Bertolli/Five Brothers: *Per ½ Cup*

	C	F	Cb
Creamy Alfredo	200	18	6
Italian Sausage	100	3	15
Olive Oil & Garlic	90	3	14
Olive w. Sundried Tomato	100	4	13
Marinara; Rst Red Pepper, average	80	2	13
Traditional Basil Pesto	270	27	4

Buitoni

Pasta Sauce: *Per Serving*

	C	F	Cb
Alfredo, ¼ cup, 2.2 oz	140	12	4
Light Alfredo, ¼ cup	80	5	5
Marinara, ½ cup	70	3	10
Pesto: w. Basil, ¼ cup, 2.2oz	300	28	6
w. Sundried Tom., ¼ cup, 2.2 oz	200	17	6
Roasted Garlic Marinara, ½ cup	60	1.5	10
Tomato Herb Parmesan, ½ cup	130	8	10
Bruschetta Sauce, avg., 2 Tbsp	30	2	2

Carb Options: *Per Serving*

	C	F	Cb
Alfredo, ¼ cup	110	10	2
Barbeque varieties, 2 Tbsp	10	0	3
Double Cheddar, ¼ cup	90	8	2
Garden Style, ½ cup	80	4.5	7
Hickory Barbecue, 2 Tbsp	10	0	3
Marinades: Italian Garlic, 1 Tbsp	0	0	0
Steak, 1 Tbsp	5	0	1

Catelli

	C	F	Cb
Garden Select Pizza Sauce, 1 fl.oz	15	0.5	2.5
Meat Sauce, ½ cup, 4 oz	85	2.5	11

Garden Select 6 Vege Recipe Sauce: *Per ½ Cup*

	C	F	Cb
Parmesan & Romano	80	2.5	12
Thick & Chunky, Tomato Basil Blast	70	1.5	13
Other varieties, avg.	80	1.5	13

Cento: *Per Serving (½ Cup)*

Sauces:	C	F	Cb
Passata Tomatoes	40	0	6
Pasta, all natural	50	3	3
Pizza, fully prepared	25	0	5
Tomato: Arrabbiata; Vodka	70	3	6
Marinara; Puttanesca	115	9	6
White Clam	165	13	5

Classico: *Per ½ Cup Unless Indicated*

	C	F	Cb
Homestyle Meat Selections Sce, ½ c.	125	5	14

Signature Recipes Sauce: *Per Serving*

	C	F	Cb
Alfredo varieties, avg., ¼ cup	110	10	3
Cabernet Marinara w. Herbs, ½ cup	60	2	10
Fire Roasted Tomato & Garlic, ½ cup	50	0.5	10
Florentine Spinach & Cheese, ½ cup	80	5	10
Mushrooms & Ripe Olives, ½ cup	60	1	11
Pesto, Sun-Dried Tomato, ¼ cup	90	5	8
Pesto, Traditional Basil, ¼ cup	230	21	6
Rstd Chicken w. Parm. & Garlic, ½ c.	90	2	13
Spicy Red Pepper, ½ cup	60	1.5	7
Spicy Tomato & Pesto, ½ cup	90	4	11
Sun-Dried Tomato, ½ cup	80	3	11

Traditional Favorites Sauce: *Per ½ Cup*

	C	F	Cb
Four Cheese	90	5	10
Italian Sausage w. Peppers & Onions	90	2	13
Roasted Garlic; Triple Mushr., avg.	80	3	11
Other varieties, average	70	1	12

Contadina: *Per ¼ Cup*

	C	F	Cb
Pizza Sauce: Flavored w. Pepperoni	35	1	5
Original; Four Cheese, avg.	30	0.5	5
Cooking Sauce: Sweet & Sour, 1 T.	40	1	8
Tomato Sauce, avg., ¼ cup	20	0	4

Del Monte

Spaghetti Sauces: *Per ½ Cup*

	C	F	Cb
w. Four Cheeses	70	1.5	15
w. Meat/Mushrooms, average	60	1	14
Other varieties, avg.	75	1	16
Chunky Sauce: Garlic & Herb	60	1.5	11
Italian Herb	60	1	12
Sloppy Joe Sauce, Original, ¼ cup	50	0	11

Dominick's: *Per ½ Cup*

	C	F	Cb
All Natural: Garl. & Onion; Marinara	80	4	10
Mushr. & Olive; Tomato & Basil	80	1	8
Italian Classics: Four Cheese	80	2.5	12
Portabella Mushroom	60	2	9
Puttanesca	70	3	10
Spicy Roasted Garlic	70	2	10
Sun Ripened Tomatoes	80	4	8
Tomato Basil	50	1	8

Brands (Cont)

	C	F	Cb
Enrico's			
Sicilian	80	2.5	13
Traditional Italian Style, 3.5 oz	60	1.5	12
Mushroom Onion, ½ cup, 4.4 oz	70	1.5	13
Other varieties, ½ cup, 4.4 oz	60	1	12
Emiril's			
Pasta Sauces: *Per ½ Cup*			
Homestyle Marinara	90	4	11
Kicked Up Tomato; Rstd Gaaahlic	70	3	9
Puttanesca	80	5	9
Roasted Red Pepper	60	3	7
Vodka Sauce	130	8	13
French's Grill & Glaze			
Honey Mustard, 2 Tbsp	90	1	18
Healthy Choice: *Per ½ Cup*			
Garlic & Herbs	60	0	13
Traditional Pasta Sauce	60	0	13
Super Chunky: Vege Primavera	60	0	13
Tomato, Mushroom Garlic	45	0	10
Heinz: *Per 1 Tbsp (Approx. ½ oz)*			
Barbecue Sauces, all flavors	35	0	9
Chili Sauce, 1 Tbsp	20	0	5
Horseradish Sauce, 1 Tbsp	75	6	2
Mustard: Pourable/Mild, 1 Tbsp	10	0.5	1
Spicy Brown	15	1	1
Seafood Cocktail Sauce	60	0	15
Steak Sauce 57	30	0	4
Tartar Sauce, 1 Tbsp	70	7	2
Tomato Ketchup	20	0	5
Worcestershire Sauce, 1 Tbsp	10	0	1
Hunt's			
BBQ Sauce: Original, 2 Tbsp	60	0	15
Hickory & Brown Sugar, 2 T.	60	0	15
Manwich Sloppy Joe Sce, ¼ cup	30	0	6
Family Favorites, avg., 2 oz	30	0	6
Spaghetti Sauce: *Per ⅙ Can (26.5 oz)*			
Traditional, 4.4 oz	50	0	10
Meat Sauce, 4.4 oz	60	0	11
Light Sauce, 4.4 oz	45	0	9
KC Masterpiece: *Per Tablespoon*			
Marinades: Garlic & Herb	30	1	5
Honey & Teriyaki	40	0.5	9
Original BBQ	60	0	15
Knorr			
Classic Sauce: *Per 2 Tbsp (Prepared)*			
Bearnaise	20	0	4
Hollandaise	20	0	4
Classic Gravy, avg., ¼ cup, prepared	25	0	4

Kraft	C	F	Cb
CarbWell Sauce, 2 Tbsp	15	0	3
Sauce: Cocktail, 1 Tbsp	30	0.3	6
Horseradish, 1 tsp	20	1.5	1
Sandwich Spread & Burger, 1 T.	45	3.5	2
Sweet 'n Sour, 1 Tbsp	30	0	7
Tartar: 1 Tbsp	70	6	4
Lemon & Herb, 1 Tbsp	75	8	0.5
Fat-Free Tartar, 1 Tbsp	12	0	3
Barbecue Sauces: Average, 2 T.	50	0.5	10
Las Palmas			
Red Chile Sauce, ¼ cup, 2 oz	20	0.5	2
Enchilada Sauces: Green Chile	25	1.5	3
Hot/Original, ¼ cup, 2 oz	15	0.5	2
Lawry's 30 Minute Marinade: *Per Tbsp*			
Caribbean Jerk	25	0	5
Lemon Pepper	10	0	2
Mesquite	5	0	1
Thai Ginger; Herb & Garlic	10	0	2
Other varieties, average	20	0	3.5
Packet Seasonings: *Per 2 teaspoons (Dry)*			
Fajitas; Taco, average	10	0	3
Average other flavors	20	0	4
McCormick Sauce Mixes			
Golden Dipt Marinade: *Per Tablespoon (Dry)*			
Cajun Style	60	4.5	2
Garlic Herb	50	5	1
Ginger Teriyaki	60	3	5
Honey Mustard	25	0	4
Honey Soy	30	0	7
Lemon Herb	80	8	0
Lemon Pepper	25	2	1
Mesquite; White Wine, avg.	10	0.5	1
Grill Mates Grilling Sauces: *Per 2 Tablespoons*			
Hickory BBQ	80	0.5	17
Mesquite; Teriyaki, avg.	60	0.5	12
Montreal Steak	35	0	7
Grill Mates Marinades, avg., 2 Tbsp	60	0	15
Pasta Sauce Mixes: *Per Serving (Dry)*			
Creamy Garlic Alfredo, 2 Tbsp	90	6	4
Four Cheese Italian, 1⅓ Tbsp	40	1.5	5
Italian Style Spaghetti, 1⅓ Tbsp	35	0	7
Pesto Pasta, 2 tsps	10	0	1
Thick & Zesty Spaghetti, 1 Tbsp	25	0	6
Tomato Basil, 1 teaspoon	25	0	5
Finishing Sauce: *Per ¼ Cup (Prepared)*			
Creamy Mushroom	70	5	3
Honey Mustard	120	1	25
Red Burgundy Wine for Beef; Rst Beef	30	1	3
Roasted Chicken Gravy w. Herbs	50	2.5	4

Updated Nutrition Data ~ www.CalorieKing.com
Persons with Diabetes ~ See Disclaimer (Page 24)

Sauces ~ Pasta, Cooking (Cont)

Brands (Cont)

	C	F	Cb
Monterey			
Pesto Sauce, ¼ cup, 2 oz	280	28	4
Mr Yoshida's			
Original Gourmet, 2 Tbsp, 30ml	90	0	20
Hawaiian Sweet & Sour, 2 Tbsp	70	0	18
Muir Glen: *Per ½ Cup (125g)*			
Organic Pasta Sauce:			
Mushr. Marinara; Portobello Mushr.	50	0	11
Other varieties, average	50	1	11
Newman's Own: *Per ½ Cup*			
Bombolina (Tomato & Basil)	90	4.5	13
Five Cheese	80	3	10
Fra Diavolo	70	3	10
Marinara; Sockarooni	70	2	12
Roasted Garlic & Peppers	70	2.5	11
Vodka	110	5	11
Old El Paso			
Enchilada Sauce: Green Chile, ¼ cup	20	1	3
Other varieties, ¼ cup	25	1	3
Sauce Mixes, 2 teaspoons, 4g	10	0	2
Picante Sauce, all varieties, 2 Tbsp	10	0	2
Taco Sauce, all varieties, 1 Tbsp	5	0	1
Salsas: Make Mine Medium, 2 Tbsp	10	0	2
Wild for Mild, 2 Tbsp	10	0	2
Thick N' Chunky varieties, 2 Tbsp	10	0	3
Pace: *Per 2 Tbsp*			
Picante Sauce	10	0	2
Chunky Salsa, average all types	10	0	2
Salsa Con Queso	90	6	6
Prego: *Per ½ Cup*			
Pasta Sauce: Marinara	100	5	11
Diced Onion & Garlic	120	4.5	18
Flavored w. Meat	130	5	19
Italian Sauasge & Garlic	120	5	16
Mini Meatball	150	6	20
Mushroom & Garlic	110	2	20
Mushroom Parmesan	130	3.5	22
Organic varieties, average	90	2.5	19
Roasted Garlic Parmesan	100	1	20
Three Chse; Tom. Basil & Garlic, avg.	90	1.5	17
Other varieties, average	120	3.5	19
Chunky Garden: Combination	90	1.5	17
Mushroom Supreme	120	4	19
Other varieties, average	110	3.5	17
Hearty Meat: Three Meat Supreme	170	10	13
Other varieties, average	160	8	15

	C	F	Cb
Premier Japan (Organic)			
Garlic/Ginger/Wasabi Tamari, 1 T.	10	0	2
Thai Soynut, 1 Tbsp	25	2	2
Ragu: *Per ½ Cup (Unless Indicated)*			
Pizza Quick Sauce: *Per ¼ Cup*			
Traditional	40	2	4
Homemade Style	30	1	4
Thick & Zesty	40	1.5	5
Cheese Creations: *Per ¼ Cup*			
Classic Alfredo	110	10	3
Double Cheddar	100	9	3
Light Parmesan Alfredo	70	5	3
Chunky Gardenstyle: *Per ½ Cup*			
Mushroom & Green Pepper	100	3	16
Other varieties, average	110	3	18
Light varieties, average	50	0	10
Old World Style: Marinara	80	4.5	8
Meat Sauce	80	4	7
Mushroom; Traditional	70	3	8
Organic: Garden Veggie	80	2.5	12
Cheese; Traditional	80	3	11
Rich & Meaty: Classic Italian Style	150	10	9
Mama's Meat Sauce	130	8	8
Sausage, Peppers & Onions	155	10	8.5
Robusto!: 7-Herb Tomato	80	3.5	9
Chopped Tom., Olive Oil & Garlic	95	5	10
Parmesan & Romano	90	3.5	10
Sauteed Beef, Onion & Garlic	90	5	9
Sauteed Onion & Garlic	80	4	9
Rainforest Organic			
Ginger Curry, 1 Tbsp	15	1	2
Papaya Pepper, 1 Tbsp	0	0	0
Rinaldi: *Per ½ Cup*			
3-Cheese	90	2	15
Original; Meat/Mushroom, avg.	80	3	12
Other varieties, average	70	2.5	12
S & W: *Per Tablespoon*			
Teriyaki, Light/Marinade	20	0	4
Safeway			
Salsa: *Per 2 Tablespoons*			
Chipotle Salsa; Sthwest Salsa, avg.	15	0	3
Peach P'apple Salsa; Salsa Verde, avg.	20	0	4
Sauce: *Per 2 Tablespoons*			
Fiesta Fajita; Rstd Tomato, avg.	15	0	2
Garlic Lovers	10	0	3
Mild Enchilada	20	0	4

Brands (Cont)

	C	F	Cb
Seeds of Change: *Per ½ Cup*	50	0.5	9
Tomato Basil Sauce	60	3.5	9
Traditional Marinara Sauce	60	3.5	6
Steel's Gourmet Sauce			
Barbeque Sce, 2 Tbsp	15	0	2
Cocktail Sce w. Dill & Lemon, 4 Tbsp	30	0	5
Rocky Mountain Ketchup, 1 oz	10	0	0
Spiced Cranberry Sce, 5 Tbsp	20	0	4.5
Sweet & Spicy, 1 Tbsp	35	2	2
The Wizard's (Organic)			
Hot Stuff, 1 Teaspoon	0	0	0
Vegetarian Worcestershire, 1 tsp	2	0	0.5
Troy's Sauces (Organic)			
Ginger Sauce, 1 Tbsp	10	0	1
Peanut Sauce, 1 Tbsp	25	1.5	2
Timpone's: *Per ½ Cup*			
Spaghetti Sauce: Classic	50	2.5	8
Family Recipe	80	3	7
Mom's	70	3	7
Tree of Life: *Per ¼ Cup*			
Tomato	50	2	9
Fat-Free Classic Tomato	40	0	9
Fat-Free Sweet Pepper	35	0	8
Verdi (Vons/Safeway): *Per ½ Cup*			
Arrabbiata	70	8	10
Four Cheese	70	3	10
Garlic & Basil	70	4	6
Marinara	60	2	10
Mushroom & Onion	60	3	6
Spicy Red Bell Pepper	50	1	9
Sundried Tomato & Olive	60	3	6
Vodka	130	10	9
Walnut Acres: *Per ½ Cup (125g)*			
Organic Pasta Sauce, average	50	1	9
Wild Oats: *Per 2 Tablespoons (1 oz)*			
Grilling Marinade: Wasabi	40	4	1
Asian Sesame	45	4.5	1
Ginger Teriyaki	30	3	1
Pasta Sauce: Funghi, ½ cup	100	3.5	4
Marinara, ½ cup	100	9	6
Norma, ½ cup	140	12	6
Puttanesca, ½ cup	120	12	8
Salsa, avg., 2 Tbsp	15	0	3

Quick Guide

Mayonnaise

	C	F	Cb
Regular			
Average All Brands, 1 Tbsp	100	11	0
Bestfoods, Kraft, 1 Tbsp	100	11	0
½ cup, 4 oz	800	88	0
Light/Reduced Fat			
Kraft, 1 Tbsp	45	3.5	2
Best Foods, 1 Tbsp	45	4.5	0.5
½ cup, 4 oz	360	36	7
Hain, Safflower Oil, 1 Tbsp	100	11	0
Hellman's, 1 Tbsp	45	4.5	0.5
Spectrum: Canola Mayo, 1 Tbsp	100	11	0
Light Canola Mayo Eggless, 1 Tbsp	35	3.5	0
Fat Free			
Kraft: 1 Tbsp	10	0	2
½ cup, 4 oz	80	0	16
Smart Beat, 1 Tbsp	10	0	3
Sugar Free: Dukes Mayo, 1 Tbsp	100	12	0

Mayonnaise Style Dressing

	C	F	Cb
BAMA Dressing, 1 Tbsp, ½ oz	50	4	3
Best Foods Sandwich Spread, 1 T.	60	5	2
Gourmayo (French's), 1 Tbsp, ½ oz	50	5	2
Miracle Whip Salad Dressing:			
Regular, 1 Tbsp, ½ oz	40	3.5	2
Light, 1 Tbsp, ½ oz	30	2	3
Free, 1 Tbsp, ½ oz	15	0	2
Nayonaise (Nasoya)			
(Tofu Base/Dairy Free/Eggless)			
Regular, 1 Tbsp, ½ oz	35	3.5	1
Fat-Free, 1 Tbsp, ½ oz	10	0	2

"Take two of these and call me in the morning"

Salad Dressings

Quick Guide

Salad Dressings
Average All Brands
Per 2 Tbsp (Approx 1 fl.oz)

	C	F	Cb
Balsamic Vinaigrette: Reg., 1 oz	90	9	3
Light, 2 Tbsp, 1 oz	45	4	5
Fat Free, 2 Tbsp, 1 oz	25	0	6
Blue Cheese: Regular, 2 Tbsp, 1 oz	150	16	2
Regular, ¼ cup, 2 oz	300	32	4
Light, 2 Tbsp, 1 oz	30	1	5
Caesar: Regular, 2 Tbsp, 1 oz	155	17	1
Regular, ¼ cup, 2 oz	310	34	2
Light, 2 Tbsp, 1 oz	70	8	5
Coleslaw: Regular, 2 Tbsp, 1 oz	125	11	8
Regular, ¼ cup, 2 oz	245	21	15
Light, 2 Tbsp, 1 oz	110	7	14
French/Italian: Regular, 1 oz	150	14	5
Regular, ¼ cup, 2 oz	290	28	10
Light, 2 Tbsp, 1 oz	65	4	9
Fat/Oil-Free, 2 Tbsp, 1 oz	40	0	10
Ranch: Regular, 2 Tbsp, 1 oz	145	16	2
Regular, ¼ cup, 2 oz	290	31	4
Light, 2 Tbsp, 1 oz	80	3	7
Fat-Free, 2 Tbsp, 1 oz	50	0.5	11
Thousand Island: Regular, 1 oz	120	11	5
Regular, ¼ cup, 2 oz	230	22	9
Light, 2 Tbsp, 1 oz	60	4	7
Fat-Free, 2 Tbsp, 1 oz	40	0.5	10

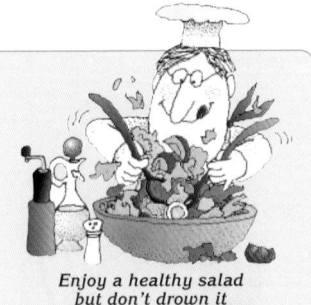

*Enjoy a healthy salad
but don't drown it
in high-fat salad dressings.
Use 'light' dressing to halve
the fat and calories.*

Brands ~ Salad Dressings

Per 2 Tbsp (Approx 1 fl.oz)

	C	F	Cb
Annie's Naturals			
Cowgirl Ranch, 2 Tbsp	120	11	3
French; Goddess, avg.	90	9	3
Organic: Buttermilk	70	7	1
No-Fat Yogurt	20	0	3
Red Wine & Olive Oil	160	17	1
Thousand Island	90	7	5
Roasted Red Pepper	70	6	3
Shiitake & Sesame	120	13	1
Tuscany Italian	80	7	5
Vinaigrette:			
Balsamic; Cilantro & Lime, 2 T.	100	10	3
Low-Fat: Honey Mustard	45	2	6
Gingerly	40	2	4
Raspberry	35	1.5	5
Bernstein's			
Creamy Caesar, 2 Tbsp	120	13	1
Fat-Free Cheese & Garlic Italian	10	0	2
Italian	110	12	1
Olive Oil Vinaigrette	90	9	3
Restaurant Recipe Italian	120	12	1
Other varieties, avg., 2 Tbsp	110	11	2
Light Fantastic: Cheese Fantastico	25	1.5	3
Roasted Garlic Balsamic	45	3.5	3
Best Foods			
Dijonnaise, 1 tsp	5	0	1
Mayonnaise: Reduced Fat, 2 Tbsp	40	4	4
Light, average., all varieties	90	9	1
Real Mayonnaise, average	90	10	0
w. Lime Juice, 2 Tbsp	180	20	0
Bob's Famous			
Blue Cheese, Lite, 2 Tbsp	80	8	1
Ranch Country, 2 Tbsp	150	16	1
Roquefort; Blue Chse	140	15	1
Thousand Island	140	14	4
Brianna's			
Blue Cheese, 2 Tbsp	120	11	5
Blush Vintage	120	7	14
French Vinaigrette, 2 Tbsp	180	19	1
New American	160	17	6
Rich Santa Fe Blend	25	0	5
Zesty French	150	15	4
Other varieties, avg.	155	14	8

Salad Dressings (Cont)

Per 2 Tbsp (Approx 1 fl.oz)

	C	F	Cb
Carb Options: Italian	70	8	0
Ranch	150	17	0
Cardini's			
Caesar, 2 Tbsp	160	17	1
Fat-Free Caesar	40	0	9
Light Caesar	80	7	5
Honey Mustard	140	13	5
Parmesan Ranch	150	15	2
Poppyseed w. Shallots	160	14	8
Southwest Caesar	140	14	3
Vintage White Wine	110	12	1
Other varieties, avg.	125	13	1
El Torito: Cilantro Pepita Caesar	140	14	1
Emeril's: *Per 2 Tbsp*			
House Herb Viniagrette	100	10	1
Kicked Up French	80	5	8
Girard's: *Per 2 Tbsp*			
Blue Cheese Vinaigrette	100	10	3
Caesar	140	15	1
Lite Caesar	70	8	5
Champagne	150	16	1
Lite Champagne	60	5	2
Chinese Chicken Salad	120	11	6
Greek Feta Vinaigrette	110	11	1
Olde Venice Italian	120	13	2
Shiitake Chardonnay	100	9	4
Spinach Salad	70	2	4
Fat-Free: Balsamic/Red Wine, avg.	25	0	6
Caesar	40	0	9
Raspberry	50	0	13
Hidden Valley: *Per 2 Tbsp*			
Regular Ranch: Italian Ranch	140	14	2
Old-Fashioned Buttermilk Ranch	140	14	2
Spicy Ranch	150	16	2
Bacon Ranch	140	14	1
Cracked Peppercorn Ranch	120	12	2
Cole Slaw	150	15	5
Light, Original Ranch	80	7	3
Fat-Free, Original Ranch	30	0	6

	C	F	Cb
Ken's Steak House Dressings: *Per 2 Tbsp*			
Balsamic & Basil Vinaigrette	110	12	1
Chunky Blue Cheese	140	16	1
Country French	150	12	10
Creamy Caesar	160	18	0
Peppercorn Ranch	180	19	1
Ranch	140	15	2
Italian w. Aged Romano	110	12	1
Thousand Island	140	13	4
Lite: Caesar/Olive Oil Vinaigrette, avg.	70	6	3
Ranch	80	6	6
Kraft			
Regular Dressings: *Per 2 Tbsp*			
Honey Dijon	110	10	6
Coleslaw	110	9	7
Creamy Italian	110	11	2
Creamy French	160	15	5
Roka Brand Blue Cheese	130	13	2
Thousand Island, avg.	120	10	5
Kraft Free (Fat-Free): Italian	15	0	4
Caesar Italian	50	0	10
Carb Well: Classic Caesar, 2 Tbsp	110	11	0
Italian	20	1.5	0
Ranch	60	6	0
Roka Blue Cheese	120	13	0
Light: Buttermilk Ranch	60	6	0
Italian, 2 Tbsp	20	1.5	0
Light Done Right!: Italian	40	3	3
Ranch	60	6	0
Other varieties, avg.	80	4.5	9
Special Collection: Caesar Italian	100	10	2
Balsamic Vinaigrette	90	8	4
Sweet Honey Catalina; Poppyseed	130	11	8
Other varieties, avg.	60	5	1
Seven Seas, all varieties	90	9	2
Kroger			
Poppy Seed	200	8	32
Real Mayonnaise	100	11	0
Zesty Italian	90	9	3
Lite: Zesty Italian	35	2	4
Ranch	70	6	3
Fat-Free, avg., 2 Tbsp	30	0	8

Salad Dressings (Cont)

Salad Dressings (Cont)

Per 2 Tbsp (Approx 1 fl.oz)	C	F	Cb
Litehouse: Caesar	130	13	2
Chunky Bleu Cheese	150	16	1
Coleslaw	100	8	8
Jalapeno Ranch	120	12	1
Lite Bleu Cheese	70	6	2
Other varieties, avg.	120	12	2
Maple Grove: *Per 2 Tbsp (1 fl.oz)*			
Balsamic Vinaigrette	50	3	5
Regular: Honey Mustard	120	9	9
Sweet & Sour	110	7	12
Fat Free: Balsamic Vinaigrette	35	0	9
Caesar Vinaigrette; Greek, avg.	10	0	3
Dijon; Poppyseed, avg.	40	0	10
Other varieties, avg.	25	0	6
Low Carb: Dijon	70	8	1
Balsamic; Raspberry Vinaigrette	5	0	1
Lite: Caesar	40	4.5	5
Honey Mustard	80	5	9
Marie's: *Per 2 Tbsp*			
1000 Island	160	15	4
Blue Cheese	170	19	0
Caesar	170	19	1
Honey Mustard	140	12	6
Poppy Seed	150	13	8
Ranch (15.5 fl.oz ctn), 2 Tbsp	170	19	1
Premium: Spinach Salad, 2 Tbsp	70	1.5	2
Italian Cheese Blend	180	20	12
Nasoya: *Per 2 Tbsp*			
Vegi Dressing (Tofu Base/Dairy Free):			
Thousand Island	60	5	2
Other flavors	65	7	1
Nayonaise: Regular, 2 Tbsp, 1 oz	70	7	2
Fat-Free, 2 Tbsp, 1 oz	20	0	4

Newman's Own: *Per 2 Tbsp*	C	F	Cb
Balsamic Vinaigrette, 2 Tbsp	90	9	3
Caesar; Olive Oil & Vinegar	150	16	1
Family Recipe Italian	120	13	1
Parmesan Italiano	140	14	2
Ranch	140	15	2
Two Thousand Island	140	14	4
Lighten Up: Light Italian	60	6	1
Light Raspberry & Walnut	70	5	7
Light Balsamic Vinaigrette	45	4	1
San-J: *Per 2 Tbsp*			
Tamari Peanut, 2 Tbsp	70	2.5	8
Tamari Sesame	45	2	5
Tamari Vinaigrette	45	3	4
Fat-Free, Tamari Mustard	25	0	5
S & W: *Per 2 Tbsp (1 oz)*			
Light: Italian	35	0	8
Red/White Wine; Raspberry Blush	40	0	10
Seeds of Change: *Per 2 Tbsp (1 oz)*			
Balsamic/Greek Feta Vinaigrette	60	4.5	5
Italian Herb Vinaigrette	60	4.5	5
Spectrum			
Fat Free: Creamy Dill/Garlic	25	0	4
Sweet On. & Garlic; Tstd Sesame	15	0	3
Low-Fat: Honey Dijon	35	2	4
Zesty Italian	30	2	1
Organic: Greek Goddess, 2 Tbsp	110	11	1
Balsamic Vinaigrette	80	8	3
Provencal Garlic Lovers	50	5	2
Rocky Mountain Ranch	130	14	1
Steel's (Sugar-Free)			
Honey Mustard, 2 Tbsp	95	7	2
Sweet Ginger Lime, 2 Tbsp	75	7	1

**For full nutritional data and product updates
check the database of the author's website
www.CalorieKing.com**

Salad Dressings (Cont)

Per 2 Tbsp (Approx 1 fl.oz) **C** **F** **Cb**

Subway Select: *Per 2 Tbsp (1 oz)*

	C	F	Cb
Premium Collection: Fat-Free Italian	35	0	7
Ranch	100	11	0.5
Atkins Sweet as Honey Mstd, 2 T.	100	11	0.5

T. Marzetti's: *Per 2 Tbsp (1 oz)*

	C	F	Cb
Asiago Peppercorn	160	16	1
Asian Ginger	120	12	4
Baja Ranch	150	15	2
Buffalo Blue Cheese	140	15	1
Chunky Blue Cheese	150	15	2
Honey Balsamic	120	11	5
Original Slaw	170	16	6
Ranch	160	17	2

Toby's: *Per 2 Tbsp (1 oz)*

	C	F	Cb
All varieties, average	120	12	1.5

Walden Farms

	C	F	Cb
Fat-Free, Calorie Free Range, 2 Tbsp	0	0	0

Wild Oats: *Per 2 Tbsp (1 oz)*

	C	F	Cb
Balsamic Vinaigrette	100	10	2
Caesar Style	100	10	2
Ranch	110	11	2
Sesame Goddess	100	10	2
Soy Ginger	50	5	3
Tuscany Italian	100	11	0.5

Per 2 Tbsp (Approx 1 fl.oz) **C** **F** **Cb**

Wishbone

	C	F	Cb
Regular: 5 Cheese Italian	120	10	6
Chunky Blue Cheese	150	15	2
Creamy Caesar	170	18	1
French: Deluxe French	120	11	5
Sweet 'N Spicy	100	12	6
Italian: Regular	90	8	3
House Italian	100	10	3
Robusto Italian	90	8	3
Ranch: Original	160	13	2
w. Garlic/Spring Onion	130	14	2
Red Wine; Balsamic Vinaigrette	50	5	3
Russian, regular	120	6	14
Thousand Island	130	12	5
Fat-Free: Chunky Blue Cheese	35	0	7
Italian	20	0	4
Ranch	30	0	7
Dressing & Marinades: Asian	70	5	5
Balsamic Olive Oil & Herbs	50	5	3
Lemon Garlic & Herb	70	5	5
Tangy Honey Mustard	80	6	7
Ranch Up!	140	15	2
Just 2 Good!: Blue Cheese	50	2	6
Classic/Creamy Caesar; Ranch	50	2	7
Country Italian; Italian	30	1.5	7
Parmesan Peppercorn Ranch	50	2	7
Thousand Island	50	2	9
Salad Spritzers: All flavors,			
10 sprays (¼ fl.oz) for 1 cup salad	10	1	1

MINIMAL EXERCISES FOR LAZY SLIMMERS!

1 After finishing your meal, place both hands on edge of table and P-U-S-H back hard!

2 Shake your head vigorously from side to side, every time you are offered a second helping of rich food.

Breakfast Cereals

Quick Guide

Cooked Cereals

	C	F	Cb
Buckwheat Groats, roasted:			
Dry, ½ cup, 3 oz	285	2	61
Cooked, 1 cup, 6 oz	155	1	34
Bulgur: Dry, ½ cup, 2½ oz	240	1	53
Cooked, 1 cup, 6½ oz	150	0.5	34
Corn/Hominy Grits:			
Dry, ¼ cup, 1.4 oz	145	0.5	31
3 Tbsp, 1 oz	110	0.5	23
Cooked, ¾ cup, 6½ oz	110	0.5	23
Instant, 1 pkt, dry, 0.8 oz	75	0	18
w. Imitation Bacon Bits, 1 oz	100	0.5	22
Cream of Rice, ckd, ¾ cup, 6½ oz	95	0	21
Cream of Wheat:			
Regular, ¾ cup, 6½ oz	100	0.5	21
Quick, ckd, ¾ cup, 6½ oz	95	0.5	20
Instant, ckd, ¾ cup, 6½ oz	110	0.5	24
Farina, Cooked, ¾ cup, 6 oz	85	0	18
Millet, dry, ¼ cup, 1¾ oz	190	2	36
Oat Bran: Raw, ⅓ cup, 1 oz	70	2	19
Cooked, ½ cup, 3¾ oz	45	1	13
Oatmeal: Dry, ⅔ cup, 1 oz	105	1.5	18
Regular, ¾ cup, 6 oz	110	2	19
1 cup, 8 oz	145	2.5	25
Instant: Regular, dry, avg., 1 oz	105	1.5	18
Flavored, dry, average, 1½ oz	150	2	32
Wheat Hearts, 1 oz dry, ¾ c. ckd	110	0.5	24

Brans, Wheatgerm, Add-Ons

	C	F	Cb
Bran: Wheat, unprocessed,			
1 Tbsp, 3g	5	0	2
Rice Bran: Raw, 1 Tbsp, 5g	15	1	2.5
¼ cup, 1 oz	95	6	15
Oat Bran: Raw, 1 Tbsp, 5g	10	0.5	4
⅓ cup, 1 oz	70	2	19
Wheat Germ: Raw, 1 Tbsp, ¼ oz	25	0.5	4
¼ cup, 1 oz	105	3	15
Fruit: Dried, average, 1 oz	70	0	18
Banana, ½ medium	55	0	14
Prunes in Syrup (5), 3 oz	90	0	23
Honey, 1 Tbsp, ¾ oz	65	0	17
Lecithin Granules, 1 Tbsp, 10g	55	4	0.5
Nuts, Almonds (6), ¼ oz	40	1	1.5
Bee Pollen Granules, 1 T., 8g	25	1	2
Psyllium Husks, 1 Tbsp, 5g	15	0	4

Hot/Cooked Cereals ~ Brands

Per Serving	C	F	Cb
Albers Grits, ¼ cup, 1.4 oz	140	0.5	31
Bobs Red Mill-10 Grain, ¼ c., 40g	140	1	28
Country Choice Oats, 1 pouch, avg.	110	2	19
Dr McDougall's			
Oatmeal: Per Package			
& Barley, Peach Raspb., 3 oz	300	4	62
& Wheat, Apple Cinn., 2.32 oz	250	3	50
Organic, Maple 4 Grain, 2.57 oz	260	3	52
Organic Instant Oatmeal: Per Packet			
Original, 1 oz	120	2	21
Light Apple Cinnamon, 1.95 oz	120	1.5	24
Light Maple Brown Sugar, 1.34 oz	150	2	28
4 Grains w. Maple Sugar, 2.2 oz	220	2	44
Erewhon: Barley Plus, ¼ c., 1.7 oz	170	1	37
Brown Rice Crm, ¼ cup, 1.6 oz	170	1	36
Instant Oatmeal, 1.2 oz pkg, avg.	130	2.5	25
McCann's Instant Irish Oatmeal			
Apple & Cinnamon, 1.23 oz	130	1.5	27
Maple & Brown Sugar, 1.5 oz	160	2	32
Original, 1 oz pkg	100	1.5	18
Steel Cut Oats, ¼ cup, 1.4 oz	150	2	27
Mother's Oat Bran, ½ cup, 1.4 oz	150	3	25
Nabisco: Cream of Wheat, 1 oz	120	0	23
Malt-O-Meal: Orig., 3T., 1.2 oz	120	0.5	25
Maple Brown Sugar, ¼ cup	170	0	37
Natures Path: Apple Cinn.1.7 oz	190	2	38
Average other varieties	200	4	40
Quaker: Oatbran, ½ cup, 1.4 oz	150	3	25
Honey Nut, 1 cup, 1.5 oz	170	3.5	31
Maple Brown Sugar, 1.9 oz ctn	160	2	33
Multigrain, ½ cup, 1.4 oz	135	1.5	29
Old Fashioned Oats, ½ cup, 1.4 oz	150	3	27
Sun Country Quick Oats, ½ c.,1.4 oz	150	3	27
Grits: Reg. all types, 1 pkg, avg.	130	0.5	29
Instant, all types, 1 pkg, 1 oz	100	0	22
Instant Oatmeal: Per Package			
Oatmeal Regular, 1 oz	100	2	19
Bakery Favorites, avg., 1½ oz	160	2	31
Fruit and Cream, avg. all flavors	130	2.5	26
Oatmeal Express, avg. all flavors	200	2.5	42
Supreme, avg. all flavors	160	3	31
Silver Palate Oatmeal, ⅓ c., 40g	160	3	26
Uncle Sam Oatmeal, 1.2 oz	130	3	24

Quick Guide

Cold Cereals
Average All Brands

	C	F	Cb
Bran Flakes, ¾ c., 1 oz	95	0.5	24
Corn Flakes, 1 c., 1 oz	100	0	24
Granola, ¼ c., 1 oz	150	7.5	16
Oat Bran Cereal, ½ cup, 1½ oz	145	3	25
Puffed Rice, 1 cup, ½ oz	55	0	13
Puffed Wheat, 1 cup, ½ oz	45	0	10
Raisin Bran, ½ cup, 1 oz	90	0.5	22
Rice Crisps, 1 cup, 1 oz	105	0.5	24
Shredded Wheat, 1 bisc., 1 oz	85	0.5	20
Sugar-frosted Flakes, ¾ c, 1 oz	115	0	28
Wheat Flakes, ¾ cup, 1 oz	105	1	24

Breakfast Bars: *See Page 137*

Ready-To-Eat Cereal

	C	F	Cb
Arrowhead Mills			
Amaranth, 1 c., 1.2 oz	140	2	26
Bran Flakes, 1 cup, 1.2 oz	140	2.5	24
Corn Flakes, 1 cup, 1.2 oz	120	0	27
Kamut Flakes, 1 cup, 1.1 oz	120	1	25
Maple Buckwheat Flake, 1 c., 1½ oz	170	1	35
Multi Grain Flakes, 1 cup, 1½ oz	170	2	33
Nature O's, 1 cup, 1.1 oz	130	2	25
Oat Bran Flakes, 1 cup, 1.2 oz	140	2.5	24
Puffed Corn/Rice, avg., 1 c., 0.6 oz	60	0.5	13
Puffed Kamut, 1 cup, ½ oz	50	0	11
Puffed Millet/Wheat, 1 cup, 0.6 oz	60	0.5	11
Rice Flakes, 1 cup, 1.7 oz	180	1	40
Shredded Wheat, 1 cup, 1.7 oz	190	1	38
Spelt Flakes, 1 cup, 1.1 oz	120	1	24
Atkins			
Morning Start: Blueberry, ½ cup	90	2	12
Crunchy Almond Crisp, ½ cup	90	2	10
Triple Berry, ½ cup	90	2	10
Back to Nature			
Energy Start:			
Hi-Protein Crunch, ½ cup 1.7oz	170	1.5	28
Organic Oat & Soy Crisp, ¾ c. 1.9oz	200	3	37
Granola: Apple Blueb., ½ cup 1.9oz	200	2.5	39
Apple Cinn.; Classic, ½ c. 1.8oz	180	2.5	36
Apple Strawberry, ½ cup 1.9oz	190	2.5	37
Cranberry Pecan, ½ cup 1.6oz	180	5	35
French Vanilla, ½ cup 1.9oz	220	6	35
Hi-Protein, ½ cup 2.2oz	260	6	41
Raisin, ½ cup 1.9oz	190	2	35

	C	F	Cb
Back to Nature (Cont)			
Heart Basics,			
Banana Nut Multibran, ¾ cup 1.9oz	170	1.5	46
Flax & Fiber Crunch, ¾ cup 1.8 oz	180	2.5	37
Hi-Fiber Multibran, ¾ cup 1.7oz	140	1	40
Organic Apple Cinn. Harvest, ¾ c.	180	1.5	45
Muesli, ¾ cup 2.3 oz	230	4	48
Barbara's Bakery			
Alpen Original, ⅔ cup, 1.9 oz	200	3	40
Breakfast O's, 1 cup, 1¼ oz	120	2	22
Brown Rice Crisps; Corn Flakes, 1 c.	115	1	25
Crispy Wheats/Soy Essence, ¾ cup	110	0.5	25
Fruity Punch; Puffins, ¾ cup, 1 oz	110	1	26
Grain Shop, ¾ cup, 1½ oz	120	1	36
Honey Crunch 'n Oats, ⅔ cup, 1 oz	110	1.5	25
Shredded Oats, 1¼ cup, 2 oz	220	2.5	46
Shred. Spoonfuls; Toasted O's, ¾ cup	120	1.5	24
Shredded Wheat, 2 biscs., 1.4 oz	140	1	31
Wild Puffs Caramel, ¾ cup, 1.1 oz	110	1	25
Bob's Red Mill			
Heartland's Ceros, Gluten-Free:			
Original Flavored, 1 cup, dry	120	0	24
Cinnamon Flavored, 1 cup, dry	110	0	23
Breadshop			
Granola: Triple Berry Cr., ⅔ cup	210	8	34
Cinnamon Raisin ½ cup, 1.9oz	220	6	37
Crunchy Oat Bran w. Alm., ½ cup	210	8.5	31
Honey Gone Nuts, 1.8oz	240	10	33
Mocha Almond Crunch, ½ c., 1.7oz	210	7	34
Pralines 'n Cream, ½ c., 1.7oz	210	7	34
Raspberry 'n Crm, ½ cup, 1.8oz	220	7.5	34
Super Natural w. Alm.,½ cup	220	9	31
Triple Berry Crunch, ½ cup 1.8oz	220	7	34
Vermont Maple, ½ cup 1.8oz	210	7	33
Cascadian Farms			
Honey Nut O's, 1 cup, 1 oz	120	2	24
Multi-Grain Squares, ¾ cup, 1 oz	110	1	25
Oats & Honey Granola, ⅔ c., 2 oz	230	6	42
Purely O's, 1 cup, 1.1oz	110	2	22
Hearty Morning, ¾ cup, 1.9 oz	200	3	43
Raisin Bran, 1 cup, 1.9 oz	180	1	43
Dr McDougall's: Muesli, 1½ oz	160	1	31
Ener-G			
Crumbles, ¼ cup, 1.1 oz	100	3	16
Rice Bran, ½ cup, 2.4 oz	220	14	34

Breakfast Cereals (Cont)

Ready-To-Eat (Cont)

	C	F	Cb
Erewhon			
Aztec, 1 cup, 1 oz	110	0	26
Corn Flakes, 1¼ cups, 2 oz	210	2.5	45
Crispy Brown Rice: 1 cup, 1 oz	110	0	25
w. Mixed Berries, 1 cup, 1 oz	120	1	27
Gluten Free, 1 cup, 1 oz	110	0.5	25
No Salt Added, 1 cup, 1 oz	110	0	25
Kamut Flakes, ⅔ cup, 1 oz	110	0	25
Raisin Bran, 1 cup, 1.8 oz	170	1	40
Rice Twice, ¾ cup, 1 oz	120	0	26
General Mills (Big G)			
Basic 4, 1 cup, 1.9 oz	210	3	44
Boo Berry, 1 cup, 1.1 oz	130	1	29
Cheerios: Regular, 1 cup, 1 oz	100	2	20
Apple Cinnamon, ¾ c., 1 oz	120	1.5	25
Berry Burst, all types, ¾ c., 1 oz	120	1.5	25
Frosted, ¾ cup, 1 oz	110	1	23
Honey Nut, ¾ cup, 1.2 oz	120	0.5	28
Multi-Grain, 1 cup, 1 oz	110	1	23
Chex: Corn, 1 cup, 1 oz	120	0.5	26
Honey Nut, ¾ cup, 1.1 oz	120	0.5	28
Multi-Bran, ¾ cup, 2 oz	160	1.5	39
Rice, 1 cup, 1 oz	100	0.5	23
Wheat, 1 cup, 1.7 oz	160	1	38
Cinnamon Tst Crunch, ¾ c., 1 oz	130	3	25
Cocoa Puffs, ¾ cup, 1 oz	110	1.5	26
Cookie Crisp; Count Choc, ¾ c., 1 oz	110	1.5	25
Country Corn Flakes, 1 cup, 1.1 oz	120	0.5	28
Fiber One, ½ cup, 1 oz	60	14	25
Fiber One Honey Clusters, 1¼ cup	160	1.5	42
French Toast Crunch, ¾ c., 1 oz	130	3	24
Golden Grahams, ¾ cup, 1 oz	120	1	26
Honey Nut Clusters, 1 cup, 2 oz	210	1	49
Kix: 1¼ cup, 1.1 oz	110	1	25
Berry Berry, ¾ cup, 1 oz	100	1.5	22
Lucky Charms, avg., ¾ cup, 1 oz	110	1	22
Oatmeal Crisp, Almond, 1 c., 2 oz	240	5	46
Raisin Nut Bran, 1¼ cups, 2 oz	180	3	38
Reese's Puffs, ¾ cup, 1 oz	120	3	22
Total: Honey Clusters, ¾ cup, 1.7 oz	170	2	37
Raisin Bran, 1 cup, 2 oz	160	1	40
Whole Grain, ¾ cup, 1 oz	100	0.5	23
Trix, avg., 0.63 oz pkt	110	1.5	21
Wheaties, ¾ cup, 1 oz	100	0.5	22

	C	F	Cb
Health Valley			
Amaranth Flakes, ¾ cup, 1 oz	100	0	23
Corn Flakes, ¾ cup, 1.1 oz	110	1	24
Cranberry Crunch, 1 cup, 1.8 oz	190	3	38
Crunchy Flakes: 'n Raisins, ¾ c., 1.2 oz	110	0.5	28
'n Strawberries, ¾ cup, 1.1 oz	100	0.5	25
Crunch-Ems!, avg., 1 cup, 1 oz	110	0	27
Fiber 7, Multigrain Flakes, 1 cup, 1.7 oz	160	1	37
Golden Flax, serving, ¾ cup, 1.8 oz	190	3	38
Granola, ⅔ cup, 2 oz	190	2	42
Heart Wise, 1 cup, 55g	200	3	37
Oat Bran Flakes: ¾ cup, 1 oz	110	1	19
w. Raisins, ¾ cup, 1 oz	110	0.5	23
Kashi			
7 Whole Grain: Flakes, 1 cup, 1.7 oz	180	1	41
Honey Puff, 1 cup, 1.1 oz	120	1	25
Nuggets, 1 cup, 1.9 oz	210	1.5	47
Pilaf, ½ cup, cooked	170	3	30
Puffs, 1 cup, ½ oz	70	0.5	15
GoLEAN: 1 cup, 1.8 oz	140	1	30
Crunch!, Honey Alm. Flax, 1 c., 1.8 oz	200	5	34
Good Friends: 1 cup, 1.8 oz	170	1.5	41
Cinna-Raisin Crunch, 1 c., 1.7 oz	170	1.5	41
Granola: Mountain Medley, ½ cup	220	7	37
Orchard Spice, ½ cup, 1.9 oz	220	7	37
Heart to Heart:			
Honey Toasted Oat, ¾ cup, 1.2 oz	110	1.5	25
Oat Flakes & Blueb. Clusters, ¼ c	200	2.5	42
Oatmeal: Apple Cinn., 1.5 oz pkg	160	2	33
Golden Brown Maple, 1.5 oz pkg	160	2	33
Raisin Spice, 1.5 oz pkg	150	2	33
Mighty Bites: Honey Cr. Cereal, 33g	110	1.5	23
Cinnamon, 1 cup, 1.2 oz	120	1.5	33
Organic Promise:			
Autumn Wheat, 1 cup, 1.9 oz	190	1	45
Cinnamon Harvest, 1 cup, 1.9 oz	190	1	44
Strawberry Fields, 1 cup, 1.1 oz	120	0	28

> *Life is what happens
> to you while you're busy
> making other plans.*
> ~ John Lennon

Ready-To-Eat (Cont)

	C	F	Cb
Kellogg's			
All-Bran: Bran Buds, ⅓ cup, 1.1 oz	70	1	24
Extra Fiber, ½ cup, 0.9 oz	50	1	20
Original, ½ cup, 1.1 oz	80	1	23
Yogurt Bites, 1¼ cups, 2 oz	190	3	44
Apple Jacks, 1 cup, 1.2 oz	120	0.5	28
Complete Oat Bran Flakes, ¾ cup	110	1	23
Complete Wheat Bran Flakes, ¾ cup	90	0.5	23
Corn Flakes, Original, 1 cup, 1 oz	100	0	24
Corn Pops, 1 cup, 1 oz	120	0	28
Cracklin' Oat Bran, ¾ cup, 1.8 oz	200	7	35
Crispix, Original, 1 cup, 1 oz	110	0.5	25
Crunch: Caramel Nut, 1¼ cups	210	3.5	41
Raisin Bran, 1 cup, 1.9 oz	190	1	45
Toasted Honey, 1¼ cups, 2 oz	220	1.5	50
Crunchy Blends:			
Low-Fat Granola: w. Raisins, ⅔ cup	230	3	49
no Raisins, ½ cup	190	2.5	40
Mueslix, ⅔ cup, 2 oz	200	3	40
Froot Loops: Original, 1 cup, 1.1 oz	120	1	26
Marshmallow, 1 cup, 1.1 oz	120	1	27
Frosted Flakes, 1 cup, 1.1 oz	110	0	27
Fruit Harvest, Banana Berry, ¾ cup	120	2	25
Honey Smacks, ¾ cup, 1 oz	100	0.5	24
Mini Swirlz Cinnamon Bun, 1 cup	120	2	25
Mini-Wheats: Frosted Big Bite (5)	180	1	41
Frosted Bite Size (24), 2.1 oz	200	1	48
Frosted Vanilla Creme (24), 1.8 oz	180	1	43
Nutri-Grain Bars: *See Page 137*			
Product 19, 1 cup, 1 oz	100	0	25
Raisin Bran: Regular, 1 c., 2.1 oz	190	1.5	45
Rice Krispies: Original, 1¼ cup	120	0	29
Berry, 1 cup, 1.1 oz	120	1	27
Frosted, ¾ cup, 1.1 oz	110	0	27
Cocoa; Treats, avg., ¾ cup, 1.1 oz	130	2	26
Smart Start: Antioxidants, 1 cup	190	0.5	43
Healthy Heart, 1¼ cup, 2.1 oz	230	3	46
Smorz, 1 cup, 1.1 oz	120	2	25
Special K: Original 1 cup, 1.1 oz	120	0.5	22
Fruit & Yogurt, ¾ cup, 1.1 oz	120	1	24
Low Carb Lifestyle, ¾ cup, 1 oz	100	3	14
Red Berries, 1 cup, 1.1 oz	110	0	25
Vanilla Almond, ¾ cup	110	1.5	25

	C	F	Cb
Malt-O-Meal			
Apple Zings, 1 cup, 1.1 oz	130	1	30
Balance ¾ cup, 1.1 oz	120	1	26
Cinnamon Toasters, ¾ c., 1 oz	130	3.5	24
Choc Mateys, 1 cup, 1 oz	120	1	24
Coco Roos/Dyno-Bites, ¾ c., 1 oz	120	1.5	26
Frosted Flakes, ¾ cup, 1.1 oz	120	0	28
Frosted Mini Spooners, 1 c., 1.9 oz	190	1	45
Golden Puffs, ¾ cup, 1 oz	110	0	24
Mother's			
Cinnamon Oat Crunch, 1 cup. 2.1 oz	230	3	48
Cocoa Bumpers, 1 cup, 1.2 oz	120	0.5	29
Groovy Grahams, 1 cup, 1 oz	100	0.5	24
Honey Round-Ups, ¾ cup	110	0.5	25
Peanut Butter Bumpers, 1 cup, 1.2 oz	130	2.5	26
Toasted Oat Bran, ¾ cup, 1.1 oz	120	1.5	24
Nature's Path			
Corn Flakes, all types, ¾ cup, 1 oz	110	1	24
Eight Grain, ¾ cup, 1.1 oz	100	1	24
Flax Plus Multigrain, ¾ cup, 1 oz	110	1.5	23
Heritage, all types, ¾ cup, 1 oz	100	1	24
Honeyed Raisin Bran, ¾ cup, 1 oz	180	1	43
Multigr. Oatbran Flakes, ¾ c., 1 oz	110	1	24
Toaster Pastries (1), 1.83 oz, avg.	210	4.5	39
Granola: Ginger Zing; Hemp, 1 oz	140	5	21
Heritage Muesli w. Hazelnuts, 1.7 oz	210	3.5	41
Pumpkin Flax Plus, ½ cup, 1 oz	140	5	20
Average, other varieties	135	4	21
Kamut Crisp Flakes, ¾ cup, 1 oz	100	0.5	23
Power Breakfast, 1 cup, 2 oz	190	2.5	40
New England Natural Bakers			
Muesli, ½ cup, 2.1 oz	220	5	40
Granola: Almond Raisin Crisp, ½ c.	220	9	36
Apple Sunrise, ½ cup	210	7	34
Berry Good, ⅔ cup, 2.1 oz	250	6	44
Grateful Date, ½ cup, 1.7 oz	210	7	33
Honey Crunch; Pecan, ½ cup	285	13	37
Low-Fat Granola, ½ cup, 1.7 oz	200	2.5	41
Maple Almond Date, ½ cup	280	11	39
Save The Forest: Chocolate Mix	160	10	18
Fruit & Nut Mix, ½ cup, 2.1 oz	270	12	35
Nut Granola, 2 cup, 2.1 oz	270	12	35
Granola: Absolutely Nuts, ⅔ cup	220	9	30
Raspberry Razzmatazz, ¾ cup	250	9	37

Breakfast Cereals (Cont)

Ready-To-Eat (Cont)

	C	F	Cb
New Morning			
Cocoa Crispy Rice, ¾ cup, 1 oz	120	0.5	26
Cocomotion, ¾ cup, 1 oz	100	0.5	22
Fruit-e-O's, Organic, 1 cup, 1 oz	120	1.5	25
Oatios: Apple Cinn., Organic, 1 c., 1 oz	120	1	18
Honey Almond, 1 cup, 1 oz	120	1	17
Oatios, Original, 1 cup, 1 oz	110	2	22
Nutritious Living			
Hi-Lo, all types, ½ cup, 1 oz	90	1.5	11
Post			
Alpha Bits, 1 cup, 1 oz, 1.1 oz	120	1	27
Bran Flakes, ¾ cup, 1 oz	100	0	24
Carb Well: Cinnamon Crunch, 1 oz	110	2	14
Golden Crunch, 1 oz	110	1	14
Cocoa Pebbles, 1 oz	110	1.5	26
Fruit & Bran, 1 cup, 2 oz	195	3	43
Fruity Pebbles, 1¼ cup, 1 oz	110	1	26
Golden Crisp, ½ cup, 1 oz	115	2	26
Grape-Nuts, ½ cup, 2 oz	200	1	48
Grape-Nuts Flakes, ½ cup, 1 oz	110	1	24
Grape-Nuts O's, 1.1 oz	120	0	28
Honey Bunches of Oats, ¾ c., 1 oz	120	1.5	25
Honey-Comb Strawb. Blasted, 1 cup	120	1	26
Oreo O's w. M'mallow Bits, ¾ c., 1 oz	110	2	23
Raisin Bran, ⅔ cup, 2 oz	190	1	46
Selects: Banana Nut Crunch, ½ c.	240	6	44
Blueberry Morning, 1 cup, 2 oz	220	3	45
Cranberry Almond Crunch, 2 oz	200	3.5	39
Maple Pecan Crunch, ¾ cup, 2 oz	220	6	40
Great Grains: Crunchy Pecan, ⅔ c.	220	6	38
Raisins Dates Pecans, ⅔ c.	210	4.5	39
Shredded Wheat: Frosted, 1.8 oz	180	1	43
Honey Nut, 1 cup, 1.8 oz	190	1.5	44
Original, 1.6 oz	170	1	40
Shredded Wheat & Bran, 2 oz	200	1	49
Waffle Crisp, 1 cup, 1 oz	120	2.5	25
Quaker			
Oat Bran, ½ cup	150	3	25
100% Natural Granola: ½ cup	205	6	35
Low-Fat: ⅔ cup	215	3	45
w. Raisins, ½ cup	215	6	38
Captain Crunch: Regular, ¾ c., 1 oz	110	1.5	23
Crunch Berries, ¾ cup, 1 oz	100	1.5	22
Peanut Butter, 1 oz	110	2.5	21

Quaker (Cont)

	C	F	Cb
Crunchy Corn Bran, 1 cup, 1 oz	90	2.5	23
Honey Graham Oh's, ¾ cup	110	2	23
Life, all types, ¾ cup, 1.1 oz	120	1.5	26
Instant Oatmeal: See Page 94			
Bars: See Page 140			
Sweet Home Farm			
Honey Nut Granola, ½ cup, 1.9 oz	200	7	34
Low-Fat Granola, ½ cup, 1.9 oz	180	3	38
Trader Joe's			
10 & 10 Cereal, ¾ cup, 1.7 oz	170	3	31
Banana Nut Clusters, 1.9 oz	240	8	40
Cornflakes, 1 cup, 1 oz	110	0	26
Cranberry Almd Clusters, 1 c., 2 oz	220	5	40
Crunch: Cherry Almond, 1 c., 2 oz	230	5	43
Van. Almd/Maple Pecan, 1 c., 2 oz	220	6	38
Essentials, 1 cup, 2 oz	170	3	37
Flakes n'Fruit, 1 cup, 1.1 oz	120	0.5	25
Frosted Flakes, ¾ cup, 1 oz	110	0	27
Golden Flax Cereal, ¾ cup, 1.7 oz	200	3.5	37
High Fiber Cereal, ⅔ cup, 1.1 oz	80	0.5	34
Honey Nut O's, ¾ cup, 1 oz	120	1.5	24
Joe's O's, 1 cup, 1 oz	110	1.5	22
More & Less Apple Cinn., ⅔ cup	100	1.5	12
Morning Lite, 1 cup, 1.4 oz	130	2	32
Muesli Cereal Blend, ¾ cup, 2 oz	200	2.5	42
Oat Bran Flakes, avg., 1 cup	200	1.5	45
Raisin Bran, 1.9 oz	170	1	44
Shred. Wheats, Bite Size, 1 c., 1.7 oz	180	1	38
Soy Flax Clusters, 1 cup	190	3	38
Touch of Honey, ⅔ cup, 1 oz	120	1.5	25
Triple Berry O's, ¾ cup, 1 oz	110	1	25
Toasted Oatmeal Flakes, ¾ c., 1.1 oz	110	1	23
Very Berry Clusters, 1 cup, 1.9 oz	230	5	42
Uncle Sam			
Cereal w. Real Mixed Berries, 1 cup	190	4.5	39
Original, ¾ cup, 1.5 oz	190	5	38
Weetabix: 2 biscuits, 1.3 oz	120	1	28
Weight Watchers			
Banana Almond Medley, ¾ cup	170	3	31
Cinnamon Cluster Crunch, ¾ cup	150	1	32
Flakes'n Fiber, ½ cup, 1.1 oz	90	2	17
Honey Almond Crisp, ¾ cup, 1½ oz	140	2	32
Puffed Vanilla Wheat, 1 cup, 1.1 oz	110	0.5	25

Grains & Flours   **C**   **F**   **Cb**

Per ½ Cup (8 level Tbsp)

	C	F	Cb
Amaranth Flour, ½ cup, 3½ oz	365	6.5	65
Arrowroot Flour, ½ cup, 2¼ oz	230	0	56
Barley: Regular, ½ cup, 2.6 oz	255	1	55
Pearled, raw, 3½ oz	350	1	78
Buckwheat: Regular, ½ c., 3 oz	290	3	61
Groats: Roasted, dry, ½ c., 2.9 oz	285	2	62
Roasted, cooked, 3½ oz	80	0.5	17
Flour, whole-groat, ½ cup, 2 oz	200	2	42
Bulgur: Dry, ½ cup, 2½ oz	240	1	53
Cooked, ½ cup, 3.2 oz	75	0.5	17
Carob Flour, ½ cup, 1.8 oz	115	0.5	46
Corn Kernels avg., cooked, ½ cup	80	1	18
Corn Bran, ½ cup, 1.3 oz	85	0.5	34
Corn Flour/Masa, ½ cup, 2 oz	215	2.5	43
Corn Grits: Dry, ½ cup, 2¾ oz	290	1	62
Cooked, ½ cup, 4¼ oz	70	0.5	15
Corn Germ, toasted, ½ cup, 4 oz	100	1.5	22
Cornmeal: Average all Types,			
3 Tbsp, 1 oz	105	0.5	22
½ cup, 2½ oz	255	1	54
Mixes: same as above	230	1	48
Made Up, ½ cup, 4.8 oz	95	0.5	20
Cornstarch: 1 Tbsp, 8g	30	0	8
½ cup, 2¼ oz	245	0	58
Couscous: Dry, 1 oz (yield 3 c. ckd)	110	0	22
1 cup cooked, 5½ oz	175	0.5	37
Farina: Dry, ½ cup, 3.1 oz	325	0.5	69
Cooked, ½ cup, 4.1 oz	55	0	12
Flaxseed: Seeds, 1 Tbsp, 8g	45	3.5	2
Ground, 2 Tbsp, 8g	60	4.5	4
Garbanzo (Chick Pea), ½ c., 1.6 oz	180	3	27
Kuzu Root Starch, 1 Tbsp, 10g	35	0	9
Matzo Meal, ½ cup, 2.2 oz	230	0.5	48
Millet: Raw, ½ cup, 3½ oz	380	4	73
Cooked, ½ cup, 2.4 oz	105	1	21
Oat Bran: Raw, ⅓ cup, 1.1 oz	75	2	21
Cooked, ½ cup, 3¾ oz	45	1	13
Oats, rolled/oatmeal:			
Dry/Groats, ½ cup, 1.5 oz	160	3	28
Cooked, ½ cup, 4.2 oz	75	1	13
Polenta: *See Cornmeal*			
Potato Flour, ½ cup, 2.8 oz	285	0.5	66
Psyllium Husks, 1 Tbsp (5g)	20	0	4
Quinoa: Dry ½ cup, 3 oz	320	5	59
Cooked, ½ cup, 3¾ oz	130	2	24

Grains & Flours (Cont)   **C**   **F**   **Cb**

Per ½ Cup (8 level Tbsp)

	C	F	Cb
Rice Bran, ½ cup, 2 oz	180	12	28
Rice Flour, ½ cup, 2¾ oz	290	1	63
Rice Polish, ½ cup, 3½ oz	360	0.5	80
Rye Flour: Dark, ½ cup, 2.3 oz	210	2	44
Medium, ½ cup, 1.8 oz	180	1	40
Light, ½ cup, 1.8 oz	190	1	41
Rye Grain: ½ cup, 3 oz	280	2	59
Flakes, ¼ cup, 1 oz	100	0.5	21
Semolina, ½ cup, 3 oz	300	1	61
Sorghum, ½ cup, 3.4 oz	325	3	72
Soy Flour:			
Defatted, 1 cup, 3½ oz	330	1	38
Low-Fat, 1 cup, 3 oz	325	6	33
Full-Fat, 1 cup, 3 oz	365	17	29
Soy Meal, defatted, 1 cup, 4.3 oz	415	3	49
Spelt Flour, ½ cup, 2 oz	190	1	41
Tapioca, pearl: Dry, ½ cup, 2.7 oz	270	0	67
3 Tbsp, 1 oz	100	0	25
Teff (Seed) Flour, 2 oz	215	2	42
Tortilla Flour Mix, ½ cup, 2 oz	220	6	37
Triticale: ½ cup, 3.4 oz	325	2	70
Flour, whole-grain, ½ c., 2.3 oz	220	1	48
Wheat Bran, unproc., ½ cup, 1 oz	65	1	19
Wheat Flakes, ½ cup, 1½ oz	160	1	35
Wheat Germ: Raw, ¼ cup, 1 oz	105	3	15
Toasted, ¼ cup, 1 oz	110	3	14
Wheat Flour:			
White, All Purpose/Self-Rising,			
1 level Tbsp, 0.6 oz	60	0	13
½ cup, 2.2 oz	230	0.5	48
1 cup, 4.4 oz	455	1.5	95
Whole Wheat, 1 cup, 4.2 oz	405	2	87

Rice

White Rice

	C	F	Cb
Raw: Short/Med. Grain, 1 c., 7 oz	715	1	158
Long Grain, 1 cup, 6½ oz	675	1	148
Glutinous, 1 cup, 6½ oz	685	1	151
Cooked Rice (Boiled/Steamed):			
Short/Medium Grain:			
½ cup, 3¼ oz	135	0	30
1 cup (½ Pint), 7.2 oz	270	0.5	59
2 cups (1 Pint), 13 oz	480	1	106
Long Grain: ½ cup, 2¾ oz	105	0	22
1 cup, 5½ oz	205	0.5	44
Glutinous/Sticky, ckd 1 c., 6 oz	170	0.5	37
Parboiled, cooked, ½ cup, 3 oz	105	0.5	22
Precook./Instant: Dry,½ c., 3½ oz	370	0	80
Cooked, ½ cup, 3 oz	90	0	20
Wild Rice: Raw, 1 cup, 5½ oz	570	2	120
Cooked, 1 cup, 5¾ oz	165	0.5	35

Brown Rice

	C	F	Cb
Average of Short or Long Grain			
Raw/Dry: ½ cup, 3¼ oz	340	2.5	71
1 cup, 6½ oz	685	5.5	143
Cooked: ½ cup, 3½ oz	110	1	22
1 cup, 7 oz	220	2	46

Rice Dishes

	C	F	Cb
Chinese Fried Rice:			
½ cup, 2½ oz	140	4.5	21
1 cup, 5 oz (½ Pint)	280	9	42
2 cups, 10 oz (1 Pint)	565	18	84
Mexican Rice: 1 cup	500	12	90
Taco John's, 1 serving (6 oz)	250	5	45
Taco Time, 1 serving (4 oz)	160	2	30
Rice-A-Roni: See Page 74			
Rice Pilaf: Restaurant, 1 cup	275	7.5	46
O'Charley's, 1 order	200	5	31
Rice w. Raisins/Pinenuts, 1 cup	400	11	60
Risotto, 1 cup	420	12	70
Saffron Rice *(Koo Koo Roo),* 4 oz	175	7	25
Spanish Rice: 1 cup	390	9	72
El Pollo Loco, small, 5 oz	160	1	35
Taco Cabana, 4 oz	180	5	30
Sticky Rice *(Koo Koo Roo),* 5 oz	155	0.5	34
Sushi Rice: 1 Tbsp	25	0	5
1 cup, 5.2 oz	390	0	77
Uncle Ben's: See Page 76			

Pasta ✦ Spaghetti ✦ Noodles

- Macaroni includes all shapes and sizes; (e.g. spaghetti, fettuccini, shells, tubes, ziti, twists, sheets, cannelloni, manicotti, elbows).
- All regular macaroni products have the same cals/fat/carb. on a weight basis.
- 1 oz Dry = approx. 2½ -3 oz cooked.

Dry Spaghetti/Macaroni

	C	F	Cb
1 oz quantity	105	0.5	21
1lb box/pkg., 16 oz	1685	7	339
Elbows, 1 cup, 3¾ oz	380	2	80
Shells, small, 1 cup, 3¼ oz	330	1.5	69
Spirals, 1 cup, 3 oz	305	1.5	64

Cooked Spaghetti/Macaroni

	C	F	Cb
Plain, All Types (no added fat):			
Firm/Al Dente (8-10 mins.), 1 oz	42	0.5	8.5
Medium (11-13 mins.), 1 oz	37	0.5	7.5
Tender (14-20 mins.), 1 oz	32	0.5	7
(Longer cooking increases water absorbed)			
Spaghetti, ½ cup, 2 ½ oz	90	0.5	18
Medium serving, 1 cup, 5 oz	225	1.5	44
Large (restaurant), 2 c., 10 oz	450	3	88
Elbows/Spirals, 1 cup, 5 oz	220	1.5	43
Small Shells, 1 cup, 4 oz	180	1	36
Protein-fortified: Dry, 1 c., 3⅓ oz	350	2	63
Cooked, 1 cup, 5 oz	230	0.5	45
Spinach/Vegetable: Dry, 1 c., 3 oz	310	1	61
Cooked, 1 cup, 5 oz	180	0.5	38
Whole-wheat: Dry, 1 c., 3¾ oz	365	1.5	79
Cooked, 1 cup, 5 oz	175	1	37

Fresh Pasta (Refrigerated)

	C	F	Cb
Plain/Spinach/Tomato, average:			
As purchased, 4.5 oz	370	3	70
Cooked, 1 cup, 5 oz	185	1.5	35
Home-made, without egg:			
Cooked, 1 cup, 5 oz	175	1	35
Buitoni			
Cut Pasta: Angel Hair, 1¼ cups	230	2.5	43
Fettuccine, 1¼ cups	260	3	56
Linguine, 1¼ cups	240	2.5	45
Spinach Fettuccine, 1¼ cups	260	3	45
Ravioletti, Three Cheese, 1 c., 90g	270	5	43

	C	F	Cb
Buitoni (Cont):			
Ravioli: Chkn & Rstd Garlic, 1¼ cup	330	10	47
Classic Beef, 1¼ cup	350	10	49
Four Cheese, 1⅓ cups	315	10	43
Light Four Cheese, 1¼ cups	260	4.5	41
Whole Wheat Four Chse, 1¼ cups	320	11	40
Tortellini: Herb Chkn, 1 cup	350	10	52
Spinach Cheese, 1 cup	320	7	49
Three Cheese, 1 cup	320	7	50
Tortellini: Chse & Rstd Garlic, 1 c.	270	8	37
Portabello Mushr. & Chse, 1 cup	290	6	49
Other varieties, avg., 1 cup	330	10	47
Pasta Sauces: See Page 86			

Noodles

	C	F	Cb
Plain/Egg: Dry, 1 oz	110	1.5	20
1 cup, 1⅓ oz	145	1.5	27
Cooked: 1 oz	40	0.5	7
½ cup, 2¾ oz	110	1.5	20
1 cup, 5½ oz	220	3.5	40
Stir-Fried: 1 cup, 5½ oz	270	9	40
2 cup serving, 11 oz	540	18	80
Yolk Free (Cooked): *Per Cup*			
'No Yolks' *(Foulds)*, 2 oz	210	0.5	41
Passover Gold *(Manischewitz)*	200	0	41
Chinese: Cellophane/Rice, dry, 1 oz	100	0	25
Chow Mein/hard, dry, 1 oz	150	9	16
Ramen Noodles: See Page 73			
Japanese: Soba, dry, 1 oz	95	0.5	21
cooked, 1 cup, 4 oz	115	0.5	24
Somen, dry, 1 oz	100	0.5	21
cooked, 1 cup, 6 oz	230	0.5	49
Japanese Style Pan Fried:			
Maruchan's Yaki-Sobu, 5.6 oz cup	260	3	50
Rice Noodles: Dry, 3.5 oz	365	0.5	83
Cooked, 1 cup, 6.2 oz	190	0.5	44
Stir Fry *(Yakisoba)*, 3.5 oz serving	430	6	52
Thai Kitchen: See Page 75, 83			
Udon *(Chikara)*, avg., 7.5 oz pkt	250	1	52

Egg Roll Skins/Won Ton

	C	F	Cb
Egg Roll Skins:			
(Fortune) 1 wrapper, 0.8 oz	65	0.5	15
Won Ton Wrappers:			
(Nasoya) 8 wrappers, 2.1 oz	160	0.5	31
Egg Roll/Spring Roll Wrapper:			
(Dynasty) 3 wrappers, 2.1 oz	170	1	36

Breads

Note: Most breads have similar calories on a weight basis. However, volume may vary.

For example, 1 oz of bread may equal 1 slice regular bread or 2 slices of a lighter bread.

It is best to weigh bread used and calculate using: 1 oz bread = 70 calories, 14g carb.

Quick Guide

Bread	C	F	Cb
White or Wheat ~ Average Per Slice			
Thin or Light, ¾ oz	50	0.5	10
Sandwich slice, 1 oz	70	1	14
Thick or Large slice, 1½ oz	105	1.5	21
Thick/Home-made, 2 oz	140	2	28
Extra Thick/Home-made, 3 oz	210	3	42
Whole Loaf, 16 oz	1120	16	224
Whole Loaf, 24 oz	1680	24	336
With Seeds or Nuts:			
Sandwich slice, 1½ oz	130	5	18
Thick slice/Home-made, 2½ oz	215	8	30
Toast ~ Has same calories as bread used			
1 Slice (1 oz fresh)			
w. 2 tsp regular spread	140	9	12
w. 2 tsp "light" spread	105	5	12
w. 1 Tbsp regular spread	170	12	12
w. 1 Tbsp "light" spread	120	7	12

Breads

	C	F	Cb
12-Grain, 1½ oz slice	110	1.5	22
Batard (8 oz), thick slice, 2 oz	150	0.5	28
Bran style/Dark, 1 oz slice	70	1	14
Bread w. Soy Isoflavones, 1.2 oz	80	2.5	13
Buttermilk, average, 1½ oz slice	110	1	22
Caraway Rye, 2 oz slice	150	2	28
Challah, ¾ oz slice	85	1.5	17
Chapati, 1 oz	110	3	18
Ciabatta, 1 slice, 2 oz	130	1	26
Corn Bread, average, 1 pce, 3 oz	220	6	37
Cracked Wheat Sourdough, 1½ oz	130	0.5	27
Croissants: *See Page 113, 173*			
Crustless Bread, regular slice ¾ oz	40	0.5	8.5
Crusts Only, regular slice, ¼ oz	30	0	7
English Toasting, slice, 2 oz	140	1.5	27
'Enriched' Breads, average, 1 oz sl.	60	1	12
Flax & Sunflower Round, 1.2 oz	90	2	18

Breads (Cont)

	C	F	Cb
Foccacia: Plain, 2 oz portion	150	2.5	28
Cheese & Garlic; Pesto, 2 oz	160	6	21
Tomato & Olive, 2 oz	150	5	21
French Stick/Baguette, 1 oz slice	70	1	15
French Toast, 1 slice, 1.6 oz	140	2	26
Sticks *(Aunt Jemima)*, 1 pce, 1 oz	90	2	17
Garlic Bread/Toast:			
Small slice + 1 tsp spread, ¾ oz	80	5	7
Med. slice + 2 tsp spread, 1½ oz	160	10	14
Thick slice + 3 tsp spread, 1.8 oz	220	14	20
Pepperidge Farm, 1 slice, 1.4 oz	160	10	15
Hemp Bread, 1.2 oz	95	2	12
Italian Bread, 2 oz slice	140	1	28
Light Bread, avg., 0.8 oz slice	40	0.5	8
Lower Carb (higher Protein/fiber),			
average all brands, 1 oz	60	1.5	9
MultiGrain, 1 slice, 1.3 oz	60	1.5	17
Nut/Health Nut, 1.35 oz slice	90	1.5	18
Oatmeal/Oatbran Bread, 1½ oz	90	0.5	19
Pita: Average all types,			
Small (4" diam) 1.1 oz	90	0	18
Large (6½" diam) 2 oz	140	1.5	27
Extra Large (9" diam) 4 oz	300	1.5	60
Popovers (1), no butter	130	2	18
Poppyseed (Vienna), 0.8 oz sl.	55	1	10
Pumpernickel: Large slice, 1.35 oz	80	0	15
Cocktail/Party size	30	0.5	6
Raisin Bread, 1 oz slice	80	1.5	14
Raisin Walnut, 1 oz slice	70	0.5	15
Roman Meal, 1.1 oz slice	80	1	15
Rye: Average, 1 thin slice, 1 oz	80	1	14
1 thick slice, 2 oz	150	2	25
Cocktail size, 0.4 oz	25	0.5	4
Sandwich Bread, 1 oz slice	70	1	12
Sandwich Pockets, 2 oz	140	1.5	25
Sourdough, 1½ oz slice	120	1	25
Sourdough French, 1 oz	75	0	14
Spelt, 1.6 oz	130	1	26
Sprouted 7-Grain, 1.5 oz slice	110	0.5	18
Squaw, 1.1 oz slice	85	0.5	13
Sweet Hawaiian Bread, 1.3 oz	110	2	19
Tacos/Tortillas: *See Page 104*			
Turkish/Middle Eastern, 1 oz sl.	80	1.5	16
Wheat-Free Breads: Spelt, 1.6 oz	130	1	26
Healthseed Rye, 1.6 oz	90	1	20
Kamut, 1.6 oz	80	2	16
Millet, 1.5 oz	100	1	20

Breads ◆ Bread Rolls ◆ Croutons

Bread Brands

	C	F	Cb
Controlled Carb Gourmet			
High Fiber, 1 slice, 1 oz	80	2.5	11
Zero Net Carb Bagel, 1 oz	120	2	14
Ener-G: Gluten-Free Breads			
Brown Rice Bread, 1 slice, 1.3 oz	130	6	18
Light Brown Rice, 1 slice, ¾ oz	50	2	7
Corn Loaf, 1 slice, ¾ oz	40	1.5	8
Light Tapioca, 1 slice, ¾ oz	45	1.5	7
Ezekiel			
Low Carb: Wheat, 0.8 oz	70	4	4
Savory Herb, 0.8 oz	60	2.5	4
Genesis 1: 29, 0.8 oz	80	2	14
Nature's Path: *Per Slice (2 oz)*			
Manna: Carrot Raisin; Millet Rice	130	0	28
Cinnamon Date	150	0	29
Fruit & Nut	140	1	27
Multigrain	130	0	26
Sun Seed	160	2	29
Whole Rye	150	0	32
Oroweat: *Per Slice*			
100% Whole Wheat, 1.3 oz	100	2	19
Sugar Free Whole Grain, 1 sl., 0.8 oz	50	1	9
Pepperidge Farm: *Per Slice*			
100% Whole Wheat, Thin	70	1	12
Carb Style 7-Grain	60	1.5	8
Cinnamon Swirl	80	1.5	15
Farmhouse Soft	110	2	19
Light Style, average	45	0	9
Raisin Cinnamon Swirl	80	1.5	15
Ralph's, Breakfast Bread: *Per Slice (2 oz)*			
Cranberry Orange, 1 sl., 2 oz	180	4	32
Wild Berry, 1 sl., 2 oz	180	3	33
Sara Lee: *Per Slice*			
Delightful White, 0.8 oz	45	0.5	9
Honey Wheat, 1 oz	80	1	16
Heart Healthy Multi-Grain, 1.4 oz	100	1.5	19
Schwan's: *Per Serving*			
Cheese & Herb Biscuits (1), 34g	110	6	11
Chse Stuffed Bread w. Sauce, 2 oz	160	5	20
Five Chse Garlic French Bread (1), 96g	330	20	26
French Baguette Bread, ¼ loaf, 49g	130	0	25
Garlic Texas Toast, 2 oz	190	10	20
Southern Style Biscuits (1), 2.2 oz	200	10	23
Trader Joe's			
Fat-Free Multi-Grain, 1.1 oz	70	0	15
Mom's White, 1.1 oz	90	1	15
Seeded Harvest, 1 oz	65	1	12
Pumpernickel, 1.3 oz	100	0	21
Wonder: Sandwich, 1 slice, 1 oz	60	0.5	13
Light Wheat, 1 slice, ¾ oz	40	0.5	9

English Muffins

	C	F	Cb
Average All Brands			
Plain/Whole wheat, 2 oz	130	1	25
Raisin-Cinnamon, 2 oz	140	1	28

Bread Rolls & Buns

	C	F	Cb
6" Roll, Plain, average 2½ oz	200	1	38
Brown 'n Serve, average, 1 oz	70	1	13
Ciabatta Roll, 3½ oz	230	4	41
Concha (Mexican Sweet Bread), 3 oz	400	19	50
Dinner Rolls: 1 small, 1 oz	90	1.5	17
1 medium (3" diam),1½ oz	110	1	23
Frankfurter/Hot Dog: 1¼ oz	110	1.5	21
1½ oz size	130	2	25
French: 1 medium, 1.3 oz	110	1.5	22
1 large, 3 oz	230	2.5	42
Hamburger: Regular, 1½ oz	110	1.5	22
Large, 3 oz	210	3	40
Hoagie/Submarine, Plain, 2⅓ oz	200	1	38
Kaiser Roll, 2 oz size	200	2.5	35
Onion Roll, 2.4 oz size	180	2.5	34
Party Roll, 0.6 oz	45	0.5	9
Sandwich Roll, 2.6 oz size	190	1.5	37
Sourdough Roll, 1¼ oz	110	1	21
Sweet Rolls, 1 oz	100	2	20
w. Icing, average	160	6	20
Wheat Roll: Small, 1.2 oz	100	1	17
Medium, 1¾ oz	130	1	23

Breadsticks, Croutons

	C	F	Cb
Breadsticks: Salt Sticks, plain, 1 oz	110	1	20
Fresh baked (1), 2 oz	180	2.5	34
Stella D'oro: Sesame (1)	50	2	7
Original, 1 piece	45	1	7
Croutons: Seasoned, 2 Tbsp, ¼ oz	35	1.5	4
9 small or 6 large, ¼ oz	35	1.5	4
Fat-Free (*Pepp. Farm*), 2 Tbsp	30	0	5

Bread Products

	C	F	Cb
Bread Crumbs, dry:			
Plain or seasoned, 1 oz	110	1.5	20
1 cup, 3½ oz	385	5	70
Corn Flake Crumbs, 1.1 oz	120	0	29
Graham Cracker Crumbs, 1 oz	110	2.5	20
Keebler, 3 Tbsp, ½ oz	70	1.5	13
Bread Dough: Frozen, 1 slice, 2 oz	140	2	26
Refrigerated, French, 1" slice	60	1	13
Wheat/White, 1" slice	80	2	14
Coating Mixes: Avg., 2 Tbsp., 1 oz	100	0.5	20
Stuffing: Average, dry mix, 1 oz	110	1	20
Made-up, ½ cup, 4 oz	180	9	11

Quick Guide

Bagels
Average All Brands

	C	F	Cb
Plain/Onion:			
1 mini/bagelette, 1 oz	75	0.5	15
1 small bagel, 2 oz	145	1	29
1 medium bagel, 3 oz	230	1.5	45
1 large bagel, 4 oz	285	2	56
Bagel Chips *(New York Style)*,			
4 slices, ¾ oz	100	4.5	12
Pizza Bagel Bites, 4 pces, 3.1 oz	200	6	29
Bagel Bites *(Ore-Ida)*, 4 pces	190	7	25
Bagel Crisps *(New York Style)*, 7 pces	140	6	17

Bagel Brands

	C	F	Cb
Controlled Carb Gourmet			
High Fiber Bagel (1), 2 oz	160	5	22
Individual Wrapped (1), 2 oz	80	6	20
Zero Net Carbs (1), 2 oz	60	1	7
Costco Bakery: Plain, 4 oz	300	1	61
Everything, 4 oz	330	3.5	62
Enjoy Life, all types, 3.2 oz	270	6	50
Lenders: Original, frozen, 2 oz	140	0.5	29
New York, frozen, 3.3 oz	230	1	47
Plain, refrigerated, 2.9 oz	210	1.5	42
Oroweat: Oatmeal, 3.4 oz	270	4	49
Whole Wheat, 3.4 oz	250	1.5	52
Sara Lee: Mini, average, 1.3 oz	100	0.5	21
Toaster Size, all types, 2.2 oz	160	1	34
3.5 oz Size (95g): Plain, 3.4 oz	250	1.5	53
Other flavors, avg., 3.4 oz	260	1	54
Healthy Heart, 3.3 oz	220	1.5	47
4 oz Size: Apple Cinnamon	310	1.5	64
Banana Walnut	350	7	61
Cranberry Orange	310	1.5	64
Western: All flavors, avg., 2 oz	110	0	25
Bagel Sandwiches: *See Page 173*			
Fast-Foods: *See Page 183*			

Bagel Sandwiches: *See Page 173*
Fast-Foods: *See Page 183*

Bagel Spreads

	C	F	Cb
Cream Cheese:			
Plain: 2 Tbsp, 1 oz	80	8	2
2 oz mini-tub	160	16	4
Reduced Fat: 2 Tbsp, 1 oz	60	5	2
2 oz mini-tub	120	10	4
Flavors: Lox, 1 oz	75	6	1
Raisin Walnut, 1 oz	90	6	8
Strawberry, 1 oz	60	3	7
Sundried Tomato, 1 oz	80	7	2
Vegetable, 1 oz	60	6	1

Rice Cakes

	C	F	Cb
Average All Types/Brands:			
Regular size, 1 cake, 9g	35	0	7.5
Hain, Mini, average, 9 pieces	70	2	12
Lundberg, all types, 15g each	60	0.5	14
Quaker, Large, all flavors, 13g each	50	0	11
Westbrae, 1 cake, 7g	25	0	5

Taco Shells & Tortillas

	C	F	Cb
Tacos: Mini Size (1)	25	1.5	2
Regular size, all types (1)	50	2	7
Super Size (1)	90	4	13
Salad Shell, flour *(Del Oro)*, 1.4 oz	230	17	10
Tortilla (Soft Taco), each	85	2	15
Corn Tortilla: 6", 1 oz each	55	0.5	22
Flour Tortilla: 8", 1.75 oz	145	3	26
Low-Fat	110	1.5	22
Burritos, 1 tortilla, 2.3 oz	190	5	32
Low-Fat	110	1.5	22
Tostada Shells, each	55	3	6
La Tortilla Factory			
Fat Free Flour Tortillas:			
Burrito size, 2.5 oz	120	0.5	34
Soft Taco, 1.8 oz	90	0	24
Low Carb Low-Fat Tortillas:			
Large, 1.26 oz	80	3	19
Original; Flavors, 1.26 oz	50	2	11
Mission Foods			
Tortillas: *Per 6" Tortilla*			
Flour, 1 oz	80	1.5	13
Low Carb Flour, 1 oz	80	2	12
Low Carb Whole Wheat, 1 oz	80	2	12
White Corn, 0.8 oz	45	0.5	8.5
98% Fat-Free Burrito, 10", 2.4 oz	180	1.5	37

Rev. Dr Robert Schuller

Inch by inch
Life's a cinch

You'll never win
If you don't begin!

Crispbreads

	C	F	Cb
Per Crispbread/Cracker			
Ak-Mak: Sesame, 5 crackers, 1 oz	115	3	19
Finn Crisp: Original, rye, 1	35	0	7
Other types, 1 crispbread	19	0	3
Kavli Norwegian: Thin (3)	50	0	11
Thick, 2 crispbreads	60	0.5	12
Malsovit Meal Wafers, 1	75	4	7
New York Flatbread Crisps, 1	35	0	7
Ry-Krisp: Natural, 1 crispbread	25	0	5
Seasoned, 1 crispbread	30	0	5
Sesame, 1 crispbread	25	1	5
Ryvita: Dark/Light, 1 piece	26	0	4
WASA: Delikatess (1)	25	0	5.5
Fiber (1); Sesam (1)	30	1	5
Original (1)	35	0.2	7.5
Runda (1)	55	1.5	9
Wheat Dore (1)	50	1	9
Westbrae Rice Wafers (7), 15g	50	0	11

Matzos

Manischewitz

	C	F	Cb
Egg 'n Onion Matzo, 1 oz	100	1	23
Grape Matzo, 1 oz each	110	0	25
Mandelin, 9 pieces	35	2	4
Matzo Meal, ½ cup	130	0	28
Matzo Farfel, 2.7 oz	180	0.5	60
Passover Egg Matzos, 1.1 oz	120	0	28
Spelt Matzos (1)	110	1	20
Tim Tam Crackers (10)	130	4	22
Tim Tam Everything (10)	130	5	19
Thin Salted Tea Matzos, 0.9 oz	100	0	22
Unsalted; Whole Wheat, 1 oz	110	0	24
Crackers: Miniatures (12)	110	0.5	25
Passover Egg Matzo (11)	110	0	20

Quick Guide

Crackers	C	F	Cb
Average All Brands: Per Cracker			
Cheese Crackers: Plain, 1" square	5	0	0.5
Small, octagonal	10	0	1
Round (2" diam.)	15	0	1.5
Sandwich (Peanut Butter)	35	1.5	4
Graham, 2½" square, 1 cracker	30	0.5	5
Melba Toast, plain, 1 piece	20	0	4
Oyster & Soup Crackers, ½ oz	60	2	10
(40 small oysters/20 lge hexagons)			
Rice Crackers: 1 small	9	0	2
Rice Snacks, Oriental-Style, ½ oz	70	3.5	9
Saltines, 5 crackers	65	2	11
Snack-type, 1 round cracker	15	0	1.5
Soda Crackers *(Saltine),* 2	25	1	4.5
Water Cracker *(Carr's):* Regular, 1	30	0	7
Small, 1 cracker	15	0	4
Wheat, thin, 1 cracker	9	0.5	1.5
Zweiback Toast, 1 piece	30	0	5

Quick Guide

Cookies	C	F	Cb
Average All Brands: Per Cookie			
Biscotti: Small, 0.5 oz	70	3	10
Regular, 1 oz	140	6.5	18
Chocolate Chip Cookies:			
Small/Thin 0.5 oz	50	2.5	7
Regular, 1 oz	100	5	14
Large, 2.3 oz *(Mrs Fields)*	280	13	40
Jumbo, 4 oz	545	26	76
Oatmeal/Oatmeal Raisin:			
Small/Thin 0.5 oz	65	2.5	10
Regular, 1 oz	130	5	20
Large, 1.7 oz *(Mrs Fields)*	180	7	29
Jumbo, 4 oz	510	20	78
Peanut Butter:			
Small/Thin 0.5 oz	70	3.5	9
Regular, 1 oz	140	7	18
Large, 2.3 oz *(Mrs Fields)*	310	16	34
Jumbo, 4 oz	540	27	67
Low-Fat Cookies			
Choc Chip (Low-Fat), ½ oz (1)	45	1.5	7.5
Oatmeal Raisin (Fat-Free), 1 oz (1)	95	0.5	22
Peanut Butter (Low-Fat), 1 oz (1)	105	5	15

VISITING
HOURS
6 A.M. TO 7 P.M.

Crackers ✦ Cookies (Cont)

Brands
	C	F	Cb

Per Cookie/Cracker (Unless Indicated)

Archway
	C	F	Cb
Apple/Date-filled Oatmeal, avg.	95	3	16
Frosty Lemon/Orange	110	4.5	18
Ginger Snaps, Regular/Iced (5)	150	5	23
Molasses (1)	110	3.5	19
Oatmeal	110	4	18
Oatmeal Raisin	100	3	18

Atkins
Endulge Crisps (1), average	130	10	15

Austin
Cookies: *Per Package*
Sandwiches: Lemon OHs!	240	10	35
Vanilla Cremes	160	7	24

Crackers: *Per Package*
Cheese w. Cheddar Cheese	210	10	26
Cheese w. Cheddar Jack Cheese	200	11	23
Cheese w. Peanut Butter	200	10	23
Crispy w. Cream Cheese & Chives	200	10	24
Dolphins & Friends Cheddar (60)	140	5	20
Sandwiches: Chse & Peanut Butter	170	7	24
Grilled Cheese Flavored	200	10	24
PB & J Flavored	200	10	24
Toasty Crackers w. Peanut Butter	200	10	23
Wheat Crackers w. Cheddar Chse	200	10	24
Zoo Animals (16)	130	2	25

Baker's: *Per Cookie (3 oz)*
Peanut Butter	320	10	52
Peanut Butter & Jelly	310	9	55
Vegan Peanut But. Choc. Chunk	320	11	53
Other varieties, average	320	6	58

Barbara's Bakery
Cookies: Fig Bars, avg. (1)
Cookies: Fig Bars, avg. (1)	60	0.5	14
Animal Cookies, Vanilla (8)	120	4.5	18
Crisp Cookies (1), average	80	4	9
Snackimals (10), average	120	4	19
Crackers: Cheese Bites (22), 1 oz	120	3	20
Organic Go Go Grahams (8) avg.	130	4	22
Rite Lite Rounds (5), average	60	2	11
Wheatines (4), average	60	1	11

Brent & Sam's
Cookies: Chocolate Chip (2)
Cookies: Chocolate Chip (2)	120	6	16
Chocolate Chip Pecan (2)	130	8	14

Carr's
	C	F	Cb
Crackers: Table Water (5)	70	1.5	13
Whole Wheat (2)	80	3.5	11
Cookies: Bisc. for Tea (2)	140	6	20
Chococcines (3)	150	9	16
Ginger Lemon Cremes (2)	130	5	20
Hob Nobs (2)	140	6	19
Imperials: Milk Chocolate (2)	140	7	18
Dark Choc (2)	150	7	19
Petites Bijoux (4)	140	5	21

Cookies &
Cookie Bars: M&M's (1)
Cookie Bars: M&M's (1)	170	9	20
Milky Way (1); Snickers (1)	180	11	21
Twix w. Peanut Butter (1)	160	9	17
Twix (1)	180	10	21

Country Choice
Ginger Snaps (5)	120	5	19
Sandwich Cremes (2), avg.	130	5	19
Soft Baked: Peanut Butter (1)	100	5	13
Avg. other varieties (1)	100	4	16
Vanilla Wafers (7)	120	5	19

Dove
Cookies: *Per Serving*
Beyond Chocolate Chunk (1)	110	5	13
Chocolate Walnut Oasis (1)	110	6	13
Chocolate Walnut Rendezvous (1)	110	6	13
Milk Chocolate Moment (3)	160	9	20
Mint Chocolate Serenade (3)	160	8	19
Toffee Chocolate Thrill (3)	160	8	20

Entenmann's
Soft Baked (1), avg., all flavors	100	5	13

Estee (Fructose Sweetened)
Chocolate Chip	40	2	5
Coconut Cookies	35	1.5	5

Famous Amos
Chocolate Chip (4)	150	7	19
Chocolate Chip, Snack Size (4)	160	6	25
Choc Chip & Pecan (4)	150	8	18
Chocolate Creme Sandwich (3)	160	6	25
Oatmeal Choc Chip & Walnut (4)	140	7	18
Oatmeal Raisin (4)	140	6	20
Peanut Butter (4)	160	7	22
Peanut Butter Creme S'wich (3)	160	7	22
Vanilla Creme Sandwich (3)	170	7	25
Low-Fat: Gingersnaps (1 pkg)	200	3	44

Per Cookie/Cracker (Unless Indicated)

	C	F	Cb
Girl Scouts			
Cookies: Caramel DeLites (2)	140	7	19
All Abouts (2); Cafe Cookies (5)	150	7	20
Cartwheels, Reduced-Fat (5)	140	4	24
Do-Si-Dos (3)	180	9	22
Lemon Coolers (5); Pastry Cremes (3)	130	4.5	22
Peanut Butter Patties (2)	150	8	16
Peanut Butter Sandwich (2)	170	6	24
Samoas (2)	150	8	19
Shortbread (4); Trefoils (4)	130	6	18
Tagalongs (2)	130	9	13
Thanks-A-Lot (2)	150	6	22
Grandma's			
Peanut Butter Sandwich Creme (5)	210	10	28
Rich 'N Chewy, Choc Chip, pkg.	270	12	38
Vanilla Sandwich Creme (5)	210	9	30
Mini Vanilla Bites (9)	150	7	22
Homestyle Big:			
Fudge Chocolate Chip (1)	170	7	27
Oatmeal Raisin (1)	180	6	30
Peanut Butter (1)	200	10	24
Chocolate Chip (1)	190	9	25
Great American Cookies			
Cookies: Original; Pecan (1)	230	12	31
Chewy Pecan Supreme (1)	230	12	31
Chewy Choc. Supreme/Sugar (1)	200	9	29
Double Fudge/ Reese's (1), avg	220	10	33
Oatmeal (1)	230	10	23
Original M&M/Reese's (1)	240	12	32
Peanut Butter/M&M (1), avg	250	13	28
Snickerdoodles (1)	240	11	33
White Chunk Macademia (1)	250	14	30
Double Doozies: Original (1)	340	17	46
M&M Big Bite (1)	340	17	46
Brownies: Cheesecake (1)	430	23	54
German Chocolate (1)	420	22	55
Iced Fudge (1)	500	23	71
Iced Fudge Nut (1)	500	27	64
Swirl Cheesecake (1)	440	23.5	56
Cookie Cakes: 16" Cookie (1)	460	22	67
16" M&M Cookie (1)	500	24	73
Heart Shaped (1)	440	21	64
Sliced Cookie Cake, 1 slice	580	27	83
Cakes, avg. 1 slice, ⅛ cake	670	30	95
Brownies: Cheesecake Brownie	400	21	48
Cheesecake Chocolate Swirl	485	25	60
Fudge	495	22	67
Fudge Nut	525	27	63

	C	F	Cb
Hain			
Cookies: Animal (9), 1 oz	110	2	16
98% Fat-Free, all types (11)	110	0	21
Crackers: Crudites (26)	120	4	21
Mini Munchees (17)	60	0.5	12
Oyster Crackers, Fat-Free (52)	60	1	12
Rich Crackers (11)	130	4.5	21
Soy Munchies (9)	60	2.5	6
Wheatettes (16)	130	3.5	21
Health Valley			
Cookies			
Biscotti Style Low-Fat, 2 cookies	120	3	23
Chocolate Chip Oatmeal (1)	100	4	14
Cookie Cremes Sandwich (2) avg.	125	5	19
Oatmeal Raisin Cookie (1)	90	3.5	14
Peanut Crunch Oatmeal Cookie (1)	100	4	14
Cookie Bars, average	200	7	33
Cafe Creations: Chocolate Chip (1)	100	5	13
Raisin Oatmeal (1)	90	3.5	15
Chunk: Chocolate/Dbl Choc. (1)	120	7	15
White Chocolate (1)	140	7	17
Fat Free, average	100	0	24
Mini: Choc. Chocolate Chip (4)	130	7	16
Other varieties (4)	120	5	16
Crackers			
Original: Amaranth Graham (6)	120	3	22
Oat Bran Graham (6)	120	3	22
Rice Bran (6)	110	3	19
Corn Bread varieties (4)	60	1.5	11
Cracked Pepper; Sesame (5)	60	1.5	10
French Onion (10)	60	1.5	10
Hershey's			
Cookies: Hershey's w. Almonds (2)	150	9	16
Almond Joy Cookies (2)	150	9	17
Reese's Cookies (2)	150	8	17
York Cookies (2)	160	9	17
Joseph's Cookies			
Sugar Free Cookies			
Brownies: Original, 1½ oz bag	150	7	26
Pecan Walnut (9 brownies)	100	5	15
Crispy Bite Size: *Per 4 Cookies*			
Chocolate Peanut Butter	95	5	13
Pecan Chocolate Chip	95	5	13
Almond; Chocolate Chip	100	5	13
Chocolate Walnut; Oatmeal Choc	100	6	14
Lemon; Peanut Butter, avg.	95	4	15
Oatmeal; Pecan Shortbread, avg.	100	5	15

Crackers ◆ Cookies (Cont)

Per Cookie/Cracker (Unless indicated)

	C	F	Cb
Keebler			
Crackers:			
Club: Original (5)	70	3	9
Reduced Fat (5)	70	2.5	12
Grahams: Original (8), 1 oz	130	3.5	22
Low-Fat varieties (8), 1 oz	110	1.5	22
Munch'ems, average (38), 1 oz	140	4.5	22
Toasted, Regular varieties (5)	80	3.5	10
Town House: Original (5)	80	4.5	9
Reduced Fat (6)	60	1.5	11
Wheatables: Reduced Fat (19)	140	4	23
Other varieties, average (17)	140	6	20
Cookies: Chips Deluxe			
Chewy (1)	80	3.5	11
Rainbow (1)	80	4	10
Chocolate Lovers; Coconut (1)	80	4.5	10
Original, 2 oz pkg	300	16	37
Rainbow Mini's 1.4 oz pkg	210	10	27
Country Style Oatmeal (2)	130	6	18
Danish Wedding (4)	130	6	18
E.L. Fudge: Original (2)	140	6	19
Double Stuffed (2)	180	9	23
S'mores Blasted (2), avg	180	9	24
Fudge Shoppe:			
Deluxe Grahams, regular (3)	140	7	17
Fudge Sticks (3), avg.	150	8	19
Fudge Stripes: Regular, avg. (3)	160	8	21
Reduced Fat (3)	130	5	21
Mini's, 1 pkg	210	10	27
Grasshopper (4)	140	7	19
Gripz, avg., 1 pouch	130	5	18
Iced Animal (6)	140	5	22
Sandies Cookies: Reduced-Fat (1)	80	3.5	11
Cookies (1) avg. all flavors	80	5	9
Right Bites, 0.7 oz pouch	100	3	17
Soft Batch (1)	80	3.5	11
Vienna Fingers: Regular (2)	150	7	24
Reduced Fat (2)	140	5	24
Wafers: Golden Vanilla Wafers (8)	140	6	21
Golden Vanilla Minis (18)	150	6	21
Reduced-Fat (8)	130	3.5	25
Vanilla Sugar (4)	160	8	21

	C	F	Cb
Kroger			
Cookies: Animal Cookies (9)	120	2.5	23
Fig Bars (2)	60	1	2
Fudgie Sticks Wafers (3)	140	8	18
Kid O's (3)	160	6	24
Crackers: Cheddar Crisps (18)	140	6	18
Socialites (12)	140	7	17
Lance			
Nekot: Peanut Butter, 1 pkg	110	11	30
S'Mores, 1 pkg	110	12	32
O Lunch, 1 pkg, avg.	230	10	34
Strawberry Cookies (5)	190	8	27
Crackers: Toasty, 1 pkg	180	9	16
Nipchee, 1 pkg	190	11	22
Toastchee: Original, 1 pkg	220	11	23
Reduced-Fat, 1 pkg	180	7	23
Malt Crackers, 1 pkg	190	10	18
Low Carb Enchantments			
Sugar Free Cookies, avg. (1), 1 oz	140	9	11
Little Debbie			
Fig Bar (1)	160	3	31
Marshmallow Pies, avg. (1)	180	7	28
Marshmallow Treats (1)	100	2.5	18
Nutty Bar (2)	310	18	32
Oatmeal Creme Pies (1)	170	7	26
Chocolate Sugar Wafer (3)	140	7	18
Vanilla Creme Wafer	130	6	19
Crackers: Chse w. P'nut Butter (4)	140	7	15
Toasty w. P'nut Butter (4)	140	7	15
Lu			
Cookies: Marie Lu (3)	160	4.5	27
Le Fondant Wafers (4)	170	10	19
Le Petit Beurre (4)	140	4	26
Le Petit Ecolier, avg. (2)	130	6	17
Shortbread (2)	140	8	16
Pim's: Chocolatier (3)	150	9	17
Orange; Raspberry (2)	100	3	17
Manischewitz			
Matzo Boards: *See Page 105*			
Biscotti: Toffee Crunch Macaroons	50	2.5	7
Cappuccino Chip	70	2.5	10
Chocolate Macaroons, each	45	2	8
Matzo Cracker, Miniatures, each	9	0	2
Tim Tam Crackers: Everything (10)	130	5	19
Original (10)	130	4	22
Whole Wheat Crackers	9	0	2

Per Cookie/Cracker (Unless indicated)

Miss Meringue

	C	F	Cb
Chocolettes (10) average	130	3.5	24
Madeleines (2) average	160	9	18
Classiques:			
Choc. Chip/Mint Choc. Chip (4)	120	1.5	25
Cappuccino/Rainbow Vanilla (4)	110	0	27
Meringue Minis: Chocolate (13)	110	0	26
Chocolate Chip (12)	130	1.5	24
Mint Chocolate Chip (13)	120	1.5	26
Other varieties (13)	110	0	27
Meringue Minis, Sugar Free (13) avg.	40	0	8

Mrs Fields Cookies: *See Fast-Foods Section*

Mother's

Butter Cookies (6)	160	8	21
Checkerboard Wafers (4)	150	9	17
Chocolate Sandwich Creme (3)	170	8	23
Chocolate Chip: Cookies (5)	160	7	21
Chocolate Chip Parade (4)	140	7	19
Cocodas Coconut (5)	160	8	21
Cookie Parade: Animal (4)	150	7	19
Circus Animal (14)	130	4.5	22
Iced Circus (6)	150	7	21
Double Fudge (2)	190	9	26
English Tea/Taffy Sandwich (2)	185	7	28
Iced Lemonade (2)	160	8	22
Peanut Butter Gaucho (2)	190	9	25
Pecan Shortbread (2)	160	9	19
Iced Raisin (2)	170	8	24
Oatmeal Cookies: Regular (2)	130	5	19
Chocolate Chip (2)	160	7	23
Oatmeal Raisin Cookies (5)	150	7	21
Striped Shortbread Cookies (3)	160	7	24
Sugar Cookies (2)	150	7	19
Sugar Free Lemon Creme (3)	160	7	23
Sugared Lemon	75	4	10
Vanilla Cremes (2)	180	7	28
Vanilla Wafers (8)	140	5	22
Bakery Wagon: Macaroons(1)	110	5	15
Peanut Butter (1)	110	6	14
Iced Oatmeal/Lemon (1)	110	4	18
Apple/Rasp. Filled Oatmeal (1)	110	3.5	17
Chocolate Chip Chunk (1)	110	4.5	16
White Chocolate Chip (3)	160	8	22
Double Thick Chocolate Chip (1)	170	8	23
Sugar Free: Chocolate Chip (4)	130	6	23
Checkerboard Wafers (6)	140	9	18
Pecan Shortbread (4)	170	11	17
Chocolate Creme (3)	130	7	23
Peanut Butter (4)	150	9	19
Oatmeal (4)	120	5	19

Murray SugarFree Cookies

	C	F	Cb
Choc Chip & Pecan (3)	160	10	18
Double Fudge (3)	140	6	23
Fudge-Dipped Wafer: Vanilla (4)	140	10	19
Shortbread (3)	140	7	21
Gingersnaps (7)	130	5	24
Lemon/Choc Cremes (3)	130	7	18
Lemon Wafers (4)	130	8	20
Oatmeal (3)	150	7	21
Peanut Butter (3)	160	10	18
Shortbread (8)	140	6	21
Shortbread Pecan (3)	170	11	18
Vanilla Sugar Wafers (4)	130	10	20

Nabisco
Cookies: *Per Serving*

Cameo Creme Sandwich (2)	130	5	21
Chips Ahoy!: Chocolate Chewy (2)	120	6	17
Chocolate Chip (3)	160	8	21
Mini Chocolate Chip Bite-Size (5)	170	8	24
Snak Saks (5)	150	8	21
Peanut Butter (1)	80	4	9
Reduced-Fat (3)	140	5	23
Soft Baked Chunky Choc. (1)	120	5	19
White Fudge Chunky (2)	80	4	11
w. 100% Whole Grain (1)	150	8	22
Ginger Snaps (4)	120	2.5	23
Lorna Doone (4)	150	7	19
Mallomars (2)	120	5	17
Morelianas, 1 oz	130	5	19
Newtons: Fig Newtons (2)	110	2	22
100% Whole Grain (2)	110	2	22
Fat-Free (2)	100	0	22
Snack Pack To Go! (2)	90	0	22
Raspberry; Strawberry (2)	100	1.5	21
Nilla Wafers: (8)	140	6	21
Reduced-Fat (8)	120	2	24
Nutter Butter: Bites (1)	170	7	24
Peanut Creme Patties (2)	160	9	17
Real Peanut Butter Sandwich (1)	90	4.5	12
Sandwich (2)	130	6	19
Sandwich Bites (10)	140	6	21
Wafers: Chocolate Stix, 1 oz	140	8	18
Chocolate Stix Bars (2)	210	11	26
Social Tea Biscuits (6)	120	4	20
Oreo: Original, 3 cookies	160	7	24
Snack pkg, 2 oz	270	12	40
Reduced-Fat, 3 cookies	150	4.5	26
Choc. Creme; Coffee'n Creme (3)	170	7	24
Double Delight: Mint'n Creme (2)	140	7	20
P'nut Butter & Choc Creme (2)	140	6	20
Double Stuf, 2 cookies	140	7	20
Fudge-Covered, 1 cookie	100	5	13
Handi-Snacks (1)	130	5	21
Mini Oreo: 9 pieces, 1 oz	140	6	21
Snack Pack, 1.2 oz (35g)	170	7	25
Uh-Oh!, 3 cookies	170	7	24
100 Calorie Packs (1) 4.8 oz	100	2	20

Crackers ◆ Cookies (Cont)

Per Cookie/Cracker (Unless Indicated)

Nabisco (Cont):	C	F	Cb
Teddy Grahams:			
Chocolatey Chip, Mini (53)	140	4.5	22
Cinnamon Snacks (24)	130	4	23
Honey Mini, Snak Saks (30)	130	4	23
Chocolate; Honey Snack (24), avg.	160	5	26
100 Calorie Packs: Cheese Nips	100	3	15
Chips Ahoy! 1 pkg	100	3	18
Fruit Snacks, 1 pkg	100	0	24
Lorna Doone, 1 pkg	100	3	16
Oreo (Thin Crisps), 1 pkg	100	2	18
Wheat Thins, 1 pkg	100	3	16
Crackers: *Per Serving*			
Barnum's Animals (10)	130	4	23
Cheese Nips Chips: Bold Cheddar (13)	140	5	20
Cheese Nips:			
Cheddar: Packs-2-Go!, 1.2 oz	170	7	22
Bag (29), 1 oz	150	7	18
Chips, avg. (13)	140	5	20
Four Cheese, 1 oz bag	150	7	18
Mini Go-Pak (53), 1 oz	150	6	19
Reduced-Fat (31) avg.	130	4.5	20
Cheddar (31), 30g	130	3.5	21
The Fairly Odd Parents, 1 oz	140	6	19
Flavor Originals:			
Better Cheddars (22)	160	8	18
Chicken in a Biskit (12)	160	8	19
Sociables Baked Savory (7)	70	3.5	9
Vegetable Thins (11)	160	9	18
Honey Maid:			
Grahams: Avg. (8)	130	3	24
Sticks (14), avg.	130	3	25
Low-Fat (8), avg.	120	1.5	26
Snack Bars: Regular (1)	150	6	24
Soft Baked varieties (1), avg.	150	4	27
Premium Saltine: Fat-Free (5)	60	0	12
Low Sodium (5)	60	1.5	11
Multigrain (5)	60	1.5	10
Original (5)	60	1.5	11
Unsalted Tops (5)	60	1.5	11
Premium, Soup & Oyster (22)	60	1.5	11
Wheat Thins: Big (11)	150	6	21
Harvest (13)	130	3.5	23
Honey; Low Sodium (16)	150	6	21
Multi-Grain (17)	130	4.5	22
Original, Packs-2-Go, 35g	170	7	23
Original (16), 31g	150	6	21
100 Calorie Packs	100	3	16
Ranch (14), 29g	140	6	19
Reduced-Fat (16), 29g	130	4	21
Toasted Chips: Multi-Grain (12)	120	4	20
Veggie (11), 28g	120	4	20
Wheatsworth, Stone Ground Wheat (5)	80	3.5	10
Zwieback, 8g	35	1	6

Per Cookie/Cracker (Unless Indicated)

Newman's Own Organics	C	F	Cb
Alphabet Cookies (10) avg.	120	3	22
Champion Chip: Chocolate Chip (4)	160	7	21
Expresso Chocolate Chip (4)	150	7	21
Wheat-Free & Dairy-Free (4)	160	8	21
Other varieties, avg. (4)	160	8	21
Fig Newman's: Fat-Free, 2 bars	120	0	28
Low-Fat, 2 bars	140	2	28
Wheat/Dairy-Free, 2 bars	120	1.5	26
Newman-O's: Original (2)	130	4.5	20
Choc. Creme (2); Mint Creme (2)	130	4.5	20
Ginger-O's (2)	120	4.5	19
Tops & Bottoms (6)	120	3	21
Wheat-Free & Dairy-Free (2)	130	4.5	21
Peek Freans			
Assorted Creme (2)	140	6	19
Nice Biscuits (2)	160	6	25
Shortcake (2)	140	7	18
Pepperidge Farm			
Cookies			
Choc Chunk:			
Chocolate Dipped Nantucket (1)	150	8	20
Dark Choc. Pecan Chesapeake (1)	140	8	15
Milk Choc.: Cashew Stowe (1)	130	6	17
Macadamia Nut Sausalito (1)	140	8	16
White Choc. Macadamia (1)	130	6	17
Other varieties, avg. (1)	140	7	18
Chocolate Delight: Rialto (1)	100	3.5	16
Other varieties, avg. (3)	180	9	21
Collection: Ginger Family (4)	160	5	26
Other varieties, avg. (2)	135	7	17
Distinctive Milano: Milk Choc. (3)	170	9	21
Other varieties, avg. (2)	130	7	16
Distinctive: Brussels (3)	150	7	21
Brussels Mint (3)	190	10	22
Chessman (3)	120	5	18
Choc Bottomed Chessman (3)	170	7	23
Geneva (3)	160	9	19
Lido (1)	90	5	10
Raspberry Chantilly (2)	120	3	23
Other varieties, avg. (3)	140	5	22
Homestyle: Gingerman (4)	130	4	21
Shortbread (2)	140	7	16
Sugar (3)	140	6	20

Per Cookie/Cracker (Unless Indicated)

	C	F	Cb
Pepperidge Farm (Cont)			
Cookies (Cont)			
Mini: Chessmen (9)	140	6	21
Brussels (3)	190	10	22
Milano (6); Mint Milano (6) avg.	160	8	18
Nantucket Dark Choc. Chunk (4)	150	8	20
Soft Baked Cookies (1) avg.	140	5	22
Sugar-Free Cookies (3) avg.	170	9	22
Crackers			
Entertaining Collection (4)	70	2.5	10
Goldfish Crisps (37) average	150	7	17
Goldfish Flavor Blasted (51) avg.	150	7	19
Goldfish Mini Sandwich (11) avg.	140	6	18
Goldfish, Original (55)	150	6	20
Snack Sticks: Three Cheese (25)	150	6	20
Pumpernickel (15)	120	1.5	22
Sesame (12)	140	6	20
Perfect Bite Cookies			
Chocolate Chip; Peanut Butter (3)	80	4.5	13
Lemon (3); Oatmeal (3), avg.	80	4	13
Pirouline: 3 rolls, average, 1 oz	150	8	18
Ritz			
Crackers: Original, ½ oz	80	4	10
Reduced-Fat, ½ oz	70	2	11
Assortment, ½ oz	80	4	10
Dinosaurs, 1 oz	130	3.5	22
Garlic Butter, ½ oz	80	4	10
Mini Bite Size Original, 1.3 oz pkg	190	9	23
Peanut Butter, 1.4 oz pkg	190	9	24
Real Cheese, 1.4 oz pkg	200	11	22
Sticks, 1 oz	150	7	19
Top'ems, ½ oz	70	3	10
Whole Wheat, ½ oz	70	2.5	11
100 Calorie Snack Mix, 1 pkg, 22g	100	3	16
Ritz Bits Sandwiches: Cheese, 1 oz	150	9	16
Cheese Go-Pak (12) 1 oz	175	9	16
Cheese Packs 2 Go!, 1.5 oz	220	13	24
Graham S'mores, 1 oz	150	6	22
Peanut Butter/& Jelly, 1 oz	140	8	16
Peanut Butter Packs 2 Go!, 1.2 oz	170	10	20
Real Cheese, 1 oz	150	9	16
Ritz Chips: Original, 1 oz	130	4.5	21
Cheddar; Sour Crm & Onion, 1 oz	130	6	19
Santa Fe Farms			
Fat Free, average (4)	80	0	18

	C	F	Cb
Snackwell's (Nabisco)			
Creme Sandwich (2) 1 oz	110	3	20
Creme Sandwich, Packs To Go!, 1 pkg	210	5	38
Devil's Food Cake, Fat-Free (1) ½ oz	50	0	12
Lemon Creme Sandwich Sugar Free (3)	130	6	24
Shortbread Sugar Free (3) 1 oz	130	5	21
Sorbee			
Sugar Free: Animal (10)	100	3	21
Chocolate Chip; Choc. Fudge (1)	110	6	15
Oatmeal (1)	110	4	16
Peanut Butter (1)	110	7	13
South Beach Diet (Kraft)			
Cookies: Peanut Butter, 1 pkg	100	5	15
Oatmeal Chocolate Chip, 1 pkg	100	5	16
Crackers, Whole Wheat, 1 pkg	100	3.5	16
Stella D'Oro			
Almond Delight, 1 oz	160	8	18
Almond Toast (3)	115	2.5	21
Anginetti, 1 oz	130	3.5	22
Anisette Sponge Low-Fat (2)	95	1	19
Anisette Toast Low-Fat (1)	125	1	27
Biscotti, average, ¾ oz	95	4	13
Breakfast Treats: Chocolate Cookie (1)	90	3	15
Original (1)	90	3	15
Original Mini, 1 oz	120	3.5	21
Viennese Cinnamon (1)	90	2.5	16
Coffee Treats: Almond Toast, 1 oz	110	2.5	19
Angel Wings, 1 oz	170	12	14
Anisette Sponge (2)	90	1	18
Anisette Toast, 1.1 oz	130	1	27
Banana Walnut Toast, 1 oz	100	2	19
Blueberry; Cinn. Toast, 1 oz	100	1	20
Roman Egg Biscuits, 1.1 oz	130	4	21
Continental Cookie Collection, 1 oz	130	4.5	20
Egg Jumbo, 1.1 oz	120	1.5	26
Lady Stella Assortment, 1 oz	130	4.5	20
Margherite (2)	130	4.5	20
Margherite Mini, 1.1 oz	150	5	24
Swiss Fudge (2) 1.1 oz	170	9	22
Striels			
Wafers: Chocolate (3)	160	9	19
Vanilla (3)	170	11	18
Kedem Tea Biscuits, all flavors (2)	32	1	6
Sunshine			
Heads & Tails, 1 pkt, 1.5 oz	210	9	28
Hi-Ho Crackers, avg. (1)	15	0.5	2
Krispy: Original; Whole Wheat (1)	10	0.3	2
Oyster & Soup, 16 crackers	60	1	11
Unsalted Tops (1)	10	0.1	1

Crackers ◆ Cookies (Cont) ◆ Refrigerated

Per Cookie/Cracker (Unless Indicated) **C** **F** **Cb**

Trader Joe's	C	F	Cb
All Butter Shortbread:			
w. Apricot/Raspberry Filling (2)	145	8	17
w. Chocolate Filling (2)	130	7	15
Brownie Bites (3)	130	6	18
Caramel Cashew Cookies	140	7	16
Cinnamon Grahams (2½ squares)	120	4	18
Chocolate: Almond Laceys (2)	170	12	16
Chip Dunkers (2)	160	7	21
Coated Choc. Chip Dunkers (2)	190	9	24
Coconut Macaroon (3)	160	10	18
Crispy Crunchy varieties (12)	150	8	13
Ginger Animal (7)	120	2	25
Lemon Crisp (5)	120	4	19
Meringues: Cappuccino (4)	110	0	26
Chocolate (4)	120	1.5	25
Fat Free (5)	110	0	27
Soft Lady Fingers (5)	100	1.5	20
Southern Style Pecan (4)	150	9	15
Swiss Almond Crunch (6)	140	8	14
Triple Ginger Snaps (6)	140	5	21
Way More Chocolate Chips (3)	160	11	14

Triscuit	C	F	Cb
Baked Whole Wheat Crackers: *Per Serving*			
Original (15) 1 oz	120	4.5	19
Thin Crisps, Original (15) 1 oz	130	5	21
Reduced-Fat (8) 1 oz	120	3	21
Cheddar (6); Rstd Garlic (8)	120	4.5	19
Deli-Style Rye (8) 1 oz	135	5	22
Garden Herb; Rosemary (6) 1 oz	120	4	20
Low Sodium, 1 oz	130	5	19

Voortman	C	F	Cb
Shortbread Cookies (2), 1.3 oz	180	10	24
Sugar Free Cookies:			
Fudge Choc olate Chip (2), 1.4 oz	180	10	26
Iced Almonette (2), 1.1 oz	150	8	17
Peanut Butter Wafers (4), 1 oz	150	7	17
Vanilla Wafers: Regular (3), 1.1 oz	140	7	20
Sugar Free (3), 1 oz	130	5	17

Wild Oats	C	F	Cb
Ginger Snaps (5)	140	5	21
Crunchy Peanut Butter (5)	150	8	16
Oatmeal Raisin (5)	130	5	21
Sandwich Cremes, avg., (3)	185	7	28
Water Crackers (4)	60	1	12
Assorted Crackers (2)	70	2	11

Zesta	C	F	Cb
Crackers: Whole Wheat (5)	60	1.5	11
Fat Free, 5 crackers	60	0	13
Original, 5 crackers	60	1.5	11
Red. Sodium; Unsalted Tops (5)	60	1.5	11
Soup & Oyster, 51 crackers	70	3	10

Thaw, Bake & Serve C F Cb

Grands! Biscuits (Pillsbury): *Per Biscuit*	C	F	Cb
Extra Rich	210	10	26
Butter Tastin'; Buttermilk, avg.	190	10	24
Reduced Fat	170	6	26
Flaky; Homestyle; Southern Style	190	9	24

Kroger	C	F	Cb
Refrigerated Cookies			
Deluxe Oatmeal Cranberry Walnut (1)	170	8	21
Deluxe Moose Tracks (1)	170	9	22
Caramel Caribou (1)	180	9	21

Pillsbury Cookies: *Per 1 oz*	C	F	Cb
Refrigerated Cookie Dough			
Big Deluxe Classics:			
Oatmeal Raisin (1)	180	7	26
Peanut Butter Cup (1)	190	9	24
White Chunk Macadamia Nut (1)	200	11	24
Other varieties (1)	200	10	25
Ready To Bake: Sugar-Free (1)	90	4	16
Chocolate Chip w. Walnuts (1)	120	7	14
Chocolate Chunk Chip (1)	120	6	15
Mini Bites Chocolate Chip (4)	120	6	15
Peanut Butter w. Reese's Pces (1)	120	5	15
S'mores (1); Choc. Candy (1)	120	5	16
Shape Sugar Cookie (2)	140	7	17
Sugar Cookie (1)	120	6	15
Refrigerated Dough: *Per 1½" Ball of Dough (1 oz)*			
Chocolate Chip/Chunk /Dble Choc	130	7	17
Oatmeal Choc. Chip; Sugar, avg.	130	6	17
Peanut Butter	120	5	17

Toll House (Nestlé)	C	F	Cb
Refrigerated Dough			
Chocolate Chip (1)	120	6	15
Chocolate Chunk/Chunk (1)	120	6	15
Fudgy Brownie (1)	190	9	26
Jumbo Chocolate Chip (1)	200	10	26
Mini Chocolate Chip (2)	120	6	15
Walnut Chocolate Chip (1)	70	6	15
Other varieties, avg. (1)	110	5	15
Ultimates Refrigerated Dough			
Chocolate Chip Lovers (1)	180	9	23
Choc. Chips & Chunks w. Pecans (1)	190	10	22
P. Butter Chips & Choc Chunks (1)	180	9	23
Triple Chocolate Decadence (1)	170	8	23
Turtle (1)	180	9	23
White Choc. Macadamia Nut (1)	190	10	22

Ready-to-Eat

	C	F	Cb
Angel Food: Plain, no oil, 2 oz	145	0	33
Plain with oil, 2 oz	145	1	27
w. Cream Frosting	255	7	45
Apple Fritters, 3 oz	360	22	38
Apple Pie: *See Pies/Tarts Page 116*			
Baklava, 1½ square, 1.75 oz	200	10	27
Banana w. Butter Cream, 2 oz	230	9	37
Black Forest, 3 oz (⅛₂)	345	11	59
Brownie, 3.7 oz	430	21	61
Bundt, 3 oz (⅛)	270	12	36
Carrot Cake: Plain, 3 oz	300	16	37
w. Cream Cheese Frosting	400	22	48
Cheesecake: Small serving, 3 oz	235	13	26
Large serving, 5 oz	395	21	44
w. Low-Fat Cheese/Fruit, 3 oz	170	4	28
Cheesecake Factory: See Fast-Foods Section			
Denny's Cheesecake, 1 slice, ⅙	580	38	51
Cherry Cobbler, 4 oz	240	8	4
Chocolate Cake: Plain, 2 oz	200	9	30
w. Chocolate Frosting, 3 oz	290	12	44
& Cream Filling, 2.2 oz	270	12	38
Chocolate Meringue, ⅙ pie	320	13	48
Churros, 1 stick, 1½ oz	125	5	18
Cinnamon Crumb Cake, 2½ oz	260	9	40
Cinnamon Roll, 3.7 oz	430	21	55
Coffee Cake, 2 oz	180	6	30
Concha: Small, 2.1 oz	240	9	33
Large (5" diameter), 5½ oz	615	23	85
Cream Cheese Crumb, 2 oz	200	9	25
Cream Puff (custard fill), 4.6 oz	335	20	30
Creme Horns, each, 3 oz	210	5	36
Croissants: *See Next Column*			
Cupcake: Plain, 1½ oz	160	7.5	23
w. Frosting	210	10	30
Danish Pastry: Small, 2½ oz	250	14	25
Large, 5 oz	500	28	50
Date Nut Roll, ½" slice, 1½ oz	180	8	27
Devil's Food, w. Frosting, 2.2 oz	210	12	38
Donut Holes, 1¼" balls, 2 oz (5)	260	15	30
Donuts: *See Page 115*			
Eclair, Choc., Cust. fill, 3½ oz	260	16	24
Fried Twinkie (1)	420	34	45
Fig Bars, average, each	160	3	31
Fruit Cake, Dark/Light, 1½ oz	140	4	26
Fudge Nut Brownie, each, 3½ oz	380	18	54
Funnel Cake (1), 9", 3 oz	380	22	40
Gingerbread: From mix, 3" sq.	210	4	41
Honey Bun, each, 2.7 oz	310	15	39
Jelly Roll, ½ roll, 1.8 oz	150	2	32
Key Lime Pie, 4.3 oz	400	25	41
Kolacky, Apricot/Rasp., ½ oz (1)	60	3.5	8
Lady Fingers, 3 oz	310	4.5	59
Lemon Cake, 4 oz piece	440	24	49

Ready-to-Eat (Cont)

	C	F	Cb
Lemon Poppy Seed Creme, 1.6 oz	180	9	23
Marble Cake, 1 slice, 4 oz	430	23	50
Mississippi Mud Pie, 4 oz	480	22	67
Mud Cake, 1 piece, 4½ oz	380	20	44
Muffins: *See Next Page*			
Orange Creme (Ring), 3 oz	310	16	39
Pineapple Upside Down, 2½ oz	230	9	36
Peach Melba, 3½ oz	300	8	52
Strawberry Creme, 4.7 oz	400	27	33
Strudel Bites, ¾ oz	60	2.5	8
Pecan Twirls, 1 piece, 1.3 oz	170	7	26
Pecan Pie, 4.3 oz	520	24	70
Pies & Tarts: *See Page 116*			
Pound Cake, 4 oz	440	24	49
Raspberry Rugulah, 1 pce, 1.2 oz	110	9	7
Scones: Blueberry, 2 oz	190	8	29
Choc Scones, 2 oz	210	10	31
Raisin Scones, 2 oz	210	9	31
Sponge: Plain, 2½ oz	220	10	33
w. Cream & Strawberry	390	12	69
w. Chocolate Icing	290	12	45
Raisin Bun, 1 bun, 2 oz	230	11	32
Raspberry Rugulah, 1 piece, 34g	110	9	7
Strudel, fruit, average, 4.4 oz	300	17	32
Sweet Roll, average, 1½ oz	150	6	23
Swiss Rolls, (2)	270	12	38
Tarts: *See Page 116*			
Tiramisu, 4.4 oz	440	22	34
Toaster Strudel, 2 oz	190	10	26
Turnovers, fruit, average, 3 oz	290	15	35

Croissants

	C	F	Cb
Average All Brands			
Plain/Butter/Cheese: Mini, 1 oz	115	6	13
Small, 1½ oz	170	9	19
Medium, 2 oz	230	12	26
Large, 2½ oz	290	15	32
Extra Large, 3 oz	330	19	37
Sweet Croissants: (aprox. 3 oz)			
Almond Filled	330	18	39
Chocolate Filled	360	19	43
Au Bon Pain: *See Page 187*			
Burger King: *Croissan'wich, See Page 194*			
Dunkin' Donuts: Plain Croissant	330	18	37
Sara Lee: All Butter, 1½ oz	170	8	20
All Butter Petite, 0.8 oz	115	5.5	13
Starbucks: *See Page 255*			
Croissants Sandwiches: *See Page 173*			

Muffins, Sweet Rolls

Quick Guide | C | F | Cb

Muffins: Ready-To-Eat
Average All Types:

	C	F	Cb
Small, 1 oz	80	3	12
Medium, 2 oz	160	6	24
Large, 3 oz	240	9	36
Extra Large, 4 oz	320	12	48
Giant, 6 oz	480	18	60
Super Size, 8 oz	640	24	96

Brands ~ Ready-To-Eat

	C	F	Cb
Awreys: Blueberry, 2.25 oz	240	12	31
Raisin Bran, 1.5 oz muffin	160	8	21
Controlled Carb Gourmet			
Almond Muffins, 3 oz	210	15	28
Entenmann's: Golden, 2.4 oz	240	12	29
Little Bites, Blueberry, 1 pouch	190	9	27
Henry's Market: Muffins, avg. (1)	460	23	57
Mini Muffins, avg. (1)	80	4	10
Hostess: Mini, 1 pouch, avg.	250	14	27
Fruit Pie/Tart, avg., 4.5 oz	475	20	68
Hearty Muffin: Blueberry, 6 oz	690	42	72
Banana Nut, 6 oz	750	48	72
Muffin Loaf: Blueberry, 3.8 oz	420	19	58
Banana Nut, 3.8 oz	460	24	56
My Favorite Muffin: Plain, 6 oz	660	30	75
Chocolate Chip, 6 oz	635	33	81
Fat Free, avg., 6 oz	325	0	78
Otis Spunkmeyer: *Per Whole Muffin (4 oz)*			
Banana Nut, 4 oz	460	22	58
Cheese Streudel	420	18	62
Wild Blueberry	420	22	52
Our Daily Muffin: Each, 3 oz	140	0.5	31
Ralphs: Banana, 5 oz muffin	730	45	68
Bran & Walnut, 5 oz	590	31	69
Fat Free, 1.65 oz	120	0	27
Sugar Free, avg., 0.8 oz	80	5	10
Starbucks: See Fast-Foods Section			
Trader Joe's: Banana, 4 oz	280	12	39
Chocolate Chip, 4 oz	430	17	65
Mini: Blueberry, 0.8 oz	110	6	12
Bran w. Raisin, 0.8 oz	80	3	15
Uncle Wally's: Rich & Moist, 4 oz	390	19	51
All Natural: Gourmet, 4 oz	280	4	28
Fat Free Gourmet, 4 oz	240	0	56
Sugar Free Gourmet, 4 oz	120	2.5	28
Weight Watchers: Blueb., 2.5 oz	180	3	38
Double Chocolate, 2.5 oz	190	4	35
Zen Bakery: Bran Muffin (1)	110	2.5	19
Oat Bran (1)	135	3	23
Blue Raspb. Oat Bran (1) 4.8 oz	270	6	46
Fast-Food Restaurants: See Page 183			

Muffin Mixes | C | F | Cb

Prepared: Per Muffin

	C	F	Cb
Archer Farms: Wild Blueberry (1)	230	8	40
Lemon Blueberry (1)	230	8	38
Betty Crocker: Apple Streusel (1)	200	6	34
Blueberry (1)	190	7	27
Choc Chip; Cinnamon Streusel (1)	220	8	30
Water Muffins: Choc Chip (1)	160	5	26
Blueb.; Lemon Poppyseed, avg. (1)	130	3.5	24
Cornbread (1)	180	6	24
Hodgson Mill: Wheat Blueberry (1)	145	1	32
Krusteaz: Fat Free, avg. (1)	140	0	32
Banana Nut; Wildberry (1)	200	10	32
Honey Cornbread (1)	120	3.5	24
Other varieties, avg. (1)	180	4.5	32
Pillsbury: Hot Roll Mix, 1 roll	130	3	21
Just Add Milk Blueb. Muffin (1)	170	5	24
Ultimate: Blueberry Streusel (1)	190	12	35
Choc Fudge Choc Chip (1)	270	13	34
Sunmaid: Honey Raisin Bran (1)	280	9	47
Trader Joe's: Pumpkin Muffin (1)	250	11	35

Sweet Rolls & Buns

Note: Weigh for actual weight as can be 10-50% higher than label weight

	C	F	Cb
Bon Appetite: Cinn. Roll, 5 oz	580	34	64
Mammoth Cinnamon Roll, 5 oz	560	28	70
Cinnabon: Classic	815	32	117
Caramel Pecanbon, 1 roll	1100	56	141
Minibon, 1 roll	340	13	49
CinnaPretzel	755	6	156
Cinnabon Stix (5) no frosting	380	21	41
Cloverhill Bakery			
Jumbo Honey Bun, 4.75 oz	540	26	70
Entenmann's: Cinn. (½) 2 oz	220	8	34
Hostess: Honey Bun, Glazed, 2.7 oz	310	15	39
Actual weight up to 3.9 oz	440	22	55
Iced/Frosted, 3.5 oz	395	5.5	50
Cinnamon Sweet Roll (1)	205	5.5	18
Little Debbie: Pecan Spinwheels, 1 oz	110	4	16
Honey Buns, 1.76 oz	220	12	26
McDonald's: Cinnamon Bun, 3.7 oz	420	18	57
Deluxe Cinnamon Bun, 5.7 oz	590	24	86
Pillsbury: Cinnamon Roll, 1.5 oz	150	5	23
Sugar Free (1) 1.5 oz	110	3.5	12
Ralph's: Cinnamon Roll, 2.5 oz	290	11	44
Trader Joe's: Cinn. Roll, 2.35 oz	250	7	44
Frosted Cinnamon Roll, 4 oz	400	9	66
Van de Kamp's: Cinn. Roll, 1.1 oz	130	7	16
Zen Bakery: Cinn. Raisin Roll, ½	100	1	21

Donutts

Quick Guide

Donuts
Average All Brands

	C	F.	Cb
Plain, 1¾ oz	210	12	25
Sugared, 1¾ oz	220	11	27
Glazed, 2 oz	250	12	34
Chocolate Iced, 2 oz	260	14	29

Brands

	C	F.	Cb
Albertson's			
Donut Holes: Assorted	150	8	18
Powdered Sugar (4) 1.7 oz	180	7	26
Gem Donuts: Plain Cake (3) 1.6 oz	190	12	20
Chocolate (3)	260	16	25
Sticky Donuts, 2.2 oz	230	10	32
Bon Appetite			
Cherry Donuts (1) 2 oz	260	15	30
Mini Donuts: Chocolate (4)	270	16	29
Powdered; Crumb, avg. (4)	240	12	32
Cloverfield			
Donut Holes (4)	260	15	30
Dolly Madison			
Regular, 1¾ oz	270	12	40
Gem varieties, ½ oz each	65	3	8
Powdered Mini, ½ oz each	60	3	8
Dunkin' Donuts			
Apple N' Spice Donut	200	8	29
Blueberry Cake Donut	290	16	35
Boston Kreme Donut	240	9	36
Chocolate Frosted Cake Donut	360	20	40
Chocolate Glazed Cake Donut	290	16	33
Cinnamon Cake Donut	330	20	34
Glazed Cake Donut	350	19	41
Jelly Filled Donut	210	8	32
Kreme Filled (Choc./Vanilla)Donut	270	13	35
Old Fashioned Cake Donut	300	19	28
Powdered Cake Donut	330	19	36
Sugar Raised Donut	170	8	22
Entenmann's			
Dark Choc. Frosted, 2 oz	280	19	28
Frosted Devil's Food, 2.3 oz	320	19	35
Glazed Buttermilk, 2¼ oz	270	14	34
Milk Chocolate Frosted, 2.4 oz	310	19	35
Powdered, 1¾ oz	230	14	25
PopEms (bite size): *Per 4 pieces*			
Glazed (4) 2 oz	240	12	31
Glazed Devil's Food (4) 2 oz	240	11	33
Popettes (bite size), 3 pcs, 1.8 oz	240	15	24

Brands (Cont)

	C	F.	Cb
Hostess			
Cinnamon Sweet Rolls, 4.2 oz	410	11	69
Dunkin Stix (3)	490	25	63
Donut Bites, 1 pouch, 2.3 oz	300	15	38
Regular: Plain, 1.4 oz	160	9	18
Chocolate Frosted, 2 oz	230	13	26
Powdered, 1.7 oz	190	9	25
Old Fashioned Glazed, 2.1 oz	240	11	33
Donettes: Frosted (3) 1.76 oz	220	13	23
Crumb (4) 2 oz	220	9	32
Powdered (4) 2.1 oz	240	12	31
Jewel: Cinnamon Spiced, 2 oz	230	15	24
Krispy Kreme			
Chocolate Glazed Cruller	290	15	37
Chocolate Iced Glazed	250	12	33
Chocolate Iced Kreme Filled	350	20	38
Chocolate Iced w. Sprinkles	260	12	38
Cinnamon Twist	230	9	33
Glazed Cruller	240	14	26
Glazed Kreme Filled	340	20	38
Maple Iced Glazed	240	12	32
New York Cheesecake	320	19	35
Original Glazed	200	12	22
Powdered Cake	280	14	37
Traditional Cake Doughnut	230	13	25
Doughnut Holes, Glazed (5)	200	11	24
Little Debbie			
Donut Sticks, 1.65 oz pkg	230	14	25
Mini Donuts, Frosted (4)	230	13	27
Tastykake			
Cinnamon, 1.8 oz	220	13	25
Mini: Frosted Rich (6)	380	22	42
Cinnamon (4) 1.8 oz	210	10	28
Powdered Sugar (6) 2½ oz	280	13	37
Van De Kamp's			
Plain (1) 1.25 oz	150	9	17
Chocolate (1) 1.4 oz	170	9	22
Powdered (1) 1.5 oz	160	8	22
Crumb (1) 1.6 oz	180	7	26
Old Fashioned Glazed: 2.3 oz	270	12	39
Chocolate, 2.3 oz	300	15	36
Glazed Choc. Donut Holes (4)	250	11	37
Mini Donuts: Powdered (3)	210	11	26
Chocolate (3)	250	15	27
Crumb (3)	200	8	28
Zingers			
Devil's/Vanilla Food, avg. (1)	155	5	26

Pies & Tarts

Quick Guide

Pies: *Average All Brands (9")*

Apple; Blueberry; Cherry:

	C	F	Cb
Small, ⅛ pie, 4½ oz	295	14	43
Medium ⅛ pie, 7½ oz	500	23	71
Large, ¼ pie, 9½ oz	640	30	92
Extra Large, ⅓ pie, 12 oz	805	37	116
Whole Pie (9"), 38 oz	2555	119	366

Other Pies: *Per Small Serving (⅛ of 8" Pie)*

	C	F	Cb
Chocolate Cream Pie	345	12	38
Custard; Coconut Custard	270	14	31
Lemon Chiffon Pie	360	14	50
Lemon Meringue	305	10	53
Pecan Pie	450	21	65
Pumpkin Pie	230	10	30
Strawberry Pie	230	9	37

Brands ~ *Per Serving*

	C	F	Cb
Denny's: Apple Pie, 7 oz	470	21	68
Chocolate Peanut Butter, 6 oz	655	39	64
Hostess: Fruit; Cherry, 4.5 oz pie	480	20	68
Lemon, 4.5 oz pie	490	22	69
Long John Silver's: Pecan Pie	370	15	23
Chocolate Cream Pie	310	22	44
Pineapple Cream Pie	290	13	39
Marie Callender's			
Cobbler, avg., ¼ pkg, 4 oz	290	15	36
Mrs Smith's: Peach Cobbler, ⅛ pie	230	10	34
Silk Pies, avg., ⅑ pie	565	40	50
Slices: Apple; Peach, 1 pce	265	13	35
Dutch Apple, 1 piece	240	10	37
Sara Lee			
Pies: French Silk Pie, 1 slice, 4.8 oz	340	21	34
Tangy Lemon Meringue Pie	220	5	41
Tropical Coconut Cream Pie	330	19	37
Cobbler Anytime Pie: Peach, 4 oz	340	17	43
Apple; Blackberry, avg., 4 oz	350	17	48
Oven Fresh Pies (9", 37 oz Box): *Per Slice (4.6 oz)*			
Apple Pie, ⅛	340	16	46
Cherry Pie, ⅛	320	14	44
Mince Pie; Blueberry Pie, ⅛, avg.	370	15	55
Pumpkin Pie, ⅛	260	11	37
Raspberry Pie, ⅛	360	16	50
Southern Sweet Potato Pie, ⅛	280	10	45
Tastykake: Fruit, average	300	11	47
French Apple	320	12	52
Coconut Creme	370	20	42
Lemon Pie	300	14	44
Van de Kamp's			
Pies: Apple; Cherry, avg., ⅛ pie	360	23	36
Pumpkin Pie, ⅛ pie	340	14	48
Pecan; Sweet Potato, ⅛ avg.	390	16	58

Pastry & Pie Crusts

	C	F	Cb
Pie Crust: Baked, 9" diameter shell			
1 Pie Shell, 6½ oz	665	44	60
2-crust shell, 11¼ oz	1660	109	150
Piecrust Sticks, 8 oz	1180	78	106
Filo Pastry: 4 sheets, 2½ oz	210	2.5	40
Athens: 5 sheets, 2 oz	180	1	37
Mini Dough Shells, 2, 8g	35	2	2
Pepp. Farm, 2 sheets, 1½ oz	120	1	25
Puff *(Pepp.Farm),* ½ sheet, 4.5 oz	510	33	42
⅛ sheet, 1½ oz	170	11	14
Bake & Fill Shell, 1.7 oz	190	13	16
Pizza Crust, ⅑ whole	80	1	17
Arrowhead Mills, Pie Crust, ⅛, avg.	110	6	14
Bisquick: Baking Mix,			
Original, ⅓ cup, 1½ oz	150	6	26
Heart Smart, ⅓ cup, 1½ oz	140	2.5	27
Betty Crocker, 9", ⅛ shell	110	7	9
Boboli: Thin Pizza Crust, ⅓, 2 oz	170	3.5	28
Original Pizza Crust, ⅛, 1.76 oz	140	2.5	24
8" Mini Pizza Crust, ½	200	5	32
Hershey's *(Keebler),* Choc Crust, ⅛	100	4.5	14
Keebler: Graham Cracker, ⅛ of 9"	110	5	14
Reduced Fat, ⅛	100	3.5	15
Shortbread Crust, ⅛	100	5	14
Graham Crackers Minis (1)	110	5	15
2 Extra Servings, ⅒ pie	130	6	18
Marie Callendars Deep Dish Pie Shell,			
⅛ pie, 1 oz	140	10	11
Mrs Smith's Deep Dish, 9" (⅛)	130	7	14
Nabisco Oreo, ⅛ of 9" crust	130	7	19
Honey Maid Graham, ⅙, 1 oz	150	8	18
Nilla Pie Crust, ⅙, 1 oz	150	8	18
Orr Brothers, Glaze for Fruit Pie, 3 oz	110	0	27
Pet-Ritz, all types, ⅛, ¾ oz	90	5	11
Pillsbury (All Ready), ⅛ pie, 1 oz	120	8	13
Trader Joe's, Pie Crust, ⅛ pie	190	13	17

Pie Filling (Canned)

Average All Brands

	C	F	Cb
Apple: ½ cup, 4¼ oz	125	0	33
21 oz Can	600	0.5	160
Apricot, 2 Tbsp	70	0	17
Blackberry, Cherry, 4 oz	120	0	28
Chocolate, Coconut, 4 oz	140	3	33
Lemon, ½ cup, 4 oz	150	2	33
Mincemeat, 4 oz	190	1	45
Peach, Strawb., Blueberry, ⅓ c., 4 oz	100	0	23
Pumpkin, 4 oz	40	0.5	9
Raisin, 4 oz	130	0	30
Raspberry, Black/Red, ⅓ cup	100	0	25

Cakes, & Pastries – Packaged

Cakes & Pastries

	C	F	Cb
Albertson's Bakery			
Butter Ring Cake, ⅛, 3 oz	310	16	39
Sock it to me Ring Cake, ⅛, 3 oz	290	12	42
Angel Food Bar Cake, ⅕	170	0	38
Cake Slices: Per Slice (1½ oz)			
Cinnamon Butter Streusel Creme	190	9	24
Butter Creme Cake	160	5	24
Lemon Creme Cake	180	9	23
Blueberry Creme Cake	170	8	22
Banquet: Cream Pies, avg., ⅓ pie	350	21	39
Bimbo			
Concha, avg., 2.1 oz	240	9	33
Homestyle Pound Cake, 2.6 oz	300	15	37
Pecan Pound Cake, 2.9 oz	330	16	41
Raisin Pound Cake, 2.9 oz	340	16	43
Buon Appetite			
Sliced Cheesecake, 4 oz	440	24	49
Sliced Marble Cake, 4 oz	430	23	50
Sliced Lemon Cake, 4 oz	440	24	49
Sliced Pound Cake, 4 oz	440	24	49
Walnut Brownie, 3.5 oz	380	18	54
Sliced Pound Cake	520	4	49
Cheese Coffee Cake, 2.2 oz	270	15	31
Banana Bread	450	25	49
Claim Jumper: Carrot Cake, 4.6 oz	450	24	54
Choc. Motherload Cake, 5.3 oz	520	27	73
Cheesecake Factory: See Fast-Foods Section			
Dolly Madison: Honey Bun, 3.75 oz	440	25	49
Cinnamon Sweet Rolls (1)	210	7	34
Dunkin' Stix, 1 stix	170	9	20
Entenmann's			
All Butter Loaf, ⅛ loaf, 2 oz	220	10	31
Cheese-Filled Crumb Coffee, 2 oz	200	9	25
Chocolate Fudge, ⅙ cake, 3 oz	260	13	39
Coffee Cake: Cheese Topped, ⅛, 2 oz	200	9	26
Bavarian Creme Coffee, ⅛, 2 oz	190	7	30
Gourmet Cinn. Rolls, ½ roll	220	8	34
Louisiana Crunch, ⅛, 3 oz	330	15	47
Pecan Danish Ring, ⅛	250	15	26
Raspberry Danish Twist, ⅛	220	11	28
Muffins/Rolls: See Page 114			
Hostess: Per Cake Unless Indicated			
Blueberry Danish, 5 oz	490	18	80
Cheese Danish, 5 oz	490	20	74
Cinnamon Streudel Cake (1)	170	6	29
Chocodiles	230	11	36
Cup Cake (1), 1.76 oz	180	6	31

Hostess (Cont)	C	F	Cb
Danish Rollers, 2 rolls, 1.9 oz	200	8	30
Ding Dongs	175	9	24
Fudge Brownie, 3oz	330	12	54
Ho Ho's, each	125	6	17
Pound Cake, 3.2 oz	120	13	45
Raspberry Zinger (1)	160	6	26
Snoballs	170	5	32
Suzy Q , 2 cakes, 4 oz	440	17	70
Twinkies, 1.5 oz	150	4.5	27
Vanilla & Chocolate Zinger (1)	160	5	26
Little Debbie			
Angel Food Cake (1) 1.4 oz	120	0.5	27
Banana Marshmallow Pie (1) 1½ oz	180	6	30
Banana Twins, 2 cakes, 2.2 oz	250	10	38
Boston Crème Rolls (1), 2.2 oz	270	12	40
Brownies (1)	290	13	40
Choc Chip Crème Pie, 1.2 oz	150	6	23
Choc Chip Snack Cake (2), 2.4 oz	300	14	42
Creme-filled Strawb. Cup Cake (1)	210	10	29
Devil Cremes (1) 1.65 oz	200	9	29
Devil Squares, 2 cakes, 2.2 oz	270	12	38
Double Chocolate Rolls, 2 cakes	280	12	41
Fancy Cakes (2)	310	15	43
Frosted Fudge , 1.5 oz cake	190	9	6
Fudge Rounds Cookie (1) 2½ oz	310	12	48
German Chocolate Cookie (1) 1.1 oz	140	7	18
Golden Cremes Cake (1)	150	9	28
Honey Buns, 1.75 oz bun	220	12	26
Marshmallow Pie (1)	180	6	30
Marshmallow Supreme (1)	140	5	22
Oatmeal Creme Pie (1)	170	7	26
Orange Cup Cake (1)	210	10	29
Pecan Spinwheels, 1 roll	100	4	16
Strawberry Shortcake Rolls, 2.1 oz	240	9	38
Swiss Cake Rolls, 2 cakes	270	12	38
Zebra Cakes, 2 cakes, 2.6 oz	330	16	47
Mrs Smith's			
Carrot Cake, ⅙, 2.9 oz	300	16	37
Cinnabon Cinn. Pecan Coffee Cake, ⅙	270	17	25
Nemo's			
Banana Cake, 3 oz	300	12	45
Chocolate Cake, 3 oz	290	12	44
Carrot Cake, 3.6 oz	380	20	46
Red Velvet Cake, 3 oz	290	11	47
Zucchini Cake, 3.6 oz	400	21	47

Cakes & Pastries (Cont)

	C	F	Cb
Pepperidge Farm			
Turnovers (Frozen): Apple, 3.2 oz	290	15	36
Raspberry, 3.2 oz	290	15	35
3-Layer Cakes: Coconut, ⅛, 2.5 oz	250	11	35
Chocolate Fudge, ⅛ cake, 2.5 oz	250	11	31
Golden, ⅛ cake, 2.5 oz	260	13	34
Fruit Squares: Apple/Blueb./Cherry	210	10	27
Rich's: Mini Eclairs (7)	335	21	32
Mini Creme Puffs (6)	290	24	15
Safeway Select			
Molton Chocolate Lava Cake, 4½ oz	440	26	50
Sara Lee (Frozen)			
Cheesecake: Per Slice			
Chocolate French, ⅕ cake	430	22	52
Choc. Swirl New York Style, ⅙	470	29	45
French Classic, ⅕ cake	410	25	41
French Strawberry, ⅙ cake	320	14	43
New York Style, ⅙ cake	350	21	35
Original Cream Cherry, ¼ cake	350	12	51
Original Cream Classic, ¼ cake	340	18	38
Original Cream Strawberry, ¼ cake	330	12	49
Cakes: Per Slice			
Coffee Butter Streusel, ⅙ cake	190	9	25
Coffee Crumb, ⅛ cake	190	8	30
Coffee Deluxe Cinnamon Rolls w. Icing (1)	320	15	41
Coffee Pecan, ⅙ cake	140	13	23
Layer Cakes: Per ⅛ Whole			
Layer Coconut, ⅛ cake, 2.8 oz	260	14	33
Layer Double Chocolate, ⅛ cake	260	13	33
Layer Fudge Golden, ⅛ cake	260	13	34
Layer Vanilla, ⅛ cake, 2½ oz	260	14	32
Pound Cakes: Per ¼ Whole			
All Butter, 2.6 oz	220	15	34
Free & Light, ¼ cake	200	4	39
Strawberry Swirl, ¼ cake	290	11	44
Bites: Per Serving			
Choc. Dipped Orig. Cheesecake (5)	100	7	8
Choc. Dipped Praline Pecan (5)	90	6	8
Triple Choc. Fudge Brownie (1)	90	4	12

	C	F	Cb
Smart Ones (Weight Watchers)			
Brownie à la Mode	190	4	33
Carrot Cake (1) 1 oz	80	2.5	16
Chocolate Cake (1) 1 oz	80	3	15
Chocolate Mousse	180	4	28
Chocolate Eclair	140	4	24
Choc. Chip Cookie Dough Sundae	170	3	34
Double Fudge Brownie Parfait	220	3	44
Double Fudge Cake	220	7	35
Key Lime Pie, 3.3 oz	190	4.5	33
Lemon Cake (1) 1 oz	80	2.5	14
Mississippi Mud Pie	160	4	27
New York Style Cheesecake	150	5	21
Tastykake: Chocolate Jnr, 3.3 oz	340	12	55
Creme Filled Koffee Kakes, 3 oz	390	19	51
Koffee Kake Junior, 2.53 oz	280	10	44
Trader Joe's			
Bakery: Apricot Tea Loaf 2 oz	160	2	34
Choc Bundt Cake, ½ cake	340	21	34
Mini Bundt Cake (1)	190	4	35
Marble Tea Loaf, ⅛, 2 oz	160	2.5	31
Plum Coffee Cake, ⅑, 2 oz	180	6	30
Mini Carrot Cake, 5 oz	400	16	58
Cupcakes: Chocolate, 3.2 oz	430	23	54
Vanilla, 3 oz	400	20	52
Frozen Dessert: Carrot Cake, ⅙, 3 oz	330	17	41
Apple Struesel, ⅓, 4.4 oz	300	17	32
Charlotte Berry Torte, ⅛, 2.8 oz	170	7	22
Chocolate Bahka, 1 roll, 2 oz	170	5	27
Choc Ganache Torte, ⅛, 3½ oz	300	17	34
Choc Lava Cake, 1 mini cake, 3.8 oz	360	23	40
Choc. Peanut Toffee Cake, ⅙, 3½ oz	440	29	36
Low-Fat Cranb. Orange Brd, 2 oz	160	2	33
Mango Passion Exotique, ⅙, 1.9 oz	150	4	30
N.Y Deli Cheesecake, ⅙, 5 oz	510	33	46
Old Fashioned Chsecake, ½₂, 4.6 oz	470	29	40
Tiramisu, ⅛, 2.2 oz	220	11	17
Tiramisu, ⅙, 3.2 oz	290	17	33
Van de Kamp's			
Angle Food Ring, ⅛ cake	130	0	29
Banana Square Cake, ¼ cake	410	18	60
Bear Claw, 1 pce, 2 oz	250	14	26
Carrot Square Cake, ¼ cake	520	33	54
Cinn. Raisin Danish, 1 pce, 2 oz	230	11	32
Crumb Cake, ⅛ cake, 2.5 oz	330	18	39
Fruit Danish, 1 pce, 2 oz	220	11	28
German Chocolate Cake, ¼ cake	290	16	36

For Extra Listings and Nutritional Data
~ See Author's Website
www.CalorieKing.com

Cakes, Cookies & Dessert Mixes

Made As Directed	C	F	Cb
Arrowhead Mills: *Per Serving (Prep'd)*			
Choc Chip	90	2	16
Cookie (1), avg. all types	90	2	16
Oatmeal Raisin	90	2	16
Wheat Free Brownie, ⅟₂₀ pkg	160	7.5	21
Aunt Jemima			
Coffee Cake, ⅛ cake, prep.	180	6	28
Banquet			
Dessert Bakes: *Per Serving (Prep'd)*			
Apple Crisp, ⅙ pkg	220	4	44
Choc. Cherry Decadence, ⅛ pkg	310	5	62
Chocolate Lava Cake, ½ pkg	370	7	73
Cherry Cobbler, ⅙ pkg	250	4	53
Peach Cobbler, ⅙ pkg	240	3.5	51
Betty Crocker			
Cakes (Super Moist): *Per ½ Cake (Prep'd)*			
Butter Recipe Yellow	250	11	35
Chocolate varieties	270	14	33
Cinnamon Swirl	280	11	42
Devil's Food	270	14	33
White	230	10	33
Other flavors, average	270	13	35
Per ⅒ Cake (Prepared): Carrot	350	16	41
Sour Cream	280	12	43
If using No Cholesterol Recipe, deduct 40 cals and 4g fat.			
Other Cakes: Pound Cake, ⅛	260	8	45
Angel Food Cake, ⅟₁₂ mix	140	0	32
Gingerbread Cake, ⅛	220	5	39
Pineapple Upside Down, ⅙	390	13	65
Sunkist Lemon Bar (1)	140	4	24
Brownie Mixes: *Per ⅟₂₀ Pkg (Prep'd)*			
Chocolate Chunk varieties	180	9	25
Dark Chocolate	170	7	24
Fudge	170	7	22
Low-Fat Fudge Brownie, ⅟₁₈	140	2.5	28
Original Supreme	160	5	27
Peanut Butter; Walnut, avg.	180	9	23
Turtle (Caramel & Pecan)	170	9	23
Cookie Mix: *Per 2 Cookies (Prep'd)*			
Rainbow Chocolate Candy	160	7	22
Other varieties, average	170	9	21
Complete Desserts: *Per ⅛ Pkg*			
Apple Crisp	270	6	53
Hot Fudge Cake	440	13	78
Peach Cobbler	290	7	55

Betty Crocker (Cont)	C	F	Cb
Dessert Bars: Almond Joy, ⅟₁₂ pkg	200	12	21
Health Toffee Bits, ⅟₁₂ pkg	190	9	27
Reeses,⅟₁₅ pkg	180	10	20
Sunkist Lemon, ⅟₁₆ pkg	140	4	24
Warm Delights: *Per Bowl*			
Cinnamon Swirl Cake	400	12	70
Fudgy Choc. Chip Cookie	340	11	58
Other varieties, average	365	11	63
Carb Monitor: *Per Serving (Prep'd)*			
Brownie: Choc Chunk, ⅟₁₆ pkg	150	9	20
Walnut (1), ⅟₁₆ pkg	160	11	20
Cookie, 2 cookies, ⅟₁₄ pkg	130	7	18
Muffin (1), ⅟₁₂ pkg	160	9	27
Muffin Mix: *See Page 114*			
Dr Oetker: *Per Serving (Prep'd)*			
Chocolate Chip Cookie Mix, ⅟₁₂	170	7.5	24
Muffin Mix, ⅟₁₂ pkg, average	170	2	30
Simple Organic Cake Mix, ⅟₁₂	255	11	32
Duncan Hines			
Angel Food, ⅟₁₂ whole	140	0	30
Boston Creme Pie, ⅟₁₂ pkg	420	19	59
Brownie Mix (low-fat recipe)			
⅟₁₈ pkg, avg. all types	170	7	25
Choc Molten Lava Cake, ⅟₁₂ pkg	310	15	43
Choc Silk Torte, ⅟₁₀ pkg	440	18	65
Cookies, all flavors, 1 cookie	65	3	8
Homestyle Cookies, avg. (2)	170	7	24
Hot Fudge Brownie Sundae, ⅑ pkg	350	14	54
Orange Dreamsicle, ⅟₁₂ pkg	410	18	57
Moist Deluxe Cake Mix:			
Average, ⅟₁₂ pkg, prepared	270	12	36
Lower Fat Recipe, ⅟₁₂ pkg, prep.	210	5	37
Ghirardelli: *Per Serving (Prepared)*			
Brownie, ⅟₁₆ pkg	180	8	26
Chocolate Chip Cookie (1)	280	13	38
Jell-O No Bake Cheesecakes: *Prep'd As Directed*			
Cherry/Strawberry, ⅑ pkg	290	10	48
Chips-Ahoy!, ⅙ pkg	360	17	48
Chocolate Silk Dessert, ⅙ pkg	290	14	37
Oreo, ⅙ pkg	370	17	51
Peanut Butter Cup, ⅛ pkg	360	21	41
Real, ⅙ pkg	350	16	48

Frostings ◆ Baking Ingredients

Cakes & Dessert Mixes (Cont)

Made As Directed	C	F	Cb
Krusteaz: Cinn. Crumb Cake, 1"	230	7	38
Lemon/Key Lime Bar, 2" bar	160	3.5	29
Bakery Style Cookie Mix: *Per Cookie*			
Chocolate Chip, 2½	140	4.5	19
Fat-Free Fudge Brownie, 2"	120	0	28
Gingerbread, ⅛ cake	210	3.5	41
Snickerdoodle	130	5	20
No Pudge			
Fudge Brownie, 1/12 pkg, prep'd.	120	0	28
Pamela's			
Ultra Chocolate Brownie, 1/16 pkg	170	8	23
Oil Free, 1/16 pkg	110	1.5	24
Robin Hood			
Angel Food Cake, 1/10 cake	160	0	38

Cake Frostings

Betty Crocker	C	F	Cb
Drizzlers, 2½ Tbsp	220	13	26
Rich & Creamy, average, 2 Tbsp	140	7	19
Whipped, all flavors, 3 Tbsp	110	5	15
Easy Flow Icing, 1 tsp	25	1	4
Duncan Hines: *Per 2 Tbsp (1.2 oz)*			
Creamy Homestyle, avg all flavors	140	6	23
Whipped, avg., 3 Tbsp	160	9	20
Pillsbury: *Per 2 Tbsp (approx. ½2 Tub)*			
Creamy Supreme: Choc Fudge	140	6	21
Classic White	140	5	22
Milk Choc	140	6	21
Vanilla; Vanilla Funfetti	150	6	25
Whipped Supreme, avg all flavors	100	5	14
Decorators, Choc., 1 Tbsp	70	2	11

> *In eating, one third
> of the stomach should be
> filled with food,
> one third with drink,
> and the rest left empty.*
>
> ~ Gitten, the Talmud

Baking Ingredients

Almond Paste:	C	F	Cb
(Marzipan), 2 Tbsp	170	7	24
Baking Powder: Regular, 1 tsp	2	0	1
Cream of Tartar, 1 tsp	8	0	2
Baking Mix *(Bisquick)* :			
Original, ⅓ cup, 1½ oz	160	5	26
Heart Smart, ⅓ cup, 1½ oz	140	2.5	27
Butter/Margarine, ½ cup, 4 oz	810	91	1
Carob Flour, ½ cup	115	0.5	46
Chocolate Baking Bars: *Average All Brands*			
Unsweetened, 1 oz	140	14	8
Grated, 1 cup, 4½ oz	680	68	36
Semi-sweet, 1 oz	140	9	16
Bitter-sweet/White Baking 1 oz	160	8	20
Chocolate Baking Chips: *Average All Brands*			
Milk Choc./Semi Sweet 1 oz	160	9	18
¼ cup, 1½ oz	240	12	30
1 cup, 6 oz	960	48	120
Mini Kisses *(Hershey)*, 1 pce	5	0.5	1
M&M's Minis, *Nestle* Morsels, 1 oz	140	8	18
Reeses Peanut Butter Chips, 1 T.	80	4	8
Cocoa Powder, Baking: *Nestle,* 1 T.	15	1	3
⅓ cup, 1 oz	80	4	12
Hershey's, 1 Tbsp	20	0.5	3
⅓ cup, 1 oz	115	3.5	21
Coconut, dried: Unsweet., 1 oz	190	18	7
Sweetened/flaked, 1 oz	130	8	15
½ cup, 1.3 oz	195	12	22
Toasted *(Baker's)*, 1 oz	170	13	13
Coconut Cream/Milk: *See Page 39*			
Cornstarch, 1 Tbsp	30	0	7
Flour, white: 1 Tbsp, 0.6 oz	55	0	12
1 cup, 4.4 oz	455	1	95
Whole Wheat, 1 cup, 4.2 oz	410	2	87
Flavor Extracts: *Average All Brands*			
Imitation, 1 tsp	10	0	2
Pure Extract, 1 tsp	20	0	4
Almond, Vanilla, 1 tsp	10	0	0.5
Fruit Pectin: Swtnd, ¼ tsp	5	0	1
Unsweetened, ¼ tsp	0	0	0
Gelatin, dry, ¼ oz pkg	25	0	0
Lemon/Orange Peel, ¼ cup	25	0	6
Rennin, 1 pkg (11g)	10	0	2
Sprinkles, all types, 2 Tbsp	120	3	23
Sugar: *See Page 123*			
Vinegar, avg. all types, 1 tsp	5	0	1
Whey, sweet, dry, 1 oz	100	0.5	21
Yeast: Active, dry, ¼ oz pkg	21	0	3
Bakers, compressed, 1 oz	30	0.5	5
Brewers; Torula, 1 oz	80	0.5	11
Fleischmann's, 0.6 oz pkg	0	0	0

Puddings, Desserts, Gelatin

Ready-To-Serve

	C	F	Cb
Instant Pudding, Reg., ½ cup	170	4	30
Reduced Calorie: *Estee*	70	0	12
Jell-O, sugar-free, ½ cup	80	2	11
Royal, sugar-free, ½ cup	100	2	17
Dr McDougall's, Rice Pudd., 3 oz	310	1.5	69
Hunt's Snack Pack: *Per 3.5oz Cup*			
Puddin' Cakes: Choc Brownie	180	7	27
German Choc Cake	160	3.5	30
Puddin Pie: Lemon Meringue	130	2.5	20
Apple; Choc Mud	170	7	26
Dessert Favorites, avg. all flavors	140	5	25
Spoonibbles, 3½ oz cup	140	3.5	25

Jell-O

	C	F	Cb
Pudding Bites, average 1 pouch	90	1.5	18
Pudding & Pie Filling: *Per ¼ Pkg*			
Cook & Serve, average, prep.	100	0	22
Instant, regular, avg.	100	0	25
Fat & Sugar Free, avg.	30	0	8
Pudding Snacks: Fat-Free, 4 oz	100	0	23
Cheesecake Snack, 4 oz	150	4.5	25
Chocolate; Creme Savers, 4 oz	160	5	28
Smoothie Snacks, 4 oz	100	2.5	18

Jewel: Chef's Kitchen

	C	F	Cb
Rice Pudding, ½ cup, 4.5 oz	230	8	35
Tapioca Pudding, ½ cup, 4.5 oz	170	8	35

Kozy Shack

	C	F	Cb
Regular flavors, avg., ½ cup	130	3	22
No Sugar Added, avg., ½ cup	90	3	10
Flan: Creme Caramel, ½ cup	150	3.5	27
Mango Sauce, ½ cup	140	4	24
Restaurant Style, ½ cup	190	6	28
Rice Pudding: Original, ½ cup	130	3	22
Cinnamon Raisin, ½ cup	140	3	24
European Style, ½ cup	130	3.5	22
Tapioca, Old Fashioned, ½ cup	130	3	23

Kraft Handi Snacks: *Per Cup (3.5 oz)*

	C	F	Cb
"Doubles", avg. all flavors	100	1	22
Chocolate Pudding Fat-Free	90	0	21
Rice Pudding	140	6	19
Vanilla Pudding	90	1	20

Kroger: *Per Container*

	C	F	Cb
Peaches & Cream w. Natural Flav.	180	2.5	36
Whipped Varieties	145	2.5	27
Manischewitz: Choc., ½ cup	110	0.5	26
Passover Gold Noodle, ½ cup	140	2	28

President's Choice

	C	F	Cb
Key Lime Pie (36 oz), ⅛ pie, 4.5 oz	435	21	56
Mississippi Mud Pie (36 oz), ⅛, 4 oz	405	22	49

Ready-To-Serve (Cont)

	C	F	Cb
Swiss Miss Pudding Snacks			
Chocolate, Low-Fat, 4 oz	140	2	27
Chocolate Vanilla Swirl, 4 oz	150	4	26
Creamy Vanilla, 4 oz	140	4.5	23
Milk/Dark Chocolate, 4 oz	160	4	28
Old Fashioned Tapioca, 4 oz	140	3.5	24

Homemade Puddings

	C	F	Cb
Apple Tapioca, ½ cup	150	0	32
Bread Pudding, ½ cup	250	8	40
Blancmange, ½ cup	140	5	19
Chocolate, ½ cup	190	6	30
Corn Pudding, ½ cup	135	4	21
Crème Brûlée, ½ cup	400	35	16
Plum Pudding, 2 oz	170	3	32
Rice with Raisins, ½ cup	200	4	38
Sponge Pudding, 3½ oz	340	16	45
Tapioca Cream, ½ cup	110	4	15
Trifle, ⅓ cup	180	7	24

Custards

	C	F	Cb
Custard Mix: Dry, ⅙ pkg	85	1	17
Prep. w. 2% milk, ½ cup	140	3.5	21
Jello Flan, w. 2% milk, ½ cup	140	2.5	20
Royal-Flan: Prep. w. 2% milk, ½ c.	130	2.5	18
Homemade Custard			
Baked: Plain, ½ cup, 4½ oz	150	7	16
w. skim milk, artif. sweetened	70	3	4
Boiled, ½ cup	165	7	18

Meringues

	C	F	Cb
Meringue Swirl, ½ cup	50	0	8
Meringue Shell, 1 oz shell	100	0	16
(Add extra calories/fat/carbohydrate for fillings)			

Jell-O · Cups · Parfait

	C	F	Cb
Gelatin Mix: *Jell-O, Royal ~ Made Up*			
Regular, all flavors, ½ cup	80	0	18
Sugar Free/Low Calorie, ½ cup	8	0	0
Creme Gelatin/Parfait: *Per ½ Cup*			
Ida Mae, ½ cup	60	2	10
Winky: Strawberry (109g)	110	1.5	22
Rainbow (130g)	100	0	24
Reser's, Dessert Parfait (110g)	100	2	19
Mrs Crockett's Kitchen, Str. Parfait	160	4	26
Gel Snacks *(Jell-O):* Regular, 3.5 oz	70	0	17
Sugar Free, 3.2 oz	10	0	1
X-Treme Cups, 2.5 oz	100	0	24
X-Treme Sticks, 2.2 oz	60	0	16

Quick Guide | C | F | Cb |

Pancakes

Plain: *Average All Types*

	C	F	Cb
Small (3" diam.), ¾ oz	50	2	6
Medium (4" diam.), 1¼ oz	85	3.5	11
Large (5" diam.), 2½ oz	175	7.5	22

Add Extra for Syrups/Butter

	C	F	Cb
Pancake Syrup: Regular, 1 Tbsp	50	0	13
¼ cup, 4 Tbsp	210	0	52
Lite, 1 Tbsp	25	0	6
¼ cup, 4 Tbsp	100	0	26
Butter/Margarine: Regular, 1 T.	100	11	0
Whipped, 1 Tbsp	70	7.5	0

Waffles

	C	F	Cb
Homemade: 7" waffle, 2½ oz	245	13	26
From Mix: 7" waffle, 2½ oz	205	8	28

Frozen Breakfasts

Aunt Jemima

	C	F	Cb
Pancakes: Buttermilk (3)	200	3.5	37
Homestyle (3)	200	3.5	37
Low-Fat (3)	190	2.5	35
Whole Grain (3)	230	6	38
Mini Pancakes (11)	240	4	46

Frozen Breakfasts:

	C	F	Cb
French Toast, Cinnamon, 2 slices	220	6	34
French Toast, Homestyle, 2 slices	240	6	39
French Toast, Sticks, 5 sticks	330	11	54

Eggo *(Kellogg's)*

	C	F	Cb
French Toast: Toaster Swirlz, set of 4	120	3	20
French Toast Sticks, avg., (2)	220	6	38
Stuffed French Toaster Sticks (2)	310	7	55
Pancakes: Buttermilk, 3 pancakes	280	9	44
Jungle, 3 pancakes	280	6	46
Nutri-Grain, 3 pancakes	240	7	40
Minis, 11 pancakes	260	8	42

Farm Rich

	C	F	Cb
French Toast Sticks, avg. (5)	300	14	40

Pillsbury

	C	F	Cb
Pancakes: Mini, average, (14)	425	7	88
Chocolate Chip (3)	270	5	50
French Toast Sticks (6)	360	7	69
Dunkables Cinn. Bites/Icing (3)	140	4.5	23
Toaster Strudel, avg. (1)	190	9	26

Krusteaz

	C	F	Cb
Pancakes: Mini (12)	220	2.5	43
Buttermilk (3)	280	4	52
French Toast: Average, 1 slice	115	2.5	18
Sticks, 4 sticks	230	5	41

Restaurant-Style: *See Fast-Foods Section*
Frozen Egg Breakfasts: *See Page 47*

Restaurant-Style: *See Fast-Foods Section*
Frozen Egg Breakfasts: *See Page 47*

Pancake Brands | C | F | Cb |

	C	F	Cb
Atkins: All-Purpose, 2 tsp. dry mix	30	0	5
Bake Mix, ¼ cup dry mix	80	0.5	8
Aunt Jemima			
Buckwheat, 4 x 4" pancakes	170	6	26
Buttermilk, 4 x 4" pancakes	180	6	25
Original Complete, 2 x 4" pancakes	160	1.5	32
Original, 4 x 4" pancakes	250	8	37
Whole Wheat Blend, 3 x 4" pancakes	200	6	29
Betty Crocker Pancake Mixes			
Complete Original/Buttermilk, 3	200	2.5	40
Bisquick (Shake 'N Pour), 3	200	3	38
CarbSense: 2 pancakes prep.	320	15	9
Hungry Jack Pancakes			
Mixes: *Per ⅓ Cup (Prepared)*			
Buttermilk, Complete, 3 x 4"	150	1.5	31
Original, w. 2% Milk, Oil, Egg	250	8	37
w. Skim Milk, Oil, Egg Whites	180	1	37
Extra Lights: Complete (3)	150	2	30
Potato Pancakes, 2 Tbsp mix	70	0	15
Microwave (frozen): Pancakes (3)	270	4.5	51
Krusteaz: No Sugar, prepared,			
3 x 4" pancakes	180	5	23
Northern Pines: 3 x 4" pancakes	380	7	71

Frozen Waffles | C | F | Cb |

	C	F	Cb
Aunt Jemima: Buttermilk (2)	200	5	33
Homestyle (2); Blueberry (2)	190	5	32
Low-Fat (2)	160	2.5	30
Eggo *(Kelloggs):* Minis, avg. (3)	250	8	39
Original: Chocolate Chip (2)	210	7	32
Cinnamon Toast (3)	290	10	46
French Vanilla (2)	200	8	27
Other varieties, avg. (2)	190	6	30
Flip Flops, avg. (2)	190	6	29
Homestyle: Original (2)	180	6	27
Lego (2)	190	6	30
Nutri-Grain: Average (2)	170	4.5	27
Low-Fat (2)	140	2.5	28
Special K, 99% Fat-Free (3)	190	1	35
Waf-Fulls (2)	150	5	27
GO-LEAN *(Kashi):* Average (1)	90	1.5	16
Hungry Jack: Blueberry, 1 waffle	105	4	15
Buttermilk; Homestyle (1)	95	3	15
Nature's Path: Average (1)	120	4	18
Lifestream; Gorilla; Koala, avg.	110	3.5	19
Other varieties, avg. (1)	120	4	17
Pillsbury: Waffles, avg. (1)	90	2.5	15
Waffle Sticks (6) & syrup	340	7	64
Van's: Belgian Original (1)	85	2	15
97% Fat Free (1)	90	1	15
Mini Homestyle (8), avg.	120	4	20

Sugar

	C	F	Cb
White Sugar, granulated:			
1 level teaspoon, 4g	15	0	4
1 heaping teaspoon, 6g	25	0	6.5
1 cube, ½"	24	0	6.5
Single portion, 1 packet	25	0	6.5
1 Tablespoon, 12g	48	0	12
1 ounce, 1 oz	110	0	20
1 cup, 7 oz	770	0	200
1 pound	1760	0	464
Brown Sugar: 1 Tbsp, 13g	50	0	13
1 ounce, 1 oz	109	0	28
1 cup, not packed, 5 oz	540	0	140
1 cup, packed, 7¾ oz	845	0	218
Powdered/Confectioners:			
Sifted, 1 cup, 3½ oz	385	0	98
Unsifted, 1 cup, 4¼ oz	460	0	117
Cinnamon Sugar, 1 tsp	15	0	4
Dextrose, 1¼ tsp	15	0	4
Fructose: Dry, 1 tsp	15	0	4
Liquid, 1 oz	80	0	21
Glucose, 1 oz	110	0	27
Glucose Tablets (1)	20	0	5
Palm Sugar, 3 Tbsp, 12g	45	0	11
Piloncillo (Brown Sugar), 3oz cone	325	0	81
Turbinado Sugar, 2 Tbsp, 1 oz	110	0	27
Unrefined Cane Sugar, 1 oz	110	0	27

Sugar Substitutes

	C	F	Cb
DiabetiSweet, 1 teaspoon	9	0	4
(Carbohydrate as Sugar Alcohol)			
Equal: Tablet/Liquid	0	0	0
Granulated, 1 pkg	4	0	1
Powdered, sachet, 0.04 oz	0	0	0.5
Sugar Lite, 1 tsp	8	0	2
NutraSweet Spoonful, 1 tsp	2	0	0.5
Nutra Taste; Sweet One, 1 pkt	0	0	0
PerfectSweet, 1 tsp	15	0.5	1
Shugr (Swiss Diet), 1 tsp	0	0	0
Sorbitol, 1 oz	110	0	27
Splenda: Powder, 1 cup	96	0	24
Sachet, sachet	0	0	0.5
Granular, 1 tsp	5	0	1
Sugar Blend, for Baking, ½ cup	385	0	96
Stevia, 1 pkt	0	0	0
Sugar Twin: 1 pkt	3	0	0
Sugar Substitute, 1 tsp	2	0	0
Sweet 'N Low, 1 pkt	0	0	1
Walgreens Wal-Sweet, 1 pkt	0	0	0
Weight Watchers; Whey Low, 1 tsp	4	0	1

Honey, Jam, Preserves

	C	F	Cb
Average All Brands			
Honey: 1 tsp, ¼ oz	22	0	5.5
1 Tbsp, ¾ oz	65	0	17
1 ounce, 1 oz	86	0	23
1 cup, 12 oz	1030	0	269
Single Portion, ½ oz pkg	43	0	11
Jams/Jellies/Marmalade/Preserves:			
Regular, 1 tsp, ¼ oz	18	0	5
1 Tbsp, ¾ oz	65	0	16
1 ounce	90	0	22
Single Portion, ½ oz pkg	38	0	11
Apple/Fruit Butters, 1 T., 0.6 oz	20	0	6
Fruit Spreads: Regular, 1 tsp	16	0	4
Low Sugar, 1 tsp	8	0	2
Low Cal. (Featherweight), 1 tsp	8	0	2
Jelly: Regular, average, 1 tsp	18	0	4.5
Imitation, Low Calorie, 1 tsp	4	0	1

Syrups, Molasses

	C	F	Cb
Syrups: *Average All Brands*			
(Corn/Rice/Maple/Pancake/Sundae/Waffle)			
Includes Aunt Jemima, Cary's, Karo, Hershey's,			
Hungry Jack, Log Cabin, Mrs Butterworth's			
Regular/Dark/Light Color:			
1 Tbsp, ½ fl.oz	55	0	14
¼ cup (4 Tbsp)	220	0	55
Single Portion, 1½ oz pkg	170	0	42
Lite: 1Tbsp	25	0	6
¼ cup (4 Tbsp)	100	0	25
Sugar-Free: *Cary's,* 2 Tbsp, 1 oz	18	0	5
Cozy Cottage, 2 Tbsp, 1 oz	10	0	3
Da Vinci, 2 Tbsp, 1 oz	5	0	1
Honey Cream Syrup, ¼ c., 2 oz	220	0	55
Molasses: Dark/Light: 1 T., ¾ oz	55	0	14
1 cup, 11½ oz	880	0	224
Blackstrap: 1 Tbsp, ¾ oz	47	0	13
1 cup, 11½ oz	750	0	208

Ice Cream Toppings

	C	F	Cb
Average All Types & Brands			
(Hershey's, Kraft, Smuckers)			
Butterscotch, Caramel, 2 Tbsp	140	1	30
Chocolate: Hot Fudge, 2 Tbsp	140	4	22
Fat Free Chocolate, 2 Tbsp	100	0	23
Pineapple, Strawberry, 2 Tbsp	110	0	28
Smuckers: Guilt-Free/Lite, 2 T.	100	0	24
Magic Shell, 2 Tbsp	210	15	18
Milky Way, 2 Tbsp	130	3.5	24

Quick Guide

Chocolate
Average All Brands
Milk Chocolate, regular:

	C	F	Cb
Plain/Nuts/Fruit, average, 1 oz	150	10	13
1½ oz Bar	225	15	23
2 oz Bar	300	20	30
4 oz Block	600	40	60
8 oz Block	1200	80	120
1 Pound, 16 oz	2400	160	240
Dark/White Chocolate, 1 oz	150	10	16
Sugar Free *(Hershey's)* 1 pce, 0.3 oz	40	3	5

Chocolate-coated:

	C	F	Cb
Almonds, 5-6, 1 oz	160	11	14
Clusters, Nut, 3 pces, 1.2 oz	200	18	16
Coffee Beans, 1.4 oz	180	9	22
Creme/Cordial Centers, 1 oz	120	5	20
Fudge, 1 oz	125	4	20
Macadamias, 9 pces, 1.3 oz	220	15	18
Mints, 1 med., ½ oz	55	1	11
Nougat & Caramel, 1 oz	125	5	18
Peanuts, 12 med., 1 oz	145	9	14
Raisins, 28 med., 1 oz	110	4	19

Cooking Chocolate:

	C	F	Cb
Sweet/Semi-sweet, 1 oz	160	9	18
Chips, 1 Tbsp, ½ oz	70	4	9
Unsweetened, 1 oz	140	15	8
Dipping Choc *(Bakers)*, ½ oz, 1T.	80	5	9
Carob: Plain, 1 oz	150	9	16

Brands & Generic

Per Piece/Serving

	C	F	Cb
Abba Zaba, 2 oz bar	250	5	48
Absolutely Almond, 2.5 oz bar	380	23	40
Aero Bar *(Nestlé)* 1.45 oz bar	210	13	26
After Dinner Mints, 1 small	25	1.5	3
After Eight Mint *(Nestlé)*, each	35	1	6
Air Head, 1 bar, 15.6g	60	0	15
Allen Wertz: Simply Sugar Free			
Coffee Time (decaf), 4	45	1.5	8
Coffee Toffee, 6	120	3	23
Other types, 4	120	2.5	24
Almond Joy: 1.6 oz bar	235	13	29
King Size, 4 pces, 3.1 oz	450	24	54
Snack, 17g	80	4.5	10
Swoops, 1 cup, 1.26 oz	200	12	21
Almond Roca: 3 pces	220	15	17
Sugar Free, 3 pces	150	15	16
Almonds, sugar-coated (15), 40g	175	4	29
Almond Clusters *(Trader Joe's)*, 2 pce, 1.2 oz	210	14	5

Brands & Generic (Cont)

Per Piece/Serving

	C	F	Cb
Altoids *(C & B)*, 10 pces	10	0	2
Amazin' Fruit, 1 bag, 1.9 oz	180	0	41
Andes: Creme de Menthe; Cherry Jubilee			
Choc covered Patty, (3), 1.4 oz	200	13	22
Thins, avg. all flav., (8), 1.4 oz	200	13	22
Anthon Berg: Cognac, each	180	8	25
After Dinner Sweet:			
Marzipan w. Madeira, 1.4 oz	175	7.5	26
Marzipan Brod	120	7	13
Asteroid *(Nestlé)* 1.9 oz	260	10	40
Atomic Fireball, 1 piece	4	0	1
Baby Ruth: King Size, 3.7 oz bar	480	24	66
2.1 oz bar	280	14	39
Fun size, 2 bars	170	8	24
Minis, 4 bars	200	9	30
Carb Select, 2 bars	180	8	26
Baci *(Perugino)*: 1 pce, ½ oz	75	6	7
Bar, 1.58 oz	230	15	27
Barley Sugar, 1 pce, 0.2 oz	25	0	6
Baskin-Robbins: 3 pce, 0.5 oz	60	1	13
Sugar Free, 4 pces	40	1	15
Big Hunt, 2 oz	230	3	47
Bit-O-Honey, 1.7 oz	180	3.5	38
Chews, 6 pces, 1.4 oz	150	3	32
Blow Pops, each	50	0	14
Bon Bons, 2 pieces	45	0	12
Boston Baked Beans, 11 pces, 15g	70	2.5	10
Brach's: Almond Supremes (11)	220	13	22
Butterscotch Hard (3), 0.6 oz	70	0	17
Caramel Clusters (2), 36g	180	10	20
Choc Bridge Mix (16), 1.3 oz	190	8	29
Circus Peanuts (6), 1.4 oz	160	0	39
Double Dippers (14), 1.4 oz	210	12	23
Golden Butter Toffee (3), 0.6 oz	80	2	15
Malted Milk Balls (15), 1.3 oz	190	7	30
Milk Maid Caramel (4), 1.37 oz	160	4.5	27
Orange Slices (3), 45g	150	0	38
Breath Savers, all types, each	5	0	2
Brite Crackers, 1 bag, 1.5 oz	140	0	32
Bubble Gum: See 'Gum' Page 131			
Buncha Crunch, ⅓ cup, 1.4 oz	180	8	26
Burnt Peanuts, 15 pces, 40g	70	3	10
Butterfinger: 2.1 oz bar	270	11	43
King Size, 3.7 oz bar	480	18	75
Fun size, each	85	3.5	14
Giant, 5 oz	680	32	96
Beast, 140g	640	24	100
On The Go, 4 bars	180	9	29
Mini, each	45	1.5	7
Snack (4) 1.4 oz	180	7	29
Stix, 1 stick, 17g	90	4.5	11

HERSHE... Reese's JOLLY RANCHER

Brands & Generic (Cont)

Per Piece/Serving

	C	F	Cb
Butterfinger (Cont):			
Crisp Bar: 1.76 oz bar	250	13	33
King Size, 90g	500	28	62
Minis, 4 pieces	220	11	29
Butterfinger B.B.'s, 1.7 oz bag	220	9	34
Buttermints, 7 pces, 13g	50	0	12
Butterscotch: 3 pces	70	0	19
Buttons (Walgreens), 3, 18g	70	0	17
Chips (Hershey's), 1 Tbsp	80	4	10
Discs (Sathers), 3 pces	70	0	17
Cadbury (Hershey's): Creme Egg (1)	170	6	28
Dairy Milk, 10 pces, 40g	220	12	24
Mini Eggs, 12 pces, 40g	190	8	28
Candy Apple, medium, 6.5 oz	280	0	60
Candy Cane, medium, 5", ½ oz	50	0	13
Candy Corn, 1 oz	100	0	26
Candy Jar Mix (Jewel), 3, 17g	70	0	17
Candy Necklaces, 20g each	80	0	20
Caramels: each	40	1	8
Chocolate, each	25	0.2	6
Creams: 3 pces, 1¼ oz	130	3	23
2.75 oz pkt, 5 pces, 1½ oz	160	3.5	30
Caramel Nips: 2 pces	60	1.5	11
Chocolate Parfait, 2 pces	60	2	11
Peanut Butter, 2 pces	60	2	11
Sugar Free Caramel, 2 pces	60	1.5	12
Caramel Popcorn, ⅔ cup	150	6	23
Caramello (Hershey's), 1.6 oz bar	210	10	29
Snack, 0.66 oz	80	4	11
Cadbury: 6 pces	200	9	27
Kingsize, 2.7 oz bar	360	16	49
Certs, Breath Mints, 1 pce	5	0	2
Charleston Chew: 1 bar, 60g	260	7	49
Minis, 2 bars, 24g	110	4	17
Chew-ets Peanut Chews:			
Original, 6 pces, 56g	260	13	25
Chocolate, 6 pces	270	14	34
Chews, 1 roll	120	1	28
Chick O Stick, 2 oz	260	6	44
Chocolate Mints (Hershey's), each	10	0.1	2
Chocolate Parfait Nips, 2 pces	60	2	11
Chuckles Jelly: each	35	0	9
Jujubes (Hershey's), 55 pces, 40g	110	0	28
Chunky Bar (Nestlé): 1.4 oz	190	11	24
King Size, 2½ oz	340	19	43
Giant, 5 oz	680	40	84
Chupa Chups, 1 pce, 0.42 oz	35	0	8
Cinnamon Bears (Walgreens), 5	130	0	34
Cinn. Buttons (Walgreens), 3 pce	70	0	17

Per Piece/Serving

	C	F	Cb
Cinnamon Disks (Walmart), 3 pces	70	0	19
Cinnamon Drops (Sathers), 19 pce	150	0	36
Circus Peanuts, 6 pces, 42g	160	0	39
CocoaVia Crunch Bars, 0.7 oz	90	5	11
Coconut Stacks, 8 pieces	260	13	37
Coffee Go Coffee/Cappuccino, ea.	18	0.4	4
Coffee Rio-Gold, each	15	0.5	3
Collard & Bowser, Eng. Toffee (2)	80	4	12
Conversation Hearts (Necco), 1 lge	10	0	4
Cote d'Or: Bouchee, each	130	8	12
Chokotoff, each	210	9	30
Nougatti	150	8	19
Bar & Nuts, 1.3 oz	220	18	12
Cotton Candy, 1 oz	110	0	28
Cough Drops: See Page 131			
Cracker Jack, ½ cup, 1 oz	120	2	23
Creme Savers: See Lifesavers			
Crisped Rice: Almond, 1 bar	130	6	18
Choc Chip, 1 bar	115	4	18
Crows, 12 pieces, 1.5 oz	140	0	35
Crunch: 5 oz bar	680	36	96
King Munch, 2.75 oz bar	380	20	52
1.55 oz bar	220	22	30
Fun size, each	90	4.5	13
King Kong, 3½ oz	480	24	66
w. Caramel: 1.52 oz	200	10	28
King Size, 2.7 oz	370	19	51
Minis, 6 pces, 37g	180	9	25
Pieces, ⅓ cup	180	8	26
White Bar, 1.4 oz bar	220	13	23
Stix, avg., 1 stick	90	6	12
Sugar Free, 4 bars	170	13	21
Dots, 12 dots, 1.5 oz	140	0	35
Double Dip Stick, 1 stick	16	0.5	3
Dove: Promises, 5 pieces, avg.	220	13	24
Single: 1 bar, 1.3 oz	200	12	22
Dark Choc, avg., 1.3 oz	190	12	22
w. Caramel, 5 pieces	220	11	24
Milk/Rich Dark Bar, 5 pces	200	12	24
Choc-covered Almonds, 13 pces	215	15	19
Dum Dum Pops (Spangler), 1 pop	25	0	5
Endulge (Atkins): Per Serving			
Caramel Nut Chew Bar, 34g	140	7	14
Peanut Caramel Cluster, 34g	110	6	9
Advantage: Original, avg., 60g	230	10	22
Caramel, avg., 44g	160	8	17
English Toffee, 1 pce	48	3	5
Eda's Sugar Free, all flav., 5, ½ oz	40	0	15

Candy, Chocolate (Cont)

Brands & Generic (Cont)

Per Piece/Serving	C	F	Cb
5th Avenue: 2 oz bar	270	13	35
King Size bar	480	24	60
Snack Size, 0.58 oz	80	4	10
Fanny May: Single Wrapped Pieces			
Mint Meltaway Patty, 3 pces, 40g	230	15	30
Pixie, 2 pces, 45g	240	14	26
Trinidad, 1 pce, 42.5g	310	12	25
Fast Break (Reese's): 2 oz bar	270	13	34
King Size	480	24	60
Ferrero Rocher: each	75	5	6
3 pces, 1.3 oz	220	15	17
Fifty 50 Snack Bars:			
Peanut Butter, 2	190	14	17
Almond Choc., 7 pce, 1½ oz	200	17	18
Crunch Choc., 7 pce, 1.1 oz	190	16	19
Dark Choc, 40g	170	14	21
Milk Choc., 3 pce, ½ bar, 43g	190	16	19
Mini Bars, 8 bars, 1 oz	140	9	16
Fluffy Stuff (Charms), 0.6 oz bag	70	0	17
Fondant: Choc-coated, 1.2 oz	120	3	27
Mint, 1 oz	105	0	27
Fran's: Gold Bar, 45g	250	14	17
Gold Bites (Almonds), 23g	120	7	13
Frootsies, 12 pces	140	3	29
Fruit Crystals (Walgreens), 3 pces	70	0	17
Fruit Drops, each	6	0	1
Fruit Gems (Sunkist), 3, 1.2 oz	105	0	26
Fruit Leathers, average, 0.5 oz	45	0	12
Fruit Pastilles, 1 roll, 1.4 oz	100	0	26
Fruit Rolls, 1 roll	70	0	17
Fruit Roll-Ups, ½ oz	50	1	12
Fruit Runts (Walgreens), 12 pces	60	0	14
Fudge: Chocolate/Vanilla (1), 21g	90	5	13
with Nuts (1), 21g	100	6	12
Choco. Marshmallow, 1 oz	120	5	19
w. Nuts, 1 oz	115	3	19
Peanut Butter, 1 oz	115	3	19
Ghirardelli:			
Squares: Dark Choc. (4), 43g	220	17	23
Other varieties (3), 45g	215	12	28
3 oz Bars: Dark Choc., 12 pieces	440	34	46
Other varieties, avg., 12 pces	440	28	52
Intense Dark: Twilight, 3 pces	200	17	17
Other varieties, avg., 3 pces	200	15	21
Godiva: Hearts, 7 pieces, 1.4 oz	210	13	23
Bars: Milk/Dark, avg., 1½ oz	230	14	24
Extra Dark 72%, 1½ oz	230	17	18
Sugar Free Bars, avg., 1½ oz	200	15	24
Assorted Chocs: 2 pieces, 31g	160	10	17
Sugar Free, 3 pieces	200	15	23
Bouchee au Chocolate, 2 pces	220	13	23
Chocolate Pretzels, 6 pces, 1.4 oz	200	10	26

Per Piece/Serving	C	F	Cb
Go Lightly: Box Candies, 2-3 pces	220	16	28
Bags: Assorted Taffy, 5 pieces	130	3	36
Vanilla Caramels, 5	150	6	31
Super Free Creme Crunch (4)	150	5	33
Goobers Peanuts, 1 pkg, 1.4 oz	200	13	21
Good & Plenty (Hershey's): 50g	170	0	43
Snack Size, 1 box, 17g	60	0	14
GooGoo Cluster, 1 bar, 1.75 oz	240	11	32
Gum Drops: 1 small, 9g	10	0	7.5
5 pces, 44g	150	0	37
Gummi Bears, 9 bears, 42g	120	0	29
Gummi Novelties (Walgreens), 6	120	0	22
Gummi Savers, 10 pieces	120	0	30
Gummi Sweet Tarts, 1 bug, 1.5 oz	150	0	34
Gummi Watch, 1	105	0	24
Gummi Worms (1), 8g	25	0	6
Guylian: Milk Choc., 8 squares, 1 oz	120	9	16
Dark Choc., 8 squares, 1 oz	130	9	16
Guylian Twists, 4 pces, 35g	200	3	17
Halvah (Joyvah): Plain, ½ bar, 2 oz	390	25	18
Choc.coated Sesame, ½ bar, 2 oz	380	23	20
Hard Candy: All flavors, 16g	60	0	15
1 regular piece	20	0	5
Heath: Original, 39g	220	12	24
Bites, 15 pces, 39g	210	12	24
King Size, 2.8 oz	430	25	49
Minis, 6 pces	240	14	27
Hershey's:			
Milk Chocolate: 1.55 oz bar	230	13	25
Cookies 'n' Creme, 1.55 oz bar	230	12	25
Snack, 0.6 oz	90	5	10
Kingsize, 2.6 oz bar	400	23	42
7 oz bar, ⅛ bar	200	12	21
w. Almonds, 1.45 oz bar	220	14	20
w. Almonds King Size	400	23	40
Crisp Bits, 5 squares, 40g	200	10	25
Bites, York (15)	160	3	33
Cacao Reserve:			
Milk Choc. (35% cacao), 1.8 oz	310	22	25
Dark Choc. (65% cacao), 1.8 oz	290	22	23
Candy-Coated Eggs:			
Milk Choc (4), 0.6 oz	90	4	12
w. Almonds (4) 0.6 oz	100	6	9
Extra Dark, avg. all var., 4 pces	210	13	21
Hugs: Regular (1), 4.5g	25	1.5	2.5
Regular (9), 40g	210	12	23
w. Almonds (9), 40g	230	14	21
Kissables: Avg. all var., 39 pces	205	10	28
Snack Size, 13g	65	3	9
Kisses, avg. all var. (1)	25	1.5	3
Miniatures: 5 pces, 1.5 oz	230	13	26
Kisses, 1 bag	420	24	44
Nuggets Snack, 4 pces	215	13	22

Brands & Generic (Cont)

Per Piece/Serving	C	F	Cb
Hershey's (Cont):			
Pot of Gold Chocolate:			
Nut Clusters, avg. all, 3 pieces	245	15	24
Nut Assortment, 1.5 oz	140	7	21
Caramel Assortment, 1.5 oz	200	9	28
Creme Assortment, 1.5 oz	170	4	32
Mint Assortment, 1.5 oz	200	10	26
Truffle Assortment, 1.5 oz	200	9	27
Sugar Free Assortment, 1.5 oz	180	16	22
Smart Zone, avg. all varieties, 50g	205	7	24
Snack Barz	115	5	17
Special Dark Choc.: 1.45 oz bar	220	13	24
King Size, 72g	400	22	44
Snack Size, 14g	70	4.5	9
Sticks, avg. all varieties, 11g	60	3	7
Swoops, avg., 1 pce, 1.26 oz	190	11	20
Whoppers, 10 pieces	100	3.5	16
Sugar Free: Choc. Candy (5)	170	13	28
Dark Chocolate Candy (5)	190	15	23
Chocolate w. Almonds (5)	180	14	23
Peanut Butter Cups Minis (5)	170	12	24
York Peppermint Patties, 3 pces	110	45	28
Honeycomb: Plain, 1 oz	115	0	27
Choc-coated, 2 pces	180	7	31
Hot Tamales: 1 box, 60g, 2.1 oz	220	0	55
Sathers, 20 pces, 1.4 oz	150	0	36
Ice Blue Mints (Walgreens), 3, 17g	70	0	17
Jawbreakers (Sathers), 15, 17g	70	0	17
Jellies, 3 medium, 1 oz	130	0	33
Jells Raspberry (Joyva), 3 pces, 44g	160	0	38
Jelly Beans: Small, 22 beans, 1 oz	100	0	24
Regular, 13 beans, 40g	150	0	37
1 bean	10	0	3
Sugar Free, 35 beans	110	0	36
Jumbo, 1 bean	20	0	5
Jewel, 13 beans, 1.4 oz	140	0	36
Sathers/Walgreens, 13 pces	150	0	37
Wonderbeans, 33 beans	100	0	24
Jelly Bellys: each	4	0	1
35 pces, 1.4 oz	140	0	37
Sugar Free Beans/Sours (37), 1.4 oz	100	0	36
Sugar Free Fruit Slices, 8 pces, 1.4 oz	60	0	30
Jelly Rings (Jewel), 5 pces, 42g	120	0	30
Jolly Rancher: Candy (3)	70	0	17
Fruit Chews (6), 1.4 oz	150	1.5	33
Gummies, 10 pces, 39g	120	0	29
Hard Candy (3), 18g	70	0	17
Lollipops, 1 pce, 0.6 oz	60	0	16
Sugar Free, 4 pces, 0.5 oz	35	0	13
Junior Caramels: 13 pces, 42g	190	6	33
Mini, 2 boxes, 24g	110	3	19

Per Piece/Serving	C	F	Cb
Junior Mints: 52g box	220	4	45
16 pces, 1.4 oz	170	3	35
Juicefuls: Red Raspb., (3), 0.6 oz	60	0	15
Assorted Fruits, 1 pce	20	0	5
Jujubes, all types (55), 40g	110	0	28
Juju Bears, 5 pces	130	0	34
Juju Mix (Sathers), 11 pce, 1½ oz	150	0	36
Jujyfruits, 16 pces, 40g	120	0	32
Kit Kat: 1.5 oz bar	220	11	27
Big Kat, 1.94 oz	290	15	35
Bites, 15 pces, 39g	200	10	25
Caramel Bar (1)	210	10	26
Extra Krispy Bar (1)	240	12	29
King Size, 3 oz bar	440	22	54
Miniature, 5 pces	230	12	27
Multipack/Snack Bar (3), 42g	220	11	27
Triple Choc Snack Bar (1), 14g	75	4	9
White Choc Bar, 1½ oz	220	12	26
Minis, 5 pces	230	12	27
Krackel: 42g bar	210	11	26
Snack size, 0.6 oz	85	4.5	17
Kraft: Caramels, (5), 40g	160	3.5	30
Kudos: See Page 139			
Lance: Peanut Bar, 1.8 oz pkg	240	14	22
Lemon Drops (3) ½ oz	50	0	14
Sugar Free (Walgreens), 4, 13g	25	0	13
Lemonhead, 10, ½ oz	50	0	14
Licorice: Average all types, 1oz	100	0	25
Bites (Switzer), each	10	0	3
Chews (Panda), each	10	0	3
Tid Bits, each	5	0	1
Twists: Black/Red, avg. 1 pce	35	0	8.5
Sugar Free, 1 pce	13	0	2.5
American Licorice Co.: Laces, 1	35	0	8
Jumbo Rope, 2 pces	140	0	34
Red Bites, 1.4 oz	140	0	33
Snaps, 31 pces, 40g	140	0.5	33
Stick, (1) 0.5 oz	35	0	8.5
Super Red Ropes (1), 66g	240	0	54
Superstring, 1⅓ pces	140	0	34
Vines, 2 pces	70	0	17
Sugar Free Red Twists (7)	90	0	25
Lifesavers: Large size, 1 candy	15	0	3.5
Regular, all flavors, 1 candy	10	0	2.5
1 Roll (14 candies), 1.14 oz	140	0	35
Creme Savers: 3 pces	60	0	11
Sugar Free, 4 pces	35	0	14
Gummi Savers (10), 39g	130	0	30
Fruit Lollipops (1), 0.4 oz	40	0	10
Peppermint (4)	60	0	15
Fruit Splosion, 10 pces	130	0	30
Sugar-Free Delites: Per Candy			
Orchard Fruits; Summer Blend	7	0	2.5
Butter Toffee; European Collect.	10	1	2.5

Brands & Generic (Cont)

Per Piece/Serving	C	F	Cb
Lik-m-aid (Nestlé), Wonka Fun Dip, 1 pkg	50	0	13
Lindt: Lindor, Balls, average (1)	75	6	5
Milk Chocolate, 12 pces, 40g	230	16	18
Truffles (3)	220	17	16
Lollipops, each, 11g	45	0	11
Look! Bar, 1.5 oz	190	6	33
M & M's: Plain, 1.7 oz pkg	235	10	34
Milk Chocolate, 1 pce	5	0.1	0.5
20 pces, 0.6 oz	70	3	10
¼ cup, 1.8 oz	255	11	37
Dark Choc.: 3.14 oz pkg	440	20	60
Fun Size, 18g pkg	90	4	13
Almond Choc., 1.3 oz pkg	190	10	22
Crispy, 1.6 oz	225	9	34
Minis, Mega Tube, 1.1 oz tube	150	7	21
Mega: Milk Choc (27), 1.5 oz	210	9	30
Peanut (12), 1.4 oz	210	11	24
Peanut: 1.92 oz pkg	280	14	33
Fun Size, 18g pkg	90	4.5	11
Peanut Butter 1.6 oz pkg	245	14	26
Mamba, 9 pces, 1½ oz	170	2.5	36
Marathon (Snickers) Bar, 1.9 oz	220	7	26
M.Azing: 1 bar, 1.5 oz	230	12	27
Peanut Butter (1), 1.5 oz	230	13	25
Marshmallow Egg, 1 egg, 1 oz	120	3	22
Marshmallows: Firm/Soft, 1 oz	90	0	23
Regular size, 4 pces, 33g	100	0	24
Mini-Marshmallow, ⅔ c., 30g	100	0	24
Choc-coat. Twists (Joyva), each	95	2	10
Fluff, 2 Tbsp, 18 g	60	0	15
Kraft: Mini, ½ cup, 30g	100	0	24
Creme, 2 Tbsp	45	0	11
Jet-Puffed, 5 pces, 30g	100	0	24
Funmallows, ⅔ cup, 30g	100	0	24
Miniature, ⅔ cup, 30g	100	0	24
Marzipan, 2 Tbsp, 39g	160	4	29
Mauna Loa: Choc., 50g	280	19	24
Choc. coated Macadamias 57g	220	15	19
Mexican Hats (7), 38g	120	0	30
Mentos: Regular (1)	10	0	3
Sugar Free (1)	5	0	2.5
Mike & Ike: 1 pkg, 1.1 oz	120	0	28
23 pces, 40g	140	0	36
Milkfulls (Storck), 6 pces, 1.4 oz	170	3	35
Milk Chocolate: *See Hershey's*			
Milk Duds (Hershey's), 13 pces	180	7	28

Per Piece/Serving	C	F	Cb
Milky Way: Midnight Bar, 1.75 oz	225	10	33
Regular Bar, 58g	250	10	41
Fun size, 2 bars, 34g	150	6	24
Milky Way To Go, 51g	230	9	36
Miniatures: (5) 32g	205	9	30
Midnight Minis (5), 41g	190	7	29
Pop'ables (13) 39g	180	7	28
Mints: Uncoated, 7 pces	60	0	17
1 small mint (¾" diam.)	4	0	1
1 large mint (1½" diam.)	10	0	2
Mon Cheri (Ferrero), 4 pces, 45g	260	18	20
Mounds: 49g bar	240	13	31
Snack, 0.68 oz	90	5	11
King Size, 3½ oz bar	490	26	58
Minis, 41g	200	11	24
Mr Goodbar: 48g bar	270	16	27
King Size, 2.6 oz bar	400	24	40
Snack, 17g	80	4.5	10
Bites (25), 40g	230	14	21
Mrs Fields Choc, 2 pieces, 33g	160	8	22
Necco Candy Wafers (40) 57g	220	0	56
Nestle Toll House, 1 pce, 1 oz	120	5	18
Neuhaus, average all types	80	5	7
Newman's Own:			
Caramel Cups, 3 pces, 1.2 oz	160	9	21
P'Nut B. Cups (Milk/Dark), 3, 1 pkg	180	12	19
Sweet Dark Choc Bar, 79g	400	26	48
Nibs, all types, 1 pouch, 63g	215	2	49
Nips (Nestle), all flavors, 2, 14g	60	2	11
Nite Bite (Glucose Bar)	100	3.5	15
Nougat, 3 pces, 1 oz	150	2.5	32
Chocolate Covered, 1 oz	125	4	22
Now & Later (Nabisco), 9, 41g	120	1	29
Nutrageous Bar (Reese's): 51g	280	16	27
King Size, 3.4 oz bar	500	30	32
Oh Henry! 2 oz bar	265	13	37
100 Grand: 1.5 oz bar	180	8	29
King Size, 2.8 oz bar	350	14	57
Snack Size, 2 bars, 43g	180	8	29
Orange (Lindt), 5 slices	230	14	23
Orange Slices: Jewel, 3, 42g	140	0	35
Walgreens, 3, 43g	150	0	36
Pastel Mints (Walgreens), 20 pces	60	0	14
Patteez (Sweet n' Low), 4 pces	100	2	29
PayDay Bar: 51g	240	11	30
King Size, 3.4 oz bar	480	24	52
Snack Size, 0.7 oz bar	90	5	10
Avalanche, 1.8 oz bar	250	13	29
Avalanche King, 3.1 oz bar	440	24	50
Peanut Bar, 1.6 oz bar	210	14	20
Peanut Butter Cups: *See Reese's; Newman's Own*			

Brands & Generic (Cont)

Per Piece/Serving	C	F	Cb
Peanut Brittle: 1 peace, 1½ oz	220	15	20
Sugar Free (Judy's), ¾ cup, 1 oz	100	6	12
Peanuts, choc-covered, 15 pces	210	12	23
Pearson's Mint Patties, (5), 38g	150	2.5	31
Pecan Roll, ⅓ bar, 40g	190	10	24
Peppermints, 7 small, 0.5 oz	60	0	15
Brach's, 3 pces	60	0	15
Peppermint Twists (2), 14g	60	0	14
Pez, 1 roll	35	0	9
Planters: Choc. Peanuts (25) 7 oz	220	13	20
Orig. Peanut Bar, 1.6 oz	230	14	22
Hersheys, 2½ oz	390	24	34
Pop'ables: Average, 13 pces, 1½ oz	180	7	29
4.9 oz Package	630	25	101
Poprocks, 9½ g pkg	35	0	9
Pralines: Small, 0.3 oz	38	2	5
1 large piece, 1.4 oz	180	10	24
Pretzels: Choc-covered,			
Minisize (6), 38g	190	9	24
White Choc Bites (23), 40g	200	9	25
Pretzel Flipz (Nestlé), 8 pces, 1 oz	130	5	20
Raisinets: 1 pkg, 1.7 oz	205	8	34
King Size, 2.8 oz	330	13	56
Dark Raisinets, ¼ cup, 45g	130	8	32
Raspberry Cream, 2 pces, 36g	155	5	25
Reception Sticks (4)	65	2	12
Red Raspberry Dollars (10)	130	0	31
Reese's			
Peanut Butter Cups: 1½ oz	230	13	23
King size, 2.8 oz	420	24	44
Mini, 5 pces, 39g	210	12	22
Snack size, 1 pce, 21g	110	6	12
Sugar free, 2 pces, avg., 39g	170	12	24
Caramel filled, 1.4 oz	190	10	24
Big Cups: Original, 1.4 oz	210	12	21
w. Nuts: 1.4 oz	220	13	20
King size, 2.8 oz	430	26	41
w. Caramel & Nuts, 1.3 oz	190	10	21
Bites, 16 pces, 40g	220	12	23
Elvis P'nut Butter & Banana Cup, 1.4 oz	200	11	24
Reeses Pieces: 25 pces, 1.6 oz	230	11	28
King size, 3 oz	400	20	46
Reeses Sticks: 1.5 oz	230	13	23
King size, 3 oz	460	26	46
Snack size, 17g	90	5	9
Nutrageous Bar: 1.8 oz bar	280	16	27
King size, 3.4 oz bar	520	30	52
Crispy Crunchy Bar: 1.7 oz bar	260	15	26
King Size, 3.1 oz bar	480	28	48
Fast Break, 2 oz bar	280	14	34
King Size	480	24	60
Swoops, 1 cup, 1.26 oz	190	11	17
Baking Chips, 1 Tbsp, 15g	80	4.5	9

Per Piece/Serving	C	F	Cb
Rice Krispies Treats (Kellogg's):			
1 bar, average all varieties	110	3.5	19
Rice Crunchy Bars, 19g bar	70	0.5	15
Riesen: Choc. Chew, 4 pces, 36g	170	6	28
Ritter Sport, w. Hazelnuts (6), 37.5g	210	14	19
Rocky Road, 1.8 oz bar	240	11	34
Robin Eggs, Large (2); Mini (10)	100	3.5	16
Rolo: All types (3), 0.64 oz	85	4	12
Mini Bites, 19 pieces, 1.4 oz	190	9	26
Root Beer Barrels (3) 0.5 oz	70	0	17
Ross Chocolate Bar: White, 1.2 oz	180	13	19
Almond; Crunchy, 1.2 oz	180	13	18
Russell Stover Candy: Creams (1)	65	3	11
Almond Delight, 15 pces	220	18	15
Chocolate Asst., 2 pces	140	6	21
Choc-covered Nuts, 3 pces	230	16	17
Cherry Blimps, 3 pces	170	5	24
Sugar Free: Mint Cremes (3)	190	14	22
Mint Patties, 3 pces	180	11	27
Pecan Delight (2), 1 oz	130	9	5
Cups (3), 1.2 oz	170	13	16
Mint Patties, 3 pces	180	11	27
Salt Water Taffy (Brach's), 5	170	2.5	36
Seashells (Guylian), 1 shell	70	4.5	6
See's Candies: Average all Flavors			
Assorted Candy, 4 pces	210	11	28
Caramels & Chews, 2 pieces	175	10	19
Creams, 2 pieces	180	9	24
Little Pops, 4 pieces	55	2	10
Lollypops (1), 20g	80	3	15
Nut Clusters, 3 pieces	225	16	16
Sesame Crunch, 3 pces	80	4	7
Signature Treasures (Nestlé):			
Choc. Creme, 3 pieces, 1.2 oz	170	9	21
Creamy Caramel, 3 pieces, 1.3 oz	170	9	23
Dark Choc Caramel, 3 pieces	160	10	22
Milk Choc Caramel, 3 pieces	170	9	23
Peanut Butter, 3 pieces	180	12	20
Simply Lite, ½ ctn, 36 pieces	130	5	18
Simply Sugar Free: See Allen Wertz			
Sixlets (Hershey), 24 pces	90	3.5	14
Skittles: Sour, 1.8 oz bag	200	2	44
Orig./Trop./Wild Berry, 2.17 oz	250	2.5	54
Fun Size, 1 bag, 15g	60	1	14
King Size, 4 oz bag	440	4.5	102
Large bag (16 oz), ¼ cup, 1.5 oz	170	2	39
Skor Toffee Bar, 1.4 oz	210	12	24
Smarties: Candy Rolls, 1 roll	25	0	6
Giant, 2 pces, 7g	25	0	5
Smores (Hershey), 1.65 oz	240	11	31

Brands & Generic (Cont)

Per Piece/Serving	C	F	Cb
Snickers: 2.07 oz bar	280	14	35
3.7 oz bar	510	24	63
Creme Egg (1), 1.2 oz	170	10	20
King Size, ⅓ bar, 1.2 oz	170	8	21
Miniatures, 4 pieces	170	1	22
Munch Bar, 1.4 oz bar	220	15	18
Pop'ables, 13 pieces, 1½ oz	190	9	24
Cruncher, 1.56 oz	220	11	24
Cruncher To Go, 2.54 oz	350	18	45
Marathon Bar: avg., 1.9 oz bar	210	8	26
King size	440	22	60
Almond, 1.76 oz	230	11	32
Fun Size, 2 bars, 34g	160	8	21
Sno Caps, ¼ cup, 40g	180	8	30
Soft 'N Chewy Butter Toffee, ea.	30	0.5	5
Sorbee: Choc., ½ bar, 40g	200	14	20
Gummie Bears, 16 pces	120	0	30
Peanut Butter, 4 pces	210	15	19
Sour Brite Crawlers, 13 pces	140	0	31
Sour Punch: All types, 2 oz	200	1.5	46
1 straw	20	0	5
Spearmint Leaves: Jewel, 5, 40g	140	0	35
Walgreens, 4 pieces, 46g	160	0	39
Spice Drops, 12 pces, 39g	130	0	33
Spree Candies: Original, 15 pces	50	0	13
Chewy Spree, 8 pces	60	0	13
Starburst: Candy Canes, 0.5 oz	70	0	18
Fruit Chews, each	20	0.4	4
2 oz pkg	240	5	48
Jellybeans, 1.5 oz	160	0	39
Jellybean Egg, 2 oz	200	0	51
Tropical Fruit, 2.07 oz pack	240	5	49
Starlight Mints, 3 pces, 16g	60	0	15
Suckers (Walgreens), 1 sucker, 11g	45	0	11
Sugar Babies, 30 pces, 40g	180	1.5	41
Sugar Coated Peanuts, 1 oz	120	8	10
Sunbursts Sunflowers (Kimmie):			
Candy Bar Bag, 1.3 oz	145	6.5	21
Coffee Break Tube, 3 oz	330	15	48
Snack Size Bag, 10g	40	2	3.5
Sweet 'N Low: Chews, each	20	0.5	4
Coffee Cremes (1)	40	3	6
Wafer Bars, avg., 3 pieces	140	7	13
Mint Cremes, 3½ pces	120	9	22
Mint Patteez, 4 pces	100	2	29
Sweet Escapes: See Hershey's			
Sweet Tarts (Nestlé), 5 pces, ½ oz	50	0	13
Symphony: 1.5 oz bar	230	14	24
Snack: Chocolate (1), 0.6 oz	90	5	10
w. Almds & Toffee (1), .5 oz	230	14	23

Per Piece/Serving	C	F	Cb
Taffy, 1 pce, 23g	80	1	19
Take 5 (Hershey's): 1.5 oz bar	210	10	26
King Size, 2.25 oz bar	320	16	38
Marshmallow, 1.5 oz bar	180	9	22
Peanut Butter, 1.5 oz bar	220	11	23
Toffifay, 5 pieces	200	11	25
3 Musketeers: 2.13 oz bar	260	8	46
Fun size, 3 pieces	190	6	34
Miniatures, 7 pieces	170	5	32
Pop'ables (15)	180	6	31
Tang-a-Roos, 1 roll	25	0	6
Terry's Choc Orange, (5), 1.5 oz	230	12	27
Tic Tac, all varieties, each	2	0	0
Toblerone: 50g (1.76 oz) bar	255	15	30
1 bar, 100g (3.5 oz)	510	30	60
⅓ bar, 33g	170	10	20
Mini, 3 pces	200	11	24
Toffees, Regular, 1 oz	160	9	18
Toll House Bars, 1 piece, 1 oz	120	5	18
Tootsie Pops, Mini (3), 24g	90	0	23
Tootsie Roll, 2.25 oz roll	245	2	55
Trolli: Gummies, 18 pieces, 40g	110	0	26
Cherry Bombers, 10 pieces	130	0	31
Truffles: Regular, 1 pce, 12g	60	4	6
Large (Godiva), 0.75 oz	110	6.5	12
Extra Large (J.Schmidt), 1½ oz	220	13	24
Turtles (Nestlé): Avg., each	80	4.5	10
Sugar Free, 3 pieces, 38g	150	11	20
Twists (Sugar Free): Licorice; Strawberry,			
7 twists, 40g	90	0	25
Twix: 2 oz pkg	280	14	37
King Size, 3 oz pkg	405	20	52
Fun Size, 0.5 oz	80	4	10
Twix To Go	480	24	64
Minis, 3 pces, 29g	150	7	19
Caramel, 24g	130	6	16
Peanut Butter To Go	480	28	48
Peanut Butter, 1.8 oz	280	17	28
Twizzlers: Twists, 3 pieces, 38g	130	0.5	30
Bites (17), 40g	140	0.5	32
Pull 'n' Peel Cherry, 62g	210	1	47
Swedish Fish, 51g	180	0	46
Sugar Free, 3 pieces	130	1	33
Uno Bar (1), 42g	250	17	22
Velamints Sugar Free, 2 pce	5	0	1
Weight Watchers/Whitmans:			
Butter Cream Caramel, 3 pces	150	8	23
Caramel Medallions, 3 pces	150	9	26
English Toffee Squares, 3 pces	160	10	23
Mint Patties, 3 pces	150	9	24
Peanut Butter Crunch, 4 pces	180	8	31
Pecan Crowns, 3 pces	150	9	22

Brands & Generic (Cont)

Per Piece/Serving	C	F	Cb
Werther's: Original, 3 pce, 15g	60	1	13
Chewy Caramel (6), 37g	170	5	30
Caramelts (8), 40g	250	18	18
Sugar-Free, 5 pieces	40	1	14
Whatchamacallit Bar, 1.7 oz	240	11	30
King Size, 2.6 oz	370	18	46
Whitman's: Pecan Roll, 2 oz roll	300	20	26
Sampler, 3 pces, 1.4 oz	200	9	28
Assorted; Dark Chocolate, 3 pces	220	12	26
Snoopy Treats, 2 pces	190	10	24
Sucratrol Mint Pattie, 1 oz	120	7	17
Whoppers, 9 pces, 21g	100	3.5	16
Wonka: Wonka Bar (1), 1.3 oz	180	10	25
Laffy Taffy: Orig., 5 bars, 1.5 oz	160	2	36
Stretchy & Tangy, 1½ oz	165	4	33
Nerds, 1 box	240	0	42
Gobstopper: Box, 1.77 oz	650	0	182
Everlasting/Chewy, 9 pces, 15g	50	0	14
Runts Fruit Box, 1.8 oz	210	0	49
Yogurt Candy,			
Coated Raisins, 27 pces, 40g	180	8	28
York Mints: 1.37 oz patty	160	3	32
Snack size, 0.5 oz	55	1	11
Peppermint Patties (3)	160	3	33
King Size (3), 2.86 oz	320	6	66
Sugar Free, Mini (3)	110	4.5	28
Swoops, 1 cup, 1.26 oz	190	11	21
Zachary Old Fashioned Drops, 1 oz	100	0	26
Zagnut, 1.75 oz bar	230	10	31
Zero Bar: 52g	240	9	36
King Size, 3.4 oz	420	16	66
Zingos, 3 pce, 2g	5	0	2

Gum ~ Per Piece

	C	F	Cb
Bazooka, each	15	0	4
Beechies	6	0	2
Big League Chew	10	0	2
Bubble Yum	25	0	6
Sugarless	10	0	3
Candilicious	30	0	2
Carefree (Sugarless/Regular)	5	0	2
Chiclets, 1 piece	5	0	1
Clorets, 1 stick	10	0	2
Dentyne	5	0	0.5
Estee, bubble/regular	5	0	2
Extra (Wrigley's), Sugar-Free (1)	5	0	2
Freshen-Up	10	0	3
Hubba Bubba: Regular	23	0	6
Sugar-free, average	14	0	0.5
Ice Breakers, 12 pieces	0	0	0
Sonic Boom Bubble Gum	15	0	3
Sticklets	7	0	2
Super Bubble	15	0	4
Trident, Original; White	5	0	1
Wrigley's, all flavors	10	0	2

Carob Candy

Per Piece/Serving	C	F	Cb
Carob: Plain/Natural, 1 oz	160	11	9
Carob Coated: Raisins, 1 oz	130	8	15
Almonds/Peanuts, 1 oz	150	10	14
Malt Balls, 1 oz	135	8	15
Caramels, 1 oz	110	4	18
Dates, 1 oz	125	5	19
Soybeans	145	9	16
Trail/Party Mix, 1 oz	140	9	15
Carob Chips, unsweetened, 1 oz	140	7	19
Carob Bars: Plain/Nut, 1 oz	160	11	13
Fruit & Nut, 1 oz	155	10	13
Mint/Orange, 1 oz	160	11	14
Carafection: Cashew Coconut Crunch, ½ Bar, (42g) 1.5 oz	250	14	5
Caroby Natural Touch, 3 oz	450	27	36

Cough Drops

	C	F	Cb
Beech Nut, 1 drop	10	0	2
Diabetic Tussin, 1 drop	0	0	0
Halls Defense Vit. C, 1 drop	15	0	4
Halls Fruit Breezers, 1 drop	15	0	4
Halls Menthol Drops, 1 drop	15	0	4
Sugar Free, 1 drop	5	0	4
Halls Plus, 1 drop	20	0	5
Helps Cough, all flavors, 1	15	0	4
Listerine Lozenge (Amer. Chicle)	10	0	2
Luden's Throat Drops, all flavors, 1	10	0	2
Sugar Free, 1 drop	0	0	0
Pine Bros, 1 cough drop	10	0	2
Ricola: Cough Drops, 1 drop	10	0	3
Sugar-Free Lemon Mint, 2 mints	0	0	1
Rite Aid, Menthol Cough, 1 drop	10	0	3
Robitussin: Regular, 1 drop	15	0	3
Honey Cough, 1 drop	40	0	10
Sugar Free Throat, 1 drop	10	0	3
Sunny Orange Vit. C, 1 drop	15	0	3
Rolaids/Sodium Free, 1	5	0	1
Sathers Peppermint Lozenges, 1	15	0	3
Squibb Cough/Throat Loz.'s, 1	15	0	4
Sucrets (Beecham) Lozenges, 1	10	0	2
Wintergreen Loz. (Walgreens), 1	15	0	3
Cough Suppresant Liquids: See Page 142			

Popcorn

Home-Popped Popcorn

	C	**F**	**Cb**
Popping Corn Kernels:			
2 Tbsp, 1 oz	110	1	26
(makes approx. 5 cups)			
Air-popped (no oil), plain, 1 oz	110	1	22
1 cup (6g)	20	0	5
Oil-popped, plain, 1 oz	145	8	16
1 cup (11g)	55	3	6
Popcorn Oil, 1 Tbsp	120	14	0

Microwave Popcorn

	C	**F**	**Cb**
Average All Brands (Popped)			
Butter: Regular, 1 cup	35	2	4
Light, 1 cup	25	1	4
Act II Popcorn:			
Butter, 1 cup, 0.3 oz	30	2	4
5 cups, popped, 1 oz	160	10	18
Light Butter, 1 cup, 0.2 oz	25	1	4
5 cups, popped, 1 oz	110	4.5	19
Butter Lovers,1 cup, 0.3 oz	35	2.5	4
4½ cups, 1 oz	170	12	16
94% Fat-Free Butter, 1 cup	30	1.5	4.5
4½ cups, 1 oz	130	2.5	28
American Fare (K-Mart):			
Butter, 1 cup, 0.3 oz	40	2	5
3 cups, 1 oz	120	2	23
Theater Butter, 1 cup	40	2	5
3.5 cups	140	8	15
Jolly Time: America's Best, 1 cup	20	0	5
Blast O Butter: Regular, 1 cup	45	3	4
Light, 1 cup	30	1.5	4
Caramel Apple Healthy Pop, 5 c.110		2	23
Healthy Pop, 1 cup	20	0	4
Kettle Mania, 1 cup	45	3	4
Mallow Magic, 1 cup	60	5	4
Newman's Own: Butter, 1 oz	130	5	18
Light Butter Flavor, 3½ cups	120	4	19
Orville Redenbacher's: *Popped*			
Movie Theater Butter, 1 cup	30	2.5	4
4½ cups, popped, 1 oz	170	12	16
Smart Pop!: Butter, 7 cups	120	2	25
Mini Bags, 6 cups	100	2	24
Tender White, 6½ cups	130	2.5	28
Pop Secret Popcorn: *Popped*			
94% Fat Free, 6 cups	120	2	26
Jumbo Pop Butter, all types, 3½ cups	180	11	18
Light Butter, 6 cups	120	4.5	20
Movie Theater Butter, 4 cups	180	13	17
One-Step, 4 cups	180	13	17
Other varieties, avg., 4 cups	170	12	17
Smart Balance: 1 cup	20	0	6
5 cups	120	2	4

Bagged Popcorn

	C	**F**	**Cb**
Average All Brands (Ready-to-Eat)			
Regular: Plain, ½ oz pkg	80	5	8
1 oz pkg	160	10	16
4 oz pkg	640	40	64
Box (store/airport), 2 oz	320	16	32
Bag (9" high x 5" wide), 3 oz	480	24	48

Brands ~ Bagged Popcorn

	C	**F**	**Cb**
Boston's: Fat Free, ⅔ cup, 1 oz	100	0	23
Lite, 2 cup, 1 oz	140	6	19
Gourmet Super Prem., 2 c., 1 oz	160	11	13
40% Less Fat, 2¾ cup, 1 oz	140	6	17
Cracker Jack: Original, ½ c., 1 oz	120	2	23
Crunch 'N Munch: ½ cup, 1 oz	140	5	23
Buttery Toffee, ⅔ cup, 1 oz	150	6	23
Caramel w. P'nuts, ⅔ cup, 1.2 oz	140	5	22
Fiddle Faddle: Caramel, ⅔ c., 1 oz	120	3.5	22
Butter Toffee, ⅔ cup	120	4	22
Henry's			
Herb, 2½ cups	160	10	15
Kettle Corn, 2 cups	120	1.5	27
Lightly Salted, 2½ cups	160	5	21
White Cheddar, 2½ cups	170	12	14
Jay's: Fat Free Caramel Corn, ¾ cup	110	0	26
Korn Krunch: *(Kornfections Treasures):*			
Almond Pecan (Sugar Free), 1 oz	150	8	19
Orville Redenbacher:			
Popcorn Cakes, Minis, avg. (8) ½ oz	60	1	11
Drizzles, avg., ⅔ cup, 1 oz	150	7	22
Poppycock: Pecan Delight, ½ cup	140	8	12
Just the Nuts, ½ cup	160	8	20
Wild Oats, all types, 2.5 cup, 1 oz	160	5	21

Movie Theater Popcorn

	C	**F**	**Cb**
Small (7 cups): Plain	385	21	44
with Butter (3 pumps, ¾ oz)	570	42	44
Medium (15 cups): Plain	825	45	94
with Butter (4 pumps, 1 oz)	1075	73	94
Large (20 cups): Plain	1100	60	124
with Butter (6 pumps, 1½ oz)	1485	102	124
Butter: 1 Pump, ¼ oz	65	7	0
4 Pumps (2 Tbsp), 1 oz	250	28	0

Potato Chips, Pretzels, Tortilla Chips

Potato Chips/Crisps

Average All Brands	**C**	**F**	**Cb**
Regular:		
Plain or flavored, 2 chips	**15**	**1**	**1.5**
1 oz pkg (20 chips)	**150**	**10**	**15**
4 oz quantity	**600**	**40**	**60**
14 oz pkg	**2100**	**140**	**210**
Brands: *Lay's* Stax, avg. all, 1 oz	**150**	**9**	**16**
Pringles: 14 crisps, 1 oz	**160**	**11**	**14**
Large, 6 oz can	**920**	**63**	**86**
Minis, 1 bag, 0.8 oz	**120**	**7**	**13**
Selects, avg., 28 chips, 1 oz	**145**	**9**	**16**
Snack Stack, 23g tub	**140**	**10**	**12**
Ruffles, 1 oz	**160**	**10**	**14**
Tim's, avg., 15 chips, 1 oz	**140**	**9**	**15**
Reduced Fat: *Pringles,* 16 Chips, 1 oz	**140**	**7**	**17**
Sun Chips; Terra, 16 chips, avg., 1 oz	**140**	**6**	**18**
Tim's, 15 chips, 1 oz		
Low-Fat/Baked, average, 1 oz	**130**	**5**	**20**
Lay's Baked!, 15 chips, 1 oz	**120**	**2**	**23**
Ruffles Baked!: 9 chips, 1 oz	**120**	**3**	**21**
Cheddar Sour Crm, 10 chips, 1 oz	**120**	**3**	**22**
Fat Free, Pringles, 15 chips, 1 oz	**70**	**0**	**15**

Corn & Tortilla Chips

Average All Brands | | |
---|---|---|---
Corn Chips: | | |
Avg. all types, 1 oz | **150** | **8** | **18**
8 oz bag | **1200** | **64** | **144**
Doritos: 13 chips, avg., 1 oz | **140** | **7** | **18**
White Nacho Cheese, 1 oz | **150** | **8** | **17**
Fritos (Sabritones), 32 Chips, 1 oz | **160** | **10** | **32**
Tortilla Chips: Average, 1 oz | **140** | **7** | **18**
(1 oz = approx. 12 chips or 13 strips) | | |
Baked! Tostitos (15) 1 oz | **120** | **3** | **22**
Doritos: 13 chips, 1 oz | **140** | **7** | **18**
Light, 13 chips, 1 oz | **100** | **2** | **19**
Baked! Nacho Cheesier, 15 chips,1 oz | **120** | **3.5** | **21**
Garden of Eatin', 1 oz | **140** | **6** | **19**
Munchies Mix, ¾ cup, 1 oz | **140** | **7** | **18**
Padrino Reduced Fat, 14 chips, 1 oz | **130** | **4** | **20**
Stacy's, Baked, Pita Chips 14 chips, 1 oz | **130** | **4** | **18**
Utz Low-Fat Baked, 10 chips, 1 oz | **120** | **2** | **23**
Wild Oats, 14 chips, 1 oz | **140** | **5** | **19**

Pretzels

Average All Brands	**C**	**F**	**Cb**
Hard Baked Pretzels		
1 oz quantity	**100**	**0**	**22**
Sticks, thin, 2¼" (9/oz), 1	**12**	**0**	**3**
Twists, thin, ¼" thick, (5/oz),1	**25**	**0**	**5**
Dutch (2¾"x 2⅝") ½ oz, 1	**55**	**1**	**11**
Sourdough (*Snyder's*), ¾ oz, each	**100**	**0**	**22**
Brands:		
American Fare, Mini Twists, 1oz	**110**	**1**	**23**
Frito-Lay, Rold Gold:		
Braided Twists (8), 1 oz	**110**	**1**	**22**
Snyders (1), avg., 1 oz	**100**	**0**	**22**
Mini (20), 1 oz	**110**	**0**	**25**
Utz Wheels/Nuggets, 1 oz	**110**	**1**	**22**
Rold Gold: Sticks (48), 1 oz	**100**	**0**	**23**
Tiny Twists/Sticks (18), 1 oz	**100**	**0**	**23**
Sourdough Hards (1), 3/4 oz	**100**	**0.5**	**21**
Thins (9), 1 oz	**110**	**1**	**23**
Twists (8), 1 oz	**110**	**1**	**22**
Choc-coated (*Snyders*), 1 oz	**130**	**6**	**18**
White Choc covered, 7 pces, 1 oz	**140**	**6**	**19**
Yogurt (*Wild Oats*), 7 pces, 1.4 oz	**190**	**8**	**29**
Soft Pretzels (Twists) average:		
Plain: Regular, 2.2 oz	**210**	**2**	**43**
King Size, 5.1 oz	**485**	**4.5**	**99**
Big Cheese, 1.76 oz	**130**	**3**	**22**
Peanut Butter filled (*Tr. Joe's*) 1 oz	**150**	**8**	**14**
Auntie Anne's: *See Fast-Foods Section*		
Frito-Lay Pretzels		
Bitesize Twists, 23 pces, 1 oz	**140**	**6**	**19**
Braided Twists, 8 sticks, 1 oz	**110**	**1**	**22**
Cheddar Cheese Tiny Twists, 1 oz	**110**	**1**	**22**
Snyder's of Hanover Pretzels		
Rods (3), 1 oz	**120**	**1**	**24**
Homestyle (15), 1 oz	**120**	**1**	**25**
Nibblers (16), 1 oz	**120**	**0**	**25**
SuperPretzel: Soft Pretzels (1)	**160**	**1**	**34**
Softstix (2)	**130**	**3**	**22**
Soft Pretzel Bites (5)	**150**	**0.5**	**32**
Pretzelfils: Pizza (2)	**130**	**2**	**22**
Pepperjack; Mozzarella, (2), avg.	**130**	**3.5**	**21**

Snacks C F Cb

Note: Actual weight of packaged snacks is usually 5-10% more than label Net Wt. For accuracy, weigh snack and allow extra calories for any extra weight.

	C	F	Cb
Bacon Cheese Crackers, 1 oz	190	10	24
Banana Chips, ¼ cup, 13 chips, 1 oz	150	8	20
Beef Jerky (Lance), average, 1 oz	70	1	4
Beef Sticks (Frito-Lay's) 1 oz	90	7	2
Bugles, Original, 1⅓ cup, 1 oz	160	9	18
Cajun Jerky, 1 strip, ½ oz	55	1	1
Cheddar Lites (Health Valley) 1 oz	120	3	21
Cheese Crackers (Frito-Lay) 1 oz	130	6	18
Cheese Filled, 1 oz	210	11	24
Cheese Curls: 1 cup, 1 oz	150	6	19
Reduced Fat (Utz), 1 oz	140	6	18
Cheese Nips (Nabisco), 38, 1 oz	150	6	19
Cheese Puffs: Average, 1 oz	150	8	12
Lite, 1 oz	130	5	19
American Fare, 1¼ cup, 1 oz	150	9	18
Cheese Twists, 1 oz	160	10	13
Cheetos: Regular all flavors, 1 oz	160	10	13
Baked!, cheese flavored, 1 oz	130	5	19
Cheez Balls, 27 balls, 1 oz	170	12	13
Cheez It: White Cheddar, 1 pkt (26)	150	8	18
Original (27)	160	8	18
Reduced Fat (29)	130	4	20
Chex Mix (General Mills):			
100 Calorie Pouch, avg.	100	3	18
Bold Blend; Peanut, ½ cup	140	6	20
Other varieties, avg., ½ cup	135	4.5	22
Churros (Mex. Pastry) 10", 1.2 oz	140	9	12
Cinna Chips (T.J. Cinn.) 3, 1 oz	110	5	15
Combos (Oven Baked):			
Crackers, ⅓ cup, 1 oz	140	6	18
1 cup, 3 oz	420	18	54
Pretzels, ⅓ cup, 1 oz	130	4.5	19
1 cup, 3 oz	390	14	57
Cookies: See Pages 105-112			
Cool Cuts: Carrot & Ranch	60	4	5
Celery & Peanut Butter	170	14	9
Corn Chips: See Page 133			
Corn Crunchies/Spirals, 1 oz	100	1.5	21
Corn Nuts: ⅓ cup, 1 oz	130	4.5	20
1.7 oz bag	220	7.5	34
Corn Puffs: Health Valley, 2 c., 1 oz	120	1.5	25
Pirate's Booty, 1 oz	130	5	18
Wotsits (Walker), 21g, (¾ oz) pkg	110	6.5	11
Dunkin Stixs (Hostess), 3, 4 oz	490	25	63
Flavor Twists (Fritos), 1 oz	160	10	16

Snacks (Cont) C F Cb

	C	F	Cb
French's Potato Sticks ¾ c., 1 oz	180	12	16
Funyun's: Onion flavor (13), 1 oz	140	7	18
Mini, 2 oz	270	13	35
Goldfish (Pepperidge Farm) 1 oz	140	5	20
Gold-N-Chees (Lance), 1 oz	150	8	17
Handi Snacks (Kraft), avg., 1 pkg	110	5	16
Honey Mustard Onion Pieces			
(Snyder's) 1 pkg, 2 oz	280	14	36
Hot Peanuts (Lays), 3 Tbsp	190	16	6
Jerky (Beef), 1 oz stick	80	1	5
Lance Sandwich:			
Capt. Wafers; Choc-O-Mint, (4)	70	3	9
Sour Dough w. Cheddar, 1 pkg	240	15	23
Other varieties, average, 1 pkg	200	10	22
Munchies (Frito-Lay):			
Classic Mix, ¾ cup, 1 oz	140	7	18
Go Snacks Mini Mix, 2.37 oz can	310	10	48
Kids Mix, ¾ cup, 1 oz	130	4	20
Traditional Mix, ¾ cup, 1 oz	130	5	19
Munchos, 16 pieces, 1 oz	160	10	16
Nabisco: Chips Ahoy, 1.3 oz	160	8	22
Cheese Nips (38), 1 oz	150	6	19
Nutter Butter Bites (10), 35g	170	7	24
Oreo, 1.3 oz	160	7	25
Ritz Bits Go-Pak Cheese (12)	160	9	16
Ritz Bits S'Mores, 1 oz	150	6	22
Mixers, avg., 1 oz	130	4.5	19
Nibblers (Snyder's): Regular (13)	130	3	24
Fat Free (16)	120	0	25
Onion Rings (T.G.I. Friday), 1 oz	140	7	16
Oriental Mix (Rice Snacks), 1 oz	130	4	21
Rice Snacks (Wild Oats) ⅔ c. 1 oz	110	0	25
Oyster Crackers (Sunshine), 1 oz	120	2	22
Party Mix (Cheez-It) ½ c., 1 oz	130	4.5	19
Peanut Butter Nuggets (10), 1 oz	140	6	15
Pirate's Booty w. White Ched., 1 oz	130	5	18
Pita Chips, avg., (9) 1 oz	130	4	18
Popcorn: See Page 132			
Pork Skins/Rind: Baken-ets, 1 oz	160	10	0
Lance, 1 pkg	80	5	0
Potato Chips: See Page 133			
Potato Puffs, 1 oz	110	3	21
Potato Skins (TGI Friday), 1 oz	150	9	17
Potato Sticks (Ralph's), ⅔ c., 1.1 oz	170	11	15

Snacks (Cont)

	C	F	Cb
Quakes: Caramel Corn (7)	60	0	13
Apple Cinn. (8)	60	0	15
BBQ (10); Ranch (10)	70	2.5	12
Chocolate (7)	60	1	13
Nacho/Cheddar Cheese (9)	70	2.5	14
Sour Cream & Onion (10)	75	2.5	12
Rice Chips, Bar-B-Q/Onion, 1 oz	140	7	18
Sandwich Crackers (Austin): Per Pkg			
Chse Cracker w. Pnut Butter, 1.37 oz	200	10	23
Reduced Fat, 1.26 oz	170	7	24
Chse Cracker w. Cheddar, 1.37 oz	210	10	26
PB & J Cracker Sandwich, 1.37 oz	200	10	24
Santitas (Frito-Lay), 1 oz	130	6	19
Sesame Sticks (Cityfarm), 1 oz	160	11	13
Soy Crisps, avg. 1 oz	105	2	15
Soy Nuts: Dry Roasted, ¼ cup, 1 oz	130	6	9
Choc-coated, 1 oz	140	7	13
Dr Soy Soy Nuts BBQ, 1 oz	150	8	8
Sun Chips (Frito-Lay), 1 oz pkg	140	6	18
TastyKake: Koffee Kake Jnr	280	10	44
Chocolate Jnr	340	12	55
Creme Filled Koffee Kakes (2)	270	13	35
Toast/Cheese Crackers, 1 pkg	220	11	23
Tortilla Chips: See Pages 133			
Tostitos: Regular, average, 1 oz	140	7	19
Light, 1 oz	90	1	20
Trail Mix (Nuts/Seeds/Dried Fruit):			
Regular, 3 Tbsp, 1 oz	150	9	10
Tropical, 3 Tbsp, 1 oz	130	6	17
w. Chocolate Chips, 1 oz	170	9	18
Dr Soy Trail Mix, 1 oz	110	4	12
Turkey Jerky Teriyaki (Oberto), 1 oz	80	1	5
Vegetable Snacks (Snyders), 1 oz	140	7	18
Veggie Chips, 1 oz	120	4	19
Veggie Stix, 1 oz	140	7	18
Wheatables (Keebler): Orig., (17)	140	6	20
Orig., Reduced Fat (19), 1 oz	140	4	23
Honey Wheat (17), 1 oz	140	6	20
Seven Grain (17), 1 oz	140	6	20
Yogurt Raisins (Sun-Maid), 1 oz	130	6	20

Fruit Snacks

	C	F	Cb
Betty Crocker: Fruit Gushers, 25g	90	1	20
Fruit by the Foot, 1 roll, 21g	80	1	17
Fruit Roll Ups, 1 roll, 14g	50	1	12
Scooby Doo; G Force, 25g pkg	80	0	21
Kellogg's: Disney Fruit Snacks, 25g	80	0	21
Fruit Streamers, 1 Roll, 0.8 oz	80	1	17
Twistables, 23g	70	0.5	17
Yogos, 23g	90	1.5	18
Nabisco: Fruit Rolls (1), 0.74 oz	80	2	16
CapriSun Juicers, 1 pouch, 26g	80	0	19
Rugrats; Wacky Faces (1)	80	0	19
Blues Clues; Dora the Explorer (1)	60	0	14
100 Calorie Fruit Snacks, 1.1 oz	100	0	24
Sunkist: Fruit Snacks, 1 pouch	90	1	20
Fruit Smoothie Blitze, 1.3 oz	140	1	32

Vending Machines

	C	F	Cb
Brownie, frosted (Lance)	320	12	52
Cheese Balls (Lance), 1 oz	170	12	13
Choc Chip Cookies (Nabisco), 40g	190	9	27
Choc Milk, 8 fl.oz	260	9	26
Coca-Cola Classic, 12 fl.oz	150	0	40
Diet Coke, 12 fl.oz	0	0	0
Corn Chips, 1 oz	160	10	15
Hostess Sweet Roll, 2.12 oz	210	7.5	34
Donut, plain, 1¾ oz	230	15	27
Fruit Pie (Hostess), 4½ oz	480	20	68
Granola/Cereal Bars	140	3	26
Hershey's, 1.55 oz bar	240	13	25
Hot Fries (Lance), 1 oz	150	10	15
Kellogg's Rice Krispies Treat	120	4.5	20
Lance Captain's Wafers, 1 pkg	200	10	22
M & M's: Plain, 1.7 oz	240	10	34
Peanuts, 1.7 oz	250	13	30
Milk: Whole, 8 fl.oz	150	8	13
Reduced Fat, 2%, 8 fl.oz	130	5	13
Milky Way, 2 oz	260	10	41
Onion Rings, 1 oz	140	7	16
Orange Juice, 8 fl.oz	110	0	26
Peanuts, roasted (Lance), 1 oz	200	15	6
Popcorn, plain, 1 oz	160	8	16
Pork Skins, 1 oz	160	10	0
Potato Chips, 1 oz	150	10	15
Reduced Fat, 1 oz	140	7	20
Pretzels, 1 oz	110	1	23
Raisins, ½ pkg	45	0	11
Reece's Peanut Butter Cups, 1.8 oz	280	17	28
Snickers, 2.1 oz bar	280	14	35
Tortilla Chips, 1 oz	140	7	9

For Full Nutritional Data and Product Updates
~ See Author's Website
www.CalorieKing.com

Breakfast Bars ◆ Sports & Diet Bars

Note: Actual weight of bars is usually 5-10% more than label Net Wt. Weigh bar and allow extra calories.

Breakfast Bars

	C	F	Cb
Apex, Breakfast Squares, 2 oz	210	7	23
Atkins: Advantage Morning Bars,			
Crisp, avg., 1.3 oz bar	170	9	14
Cinnamon Bun, 1.4 oz bar	150	7	15
Barbara's Bakery: Nature's Choice	150	2	28
Fruit & Yogurt Bar, 1.1 oz	130	3	29
Full Circle, Fr. & Cereal, avg., 1.3 oz	135	2	26
General Mills: Milk 'n Cereal Bars,			
Cinnamon Toast Crunch, 1.6 oz	180	4	33
Other varieties, average, 1.6 oz	160	4	28
Health Valley: Bar, avg., 1.3 oz	130	2	27
Cereal Tarts, all flav. 1 bar, 1.4oz	130	2	28
Kellogg's			
All-Bran Cereal Bar, avg., 1.2 oz	130	3	26
Crunch Cereal Bar, avg., 1 oz	110	2	22
Smart Start Bars, 1.4 oz	150	2.5	30
Pop Tarts: French Ioast (1), 1.8 oz	220	8	35
Fruit/Frosted, avg., 1.8 oz	200	5	37
Low-Fat, all flavors, 1.8 oz	190	3	39
Go Tarts, avg., 1.2 oz	140	4.5	24
Market Pantry (Target), Bar, 1.4 oz	140	3	26
Nature's Path: Crispy Rice, avg.	110	3	20
Toaster Pastries, 1.8 oz	210	5	37
New England Natural Bakers			
Save the Forest Bars (1), 1 oz	120	4.5	19
Nutri-Grain Bars			
Cereal Bars, avg., 1.3 oz	140	3	26
Fruit & Nut Bar, 1.1 oz	120	3.5	22
Yogurt Bars, avg., 1.3 oz	140	3	26
Post, Honey Bunches of Oats Bar	140	4	24
Quaker			
Breakfast Cookies, 1 pce, 1.7 oz	170	4.5	33
Fruit Flavor Crisp Bar, 1.3 oz	130	2.5	26
Fruit Flavor Crisp Bites, 1 pouch	130	2.5	28
Muffin Bars, 1.3 oz	130	3.5	26
Granola Bars: See Page 140			
Russell Stover, Bar, 1.1 oz	100	5	13
Slim-Fast: Fruit Crisp, 1.3 oz	180	4.5	29
Muffin Bar, 1.2 oz	140	5	20
South Beach Diet (Kraft)			
High Protein Cereal Bars (1), 1.3 oz	140	5	15
Special K Cereal Bars, avg., 0.8 oz	90	1.5	18
Trader Joe's: Fig, 1.3 oz	120	2	18
Apple, Blueberry/Strawb., avg.	140	2.5	28

Other Bars

Per Bar

	C	F	Cb
ABB: Extreme XXL Bar, 4.9 oz	530	11	68
Steel Bar, 2.3 oz	250	4	36
AdvantEdge			
Carb Control Crisp Bar, 2.1 oz	240	8	27
Carb Control Nutrition Bar, 2.1 oz	220	7	28
Complete Nutrition Bar, 2.1 oz	240	8	27
Alpen Cereal Bars: *Per 3.5 oz Bar*			
Alpen Light (1), 0.74 oz	285	4	56
Fruit & Nut (1), 1 oz	110	3	20
Fruit & Nut w. Chocolate (1), 1 oz	125	4	20
Groove (1), 1.1 oz	140	5	21
Raspberry & Yogurt (1), 1.03 oz	120	3	21
Apex: Fix Crisp Bar, 1.4 oz	160	4	21
Fix Fruit Fuel Bar	210	3.5	36
Atkins: Endulge (See Page 125)			
Original Bar, average, 2.1 oz	220	9	22
Caramel Bar, average, 1.6 oz	180	6	17
Granola Bar, average, 1.7 oz	220	8	18
Back to Nature			
Bakery Squares, avg., 1.07 oz	125	4.5	20
Chewy Trail Mix Bar, avg., 1 oz	120	4.5	19
Fruit & Grain Bar, 1.07 oz	110	2	20
Balance: Balance Bars 1.7 oz	200	6	23
Balance Bar Bare:			
Sweet & Salty, average, 1.8 oz	210	9	23
Trail Mix, average, 1.8 oz	210	7	23
Carb Well: Caramel 'n Choc., 1.7 oz	190	7	23
Chocolate Fudge, 1.7 oz	190	6	23
Chocolate Peanut Butter, 1.7 oz	200	8	22
100 Calorie Bar, avg., 1 oz	100	4	14
Gold/Crunch Bars, avg., 1.7 oz	210	6	23
Barbara's Bakery: Granola, ¾ oz	80	2	14
Crunchy Granola, 1.5 oz	190	8	27
Fruit & Yogurt Bar, 1.1 oz	150	3	39
Bariatrix Proti-Bar: (15g Protein)			
Caramel Nut, 1.42 oz	150	4.5	15
Be: Protein Bar, 2 oz	150	2.5	22
Healthy Kids Bar, 1.53 oz	110	1.5	19
Bear Valley, Meal Pack, 3.75 oz	420	13	59
Biochem: Strive, avg., 2.1 oz	190	9	24
Greens & Whey Bar, 2.1 oz	280	12	26
Raw Foods & Whey Bar, 2.1 oz	200	4	37
Bumble Bar: Original/w. Nuts 1.6 oz	230	15	20
Chocolate crisp, 1.6 oz	200	11	25
Lushus Lemon, 1.6 oz	210	12	21
CarbRite Diet (Doctor's), avg., 2 oz	190	4	32
Caribou Coffee, Snack Bar, avg.	140	3.5	26

Note: Actual weight of bars is usually 5-10% more than label Net Wt. Weigh bar and allow extra calories.

Other Bars (Cont)

Per Bar

	C	F	Cb
Cascadian Farms (*General Mills*)			
Chewy Granola Bar, 1.3 oz	135	3	25
Champion Nutrition, SnacBar	180	3	24
Cheetah (*NutraFig*), 2.25 oz bar	210	2	43
Clif Bars: Builders Bars, 2.5 oz	270	8	30
Luna Bar, average, 1.5 oz	180	4.5	27
Mojo Bar, average, 1.5 oz	200	9	24
Nectar Bar, average, 1.6 oz	165	6	28
Z Bar, average, 1.26 oz	120	3	22
Curves (*General Mills*)			
Chewy Granola Bar, avg., 25g bar	100	3	18
Chocolate Peanut, 25g bar	100	3.5	17
Designer Supplements			
Sustain Bar, 2½ oz	300	9	35
Designer Whey			
Big Whey Bar, 3.57 oz	420	16	38
Gourmet bars, avg. all flav., 2.7 oz	260	7	7
Detour (*Next Proteins*): 2.8 oz bar	320	9	32
Core Strength, average, 1.78 oz	205	6	22
Go, 1.93 oz	210	3	34
Bikers Bars, average, 1.78 oz	210	5	29
Runner Bars, 1.78 oz	200	3.5	29
Buzz Bars, 3.03 oz	330	10	30
Oatmeal Whole Grain, 4.28 oz	460	12	58
Lower Sugar, 3.03 oz	340	10	33
Disney Magic, Chewy Granola, 1 oz	115	3	21
Dr Soy			
Protein Bar, Lemon, 1.76 oz	170	4	26
Chocolate/Peanut, 1.76 oz	190	5	25
Healthy Snacker, avg., 1.7 oz bar	180	6	28
EAS Advantage Edge			
Carb Control, average, 2.12 oz	230	8	27
Complete Nutrition, 2.12 oz avg.	240	8	28
EAS			
Champions Energy Bar, 1.42 oz	160	4.5	26
EAS Myoplex			
Deluxe Nutrition Bar, avg., 3.2 oz	350	10	36
Lite Nutyrition Bar, avg., 1.97 oz	190	4.5	26
Carb Control, 2.5 oz	260	8	25
Elev8 me: Protein & Fruit Trail,			
All Fruit Blend, 2.3 oz bar	210	3	32
Cocoa & Coconut, 2.3 oz	230	6	32

Per Bar

	C	F	Cb
Fi-Bar Nectar Granola Bars, 1 oz	120	2	26
Chewy & Nutty Bar, 1.2 oz	140	4.5	23
First Endurance, EFS Bar, 2.32 oz	250	6	40
General Mills, Fiber One Granola, avg.	145	4	28
GeniSoy: Genisoy Bars, 2.2 oz	240	4.5	35
Natural Choice, 1.6 oz	170	4.5	20
Protein Crunch, 1.6 oz	150	5	18
Soy Protein Bars, avg., 2.2 oz	235	4.5	33
Ultra Bar, 1.6 oz	160	2	27
Glenny's: Light 'n Crispy, ½ oz	60	2.5	9
Slim Carb: Double Fudge, 1.3 oz	130	2.5	13
Slim 1, 1.06 oz	100	3	21
Glucerna: Meal Replacement, 2 oz	220	7	34
Snack Bar, avg., 1.3 oz	150	4	25
Mini Snack Bar (1)	80	2.5	12
GNC ProCrunch: Choc Crisp	260	7	33
Cookies n' Cream; S'Mores	250	4	37
Peanut Butter Crunch, 2.3 oz	260	7	34
Pro Crunch Lite, 1.2 oz	140	1.5	4
Greens + Bar: + Energy, avg., 2 oz	245	10	33
+ High Protein, avg., 1.6 oz	255	12	22
Hammer Nutrition, Hammer (1)	220	9	25
Health Valley Fruit/Granola, avg.	190	5	29
Hershey's Smart Zone, avg, 50g	200	7	21
High Protein: Peanut Butter, 4 oz	300	6	33
Other varieties, average	335	8	36
HMR Benefit Bar, 1.1 oz	160	5	22
Honey Stinger: Stinger Energy (1)	180	3	28
Stinger Protein Bar, 3.2 oz	390	20	36
ISS Research: Oh Yeah, 3.03 oz	375	16	32
Natural Bar, 1.64 oz	200	7	18
Protein Wafer, 2 sticks, 1.35 oz	210	13	8
Pro 42, 3.75 oz	380	8	37
Jay Robb: Jay Protein Bar, 2 oz	230	11	24
Yammit! Energy Bar, 2 oz	250	12	35
Jenny Craig			
Anytime Bar: Oat & Honey,1.78 oz	170	4.5	32
Cookies & Crm/Peanut Butter, 1 oz	110	3	12
Choc Caramel/Peanut Butter, 1.32 oz	150	5	19
Choc Chip Snack Bar, 1.21 oz	140	3	23
Jocalat, avg. all flavors, 1.71 oz	190	11	25
Joyva Sesame Crunch, 1.1 oz	190	8	15
Joy Ride Bars: *See Next Proteins*			
Kashi Golean: Bars, avg., 2.7 oz	290	6	48
Crunchy!, avg., 1.76 oz bar	170	4.5	30
Go Lean Roll, avg., 1.9 oz	190	5	28
TLC: Crunchy Granola Bar, 1.42 oz	180	6	26
Chewy Granola Bar, 1.3 oz	140	5	19

Per Bar	C	F	Cb
Kind Fruit & Nut Bars			
Almond & Coconut	190	14	14
Fruit & Nut Delight	170	11	16
Walnut & Date	150	7	22
Kudos: Chocolate Chip, 1 oz	120	3.5	24
Peanut Butter, 1 oz	130	6	18
M&M's; Snickers, average, 0.84 oz	100	3	17
Larabar: Apple/Cherry Pie, 1.6 oz	190	8	28
Banana Cookie Dough, 1.8 oz	220	11	28
Lean Body: Cookie Bar, 3.25 oz	360	30	13
Gold, 3 oz	330	7	36
Hi Pro Granola Bar, 285 oz	340	11	39
Rockin Roll, 2.5 oz	290	16	25
Lindora: Chocolate Chip	140	5	15
Other varieties, average	150	5	16
Luna Bars: *See Clif Bars*			
Marathon *(Snickers):* Energy, 2 oz	220	7	29
Low Carb, average, 1.7 oz	170	7	19
Protein, average, 2.8 oz	290	9	40
Market Pantry *(Target)*			
Chewy Granola, 1 oz, average	120	12.5	22
Sweet & Salty Bar, 1.3 oz, avg.	150	6	23
Maximum Human Performanc			
Macrobolic, 2.5 oz	250	6	38
Probolic-SR, 2.98 oz	290	9	31
Medifast: Fit! Bar, 1.5 oz	160	5	23
Plus for Diabetics, avg., 1.5 oz	140	5	22
Met-Rx: "Big 100", 3.5 oz	360	5	50
Protein Plus, 3 oz bar	320	9	32
MLO Bio Protein: 2.85 oz	320	7	43
Extreme, 3.2 oz	370	8	43
Mojo Bars: *See Clif Bars*			
MRM Response, 2.1 oz	210	8	20
Muscle Tech: Nitro-Tech, average	280	7	30
Complete Cookie Bar, 2.7 oz	310	12	25
Complete Oat Bar, 3.4 oz	350	11	40
Myoplex: *See EAS*			
Nabisco: HoneyMaid Bars, 1.32 oz	150	6	24
100 Calorie Chewy Granola Bars:			
Chips Ahoy, 1 bar	100	1.5	22
Nutter Butter, 1 bar	100	1.5	21
Oreo, 1 bar	100	2	21
Nature Valley Granola Bars			
Chewy w. Yogurt coating, 1.42 oz	140	3.5	26
Crunchy, average, 2 bars, 1.5 oz	180	6	29
Heart Healthy: Honey Nut, 40g	160	4	28
Oatmeal Raisin, 1.42 oz	150	2	30
Sweet & Salty, average, 1.3 oz	165	8	21
Trail Mix, average, 1.3 oz	140	4	26

Per Bar	C	F	Cb
Nature's Path			
Rebound, 2 oz	190	4	33
Optimum Energy, avg., 1.97 oz	230	7	35
Flax Plus; Hemp Plus, avg., 1.2 oz	140	3	27
Granola: Apricot 'n Nut, 1.2 oz	160	5	26
Cranberry Soy, 1.2 oz	160	4	27
Next Proteins: Detour, 2.8 oz	320	9	32
Joy Ride, 2.8 oz	340	12	27
One Way, 3 oz	340	12	29
U-Turn Protein, 2.8 oz	300	8	26
NiteBite *(Time-release Glucose Bar)*			
Choc. Fudge; P'nut Butter, 0.89 oz	100	3.5	15
Now, Fivacious Bar, 1.78 oz	210	12	26
Nutiva: Hempseed, 1.4 oz	210	14	11
Flax Chocolate, 1.4 oz	200	12	19
NutriSystem Nourish, avg., 1.44 oz	125	3	20
Dessert Bar	160	4	28
Granola Bar, avg.	150	2.5	28
Nutrilite: Trim Advantage Bars,			
Protein Bars, avg., 2.1 oz	260	9	25
Meal Bars, 2.1 oz	230	7	28
XS Power Butrition, 1.6 oz	180	6	20
Odwalla Energy Bars			
Choc. Chip Peanut/Crunch, avg.	245	7	38
Super Protein, 2.2 oz	230	4.5	31
Other varieties, average, 2.2 oz	240	6	41
One Way Bars: *See Next Proteins*			
Planters CarbWell			
Peanut Butter Crunch, 1.25 oz	160	12	16
Caramel Choc Crunch, 1.35 oz	180	13	17
PR Bar average, 1.78 oz	200	6	22
Power Bar: Harvest Dip'd, avg., 2.3 oz	250	5	42
Harvest, 2.3 oz	250	5	42
Heart Healthy	240	4	42
Nut Naturals, avg., 1.6 oz	210	10	20
Pria Bars: 110 Plus	110	3	16
Carb Select, avg., 1.7 oz	170	7	22
Complete, average	170	6	22
Grain Essentials, average	165	3	30
Protein Plus: Average, 2.75 oz	300	6	48
Reduced Sugar, average	265	8	31
Triple Threat, avg., 1.93 oz	225	6	31
Power Crunch, average, 1.3 oz	220	12	10
Premier: Protein Eight, 2.4 oz	260	7	23
Premier Protein Bar, 2.5 oz	290	9	23
Odyssey Bar, avg., 2.8 oz	320	11	30
Organic, average	160	6	28
Twisted Bar, 1.6 oz	190	6	21
Promax: Average, 2.7 oz bar	290	6	40
Triple Layer Bar, 2.5 oz	290	8	36
Protein Complete, avg., 1.97 oz	180	2.5	19

Granola, Sports & Diet Bars (Cont)

Other Bars (Cont)

Per Bar	C	F	Cb
Prozone Nutrition Bar,			
Fruit Snax Bar, 1.4 oz	140	0	32
Pure Protein: See Worldwide Sport Nutrition			
Pure Fit, average, 2 oz bar	235	6	27
Quaker Chewy Granola Bars			
Chewy (Regular): Avg. 0.86 oz	100	2.5	19
Peanut Butter/Chocolate	100	3	17
Chewy Dipps: Choc Chip, 1.1 oz	140	5	22
Peanut Butter	150	7	19
Granola Bites, 1 pouch, 0.71 oz	90	3.5	14
Snack Bars:			
Chewy Granola 25% Less Sugar	100	3.5	17
Chewy 90 Cal Granola, 0.86 oz	90	1.5	19
Sweet & Salty Crunch, (2), 1.2 oz	150	6	23
Real Protein, avg., 2.75 oz bar	280	7	21
Rebar: Energy, 1.75 oz	180	8	29
Greens, 1.75 oz	160	0	38
Supplement, 1.75 oz	200	8	21
Resource, OptiSource Mini Bar	90	2.5	10
Revival Soy Bars (Direct): Per Bar			
Chocolate Temptation	270	7	32
Apple Cinnamon; Marshm. Krunch	220	3	30
Peanut Butter/Choc Pal, avg.	240	6	28
Low Carb, average all flavors	235	8	31
Slim-Fast Bars			
High Protein Meal Bars, 1.71 oz	195	6.5	20
Cookie Bar, average, 1 oz	120	3.5	19
Muffin Bar, average, 1.2 oz	140	5	20
Optima: Fruit Crisp Bars, avg.	180	4.5	29
Meal Bars, average, 2 oz	220	5	35
Snack Bars, average, 1 oz	120	4	20
Granola Bars, average	220	6	35
Lower Carb: Average	180	6	18
Snacks, average, 1 oz	120	5	18
Original: Brkfst & Lunch Bars, avg.	140	5	20
Meal-On-The-Go, average, 2 oz	220	5	35
Skippy Snack Bars, avg., 1.2 oz	170	11	17
Trail Mix Bars, average, 1.2 oz	150	7	17
SlimWhey, average, 1.1 oz	120	4	14
SoyJoy, Bar, avg., 1.07 oz	135	6	15
Solo GI, average, 1.78 oz	200	7	26

Per Bar	C	F	Cb
Special K: Granola Snack Bites, 0.82 oz	90	2	18
Meal Bar, 1.6 oz	190	6	28
Protein Snack Bar, avg., 1 oz	110	3	16
Spiru-tein (Nature's Plus), 1.4 oz	150	5	19
Supreme, 1.8 oz	170	4.5	21
Steel Bar (ABB), 2 oz	250	4	36
Strive (Biochem), avg., 2.1 oz	230	9	24
The Sports Club/LA:			
Caramel Cr./Choc P'nut (16g prot.)	200	5	22
P'nut Butter Fudge (13g prot.)	185	9	13
Think Thin! Avg., 2.1 oz	240	8	27
Green Tea, 1.76 oz	180	5	28
Organic Bar, average, 1.76 oz	155	4	23
Protein Bar, average, 2.1 oz	230	8	26
Tiger's Milk: Protein Rich, 1.25 oz	140	5	18
Peanut Butter, 1.25 oz	150	6	18
King Size Bars, 1.96 oz	230	10	28
Thorpedo Bar: Macad. Pineapple	260	14	31
Alm. Apricot & Yogurt, 2.14 oz	240	8	39
Trader Joe's: Choc. Chip, 1.25 oz	140	4	25
Joe Joe's Chewy Coated Granola	140	5	25
Nutty Choc. Granola Bar, 1.25 oz	150	8	20
Peanut Butter, 1.25 oz	160	8	20
Peanut Crunch, 1.25 oz	130	2.5	25
Sweet Savory & Tart Trail Mix Bar	140	4.5	24
Vanilla Almond Crunch, 1.25 oz	130	4	21
Tri-O-Plex: avg., 4.2 oz	430	16	45
Duo Bar, average	380	11	33
U-Turn Bars: See Next Proteins			
Usana: Fibergy Bar, 1 oz	100	1.5	23
Nutrition Bar: Oatmeal Raisin, 1.96 oz	190	3	22
Peanut Butter Crunch, 1.46 oz	150	4	20
Vyo-Pro (AST) Chocolate, 2.2 oz	200	7	24
Worldwide Sport Nutrition: Pure Protein,			
Country Berry; Choc Chip, 2.75 oz	300	8	29
Chocolate Deluxe, 2.75 oz	270	7	26
Chocolate Peanut Butter, 2.75 oz	300	9	26
Karma Bars, 1.78 oz	200	6	25
Protein Revolution	280	9	26
Xyience, X Smart Bar, 1.78 oz	270	7	33
Zoe Flax & Soy, Choc., 1.8 oz	190	7	23
ZonePerfect: Average, 1.76 oz	210	7	23
Snack Size, 0.72 oz	80	8	25

Nuts

Per 1 oz Unless Indicated

	C	F	Cb
Acorns, raw 1 oz	110	7	12
Almonds, Dried/Dry Roasted:			
Whole, 24-28 med., 1 oz	170	15	5.5
½ cup, 2½ oz	420	37	13
Chopped,½ cup, 2¼ oz	380	34	12
Sliced, ½ cup, 1⅔ oz	280	25	9
Choc. coated (5-6), 1 oz	150	10	15
Oil Rstd *(Blue Diamond)*, 1 oz	170	16	5
Honey Roasted, 1 oz	170	14	8
Almond Meal (partially defatted)			
1 cup (not packed), 2¼ oz	260	11	11
Brazil Nuts, 8 med., 1 oz	185	19	3.5
Cashews, Dry or Oil Roasted:			
14 large/18 med./26 small, 1 oz	165	14	9
½ cup, 2.4 oz	375	31	20
Honey Roasted, 1 oz	165	13	10
Chestnuts, avg. all: Dried, 1 oz	105	1	22
Raw/Fresh, 5-6 nuts, 1 oz	60	0	13
Canned, water chestnuts,			
sliced/whole/drained, 1 oz	30	0	7
Coconut: Flesh, 1 oz	100	10	4
Raw: 1 pce. (2"x2"x½"), 1.6 oz	160	15	7
½ medium (4½" diam.)	700	66	30
Dried (Desiccated):			
Unsweetened, 1 oz	187	18	7
Sweetened: Shredded, 1 oz	140	10	13
Grated, ½ cup, 1.3 oz	185	12	18
Cream (canned), ½ cup, 5.2 oz	285	26	12
Milk (canned), ½ cup, 4 oz	225	24	3
Water (center liq.), ½ c., 4¼ oz	23	0	4.5
Filberts or Hazelnuts:			
Shelled, 18-20 nuts	180	17	4.5
Chopped, ¼ cup, 1 oz	180	18	5
Ground, ¼ cup, 0.6 oz	120	12	3
Ginkgo Nuts, can., 14 med., 1 oz	32	0.5	6.5
Hickory, 30 small nuts, 1 oz	200	18	5
Macadamia Nuts, shelled:			
Raw, 7 med./14 small, 1 oz	200	21	4
½ cup, 2.3 oz	480	51	10
Dry Roasted, 1 oz	205	22	4
½ cup, 2.4 oz	480	51	9
Choc. coated, 2-3 pces, 1 oz	170	12	14
Mixed Nuts: 18-22 nuts, 1 oz	170	15	7
Planters: Dry Roasted/Honey	170	15	7
Oil Roasted, all types	180	16	7
Sweet Roasts, 26 pces, 1 oz	160	12	10
Nut Toppings: Chopped, 1 T., ¼ oz	40	4	1.5

Per 1 oz Unless Indicated

	C	F	Cb
Peanuts:			
Raw/Dried: In shell, 1 oz	117	10	3
Shelled, 1 oz	160	14	4.5
Boiled, shelled, ½ cup, 3.1 oz	285	20	19
Roasted: 30 lge./60 sml., 1 oz	165	14	6
1 cup, 5.1 oz	860	76	22
Chopped, 3 Tbsp, 1 oz	165	14	6
Planters: Cocktail, 1 oz	170	14	6
Rich Roasted in Choc., 2½ oz	220	14	19
Roasted in Shell, Salted, 1 oz	160	14	5
Dry Roasted, 1oz	160	13	6
Honey/ & Dry Roasted, 1 oz	160	13	8
Spanish Raw, 1 oz	150	13	6
Spanish Redskin, 1 oz	180	14	5
Sweet N' Crunchy, 1 oz	140	7	16
Pecans: Kernel halves, 1 oz	195	20	4
(20 Jumbo or 31 large halves)			
1 cup halves, 3.8 oz	755	78	15
Chopped, ½ cup, 2 oz	380	39	7.5
Oil Roasted, 15 halves, 1 oz	205	20	4
Honey Roasted, 1 oz	200	21	4
Pilinuts, dried, ¼ cup, 1 oz	215	24	4
Pinenuts, dried, 1 Tbsp, 10g	70	7	1.5
Pistachios: Unshelled, ½ cup, 2 oz	165	14	7
Shelled, ¼ cup, 45 nuts, 1 oz	170	14	8.5
Lance, 1.1 oz package	95	7	4
Sesame Nut Mix: *Planters,* 1 oz	160	13	9
Soy Nuts: Dry Roasted, 1 oz	130	6	9
½ cup, 3 oz	390	18	29
Dr Soy: Choc coated, 1 oz pkg	140	7	13
Flavors, average, 1 oz	150	8	8
Trail Mix: *(Planters)* Fruit & Nut, 1 oz	140	9	14
Golden Nut Crunch, 1 oz	160	11	12
Honey Nut & Caramel, 1 oz	160	10	16
Mixed Nuts & Raisins, 1 oz	150	11	10
Nut & Chocolate, 1 oz	160	10	16
Nuts, Seeds & Raisins, 1 oz	160	12	11
Spicy Nuts & Cajun Sticks, 1 oz	150	10	13
Sweet & Nutty, 1 oz	150	10	14
Walnuts:			
Black: 15-20 halves, 1 oz	175	17	3
Chopped, ¼ cup, 1.1 oz	195	18	3
English/Persian:			
14 halves, 1 oz	185	18	4
Chopped, ¼ cup, 1 oz	190	19	4
Ground, ¼ cup, 0.7 oz	130	13	3

Seeds ◆ Supplements

Seeds

	C	F	Cb
Alfalfa Seeds, sprouted, ½ c., ½ oz	5	0	1
Caraway, Fennel, 1 tsp	7	0.5	1
Cottonseed Kernels, rst., 1 Tbsp	50	3.5	2
Flax Seeds, 3 Tbsp, 1 oz	140	9	9
Lotus Seeds, dried, ½ c., ½ oz	55	0.5	10
Poppy Seeds, 1 tsp	15	1	1
Pumpkin & Squash Seeds, whole:			
Roasted/Tamari, 1 oz	150	12	4
½ cup, 4 oz	590	48	15
Dried, 142 hulled seeds, 1 oz	155	13	4
Safflower Kernels, dried, 1 oz	150	11	10
Sesame Seeds: Dried, 1 Tbsp, 9g	50	4.5	2
Roasted/Toasted, 1 oz	160	14	7.5
Sunflower Kernels/Seed:			
Dry Roasted, 1 Tbsp, 8g	45	4	2
¼ cup, 1 oz	165	14	7
Oil Roasted, ⅓ cup, 1 oz	170	14	6.5
Watermelon, dried, ¼ cup, 1 oz	150	13	4

Quick Guide

Peanut Butter: *Average All Brands*

	C	F	Cb
½ cup, 5 oz	850	70	30
1 level tsp, 6g	35	3	1.5
1 level Tbsp, 0.6 oz (17g)	105	8.5	3.5
2 level Tbsp, 1.2 oz (34g)	210	17	7
1 oz Quantity (28g)	170	14	6
Jif: Reduced Fat, 2 Tbsp	190	12	15
Creamy; Crunchy; Simply, 2 Tbsp	190	16	7
Peanut Butter & Honey, 2 Tbsp	190	15	11
Peter Pan: Plus (Vits/Mins) 2 T., 1.2 oz	190	16	6
Honey Roast, 2 Tbsp, 1.2 oz	190	14	12
Peanut Wonder, 2 Tbsp	100	2.5	13
Smucker's: Honey Swtnd., 2 Tbsp	200	16	9
Goober Grape/Strawb., 2 Tbsp	160	9	16
Skippy: Carb Options, 1 Tbsp	100	8.5	5
Reduced Fat, 2 Tbsp	190	12	15
Squeeze Stix, 1 Tube, 0.9 oz	140	12	5

Other Nut & Seed Butters

	C	F	Cb
Almond Butter, 1 Tbsp, ½ oz	100	10	3.5
Almond Butter Honey Rstd, 1 T.	90	7	5.5
Beanut Butter, 1 Tbsp, ½ oz	90	5.5	7
Cashew Butter, 1 Tbsp, ½ oz	95	8	4.5
Hazelnut Butter, 1 Tbsp, ½ oz	105	10	2.5
Pecan Butter, 1 Tbsp, ½ oz	110	10	2
Pistachio Butter, 1 Tbsp, ½ oz	90	6.5	4.5
Sesame Butter/Tahini, 1 T., ½ oz	90	8	3
Soy Nut Butter, 1 Tbsp, ½ oz	75	5	4
Sunflower Seed Butter, 1 Tbsp	95	8	4
Nutella Hazelnut Spread, 2 Tbsp	200	11	24

Supplements

	C	F	Cb
Aloe Vera Juice, undiluted, 2 fl.oz	5	0	1
Cod Liver Oil, 1 Tbsp	125	13	0
Evening Primrose Oil, capsules, 1	5	0.5	0
Fiber Supplements: Tabs, 1	1	0	0
Metamucil, 1 packet	5	0	0
Regular, 1 rounded Tbsp	34	0	8
Sugar-Free, 1 Tbsp	6	0	1
Fish Oil Capsules, average, 1	10	1	0
Flax Oil: Capsules, 2	10	1	0
Barlean's, 3 softgels	110	11	0
Garlic Tablets/Capsules, each	3	0	0
Lecithin Granules, 1 Tbsp, 10g	55	4	0.5
Protein: Powders, average, 1 oz	100	0.5	0
Tablets, 20 tabs, ½ oz	70	0	0
Seaweed: Dried, 1 oz	85	0.5	22
Soaked, drained, 1 oz	15	0.5	4
Spirulina, 1 tablet	2	0	0.5
Vitamins/Minerals: Tabs/Caps, 1	2	0	0
Vitamin E Capsules, each	5	0.5	0
Viactiv Chews (1)	20	0.5	4
Yeast: Tablets, 2 tabs	4	0	0.5
Flakes, 1 heaping Tbsp, ⅓ oz	30	0.5	4
Powder, 1 heaping Tbsp, ½ oz	50	0.5	6

Cough & Pharmaceutical

	C	F	Cb
Cough/Cold Syrups: *Per Tablespoon*			
Regular: w. sugar, 1 Tbsp	35	0	9
w. alcohol, 1 Tbsp	46	0	9
Sugar-Free *(Diabetic Tussin)*, 1 T.	0	0	0
Cough Drops/Lozenges*: See Page 131*			
Antacids: Average, 1 tablet	4	0	1
Liquid, 1 Tbsp	6	0	1
Sudafed Syrup, 1 tsp	14	0	3
Tylenol Liquid: Child, 1 tsp	17	0	4
Extra Strength, 1 tsp	11	0	3

𝒩*ut eaters are healthier and live longer say medical researchers.*

Nuts are a nutritious source of protein, antioxidants, vitamins, minerals, healthy fats and fiber.

Their fat and fiber content can help to lower blood cholesterol, but watch the quantity if overweight.

Fresh Fruit

Weights As Purchased	C	F	Cb
Acerola, 1 cup, 20 pcs, 3½ oz	30	0	7.5
Apples: Whole, average all varieties,			
1 small (4 per lb), 4 oz	55	0	13
1 medium (3 per lb), 5½ oz	70	0	17
1 large (2 per lb), 8 oz	110	0	26
1 extra large, 11 oz	150	0	36
without skin: 1 medium, 4½ oz	60	0	14
1 cup slices, 4 oz	55	0	13
Candy/Caramel Apple, 1 med., 6½ oz	245	4	54
Nut Coated, 1 medium	230	5	46
Apricots: 1 small (12 per lb)	17	0	4
1 medium (8 per lb), 2 oz	25	0	6
1 large (5-6 per lb), 3 oz	40	0	10
Avocado (w/out seed/skin):			
Avg., ½ medium, 3 oz	160	15	8
1 salad slice, ½ oz	25	2	1
Mashed/Puree, 2 Tbsp, 1 oz	50	4.5	2
¼ cup, 2 oz	90	9	5
Californian, ½ medium, 3 oz	160	14	8
Mashed/Puree, ½ c., 4 oz	190	18	10
Florida, ½ medium, 5½ oz	180	15	12
Mashed/Puree, ½ c., 4 oz	140	11	9
½ cup cubed, 3 oz	105	8	7

Note: Avocados are nutritious and contain no cholesterol. Fat is mainly monounsaturated and benefits blood cholesterol. Excellent substitute for butter or margarine.

	C	F	Cb
Banana, (weight with skin):			
1 small (6", 4 per lb), 4 oz	90	0	23
1 medium (7", 3 per lb), 5 oz	105	0	27
1 large (8"), 7 oz	120	0	30
1 extra large (9"), 9 oz	135	0	35
w/out skin, 1 oz	25	0	6
Berries: (Blueberries/Black/Boysenberries)			
½ cup, 2.5 oz	40	0	10
1 pint, 14 oz	230	1.5	58
Breadfruit, ½ cup, 4 oz	115	0	30
Cactus Pear, 1 fruit, 3½ oz	40	0	9
Cantaloupe: Flesh (no rind), 1 oz	10	0	2
1 cup pieces/balls, 5.5 oz	55	0	13
½ Circle Slices (no rind):			
1 thin (¼"), 1 oz	10	0	2
1 medium (½"), 2 oz	20	0	5
1 thick (¾"), 3 oz	30	0	7
Wedges (Length cut, no rind):			
1 thin, ⅛ medium, 2 oz	20	0	5
1 thick, ¼ medium, 4 oz	40	0	9
Whole (Weights with seeds and rind):			
½ small, 20 oz	195	1	46
½ medium, 28 oz	270	1.5	65
½ large, 2½ lb	370	2	90
Carambola (Starfruit), 1 med, 3 oz	30	0	6
Cassava, ⅓ cup, 2½ oz	115	0	27
Cherimoya, 1 cup, 5.5 oz	115	1	27

Weights As Purchased	C	F	Cb
Cherries: 8 cherries, 2 oz	35	0	9
½ lb, (30 cherries)	145	0.5	36
Clementine, 1 med., 2.6 oz	35	0	9
Coconut: Fresh,			
1 piece, 2"x2"x½", 1 oz	100	10	4.5
Shredded, fresh, ½ cup, 1.4 oz	140	13	6
Sweetened, dried, ½ cup, 1.6 oz	235	16	22
Crabapples, ½ cup slices, 2 oz	40	0	11
Cranberries, ½ cup, 2 oz	25	0	6.5
Currants, raw, ½ cup, 2 oz	35	0	8
Custard Apple, raw, 4 oz	115	1	28
Dates: See Dried Fruits			
Dragon Pearl Fruit,			
1 medium, 11½ oz	330	1.5	76
Durian, flesh, 4 oz	165	6	31
Elderberries, ½ cup, 2½ oz	55	0.5	13
Feijoas, 1 medium, 2 oz	30	0.5	5.5
Figs, green/black:			
1 medium, 2 oz	40	0	10
1 large, 3 oz	60	0	15
Gooseberries, raw, ½ c., 2½ oz	35	0	7
Grapefruit: Average all types,			
½ fruit, 10 oz (6 oz flesh)	55	0	13
1 cup sections w. juice, 8 oz	75	0	18
Grapes: Average, 1 cup, 5½ oz	105	0	28
1 small bunch, 4 oz	80	0	20
1 medium bunch, 7 oz	140	0	36
1 large bunch, 16 oz	315	0	82
Granadilla, flesh 3½ oz	95	0	23
Groundcherries, ½ cup, 2½ oz	35	0	9
Guava: 1 medium, 4 oz	80	1	16
Honeydew: 1 slice, ¾" thick, 3 oz	30	0	7
1 wedge, (⅛ of 7" diam.,			
12 oz (with rind)	80	0	20
1 cup cubes/balls, 6 oz	60	0	14
½ small (4½ lb whole)	180	0.5	45
½ medium (6lb whole)	230	1	56
Honey Murcots, 1 only, 5 oz	45	0	11
Jaboticaba, flesh, 4 oz	75	2	15
Jackfruit, flesh, ½ average, 4 oz	105	0	27
Jambos (Brazil Cherry), flesh 4 oz	35	0	8
Java-Plum, 4 plums, ½ oz	10	0	2
Jujube, 3 oz	65	0	17
Kiwifruit, 1 medium, 2.7 oz	45	0	11
1 large, 3.2 oz	55	0.5	13
Kumquats, 5 medium, 3½ oz	65	1	15
Kiwano, ½ medium, 5 oz	35	0	8
Langsat, Duku, 1 medium, 2 oz	25	0	5
Lemon, 1 medium, 3 oz	25	0	8
1 wedge, 1 oz	5	0	1.5
Peel, 1 Tbsp	4	0	1
Limes, 1 med. (2" diam.), 2.4 oz	20	0	7
Loganberries, froz., ½ cup, 2½ oz	40	0	9

143

Fresh Fruit (Cont)

Weights As Purchased	C	F	Cb
Longans, 5 fruit, ½ oz	10	0	2.5
Loquats, 4 fruit, 2¼ oz	30	0	8
Lychees, 4 fruit, 2¼ oz	32	0	7
Mamey Apple: 1 whole, 3 lb	430	4	106
¼ fruit (1 cup flesh), 7 oz	100	1	25
Mandarin: 1 small, 3 oz	35	0	9
1 medium, 4 oz	45	0	11
1 large, 6 oz	50	0	13
Mango: Flesh, ½ cup slices, 3 oz	55	0	14
1 small mango, 7 oz	90	0.5	24
1 medium, 10 oz	130	0.5	34
1 cheek, 4 oz	60	0	14
1 large, 17 oz	220	1	58
1 extra large mango, 24 oz	310	1.5	82
Melon, avg, 1 cup, cubes/balls, 6 oz	60	0	14
Monstera Deliciosa (Taxonia), Edible part, 4 oz	50	0	11
Mulberries, 20 fruit, 1 oz	15	0	3
Nashi Fruit (Asian Pear), 1 med., 7 oz	85	0	21
Nectarines: 1 medium, 4 oz	50	0	12
1 large, 5½ oz	70	0	16
Oheloberries, ½ cup, 2½ oz	20	0	5
Olives (Pickled): Green, 10 lrg, 1½ oz	60	6.5	1.5
Ripe, Greek Style, 10 med., 1 oz	70	6	4
Ripe (Black) Californian:			
1 small/medium	5	0	0.2
1 large/extra large	6	0.5	0.5
1 jumbo	7	0.5	0.5
1 colossal	11	1	0.5
Oranges: Average all varieties,			
1 small, 5 oz (with skin)	45	0	11
1 medium (3" diam.), 7 oz	85	0	21
1 large, 10 oz	130	0	33
Flesh only, 1 cup, 6 oz	85	0	21
Californian Valencia,			
1 medium (2¾" diam.), 6 oz	60	0	14
Calif. Navels (3" diam.), 7 oz	70	0	17
Sunkist Navel, large, 14 oz	130	0	30
Florida Orange, 1 medium, 7 oz	70	0	17
Peel, 1 Tbsp	0	0	0
Papaya: ½ cup, cubed, 2½ oz	30	0	7
1 medium, (5"x3" diam.), 16 oz	120	0	30
Green (unripe), ½ cup, 3½ oz	20	0	5
Passionfruit, 1 medium, 1¼ oz	35	0	8
PawPaw (see Papaya)			
Peaches: 1 small/donut, 3 oz	30	0	7.5
1 medium (4 per lb), 4 oz	45	0	11
1 large, 6 oz	65	0	16
1 extra large, 10 oz	110	0	27

Weights As Purchased	C	F	Cb
Pears, Average all types:			
1 mini, 2½ oz	35	0	8
1 small, 5 oz	75	0	18
1 medium, 7 oz	105	0	25
1 large, 9 oz	135	0	33
1 extra large, 12 oz	175	0	42
Pepino, ½ medium, 4 oz	20	0	4
Persimmons: Native, 1 oz	35	0	9
Japanese (2½"d. x 2½"h), 7 oz	120	0	30
Seedless (Maui), 1 med., 5 oz	100	0	25
Pineapple (wts without skin):			
1 thin slice (½"), 2 oz	25	0	6
1 thick slice (¾"), 3 oz	40	0	10
1 cup, diced, 5½ oz	75	0	19
1 medium, 1½ lb (peeled)	325	0	86
Wedges *(Del Monte)*, 12 oz pkg	195	0	47
Canned: *See Page 146*			
Pitanga, (Surinam-Cherry) (5), 1.2 oz	10	0	2
Plaintains, ½ cup slices, 2½ oz	90	0	22
Plums: Average all types,			
Mini/Damson, (1" diam.), ½ oz	7	0	1.5
Small (2" diam.), 2¼ oz	30	0	7
Med. (2½" diam.), 3½ oz	45	0	10
Large (3" diam.), 5 oz	60	0	14
Pluot (plum-apricot), 1 med., 5 oz	80	0	19
Pomegranate, 1 medium, 10 oz	105	0.5	25
Pummelo, flesh, ½ cup, 3 oz	35	0	9
Prickly Pear, 1 medium, 5 oz	40	0.5	10
Quince, 1 medium, 3½ oz	55	0	14
Rambutan (Rambotang), Red/Yellow, 1 medium, 2 oz	15	0	4
Raspberries, ½ cup, 2 oz	30	0	7
Rhubarb, raw, ½ cup, 2 oz	15	0	3
Sapodilla (Chico), 1 med., 7½ oz	140	2	34
Sapotes, ½ medium, 8 oz	150	0.5	38
Satsuma Tangerine, 1 med., 3 oz	45	0	11
Soursop, 1 cup pulp, 8 oz	150	0.5	38
Starfruit, 1 medium, 3 oz	30	0	6
Strawberries: 1 cup, 5½ oz	50	0.5	12
6 medium/3 large, 2 oz	20	0	4
1 pint, 14 oz	115	1	27
Chocolate Dipped, 2 medium	45	2.5	6
Sugar Apples, ½ cup pulp, 4 oz	120	0	30
Tamarillo, 1 medium, 3 oz	20	0	3
Tamarind, 1 fruit (3"x1")	5	0	1.5

Weights as Purchased

	C	F	Cb
Tangelo: 1 small, 4 oz	55	0	13
1 medium, 5 oz	70	0	17
1 large, 7 oz	95	0	23
Tangerine, 1 medium, (2½" diam.), 4 oz	50	0	13
Tangor, 1 medium, 4 oz	35	0	7
Tomatillos (3), 3½ oz	35	1	6
Tomatoes:			
1 small (2¼" diam.), 3 oz	15	0	3
1 medium (2¾" diam.), 5 oz	25	0	5
1 large (3½" diam.), 8 oz	40	0.5	9
1 extra large (3" diam.), 12 oz	60	0.5	14
Grape, 5 medium, 2 oz	10	0	2
Yellow Tear Drop, 3 medium, 1 oz	5	0	2
Cherry: 4 medium, 2 oz	10	0	2
1 cup, 5¼ oz	27	0	6
Slices (Medium Tomato):			
2 thin slices, 1 oz	5	0	1
2 medium (¼" thick), 1½ oz	7	0	2
2 thick (⅜"), 2 oz	10	0	2
Wedge, ¼ medium tomato, 1¼ oz	6	0	1
Chopped, 1 cup, 6½ oz	35	0.5	7
Fried Green Tomato, 2 slices, 2½ oz	140	11	9
Canned Tomatoes/Products: See Page 85			
Tree Tomato (Tamarillo), 3 oz	20	0	5
Ugli Fruit, Tangelo type, 5 oz	40	0	8
Watermelon: Flesh only/no rind, 1 oz	9	0	2
1 thin slice, (circle, ⅜"), 2 oz	15	0	4
1 cup cubes or balls, 5½ oz	45	0	11
10 balls, 4.3 oz	35	0	9
Regular (Long Shape):			
1 thick (1") slice (¼ circle, 4½" radius)			
9 oz with skin (5½ oz no rind)	50	1	12
1 thin (½") slice (¼ circle)	25	1	6
1 thick (1") slice (½ circle)			
18 oz with rind	100	1	22
1 whole melon (15" long, 7½"diam.)			
20 lb w. rind, (10 lb no rind)	1360	7	330
Seedless (Round Shape):			
Medium size (13 lb, 8¼" diam.)			
1 whole, 8½ lb (no rind)	1160	5	280
Wedge (⅛ whole melon),			
26 oz (with rind)	145	1	35
Flesh only (no rind), 8 oz	70	0.5	17
Mini size (6 lb, 6½" diam.),			
1 whole, 3½ lb (no rind)	480	2.5	110
Wedge (⅛ whole),			
1½ lb (with rind)	60	0.5	14
Wax Jambu (Rose Apple), 2 oz	14	0	3

Dried Fruit

	C	F	Cb
Apples, 5 rings, 1 oz	80	0	19
Apricots, 8 halves, 1 oz	65	0	16
Banana Chips, ½ cup, 1½ oz	220	14	25
Banana Flakes, 4 Tbsp, 1 oz	80	0	20
Cranberries, swtn. dr., ⅓ c., 1.4 oz	125	0.5	30
Currants, ¼ cup, 1¼ oz	100	0	25
Dates: 5 medium dates, 1½ oz	120	0	29
Large Calif.: 1 date, 0.7 oz	55	0	13
3 dates, 2 oz	170	0	39
½ cup, chopped, 3 oz	240	0	58
Date Crumbles (Bob's Redmill),			
1 oz, ¼ cup	90	0	22
Figs, 3 medium figs, 1 oz	90	0	23
Goji Berries, 3 Tbsp, 1 oz	105	1.5	24
Longans; Lychees, 1 oz	80	0	20
Mango Slices, 5 pieces, 1.4 oz	25	0	6
Mixed Fruit, 1 oz	70	0	17
Papaya Spears, 2 pieces, 1.4 oz	120	0	30
Peaches, 2 halves, 1 oz	60	0	15
Pears, 3 halves, 2 oz	140	0.5	34
Plums (Sunsweet) (5), 1.4 oz	100	0	24
Prunes (dried Plums): w. pits, 1 oz	70	0	17
1 medium (60/lb)	16	0	4
1 large (50/lb)	22	0	5
1 extra large (40/lb)	25	0	6
Without pits, 4 med., 1 oz	70	0	17
Cooked: w. sugar, ½ cup, 5 oz	155	0	38
w/out sugar, ½ cup, 4½ oz	135	0	33
Raisins: 2 Tbsp, 1 oz pkg	85	0	20
½ cup, 2.8 oz	220	0.5	56

Candied Glazed Fruit

	C	F	Cb
Apricot, 1 medium, 1 oz	70	0	17
Cherry, 3 large, ½ oz	45	0	11
Citron/Fruit Peel, 1 oz	85	0	20
Ginger, 1 oz	90	0	21
Pineapple, 1 slice, 1¼ oz	120	0	29

Fruit Leather/Rolls

	C	F	Cb
Average All Brands, 1 oz	105	1	24
Fruit By The Foot, (Betty Crocker)			
1 roll, ¾ oz	80	0	17
Fruit Gushers, (Betty Crocker), 1 oz	90	1	20
Fruit Roll-Ups, (Betty Crocker) 1 roll	50	1	12
Stretch Island, Leathers, 2 pces, 1 oz	90	0	20
Other Fruit Confectionery/Snacks/Bars: *Page 137*			

Canned/Bottled Fruit

Solids & Liquids:	C	F	Cb
Per ½ Cup (Approx. 4½ oz)			
Apples, sweetened	70	0.5	17
Apricots: In water/diet	35	0	8
In juice/lite	60	0	15
In syrup	105	0	28
Black/Blueberries: Heavy syrup	120	0	30
In light syrup	110	0	26
Cherries, pitted: in water	55	0	15
In light syrup	85	0	22
In heavy syrup	105	0	27
In extra heavy syrup	135	0	34
Maraschino, 1 oz	50	0	12
Pie, ⅔ cup, 5 oz	90	0	22
Fruit Salad: In water/diet	35	0	10
In juice/Light	60	0	16
In heavy syrup	95	0	25
Gooseberries, Light syrup	90	0	24
Grapefruit: Juice pack	45	0	12
In light syrup	75	0	20
Lychees, ½ cup, 4.5 oz	105	0	26
Mixed Fruit: In water/diet	40	0	10
In fruit juices/light syrup	70	0	18
In heavy syrup	90	0	24
Peaches (halves/slices): In water/diet	30	0	7
In juice/light	55	0	14
In light syrup	70	0	18
drained, ½ peach	55	0	14
In heavy syrup	100	0	26
Pears: In water/diet	35	0	10
In juice/light	60	0	16
In heavy syrup	100	0	26
Pineapple: All types			
In own juice	75	0	20
In heavy syrup	100	0	26
1 slice (ring), drained, 1½ oz	15	0	4
Plums: In water	50	0	14
In juice	75	0	19
In light syrup, 3 plums	85	0	22
In heavy syrup, ½ cup	115	0	30
Prunes: In heavy syrup	125	0	33
In Liqueur, ½ cup, 125g	280	0	70
Stewed in Water, ½ cup	135	0	35
Raspberries, in heavy syrup	115	0	30
Strawberries: In water	25	0	6
In heavy syrup	120	0	31
Tropical Fruit Salad: In light syrup	80	0	21
In heavy syrup	110	0	29

Fruit Snack Cups

	C	F	Cb
Dell/Take-Out: Small, 6 oz	70	0	16
Large, 12 oz	140	0	32
Yogurt & Fruit Cup, 15 oz	380	4.5	75
Del Monte Fruit Cups			
Fruit Cups: Per 4 oz Cup			
Strawberry Banana	70	0	17
Mandarin Orange Segments	70	0	17
Pineapple Tidbits	70	0	18
Tropical Fruit	70	0	18
Fruit Naturals: Per 8 oz Cup			
Pineapple Chunks	140	0	35
Red Grapefruit	120	0	30
Fruit & Gel Cups: Per 4½ oz Cup			
Mixed Fruit/Peaches in Fruit Gel	90	0	22
Lite varieties in Gel, avg.	14	0	14
Carb Clever: Per ½ Cup (4.2 oz)			
Fruit Cocktail/Pears (chunks/slices)	40	0	10
Peaches (chunks/slices)	30	0	7
Pull Top Cans: in 100% Juice, 4 oz	80	0	20
Lite varieties, 4 oz	50	0	13
Dole Fruit Bowls			
4 oz Bowls: Peaches	70	0	18
Mixed Fruit/Tropical Fruit	80	0	19
Pineapple	60	0	16
Fruit n Gel Bowls (4.3 oz): Regular	90	0	23
Reduced Sugar	60	0	16
Mott's: Healthy Harvest, 4 oz cup	50	0	13
Vons: Mixed Fruit,			
In heavy syrup, 1 cup, 4.5 oz	100	0	25
In lite syrup, 1 cup	60	0	14

Apple & Fruit Sauces

	C	F	Cb
Apple Sauce:			
Regular/sweetened, 2 Tbsp, 1 oz	20	0	6
4 oz package	85	0	22
¼ cup	50	0	13
Fruit Sauces & Purees:			
Average all fruit types, 2 Tbsp, 1 oz	25	0	6
½ cup, 4 oz	100	0	24
Mott's: Classics, avg. 4 oz	100	0	25
Apple Sauce: Original, 4 oz	100	0	24
Fruit Flavored, avg., 4 oz	90	0	23
Unsweetened, 4 oz	50	0	12
Ocean Spray: Per ¼ Cup (2½ oz)			
Jellied Cranberry Sauce	110	0	25
Whole Berry Cranberry Sauce	110	0	27

Vegetables

Vegetables

	C	F	Cb
Alfalfa Sprouts, ½ cup, ½ oz	5	0	0.5
Artichokes, Globe/French:			
1 medium, 4½ oz	60	0	13
1 large, 5.7 oz	75	0	17
Artichoke Heart (Fanci Food):			
Plain, 1 piece	8	0	1
Marinated, ¼ bottle, 1 oz	25	1.5	2
Asparagus, raw/froz.: 4 med. spears	12	0	2.5
Cuts & Tips (Del Monte), ½ cup, 4.3 oz	20	0	3
Bamboo Shoots, ckd, ½ c, 2 oz	7	0	1
Beans: Green/Snap/String, ½ c, 2 oz	17	0	4
10 beans (4" long), 2 oz	17	0	4
Dried Beans, average all types: (Kidney, Brown, Haricot, Lima, Mung, Navy, Pinto, Red, White)			
Raw: 2 Tbsp, 1 oz	95	0.5	18
1 cup, 7 oz	665	3	126
Cooked: 1 oz	35	0	7
½ cup, 3 oz	105	0	21
Bean Sprouts, avg., ½ cup, 2 oz	17	0	3.5
Beets: Raw, 1 beet (2" diam), 3 oz	35	0	8
Cooked, ½ cup, slices, 3 oz	37	0	8.5
1 beet, 2" diam., 1¾ oz	22	0	5
Beet Greens, ckd, ½ c, 2½ oz	20	0	4
Bell Pepper: See Peppers			
Bitter Melon/Gourd, ½ c pcs, 1.6 oz	14	0.3	1.5
Black Eyed Peas, ckd, ½ c., 2 oz	100	0.5	18
Bok Choy (Chinese Chard), ckd., 3 oz	10	0	1.5
Breadfruit, ¼ small fruit, 3.4 oz	100	0.2	26
Broadbeans (Fava Beans):			
Green (in pod), raw: 4 pods			
(3½ oz w. shell; 1.2 oz beans)	30	0	6
1 cup beans (no shell), 4½ oz	110	1	22
Mature Seeds: Raw, 1 c., 5.3 oz	512	2.3	87
Cooked, 1 cup, 3 oz	94	0	17
Broccoflower, ⅛ head, 3½ oz	35	0	7
Broccoli: Raw, chopped, 1 cup, 3 oz	30	0	6
3 Florets, 3 oz	25	0	5
1 Spear (5" long) 1.1 oz	10	0	2
1 Whole: Medium size, 14 oz	135	1.5	26
Large, 21 oz	203	2	40
1 Head (no stalk), 11 oz	105	1	21
1 Stalk, small (5" long), 5.3 oz	50	0.5	10
Brocco Sprouts, ½ cup, 2 oz	16	0	2
Brussel Sprouts: ckd, ½ cup, 2.8 oz	28	0.5	6
2 Sprouts, 1½ oz	15	0	3
Butterbeans, cooked, ½ cup, 3 oz	90	0	16
Cabbage, All types/colors, average:			
Raw: 1 Leaf, large, 1.2 oz	8	0	2
Shredded, 1 cup, 2½ oz	17	0	4
½ Lge Head (7" diam), 22 oz	150	1	35
Cooked, shredded, ½ cup, 2½ oz	17	0.5	3.5
Cactus (Nopal), sliced, 1 cup, 3 oz	14	0	3

Vegetables (Cont)

	C	F	Cb
Carrots: Regular thick variety,			
1 small, 4 oz	47	0	11
1 medium, 6 oz	70	0	16
1 large, 8 oz	93	0	22
Chopped, 1 cup, 4½ oz	52	0.3	12
Grated, 1 cup, 4 oz	45	0.3	11
Slices, 1 cup, 4½ oz	50	0.3	12
Sticks (4"), 4, 1½ oz	18	0	4
Long thin variety, 1 medium, 2.2 oz	25	0	6
Baby: Snack size, 3 medium, 1 oz	10	0	2.5
Snack Pack, 3 oz	30	0	7
Cauliflower: Raw: 1 cup (pces), 3½ oz	25	0	5
½ medium head, 10 oz	72	0	15
Cooked, 3 florets, 2 oz	12	0	2
Celeriac, ½ cup, raw, 2¾ oz	33	0	7
Celery: 1 large stalk, 11", 2.2 oz	10	0	2
1 small stalk, 5", ½ oz	2	0	0.5
4 Strips/sticks, ½ oz	4	0	1
Chopped, 1 cup, 3½ oz	14	0	3
Chard (Swiss), ½ cup, ckd, 3 oz	18	0	3.5
Chayote Squash, raw, 1 cup, 4½ oz	22	0	4
Chick Peas (Garbanzo Beans):			
Dry, 1 cup, 7 oz	730	12	121
Cooked, 1 cup, 6 oz	270	4	45
Chicory Greens, 1 cup, 1 oz	7	0	1.5
Chicory/Witloof: See Endive			
Chili Peppers: See Peppers			
Chinese Long Bean, sliced, 1 c., 3.2 oz	45	0	8
Chives, chopped, 1 Tbsp	1	0	0
Choy Sum, 3 oz	13	0	3
Cilantro (Coriander), 1 Cup	4	0	0.5
Collards, cooked, ½ cup, 3 oz	25	0	5
Corn, yellow/white:			
Raw: Kernels, ½ c., 3 oz	80	0.5	19
Ear (5"x 1¾"), raw, 5½ oz	153	1	37
Cooked: Kernels, ½ c., 3 oz	77	0.5	18
Cob, cooked, dr: Small, 2¼ oz	60	0.5	14
Large ear, 5½ oz	118	1	28
(Also see Frozen & Canned Corn Page 149-150)			
Courgette: See Zucchini			
Cress, Garden, raw, ½ cup, 1 oz	8	0	1.5
Cucumber: 1 whole, 11 oz	45	0.5	10
½ cup slices, 2 oz	8	0	2
Mini/Lebanese (1), 3 oz	13	0	3
Daikon Radish, ½ cup, slices, 2 oz	9	0	2
Dandelion Greens, raw, ½ cup, 1 oz	12	0	2.5
Edamame (Immature green soybeans):			
Shelled, ½ cup, 2.6 oz	110	5	8
With shells, 10 pods, 1¼ oz	30	1	3
Eggplant: Raw, ½ medium, 4 oz	27	0	7
Raw, ½ cup, 1" pieces, 1½ oz	10	0	2.5
1 slice, fried, 1 oz	75	4	10
Endive, Belgian/French: Raw,			
1 med. head (6"), 2½ oz	12	0	2.5

147

Vegetables (Cont)

Food	C	F	Cb
Fiddleheads, 3.5 oz	34	0.5	5.5
Fava Beans: *See Broadbeans*			
Fennel, 1 cup, sliced, 3 oz	27	0	6.5
Gai Choy Cabbage, ckd, 1 cup, 6 oz	20	0	3
Gai Lan (Chinese Kale), ckd, 1 cup	36	0.5	7
Garlic, 1 clove	4	0	1
Ginger: ¼ cup slices, 1 oz	20	0	4.5
Crystallized (sugared), 7 pce, 1½ oz	130	0	35
Horseradish, raw, 1 pod, ½ oz	5	0	1
Jerusalem Artichoke, raw, ½ cup	57	0	13
Jicama, raw, sliced, ½ cup, 2¼ oz	23	0	5.5
Kale, 1 cup, chopped, 2½ oz	34	0.5	7
Kohlrabi, ½ cup, cooked, 1¾ oz	17	0	4.5
Lambsquarters, chopped, 1 c., 6.3 oz	60	1.5	9
Leek, cooked, 1 whole, 4½ oz	38	0	9
Lentils, green/brown: Dry, 1 oz	100	0.5	17
Dry, 1 cup, 6¾ oz	678	2	115
Cooked, ½ cup, 3½ oz	115	0.5	20
Lettuce: 1 cup, chop./shred., 2 oz	7	0	1.5
Butterhead, 2 leaves, ½ oz	2	0	0.5
Cos/Romaine, shred'd, 1 c., 1.7 oz	10	0	1.5
Iceberg: 1 outer leaf, ½ oz	2	0	0.5
1 medium head, 15-16 oz	75	1	16
Lamb's Lettuce, 2½ oz	15	0	3
Lima Beans, baby, ckd,½ c., 3 oz	105	0	20
Lotus Root, 10 slices, ckd, 3 oz	59	0	14
Mung Bean Sprouts, ½ cup, 2 oz	16	0	3
Mushrooms: Raw, 1 medium, 0.6 oz	4	0	0.5
Raw, 1 large, sliced, ¾ oz	5	0	1
Raw, ½ cup pieces, 1¼ oz	8	0	1
Cooked, ½ cup pieces, 2½ oz	22	0.5	4
Mustard Greens, ckd, ½ cup, 1 oz	7	0	1.5
Nopal (Cactus): 1 leaf, 4½ oz	20	0	4.5
Sliced, 1 cup, 3 oz	14	0	3
Okra, cooked, ½ c., slices, 2¾ oz	18	0	3.5
Onions: Raw: 1 small, 2½ oz	29	0	7
1 medium, 4 oz	48	0	11
1 large, 5½ oz	63	0	15
1 jumbo, 16 oz	190	0.5	46
Chopped: Raw, ½ cup, 3 oz	34	0	8
1 Tbsp, 0.4 oz	4	0	1
Slices: 1 cup, 4 oz	48	0	12
1 thin slice, small, 0.4 oz	4	0	1
1 medium slice (⅛"), ½ oz	6	0	1.5
1 large slice (¼"), 1⅓ oz	16	0	4
Dehydrated flakes, ¼ c, ½ oz	50	0	12
Rings, breaded/fried, 2 rings	80	5	9
Scallions, ½ cup, 2 oz	16	0	3.5
Spring, 1 cup, chopped, 2 oz	16	0	3.5
French's Fried Onions: *See Page 72*			
Blossom/Blooming: See Fast-Foods (Chili's/Outback)			

Food	C	F	Cb
Parsley, chopped, ½ cup, 1 oz	10	0	2
Parsnips: 1 medium, 4 oz	85	0	20
Cooked, ½ cup slices, 2¾ oz	55	0	13
Peas: Raw, Green, ¼ cup, 1½ oz	30	0	5
Raw, with pods, ½ lb	70	0	13
Snow Peas, 10 pods, 1.2 oz	14	0	2.5
Split: Dry, hulled, 1 oz	97	0.5	17
Cooked, 1 cup, 7 oz	230	1	42
Peppers: Sweet, 1 medium, 4.2 oz	28	0	6.5
Bell: 1 medium, 4.2 oz	28	0	6.5
½ cup, chopped, raw, 2½ oz	20	0	4.5
1 ring (3" diam. x ¼" thick)	3	0	0.5
Chili: Green/Red, 1 oz	18	0	4.5
Habanero, 1 only, 8g	11	0	1
Pigeon Peas, cooked, ½ cup, 3 oz	94	1	21
Pimientos, 3 medium, 3½ oz	25	0	5
Poi, ½ cup, 4.2 oz	134	0	33
Pumpkin: Mashed, ½ cup, 4⅓ oz	25	0	6
Raw, 1" cubes, 1 cup, 4 oz	30	0	7.5
Pumpkin Flowers, 1 cup, 1.2 oz	5	0	1
Purslane: Cooked, ½ c., 2 oz	10	0	1
Raw, 1" cubes, 1 cup, 1.5 oz	7	0	1.5
Potatoes: Raw (with skin)			
1 Baby, Gourmet, 2 oz	45	0	10
1 Small, 6 oz	130	0	30
1 Medium, 7.5 oz	164	0	37
1 Peeled, 4 oz	90	0	20
1 Large, 8 oz	175	0	40
1 Extra large (Russet), 13 oz	284	0	65
1 Jumbo (Russet), 16 oz	350	0.5	80
Baked (no fat); large, 10 oz raw:			
Plain, with skin, 7 oz	185	0.3	42
without skin, 5½ oz	145	0	34
Garlic Potatoes, mashed, 4 oz	128	5	19
w. Skin/Toppings: + 2 tsp fat	270	8	58
+ Sour Cr./Chives, 2 Tbsp	320	6	60
+ Plain Yogurt, 2 Tbsp	260	1	60
+ Grated Cheese, 1 oz	370	6	58
+ Cottage Cheese, 2 oz	315	2	60
Mashed w. milk and fat, ½ c.	120	4.5	18
Hash Browns: w. Butt. Sce, 2½ oz	125	6	17
Homemade, ½ cup, 2¾ oz	207	10	21
Potato Skins: (w. Cheese topping),			
½ whole (8 oz baking), 4 oz	240	13	22
French Fries: Small serve, 2.6 oz	250	13	30
Medium serve, 4 oz	380	20	47
Froz., uncooked, 18 fries, 4 oz	167	5.5	23
Oven-heated, 18 fries, 4 oz	167	5.5	23
Take-Out, 1 serve, 5 oz	440	25	60
McDonald's: Small, 2.6 oz	250	13	30
Medium, 4 oz	380	20	47

Vegetables (Cont)

	C	F	Cb
Potatoes (Cont)			
Fried, 18 fries, 4 oz	167	5.5	28
Au Gratin, ½ cup, 4.3 oz	162	9	14
Pancakes, 2 small, 2 oz	120	6.5	12
Kugel, 5 oz	300	20	26
Puffs, fried, 4 puffs, 1 oz	53	2.5	8
Scalloped, ½ cup, 4¼ oz	114	5.5	15
Ore-Ida Frozen Potatoes: *See Page 150*			
Potato Salad, ½ cup, 4½ oz	180	10	14
Radicchio, 2 leaves, ½ oz	4	0	1
Shredded, 1 cup, 1½ oz	18	0	3.5
Radish: Avg., 10 only, 1½ oz	7	0	1.5
Oriental, ½ c. slices, 1½ oz	8	0	2
Rutabagas, ckd., ½ c. cubes, 3 oz	33	0	7.5
Salsify, ckd, ½ c. slices, 2½ oz	48	0	11
Sauerkraut, ½ cup, 2½ oz	13	0	3
Seaweed: Average, dried, 1 oz	7	0	2
Soaked, drained, 1 oz	15	0	4
Nori/Laver, dried, 6 sheets, ½ oz	35	0	5
Shallots, chopped, 1 Tbsp, ½ oz	7	0	1.5
Sorrel, raw, ½ cup, 4 oz	23	0.5	4
Soybeans: Mature, dry, 1 oz	118	5.5	9
Dry, ½ cup, 3⅓ oz	387	18	28
Cooked, ½ cup, 3 oz	150	7.5	8.5
(Soy Products/Tofu/Tempeh: *See Page 77*)			
Spinach: Cooked, ½ cup, 3 oz	20	0	3.5
Raw: 3 leaves/1 cup, 1 oz	7	0	1
1 Bunch, 12 oz	78	1.5	12
Creamed, avg., ½ cup, 4½ oz	187	15	8
Squash: Summer, raw, ½ c., 2½ oz	10	0	2
Cooked, ½ cup slices, 3 oz	14	0	3.5
Winter, cooked,			
Acorn, ½ cup cubes, 3½ oz	34	0	9
½ medium (10 oz raw wt.)	114	0	30
Butternut, ½ c. cubes, 3½ oz	40	0	10
¼ medium (9 oz raw wt.)	115	0	30
Spaghetti, ½ cup, 1¾ oz	16	0	3.5
Succotash, ckd, ½ cup, 3⅓ oz	110	1	23
Sweetcorn: *See Corn*			
Sweet Potatoes: Cooked with Skin (no fat)			
1 medium, 4 oz	103	0	24
No skin, mashed, ½ c., 5½ oz	125	0	29
Swedes, ½ cup, 2 oz	20	0	4.5
Swiss Chard, ckd, chopped, 1 c., 6 oz	35	0	7
Taro, cooked, ½ cup, 2⅓ oz	94	0	23

Vegetables (Cont)

	C	F	Cb
Tomatoes: 1 small (2¼" diam.), 3 oz	15	0	3
1 medium (2¾" diam.), 5 oz	25	0	5
1 large (3½" diam.), 8 oz	40	0.5	9
1 extra lge (3" diam.), 12 oz	60	0.5	14
Chopped, 1 cup, 6½ oz	35	0.5	7
Extra Listings: *Page 145*			
Tomatillo, 1 medium, 1.2 oz	10	0	2
Turnips: White, ckd, ½ cup, 2¾ oz	17	0	4
Greens, cooked, ½ cup, 2½ oz	14	0	3
Water Chestnuts: 5-6 nuts, 1 oz	56	0.5	13
½ cup slices, 2¼ oz, raw	60	0	15
Canned, 1 oz	14	0	3.5
Watercress, 10 sprigs, 1 oz	3	0	0.5
Yam: Cooked, ½ cup, 2½ oz	80	0	19
Baked, 1 medium (6") 8 oz	264	0.5	63
1 large (9") 12 oz	395	0.5	94
Yardlong Bean, 1 pod, ½ oz	6	0	1
Yucca Root, ½ cup, 3 oz	165	0.5	39
Zucchini: 1 medium, 7 oz, raw	30	0.5	6.5
½ cup slices, cooked, 3 oz	14	0	3.5

Frozen Vegetables

	C	F	Cb
Birds Eye			
Broccoli/Corn/Vegetables, ⅔ cup	50	1	9
Chopped Spinach, ⅓ cup	30	0	3
Other varieties, average, 1 cup	30	0	6
Baby: Corn & Vege Blend, ⅔ cup	50	1	9
Broccoli Florets, 3 oz	30	0	4
Corn, Pea & Bean Blend, ¾ cup	70	0.5	13
Sweet Peas, ½ cup, 3 oz	70	0	12
Whole Green Beans, 1 cup, 3 oz	35	0	5
Deluxe Vegetables: *Per Cup*			
Sugar Snap Stir Fry, 3½ oz	40	0	7
Broccoli, Cauliflower & Peppers	25	0	3
Broccoli, Carrots & Water Chestnuts	35	0	6
Steam Fresh: *Per Serving*			
Broccoli Cuts, 1 cup	30	0	4
Mixed Veges, ⅔ cup	60	0	12
Super Sweet Corn, ⅔ cup	70	1	14
Stir Fry: *Prepared (Includes Pasta)*			
Asian, 1 cup	60	1	12
Green Bean & Almonds, ¾ cup	80	4	8
Voila! Meals: *See Page 61*			
Green Giant			
Vegetables: Asparagus Cuts, ⅔ c.	20	0	3
Corn: Nibblers, ½ ear, 2.2 oz	70	0.5	14
Extra Sweet Niblets, ⅓ cup	70	1	13
Shoepeg, no sauce, ½ cup	70	1	15
Honey Glazed Carrots, 1 cup	90	3	15
Le Sueur Baby Sweet Peas, ¾ cup	60	0.5	11
Spinach, no sauce, ½ cup, 3½ oz	25	0	3

Vegetables – Frozen, Canned, Bottled

Frozen Vegetables (Cont) — C F Cb

Green Giant (Cont)

Veges In Cheese & Cream Sauce: *Prepared*

	C	F	Cb
Alfredo Vegetables, ¾ cup	70	2.5	9
Broccoli, Cauliflower, Carrots, 1 c.	50	1.5	7
Cauliflower & Cheese Sce, ½ cup	60	2.5	6
Creamed Spinach, ½ cup	70	2.5	9

Rice & Vegetables: *Per ½ Pkg (Prepared)*

	C	F	Cb
Cheesy Rice & Broccoli	135	2.5	25
Rice Medley	140	2	26
Rice Pilaf	115	1.5	22
White & Wild Rice	140	3	25

Ore-Ida (As Purchased):

French Fries:

	C	F	Cb
Country, 18 fries, 3 oz	120	4	19
Crispers 20 pces, 3 oz	210	12	23
Crispy Crunchies, 13 fries, 3 oz	160	8	20
Fast Food Fries, 27 fries, 3 oz	180	7	21
Waffle Fries, 8 fries, 3 oz	160	6	22
Golden Crinkles, 12 pces, 3 oz	130	4	17
Golden Fries, 14 pces, 3 oz	120	2.5	20
Oven Chips, 7 pces, 3 oz	160	7	22
Shoestrings, 32 pces, 3 oz	150	6	19
Steak Fries, 7 fries, 3 oz	120	3	17
Zesties, 12 pces, 3 oz	140	5	22
Hash Browns: Toaster, 2 patties	220	12	25
Potatoes O'Brien, ¾ c., 2 oz	60	0	13
Onion Rings: Gourmet, 3 pces, 3 oz	190	9	24
Onion Ringers, 6 pces, 3.2 oz	220	12	25
Sweet Potatoes: 4 oz	80	0	18
Tater Tots: 9 pces, 3 oz	150	7	22
Mini, 19 pces, 3 oz	190	10	19
Onion, 9 pces, 3 oz	160	7	22
Extra Crispy, 12 pces, 3 oz	145	7	19
Twiced Baked: Potatoes, 1, 5 oz	190	7	26

TGI Friday's

	C	F	Cb
Potato Skins, avg., 3 pces, 3½ oz	210	11	20
Wild Oats: Tater Bites, 9 pces, 3 oz	150	6	21
Shredded Hash Browns, 1 c., 3 oz	70	0	15
French Fries, 14 pces, 3 oz	110	3	17

Eat at least 5 servings of fruit and vegetables every day . . . and Enjoy Better Health!

Canned/Bottled — C F Cb

Solids & Liquid

	C	F	Cb
Artichoke Hearts (Fanci Foods):			
Plain, 1 oz (1)	8	0	1
Marinated, 1 bottle, 1 oz	25	1.5	2
Asparagus, Drained: 3 spears, 2 oz	10	0	1.5
Pieces, ½ cup, 4.3 oz	25	0.5	3
Bamboo Shoots, 1 cup, 4½ oz	25	0	4
Bean Salad, ½ cup, 4⅓ oz, no oil	90	0	20
Beans: Green, ½ cup, 2½ oz	15	0	3
Baked Beans, ½ cup, 4½ oz	120	0.5	27
Butter Beans, ½ cup, 4½ oz	90	0	16
Italian, cut, ½ cup, 4½ oz	30	0	6
Kidney Beans, ½ cup, 3½ oz	105	0.5	19
Lima Beans, ½ cup, 4½ oz	80	0	15
Pinto Beans, ½ cup, 4½ oz	105	1	19
Beets: Sliced, ½ cup, 3 oz	26	0	6
Crinkle/Pickled (Del Monte) ½ cup	80	0	20
Carrots: Sliced, ½ cup, 2½ oz	20	0	4
Honey Glazed (Del Monte) ½ cup	75	0	18
Corn: Kernels, ½ cup, 4½ oz	80	0.5	18
Creamed style, ½ cup, 4½ oz	92	0.5	23
Garbanzo/Chick Peas, ½ c., 4.2 oz	143	1.5	27
Green Chilis, diced, 2 Tbsp, 1 oz	6	0	1.5
Hearts of Palm (1), 1.2 oz	7	0	1
Mushrooms: ½ cup, 2½ oz	20	0	4
in Butter Sauce, 2 oz	20	1	3
Onions: Pickled, 1 med., ½ oz	10	0	2
Cocktail, 1 onion	0	0	0
French's Fried Onions: See Page 72			
Peas, ½ cup, 3 oz	60	0.5	10
Peppers: Hot Chili, Jalapeno, (1), 1 oz	6	0	2
Sweet, undrained, 2½ oz	13	0	3
Jalapeno, w. liq., ½ c. chopped	18	0.5	3
Fried, drain, 2 Tbsp, 1 oz	60	5	3
Salsa, average all types, 2 Tbsp	10	0	2
Sauerkraut, undrained, ½ c., 4 oz	22	0	5
Spinach, ½ cup, 3½ oz	25	0.5	3.5
Succotash: w. Cr. Style Corn, ½ c.	100	0.5	23
w. whole kernels, undrained, ½ c.	80	0.5	18
Sweetcorn: See Corn			
Sweet Potato: ½ cup, 3½ oz	90	0	24
Tomatoes, Sundr.: Natural, 5-6 pce	22	0	5
In Oil, drained, 6 pces, ½ oz	38	2.5	4
Tomato Products: See Page 85			
Vegetables, mixed, ½ cup, 4 oz	45	0	8
Yams: in Light Syrup, ½ cup, 4 oz	105	0	25
Candied, ½ cup, 5 oz	170	0	46
Zucchini in Tom. Sce., ½ c., 4 oz	30	0	8

Take-Out Salads & Vegetables

Avg. All Outlets: Per Serving	C	F	Cb
Antipasto Salad, ½ cup	135	8	13
Bean Salad, ½ cup	110	4	17
Bulgur Salad, ½ cup	70	2	12
Caesar Salad, Classic, 1 cup	200	14	15
Side Salad, no Dressing	25	0	6
Carrot Raisin: No Dressing, ½ cup	20	0	5
with Dressing, ½ cup	135	12	6
Chef Salad: Regular, no Dressing	620	37	8
w. 2 oz 1000 Island	860	61	8
Chicken Salad Platter, 6 oz	200	8	12
Coleslaw: Traditional, ½ cup	150	8	18
w. Low Cal Dressing, ½ cup	50	2	8
Corn, Mexican, ½ cup	240	12	33
Cucumber: Non-Oil Dressing, ½ c.	60	0	14
w. Oil Dressing, ½ cup	140	12	8
Eggplant Salad, ½ cup	75	4	7
Fettucini w. veges, ½ cup	135	6	16
Garden Salad, no Dressing, 1 cup	10	0	2
Greek Salad, 1 cup	105	8	7
Greek Vegetables, 1 cup	110	8	6
Lettuce, hearts, ½ head	15	0	2.5
Lobster Salad Platter, 6 oz	200	8	12
Macaroni Salad, ½ cup, 4 oz	140	6	17
Nicoise, 1 cup	450	32	19
Pasta Salad, ½ cup	200	11	19
Pineapple Coconut Slaw, ½ cup	100	9	4
Potato Salad: Dijon, 3 oz	120	7	13
w. Mayonnaise, ½ cup	215	15	17
Lowfat, ½ cup	110	1.5	21
Rice Salad, ½ cup	150	10	13
Saffron Rice, ½ cup	145	3	26
Spinach Salad, 1 cup	180	13	13
Tabouli, ½ cup	125	7	13
Three Bean Salad, ½ cup	90	4.5	12
Tomato & Mozzarella, ½ cup	180	14	10
Tortellini w. Basil Pesto, ½ cup	150	9	15
Waldorf w. Mayo, ½ cup	110	7	12
Signature Salads: *Per Serving (6 oz)*			
(Supplied to Deli's and Institutions)			
Antipasto Salad, 6 oz	510	50	4
Artichoke Salad, marinated	400	41	8
California Medley	120	7	15
Cheese Agnolotti	250	8	23
Chicken Salad	420	33	11
Crabmeat Flavored	450	38	20

Take-Out Salads (Cont)

Signature Salads (Cont)	C	F	Cb
Egg Salad	300	23	14
Fresh Button Mushroom	190	16	6
Garden Olive	630	67	3
Ham Salad	400	32	14
Prima Pasta Salad	360	30	18
Seafood Pasta Del Mar	170	10	21
Seafood with Crab & Shrimp	420	34	20
Shrimp Salad	360	32	8
Tuna Salad	450	36	14
Fast-Food Restaurants: *See Page 183*			

Fresh Salad Packs

Pre-Packaged (Supermarkets)	C	F	Cb
Dole: Caesar Kit, 3½ oz	170	15	8
Asian Crunch Kit, 3½ oz	120	6	12
Bacon Lettuce Kit, 3 oz	130	9	8
Regular Salad Packs *(no added dressing):*			
Classic Coleslaw, 3 oz	25	0	4
Classic Iceberg, 3 oz	15	0	4
Soy Cheese, 3½ oz	80	6	3
Fresh Mates: *Per ¼ Container*			
Broccoli ranch, 1½ cups	230	13	25
Cheddar Bacon Ranch, 1½ c.	370	22	35
Garden Vegetable, 1½ cups	240	14	25
Italian Herb, 1½ cups	270	12	33
Fresh Express			
Salad Kits: *Per Serving (Prepared)*			
Caesar, ⅓ kit	150	13	8
Caesar w. Light Dress., ⅓ kit	100	7	8
Caesar Supreme, ⅓ kit	170	14	8
Asian, ¼ kit	170	10	17
Taco Fiesta, ⅓ kit	110	8	7

Salad Toppings

	C	F	Cb
Bacon Bits, average, 1 Tbsp	35	2	2
Chow Mein Noodles, dry, ½ cup	120	7	13
Croutons, 2 Tbsp, 10g	40	1	7
Olives, 5 medium	25	2	0
Potato Chips, 20 chips, 1 oz	150	10	15
Sunflower Seeds, 1 Tbsp, 8 g	45	4	1.5
Tortilla Chips, 12 chips, 1 oz	140	7	19

Fruit & Vegetable Juices/Smoothies

Minute Maid **V8**

Quick Guide | C | F | Cb

Orange Juice
Average ~ Fresh or Sweetened:

	C	F	Cb
½ Cup, 4 fl.oz	55	0	13
Small Glass, 6 fl.oz	85	0	19
Regular Glass, 8 fl.oz	110	0.5	26
8¾ fl.oz Box	120	0.5	28
10 fl.oz Bottle	140	0.5	32
11½ fl.oz Can	160	0.5	37
16 fl.oz Bottle	225	1	52
20 fl.oz Bottle	280	1	64
64 fl.oz/½ Gallon	895	4	206

Juices ~ Generic

Average All Brands: Per 8 fl.oz Unless Indicated

	C	F	Cb
Aloe Vera Juice, unsweet., 2 oz	10	0	0
Apple Juice: 8 fl.oz	120	0	29
10 fl.oz Bottle	145	0.5	36
16 fl.oz	235	0.5	58
Carrot Juice: Fresh, 6 fl.oz	35	0	8
Sweetened, 6 fl.oz	75	0	17
Cranberry Juice, Cocktail/Blend	140	0	34
Fruit Blends, average, 8 fl.oz	110	0	27
Fruit Nectars, average, 8 fl.oz	140	0	36
Grape Juice, 8 fl.oz	155	0	38
Grapefruit Juice, 8 fl.oz	95	0	22
Lemon/Lime Juice: 1 Tbsp	3	0	1
1 cup, 8 fl.oz	50	0.5	16
Concentrate, 1 tsp	0	0	0
Noni Juice: *Tahitian,* 2 Tbsp, 1 fl.oz	5	0	1
Tahiti Traders, 1 fl.oz	20	0	5
Orange Juice, 8 fl.oz	110	0.5	26
Passion Fruit Juice (Fresh):			
Purple, 1 cup, 8 fl.oz	125	0	34
Yellow, 1 cup, 8 fl.oz	80	1.5	14
Papaya/Peach Nectar, avg., 8 fl.oz	140	0	36
Pear Nectar, 8 fl.oz	150	0	40
Pineapple Juice, 8 fl.oz	130	0	32
Prune Juice, 8 fl.oz	180	0	45
Strawb./Raspberry Juice, 8 fl.oz	100	0	23
Tangerine Juice, 8 fl.oz	105	0.5	25
Tomato Juice, 8 fl.oz	40	0	10
Vegetable Juice, 8 fl.oz	45	0	11
Wheat Grass Juice: 1 fl.oz 'Shot'	5	0	1
2 fl.oz 'Shot'	15	0	2

Quick Guide | C | F | Cb

Fruit Smoothies (Jamba Juice; Smoothie King)
Average All Brands

	C	F	Cb
Fruit Only: 8 fl.oz	115	0.5	29
12 fl.oz	175	1	43
16 fl.oz	230	1	58
24 fl.oz	350	1	78
Fruit + Non-Fat Milk/Soy:			
12 fl.oz	135	0	29
16 fl.oz	155	0	37
24 fl.oz	265	1	59
Fruit + Non-Fat Frozen Yogurt/Sherbet:			
12 fl.oz	200	0	47
16 fl.oz	265	0	63
24 fl.oz	395	0	95

Juice Brands | C | F | Cb

Per 8 fl.oz Unless Indicated

	C	F	Cb
Apple & Eve			
Naturally Cranberry	130	0	32
Cranberry/Raspberry Apple	120	0	26
Cranberry Grape	140	0	34
Bolthouse			
100% Juices: Carrot, 8 fl.oz	70	0	14
Passionfruit Apple Carrot	120	0	29
Valencia Orange	110	0	24
Vedge	65	0	14
Lemonade: Cranberry	130	0	33
Mango	120	0	30
Prickly Pear	140	0	34
Fruit Smoothies: *Per 8 fl.oz*			
Berry Boost	110	0	30
Blue Goodness	170	0	41
C-Boost	150	0	36
Green Goodness	140	0	33
Strawberry Banana	125	0	29
Bright & Early *(Minute Maid)*			
Orange Juice (Chilled/Frozen)	110	0	29
Campbell's			
Tomato Juice: 5.5 fl.oz can	30	0	6
11.5 fl.oz	60	0	13
Capri Sun			
Sport, all flavors, 6.75 fl.oz	60	0	16
Big Pouch: *Per 6.75 fl.oz Pouch*			
Mountain Cooler	90	0	23
Average other flavors	100	0	27
Clamato			
Tomato Cocktails, average, 8 fl.oz	60	0	11

Juice Brands (Cont)

Per 8 fl.oz Unless Indicated

	C	F	Cb
Crystal Geyser			
Juice Squeeze: *Per Bottle (12 fl.oz)*			
Blackberry Pomegranate	170	0	43
Ruby Grapefruit	150	0	36
Average other flavors	140	0	32
Dole			
100% Juice, Pineapple, 8 fl.oz	130	0	30
100% Fruit Juice Blends: *Per 6 fl.oz*			
Pine-Orange Banana	100	0	25
Pineapple Orange	90	0	22
Chilled, 100%: *Per 8 fl.oz*			
Berry Blend	140	0	35
Pineapple Juice	130	0	30
Pineapple Orange Banana	130	0	30
Average other flavors	120	0	29
Frozen Concentrates 100%: *Per ¼ Cup*			
Country Raspberry	140	0	34
Pine-Orange Ban.; Pineapple Juice	130	0	30
Average other flavors	120	0	28
Single Serve, 100%: *Per Bottle (15.2 fl.oz)*			
100% Apple, no sugar added	210	0	49
100% Blends: Cranberry	150	0	36
Grape, no sugar added	290	0	72
Orange, no sugar added	200	0	47
Pineapple Peach Mango	130	0	31
Ruby Red Grapefruit, no sug. add.	260	0	63
Strawberry Kiwi	120	0	31
Hawaiian Punch: *Per 8 fl.oz*			
Berry Blue Typhoon	120	0	29
Bodacious Berry	110	0	29
Fruit Juicy Red	120	0	30
Green Berry Rush	120	0	30
Lemonade	80	0	22
Light Hawaiian Punch, all flavors	45	0	11
Mazin Melon Mix	110	0	29
Orange Ocean	120	0	29
Tropical Vibe	110	0	29
Wild Purple Smash	110	0	29
Donald Duck			
100% Orange Jce (+Calcium), 8 fl.oz	110	0	27
Eden, Organic Apple, 8 fl.oz	90	0	24
Five Alive *(Minute Maid):* Frozen Concentrate, made up, 8 fl.oz	110	0	29
Florida's Natural			
Cranberry Apple, 8 fl.oz	110	0	27
Orange Juice, 8 fl.oz	110	0	26
Ruby Red Grapefruit Juice, 8 fl.oz	90	0	22

Per 8 fl.oz Unless Indicated

	C	F	Cb
Fuze: *Per 8 fl.oz*			
Refresh, 8 fl.oz	90	0	24
Slenderize: w. sugar, 8 fl.oz	10	0	2
no sugar, 8 fl.oz	5	0	1
Vitamin Tea	60	0	16
Goya Nectar			
Apricot Nectar, 12 fl.oz	220	0	53
Pear Nectar, 12 fl.oz can	220	0	59
Hansen's: *Per 8 fl.oz Unless Indicated*			
Fruit Juice: Apple varieties	120	0	28
Grape	160	0	40
Pomegranate	160	0	39
Juice Slam: *Per Box (6.75 fl.oz)*			
Apple	90	0	23
Other varieties, avg.	120	0	29
Smoothies: *Per Can (11.5 fl.oz)*			
Fruit flavors, regular, avg.	175	0	43
Energy Island Blast	170	0	45
Low Carb Smoothie, 11.5 fl.oz	40	0	9
Energy Smoothies: *See Page 159*			
Hawaiian Punch			
Fruit Juicy: Red, 8 fl.oz	120	0	30
Box, 8.45 fl.oz	120	0	30
Red Light, 8 fl.oz	45	0	11
Hawaii's Own			
Frozen Concentrate: *Per 8 fl.oz (Prep'd)*			
Average all varieties	110	0	28
Hi-C Juice Drinks: Average, 8 fl.oz	120	0	32
6.75 fl.oz box, average	100	0	27
Blast, 6 fl.oz pouch	100	0	26
Hood: Apple, 8 fl.oz	120	0	31
Fruit Punch	120	0	30
Orange	120	0	30
Jamba Juice: *See Fast-Foods Section*			
Juicy Juice (Nestle): *Per Box (6.75 fl.oz)*			
Grape	100	0	25
Average other flavors	100	0	24
4.23 fl.oz box, average	70	0	16
Kerns All Nectars			
Canned Juice: *Per Can (11.5 fl.oz)*			
Pear	220	0	54
Pineapple Coconut	280	8	53
Other flavors, average	210	0	52
Kool Aid			
Jammers: Sugar Jammers	10	0	2
Other varieties, 6.75 fl.oz pouch	90	0	24
L & A: Black Cherry, 8 fl.oz	180	0	45
Grape Juice Plus	160	0	40
Mixed Berry	120	0	30
Prune Juice	180	0	41
Average other varieties	140	0	32

Fruit & Vegetable Juices (Cont)

Juice Brands (Cont)   C F Cb

Per 8 fl.oz Unless Indicated

	C	F	Cb
Lakewood Organic			
Carrot Pineapple, 6 fl.oz	85	0	19
Coconut, 6 fl.oz	90	1.5	20
Cranberry/Lemonade, 8 fl.oz	90	0	22
Mango, 6 fl.oz	80	0	20
Papaya; Pure Carrot, avg., 6 fl.oz	75	0	18
Pure Cranberry, 6 fl.oz	50	0	12
Pure Pineapple, 6 fl.oz	95	0	23
Pure Prune, 8 fl.oz	165	0	40
Pure Pink Grapefruit, 8 fl.oz	90	0	22
Red Tart Cherry, 6 fl.oz	80	0	19
Super Veggie, 8 fl.oz	40	0	9
Average other varieties, 8 fl.oz	105	0	26
Langers: *Per 8 fl.oz*			
Apple Juice; White Cranberry avg.	120	0	28
Cranberry/100 Varieties, avg.	140	0	35
Cranberry Berry	135	0	34
Cranberry Grape	165	0	41
Cranberry Raspberry	150	0	36
White Grape	160	0	40
Low Carb: Apple Juice	60	0	14
Cranberry/Grape	30	0	8
Seasonal Blends: *Per 8 fl.oz*			
Summer	120	0	31
Spring; Autumn; Winter	120	0	30
Frozen Concentrate: *Per 8 fl.oz (Prepared)*			
Cranberry	120	0	35
Other flavors, average	120	0	30
Malibu Beach: *Per 8 fl.oz*			
Teas: Tropical Tea	10	0	3
Beach Peach; Oceanside	10	0	3
Juices: Malibu Mango	10	0	3
Sunset Strawberry; Redondo	10	0	3
Martinelli's			
Sparkling Juice: *Per 8 fl.oz*			
Apple-Cranberry	110	0	27
Apple-Grape	120	0	31
Cider	140	0	35
Mistic (Mega 24 fl.oz)			
Mega 24 fl.oz: Avg. all flavors, 8 fl.oz	120	0	30
24 fl.oz	360	0	90
Tropicals, all flavors, 8 fl.oz	120	0	31
Lemon Tea, 8 fl.oz	90	0	23
Grape Strawberry, 8 fl.oz	130	0	32
Watermelon Kiwi, 8 fl.oz	110	0	28
Peach Beach, 8 fl.oz	0	0	0
Diet Lemon Tea, 8 fl.oz	100	0	24

Per 8 fl.oz Unless Indicated   C F Cb

	C	F	Cb
Minute Maid			
Orange Juice, Premium, 8 fl.oz	110	0	27
Light Orange Juice	50	0	13
Heart Wise; Kids Plus	110	0	27
Lemonade, all flavors, average	120	0	28
Premium Blends, avg. all flavors	120	0	28
Simply Orange 100%	110	0	27
Tropical Punches	100	0	28
Juices to Go, average, 11.5 fl.oz	155	0	45
Boxed Juices, average, 6.75 fl.oz	90	0	25
Coolers, average, 6.75 fl.oz	90	0	25
Soft Frozen Lemonade, 12 fl.oz	300	0	75
Frozen Concentrates, 8 fl.oz (Prep'd),			
Average all varieties	120	0	29
Mott's			
Apple Juice, 8 fl.oz	120	0	29
Fruit Punch, 6.75 fl.oz	100	0	25
Grape Apple, 6.75 fl.oz	150	0	37
100% Fruit Juice Boxes: *Per Box (4.23 fl.oz)*			
White Grape	60	0	15
Average other flavors	60	0	15
Juice Paks: All flavors, 6.75 fl.oz	100	0	25
Mini Motts, 4.23 oz	60	0	15
Plus Lite Applejuice, 8 fl.oz	60	0	15
Naked Juice			
Just Juices: *Per ½ Bottle (16 fl.oz)*			
Apple, 8 fl.oz	120	0	29
Carrot	80	0	13
O-J Orange	110	0	25
Tangerine Scream	110	0	25
Fruit Smoothies: *Per ½ Bottle (16 fl.oz)*			
Antioxidants: Berry Blast, 8 fl.oz	120	0	30
Mighty Mango	120	0	30
Pomegrananate varieties, avg.	150	0.5	37
Rainforest Acai	160	1.5	30
Energy: Orange Mango Motion	120	0	30
Strawberry Kiwi Kick	110	0	27
Proteins, Protein Zone	250	4	32
Superfoods: Blue Machine, 8 fl.oz	170	0	41
Green Machine	130	0	32
Purple Machine	150	1.5	34
Red Machine	150	2	31
Well Being: Power-C, 8 fl.oz	110	0.5	27
Strawberry Banana-C	120	0	29
Tropical-C	140	0	32

Juice Brands (Cont)

Per 8 fl.oz Unless Indicated

	C	F	Cb
Nantucket Nectars			
Juice Cocktails: *Per 8 fl.oz*			
Carrot Orange Mango	120	0	28
Cranberry	130	0	33
Grapeade Guava; Orange Mango	130	0	33
Other varieties, avg.	120	0	30
100% Juice: *Per 8 fl.oz*			
Grape Juice	130	0	31
Peach Orange, organic	130	0	32
Pineapple Banana	140	0	34
Pomegranate Cherry & Apple	110	0	26
Premium Orange Juice	110	0	26
Squeezed Nectar Teas: *Per Bottle (16 fl.oz)*			
Diet Lemon Tea	0	0	1
Original Lemon Tea	80	0	22
Nectar Lemonades, avg., 8 fl.oz	130	0	32
Newman's Own			
Lemonade (Reg./Pink), 8 fl oz	110	0	27
Fruit Juice Cocktail: Gorilla Grape	140	0	34
Orange Mango Tango	150	0	37
Razzma Tazz Raspberry	120	0	28
Northland			
100% Juice: *Per 8 fl.oz*			
Cranb./Peach/Blackberry; Raspb.	140	0	34
Cranberry Grape	140	0	36
Ocean Spray *Per 8 fl.oz*			
Cranberry Juice Cocktail, avg.	130	0	33
100% Cranberry Juice, avg., 8 fl.oz	140	0	35
White Cranberry Juice, avg.	120	0	30
Cranberry Blends: *Per 8 fl.oz*			
CranApple; CranTangerine, avg.	140	0	35
CranCherry	130	0	32
CranGrape	140	0	35
CranMango/Raspberry/Strawberry	120	0	30
Light Juice Drinks: *Per 8 fl.oz*			
Light Cranberry Drinks	40	0	10
Light Ruby Grapefruit Juice Drink	40	0	10
Diet Juice Drinks, 8 fl.oz	5	0	2
Juice Cocktail: *Per 8 fl.oz*			
Ruby Red Grapefruit/Tangerine	120	0	31
White Grapefruit, 8 fl oz	100	0	21
Ruby Grapefruit Juice Drinks: *Per 8 fl.oz*			
Ruby Red Grapefruit	120	0	30
Light Ruby Grapefruit	40	0	10

Per 8 fl.oz Unless Indicated

	C	F	Cb
Odwalla			
AntioxiDance; Grapefruit, avg	90	0	23
B Berrier; Quencher	120	0	30
Carrot Juice	70	0	15
Carrot, Orange, Apple	100	0	23
Glorious Morning; B Monster	140	0	33
Mo'Beta	150	0	37
Poma Grand, average	160	0	40
Strawberry Lemonade	110	0	28
Super Protein, average	175	4	24
Wellness Echinacea	150	1	33
Smoothies: Blueberry B Monster	140	0	33
C Monster	150	0	36
Blackberry Fruitshake	150	1	36
Mango Tango	150	1	34
Strawberry Banana	150	0	36
Old Orchard: Apple Juice, 8 fl.oz	120	0	29
Frozen Concentrate: *Per 8 fl.oz (Prep'd)*			
Apple	120	0	29
Other flavors	130	0	31
Orange Julius: Original (Orange, Strawberry),			
16 fl.oz	220	1	54
20 fl.oz	270	1	68
32 fl.oz	440	1	108
Other Drinks: See Fast-Foods, Page 229			
Pom Wonderful			
100% Juice: *Per 8 fl.oz*			
Mango	140	0	36
Blueberry; Pomegranate	160	0	40
Cherry	150	0	38
Tangerine	140	0	34
R.W. Knudsen			
Fruit Juices: Apple	120	0	30
Cranberry Raspberry	130	0	32
Creamed Papaya	40	0	10
Grapefruit; Just Blueberry, avg.	100	0	24
Guava Strawberry	120	0	28
Hibiscus Cooler	100	0	25
Just Concord	160	0	40
Tomato	60	0	14
Other varieties, average	120	0	30
Sparkling Juice, avg., 8 fl.oz	120	0	30
Nectars: Coconut	140	5	27
Peach	130	0	31
Boysenberry, average	130	0	31
Very Veggie, 8 fl oz	50	0	11
Simply Nutritious: Mega C	140	0	34
Average other varieties	125	0	30

Fruit & Vegetable Juices (Cont)

Juice Brands (Cont)
Per 8 fl.oz Unless Indicated

	C	F	Cb
Ralphs			
Lemonade (Premium Juice), 8 fl.oz	110	0	29
Orange Juice, 8 fl.oz	120	0	30
Pineapple Juice, 8 fl.oz	130	0	33
ReaLemon - ReaLime (Borden)			
Lemon/Lime Juice (from concentrate)			
1 teaspoon	0	0	0
2 Tbsp, 1 fl.oz	8	0	2.5
Santa Cruz (Organic)			
Apple Juice; Cider & Spice	120	0	30
Concord Grape; White Grape	160	0	40
Orange Mango	130	0	32
Tropical Blend	140	0	33
Average other varieties	100	0	24
Nectars: Cranberry	110	0	27
Average other varieties	115	0	30
Sodas: *Per 12 fl.oz*			
Cherry	140	0	34
Concord Grape	150	0	36
Lemonade; Champagne Style	100	0	26
Raspberry Lemonade; Apricot	120	0	29
Other varieties	130	0	33
Juice Boxes: *Per 8 fl.oz*			
Lemon	120	0	29
Orange; Grape, average	100	0	24
Tropical Punch	110	0	27
Simply Orange			
Lemonade, 8 fl.oz	120	0	30
Limeade	120	0	31
Orange Juice, all varieties	110	0	26
Snapple			
Fruit Drink Blends, 8 fl.oz	120	0	29
Grapeade; Orangeade 8 fl.oz	120	0	29
Lemonade, all types	110	0	28
Diet: Snapple Apple	15	0	4
Kiwi Strawberry	20	0	5
Avg. other flavors	10	0	2
Snap.E Tom			
Tom. & Chile Cocktail, 11 oz can	80	0	16
Stonyfield Farm: *Per Bottle (10 fl.oz)*			
Peach Smoothie	250	3	49
Wildberry; Strawberry Smoothie	250	3	46
Light Smoothies, 10 fl.oz	130	0	41

Per 8 fl.oz Unless Indicated

	C	F	Cb
SunnyD			
Baja Juice: *Per 10 fl.oz Bottle*			
Berry	160	0	36
Orange	160	0	39
Orange Pineapple	160	0	39
Red Punch	140	0	36
Blends, avg., ½ bottle, 8 fl.oz	80	0	20
Originals: *Per 8 fl.oz*			
w. Calcium	140	0	35
Fruit Punch	120	0	29
Lemonade; Mango	130	0	31
Reduced Sugar	60	0	15
Smooth Style	130	0	32
Tangy Original Style	120	0	29
Sunsweet			
Prune Juice/w. Pulp, 8 fl.oz	180	0	43
Tampico: Citrus Punch, 1 cup	110	0	25
Mango/Trop. Frt. Punch, 1 cup	110	0	28
Tang			
Pouches, average all flavors (1)	90	0	24
Mix: *Prepared as Directed*			
Regular (2 Tbsp dry), 6 fl.oz	110	0	27
Sugar Free, 8 fl.oz	5	0	0
Trader Joes: *Per 8 fl.oz*			
Refrigerated: Carrot Juice	80	0	13
Ginger Limaid	120	0	31
Organic Carrots & Greens	80	0	19
Original Lemonade	110	0	27
Strawberry Lemonade	120	0	29
Strawberry Smoothie	110	0	27
Other varieties, average	110	0	25
100% Juice, all varieties	120	0	30
All Natural Pasteurized: *Per 8 fl.oz*			
Concord Grape	160	0	39
Cranberry Harvest	130	0	36
Cranberry; White Grape	130	0	36
Garden Patch; Vege -10	50	0	12
Hawaiian Pineapple	110	0	29
Just Pomegranate	150	0	37
Lemon Ginger w. Echinacea	140	0	36
Mango Lemonade	140	0	35
Mango Passion Fruit Blend	130	0	33
Rio Red Grapefruit	140	0	35
Average other varieties	125	0	30

Juice Brands (Cont)

Per 8 fl.oz Unless Indicated

	C	F	Cb
Tree Top			
Apple Reserve/Fruit Punch	120	0	31
Apple Berry/Grape	130	0	32
Apple/Spiced Cider	120	0	29
Fiber Rich: Apple	140	0	35
Apple Apricot/Orange Banana	160	0	37
Grapefruit	130	0	30
Grower's Best, Apple NSA	120	0	29
Orange	120	0	28
Orchard Blends	130	0	31
Boxes: Average, 6.8 fl.oz	100	0	26
Tropicana			
Chilled Juices: Grape	155	0	38
Cranberry; Cranberry Cocktail	140	0	34
Orchard Berry/Apple, avg.	115	0	29
Essentials: Fiber, 8 fl.oz	120	0	29
Healthy Heart	120	0	26
Healthy Kids	110	0	26
Immunity Defense; Low Acid	110	0	26
Light 'n Healthy varieties	50	0	13
Non-Refrigerated Juice Drinks: *Per 8 fl.oz*			
100% Fruit Punch	135	0	32
100% Grape	150	0	38
100% Orange; Apple; Ruby Red	110	0	27
100% Pineapple Orange	130	0	32
100% Strawberry Orange	140	0	34
Light 'n Healthy, average	50	0	14
Refrigerated Juice Drinks: *Per 8 fl.oz*			
Berry Punch	130	0	32
Fruit Punch	130	0	32
Lemonade	120	0	29
Orangeade; Peach Orchard Punch	130	0	33
Tropical Punch	120	0	31
Light varieties, average	10	0	3
Twisters: Average, 8 fl.oz	120	0	29
20 fl.oz bottle	300	0	74
Fruit Smoothies, avg., 11 fl.oz	220	0	54
V8® Juices & Drinks			
V8 100% Vegetable Juice, 5.5 fl.oz	30	0	7
1 Can, 11.5 fl.oz	70	0	14
V-8 Splash, average, 8 fl.oz	75	0	19
V-8 Splash Smoothies: Strawb. 8 fl.oz	90	0	20
Tropical Colada, 8 fl.oz	100	0	21
Diet V-8 Splash, all flavors, 8 fl.oz	10	0	3
Fusion, all flavors, 8 fl.oz	120	0	28

Per 8 fl.oz Unless Indicated

	C	F	Cb
Veryfine			
Apple Juice (100%)	110	0	27
Orange Juice (100%)	120	0	30
Walnut Acres: *Per 8 fl.oz*			
Organic: Apple	110	0	29
Apricot; Raspberry	130	0	32
Cherry	140	0	34
Cranberry	110	0	26
Incredible Vegetable	50	0	12
Other varieties, avg.,	120	0	32
Welch's: *Bottled Juices*			
100% Red Grape	170	0	42
100% White Grape	160	0	39
100% White Grape Blends: Peach	160	0	37
Other varieties	140	0	35
Tomato Juice, 8 fl.oz	50	0	10
Concentrates: *Per 8 fl.oz Made Up*			
100% Grape	170	0	42
American White Grape	160	0	39
Cocktails: *Per 8 fl.oz Made Up*			
Concord Grape Concord Red	150	0	36
Mountain Berry	140	0	34
Strawberry Breeze	130	0	33
Light Cocktails: *Per 8 fl.oz Made Up*			
Grape	70	0	18
White Grape	70	0	18
White Grape, Peach	70	0	18
Sparkling Cocktail, avg., 8 fl.oz	160	0	40
Wild Oats			
Down to Earth, average, 8 fl.oz	130	0	32

Nutrition/Energy Shakes & Drinks

Nutritional Shakes/Drinks

	C	F	Cb
180 High Energy, 8.2 fl.oz	120	0	33
180 X-3 Lime, 8 fl.oz	10	0	3
24-7 Energy: Avg, 16 fl.oz can	260	0	60
Sugar Free	0	0	0
ABB			
Energy: Turbo Tea, 18 fl.oz	150	0	38
Diet Turbo Tea, 18 fl.oz	0	0	0
Adrenalyn Stack, 22 fl.oz	25	0	6
Speed Stack, 18 fl.oz	5	0	1
Nitric Force, 22 fl.oz	10	0	2
Ripped Force, 18 fl.oz	90	0	22
Extreme Ripped Force, 22 fl.oz	100	0	24
Hi-Pro: Extreme Body RTD 50, 15 fl.oz	240	1	6
Pure Pro, 22 fl.oz	180	0.5	2
Pure Pro Shake, 11 fl.oz	170	1	5
Whey Force, 9.5 fl.oz	120	1.5	4
Power: Blue Thunder, 22 fl.oz	310	0.5	43
Carbo Force, 18 fl.oz	440	0	110
Extreme XX1, 24 fl.oz	1040	4	208
Mass Recovery, 18 fl.oz	380	0	60
AdvantEdge (EAS): *Per Container (11 fl.oz)*			
Carb Control Ready-to-Drink	110	3	2
Complete Nutrition Ready-to-Drink	200	3	28
Airforce, Nutrisoda, 250ml	10	0	1
AllSport, all flavors, 8 fl.oz	60	0	16
AMP Energy Drink, 8.4 fl.oz can	110	0	29
Tall Boy, 16 fl.oz can	220	0	58
Amway: Trim Advantage, 11.2 oz	150	3	16
XS Energy Drink, 8.4 oz	8	0	0
XS Power Protein Shake, 11 oz	220	6	4
Arizona: Caution Energy, 8.3 oz	130	0	34
Caution Energy Low Carb, 8.3 oz	10	0	3
Green Tea Energy, 8 oz	100	0	26
Lite Tea Energy, 8 oz	70	0	19
Atkins: Advantage Shake, 11 oz can	160	9	4
Bacchus Energy, 3.3 oz	60	0	15
Bally Total Fitness, Whey Pro, 1 scoop	100	1.5	2
Blast, 8.3 oz	120	0	29
Bariatrix Shakes, 1 serving	100	2	6
Anytime Drinks, 8 oz, average	90	4	4
Proti 15 Drink, avg., 1 pkg	75	1	4
Bawls Guarana, 10 fl.oz	120	0	32
Guaranexx Sugar Free, 10 fl.oz	0	0	0
Blox Energy: Citrus, 8.4 fl.oz	120	0	29
Black Cherry; Orange Rush, 8.4 fl.oz	110	0	26
Blue Sky: Blue Energy, 8.3 fl.oz	120	0	29
Blue Sport, 8 oz	45	0	12
Body Fuel (w. NutraSweet), 1 scoop	80	0	20
Bookoo Energy, 16 fl.oz can	220	0	54
Boost: Nutritional Energy, 8 fl.oz	240	4	41
Boost Plus, 8 fl.oz can	360	14	45
Boost w. Fiber, 8 fl.oz can	240	4	42
Glucose Control, 8 fl.oz	190	7	16

Per 8 fl.oz Unless Indicated

	C	F	Cb
Carboplex (Unipro) mix, ½ cup, 2 oz	210	0	52
Carnation Instant Breakfast			
Powder: 1 envelope, 1.3 oz	200	1	39
Carb Conscious, 1 envel., 21g	150	1	24
Ready-To-Drink, avg., 11 fl.oz	250	5	40
Celebrity Juice Diet, 4 fl.oz	60	0	14
CeraSport: Liquid, 11 fl.oz	70	0	17
20g package (makes 16 fl.oz)	80	0	19
Champion Lyte, Sports Drink	0	0	0
Champion Nutrition			
Heavywyt Gainer 900, 4 sc., 5.4 oz	630	10	101
Ultramet: Original, 1 pkt, 2.7 oz	280	2	24
Ultramet Lyte, 1 pkt, 2 oz	190	1	17
Ultramet Low Carb, 1 pkt, 2 oz	230	6.5	6
Citrucel Fiber Shake, 1 pkg	50	2	6
Coca-Cola Black 8 fl.oz	45	0	12
Curves Protein Drink (mix):			
Chocolate; Vanilla, 2 scoops	100	1.5	8
made with skim milk, 8 fl.oz	190	2	23
Designer Whey Protein Van., 1 scp	90	1.5	2
e10 Energy Drink, 8.4 fl.oz	5	0	0
EAS ~ *See AdvantEdge/Myoplex*			
Endura (Unipro), 2 scoops, 1.3 oz	120	0	29
Ensure: High Protein, 8 oz bottle	230	6	31
Ensure Plus, 8 fl.oz can	250	6	42
Ensure Plus, 8 fl.oz bottle	350	11	50
Ensure Regular, 8 fl.oz can	250	6	40
Glucerna, 8 fl.oz can, average	200	7	27
Weight Loss Shake, 11 fl.oz	290	11	39
High Calcium, 8 fl.oz	220	6	31
Enterex Glucose Control, 8 fl.oz			
(Carbohydrates as Maltodextrin)	237	9	27
Equaline (Albertson's)			
Advanced, 8 fl.oz	250	6	40
Plus, 8 fl.oz	350	11	50
Fruit20 (Veryfine), 8/16/20 fl.oz	0	0	0
Full Throttle, 16 fl.oz	220	0	57
Sugar Free	5	0	0
Fuze: Slenderize, 8 fl.oz	5	0	3
Refresh, 8 fl.oz	90	0	25
Vitalize, 8 fl.oz	100	0	25
Go Fast Sports: 8 fl.oz	90	0	23
Go Fast Lite, 8.3 fl.oz	20	0	14
Gatorade: Endurance, 8 fl.oz	50	0	14
All Stars, 8 fl.oz	90	0	22
Fierce/AM/Extreme, 8 fl.oz	50	0	14
Lemonade/Raspb. Lem, 8 fl.oz	50	0	14
Rain; X Factor, 8 fl.oz	50	0	14

Nutritional Shakes/Drinks (Cont)

Per 8 fl.oz Unless Indicated **C** **F** **Cb**

	C	F	Cb
Genisoy: Ultra XT, 3 Tbsp	150	1	20
Protein Powder, 3 Tbsp	130	1	17
Glaceau: Vitamin Water, 8 fl.oz	50	0	13
Smart Water	0	0	0
Glucerna Wt Loss Shakes, 11 oz	200	7	27
GNC Lean Shake, 2 scoops	180	2	30
GNC Pro Performance:			
Mega MRP: Original, 1 pkt	260	2	20
Extreme Choc., 3 scoops	290	3	11
24 Hour Pro Complex, 39g	150	5	7
100% whey Protein, 29g	130	2.5	5
500 Gram Slam RTD, 15 oz	230	1	6
Crea Drive, 45g	140	0	34
Mass XXX, 195g	750	6	124
Weight Gainer 2200 Gold, 493g	2300	16	441
Wheybolic Extreme 60, 82g	310	2	13
HMR: 70 Plus, 1 package	110	0.5	13
500	100	1	17
Hansen's: Energy Pro, 8 fl.oz	60	0	16
Energy Original, 8.3 fl.oz Can	140	0	36
Rumba, 8 fl.oz	120	0	28
Smoothies: See Page 153			
Hollywood Celebrity Diet: ½ cup	100	0	25
24hr/48hr Miracle, 4 oz	100	0	25
Impulse Energy Drink, 8.3 oz	110	0	28
Isopure Perfect, 1 pkg (88g)	300	0	25
Jarrow: Whey Protein, 1 scoop	100	1	4
Berry High, 1 scoop	20	0	5
Muscle Optimal, 2 scoops	180	2	17
Jolt CK2: *Per 23.5 fl.oz Can*			
Blue	360	0	90
Cola (Red)	300	0	75
Ultra (Green)	0	0	0
Jones: Energy, 8.4 fl.oz	130	0	32
Whoop Ass, 8.4 fl.oz	110	0	29
Kashi GoLEAN Shakes, 2 scoops	220	1	32
Knudsen: ReCharge, all flavors	70	0	18
Simply Nutritious, ½ bot., 16 fl.oz	130	0	30
Kombucha, Wonder Drink, 8.5 fl.oz	60	0	16
La Brada			
Powders: Lean Body, 79g	330	8	24
Lean Body Mass 60, 4 scoops	610	7	77
Breakfast, 92g	360	7	35
Carb Watchers, 65g	240	4	12
For Her, 49g	180	3	9
Iso Power 60, 2 scoops	290	2	7
Pro V 60, 2 scoops	315	3	12
Drink: Lean Body, (40g Pro.), 17 fl.oz	260	9	9
Lipovitan EB3, 8.3 fl.oz	110	0	28
Lost Energy Drink, 8.3 fl.oz can	100	0	26

Per 8 fl.oz Unless Indicated **C** **F** **Cb**

	C	F	Cb
Max Velocity (Albertson's), 8.45 fl.oz	120	0	33
Lite, 8.45 fl.oz	10	0	0
MDX (Mountain Dew), 8 fl.oz	120	0	32
Met-Rx: Original, 1 pkt, average	260	3	21
Protein Plus, 3 scoops	110	1	4
Nutri Shake	240	2	28
RTD 40, 15 fl.oz can	240	3	13
Metabolol: Endurance, 2 scp, 52g	200	5	24
Met, 2 scoops, 66g	200	3	40
Met Max, mix, 2 scoops	230	2.5	11
Creatinine Extreme, 2 scoops	280	0	68
Monster Energy: 16 fl.oz can	200	0	50
XXL, 24 fl.oz can	300	0	75
Lo-Carb, 16 fl.oz can,	20	0	5
MRM: Low Carb Protein, 1 scoop	120	2.5	4
Iso-bolic, 1 scoop	115	1.5	1
Whey Pumped, 1 scoop	90	1	5
Muscle Milk (Hi Protein), avg., 17 fl.oz	350	17	17
Muscle Tech Nitro: Complete	300	4	22
Cell Tech RTD, 14½ oz	300	0	75
Mass Tech Weight Gain, 5 scoops	830	5	150
Nitro Tech RTD, 15 oz	210	1	5
Myoplex: Original Shake, 17 fl.oz	310	7	20
Carb Control, 11 fl.oz	110	3	4
Deluxe Powder, 1 pkt, 2.7 oz	300	4.5	28
Lite (Ready to Drink), 11 fl.oz pkg	170	2	20
Lite Powder, 1 pkt, 2 oz	180	0.5	20
Naturade: Power Shake, 1 scoop	100	1	10
100% Soy, 2 Scoops (1.3 oz), dry	160	5	20
Protein Booster, avg., ⅓ c. dry	80	1	1
Ribo-tein, avg., 1 oz scoop	100	0.5	21
Total Soy, Orig., 1 scoop, 1.3 oz	150	2	20
Nature's Best: Isopure	300	0	25
Isopure Endurance, 3 scoops	330	0	60
Carbo Power, 16 fl.oz	400	0	100
Zero Carb, 2 scoops, 2.1 oz	220	0	3
Pro Smoothie, 15 oz	240	1.5	7
Noni: Tahitian/Pacific, 2 Tbsp	10	0	3
Noni Juice, 1 fl.oz	10	0	3
Liquid Hawaiian/Tahiti, 1 Tbsp	30	0	8
Hiro: Vitality, 8 fl.oz	10	0	1.5
Energy/Mobility, 8.5 oz	10	0	3
Nutrament (Mead Johnson), 12 fl.oz	360	10	52
NuVim, 1 cup, 8 fl.oz	10	0	2
Ny-Tro Pro 40, average	260	1	23
Optifast 800: Powder, 1 serving	160	3	20
Ready-To-Drink, Chocolate	160	3	20
Optimum Pro Complex, 2 scoops	260	3	3
Pedialyte (Abbott)	25	0	6
Pimp Juice Energy, 250ml	130	0	35
Piranha Energy (EAS), 8.4 oz	130	0	33
Pitbull Energy Drink, 1 can	110	0	28

Nutritional Shakes/Drinks (Cont)

Per 8 fl.oz Unless Indicated

	C	F	Cb
Powerade: Regular, 12 fl.oz	90	0	25
20 fl.oz bottle	160	0	41
Light, 8 fl.oz	25	0	7
20 fl.oz bottle	65	0	17
Option, all flavors, 8 fl.oz	10	0	2
PowerBar			
Recovery: Choc shake, 1 scoop	250	5	40
Vanilla shake, 10.6 oz	240	5	34
Endurance, 1 scoop, 0.7 oz	170	0	42
Power Gel, Chocolate, 1.5 oz	110	0	27
ProBalance, 8.45 fl.oz	300	41	56
Pro-Cal 100 (*R-Kane*), 1 pkt	100	1.5	7
Red Bull Energy Drink, 8.3 fl.oz	110	0	28
Sugar-Free, 1 can	10	0	3
Red Devil Energy Drink, 100ml	65	0	15
Red Jak: Energy, Reg., 8 fl.oz	120	0	31
Energy, Low Carb, 8 fl.oz	10	0	1
Resource (*Novartis*): Shake, 8 fl.oz	270	6	45
Shake Plus, 8 fl.oz	480	16	69
Health Shake: 4 fl.oz	200	4	35
No Added Sugar, 4 oz	200	9	22
Diabetishield, 8 fl.oz	150	0	30
Breeze, 237ml	250	0	54
Benefiber Juice, 4 oz	70	0	18
Revenge Pro (*Champ. Nutr.*), 1 oz	100	0.5	30
Pro-Score 100, 2 scoops	160	2	1.5
Revival Soy: Plain Soy, 1 pkg	120	3.5	3
Chocolate Day Dream, 1 pkg	240	2.5	36
Other varieties, avg., 1 pkg	225	2	33
Rhino's Energy Drink, 100ml	50	0	13
Ripe It Energy Fuel, 16 fl.oz	260	0	66
Chic (Sugar Free), 12 fl.oz	5	0	1
Rite Aid: Nutritional, 8 fl.oz	250	6	40
Plus, 8 fl.oz	350	11	50
Rockstar: Energy Drink, 8 fl.oz	140	0	31
Diet Energy Drink, 8 fl.oz	10	0	2
50% Juice, 16 fl.oz can	200	0	48
Rush Energy Lite, 8 fl.oz	0	0	0
Regular, 8 fl.oz	120	0	30
Sav-on Nut'l: Plus, 8 oz	350	11	50
Equaline Advance, 8 oz	250	6	40
High Protein, 8 oz	230	6	31
Six Star Body Fuel:			
Advanced Whey Protein, 1 scoop	110	2	3
Advanced Creatinine, 1 scoop, 57g	170	0	1
Slim·Fast			
Ready to Drink Shake:			
Original, 10.8 oz	220	3	40
High Protein, 11 oz	190	5	24
Easy To Digest, 11 oz	180	5	26
Optima Shake, 10.8 oz can	180	6	24
Low Carb Diet, 11 oz	190	9	6
Powder Shake Mix: 1 scoop	100	4	18
w. 8 fl.oz fat-free milk	200	5	30

Per 8 fl.oz Unless Indicated

	C	F	Cb
Snapple: Diet, 8 fl.oz	20	0	4
Diet Tea, 8 fl.oz	0	0	1
Iced Tea, 8 fl.oz	100	0	25
SoBe: Power, avg., 8 fl.oz	120	0	30
Fountain, 8 fl.oz	110	0	27
Ice, 8 fl.oz	110	0	27
Synergy, 11.5 oz	120	0	30
Adrenaline Rush, 16 fl.oz	260	0	65
Sugar Free, 16 fl.oz	10	0	1
Juice Elixers, 8 fl.oz	100	0	25
Lean, all flavors, 8 fl.oz	5	0	1
Life Water, 8 fl.oz	50	0	13
Lizard, avg. all types, 8 fl.oz	120	0	30
No Fear: Regular, 16 fl.oz	260	0	65
Sugar Free	10	0	1
Solaray Soytein (*Protein Energy Meal*),			
Natural, 1 heaping scoop, 24g	70	0.5	5
Flav., avg., 1 heaping scoop, 33g	110	1	12
Sparks (Alcoholic) ~ *See Page 170*			
Sport Pharma Biomax, 2 scoops	250	3.5	6
Spiru-Tein Powder, 1 scp, avg., 34g	100	0	10
Stacker 2: Protein Water, 19.4 oz	80	0	1
Sweet Success (*Nestlé*):			
Powderblend, 2 scoops, 32g	180	0	45
Vitatein Shake, 11 fl.oz can	200	3	38
Tab Energy, 10 fl.oz	5	0	0
The Sports Club/LA, PTS Protein Powder,			
Choc/Mocha/Van., 2 scoops, 1 oz	110	3	5
Twin Lab: Ultra Fuel, 16 fl.oz	400	0	100
Energy Fuel, 250ml can	0	0	0
Usana: Nutrimeal, 3 scoops, 61g	230	7	33
Fibergy, 2 scoops, average	90	1	24
SoyaMax, 2 scoops	110	1	1
Walgreens Nutritional Drinks			
Nutritional Drink, 8 oz can	250	6	40
Plus, 8 oz can	350	11	50
Theragran-m, 8 oz	250	6	40
Theragran Plus, 8 oz	350	11	50
Weider (Powders)			
Creatine ATP, ½ cup, 1.7 oz	210	0	37
Mass 1000, 1 ⅓ cups	740	4	146
Ultra Whey Pro, ⅓ cup, 1 oz	110	1.5	4.5
Dynamic:			
Muscle Builder, 2 scps, ½ c., 45g	160	1	22
Weight Gainer, 4 scps, ⅔ c.,85g	450	1	99
Worldwide: Carbo Rush, 20 fl.oz	270	0	87
Pure Protein Shakes, 11 fl.oz, avg.	160	1	2
Rapid Recovery, 20 fl.oz, avg.	275	0	32
Thermo Rage, 20 fl.oz	20	0	4
Thermo Rush, 20 fl.oz	5	0	1
Xtreme Trim, 20 fl.oz	25	0	7
Supercharged tea, 20 fl.oz	15	0	4

Quick Guide

Cola Soda Drinks
Average All Brands
Includes *Coca-Cola* and *Pepsi*

	C	F	Cb
8 fl.oz Cup	100	0	26
12 fl.oz Can	150	0	39
16 fl.oz Bottle	200	0	52
20 fl.oz Bottle	250	0	65
24 fl.oz (Pepsi)	300	0	84
1-Liter Bottle (34 fl.oz)	400	0	100
2-Liter Bottle (68 fl.oz)	800	0	200

Other Soda Drinks (Average All Brands)

	C	F	Cb
Club Soda, 12 fl.oz	0	0	0
Cream Soda, 12 fl.oz	190	0	48
Diet/Low Cal Drinks, 12 fl.oz	5	0	1
Ginger Ale, 12 fl.oz	125	0	31
Lemon Lime, 12 fl.oz	150	0	37
Orange, 12 fl.oz	180	0	45
Pink Lemonade, 12 fl.oz	180	0	45
Root Beer, 12 fl.oz	150	0	39
Tonic Water, 12 fl.oz	125	0	2
Mineral Water: Plain, 12 fl.oz	0	0	0
Sweetened/flavored, 12 fl.oz	150	0	37
w. Fruit Juice, 12 fl.oz	120	0	30
Soda Water/Seltzer: Plain/Diet	0	0	0
Sweetened/flavored, 12 fl.oz	155	0	39
w. Fruit Juice, 12 fl.oz	160	0	40
Soft Frozen Lemonade, 12 fl.oz	300	0	75

Fountain, Movie Theater & Take-Out

Average All Flavors

	C	F	Cb
Small Cup, 12 fl.oz: No Ice	160	0	40
With ⅓ Ice	120	0	30
Regular, 16 fl.oz: No Ice	215	0	53
With ⅓ Ice	160	0	40
Medium, 22 fl.oz: No Ice	295	0	73
With ⅓ Ice	220	0	55
Large, 32 fl.oz: No Ice	430	0	105
With ⅓ Ice	320	0	80

(Note: ⅓ Cup of Ice = ¼ Cup Liquid)

Soda Brands

Per 12 fl.oz Unless Indicated

	C	F	Cb
A&W: Cream Soda	180	0	46
Diet Cream Soda/Root Beer	1	0	0
Root Beer	170	0	46
Albertson's: Max Cola	165	0	44
Lemon Lime	150	0	41
Other flavors, average	180	0	48

Soda Brands (Cont)

Per 12 fl.oz Unless Indicated

	C	F	Cb
Barq's: Root Beer	165	0	45
Floatz, 12 fl.oz	190	0	51
Big Red, 12 fl.oz	150	0	38
Blue Sky: Cola; Orange Cream	160	0	43
Cherry; Raspberry; Root Beer	155	0	42
Grape; Lemon Lime; Dr Becker	130	0	36
Organic, all flavors, avg.	165	0	40
Other varieties, average	145	0	43
Bubble Up, 12 fl.oz	165	0	42
Cactus Cooler, 12 fl.oz	150	0	40
Canada Dry: Club Soda	0	0	0
Ginger Ale, all flavors	120	0	33
Tonic Water	90	0	24
Diet, 12 fl.oz	0	0	0
Clearly Canadian, average	120	0	32
Coca-Cola: *Per 12 fl.oz*			
Classic/Caffeine Free	145	0	41
Diet Coke, all flavors	0	0	0
Cherry Coke/Vanilla Coke	155	0	42
Coca-Cola Zero	0	0	0
Coca-Cola Blak, 8 fl.oz bottle	45	0	12
Country Time, Lemonade, 333 ml	180	0	35
Crush, all flavors	185	0	51
Dad's: Orange Cream Soda, 12 fl.oz	180	0	45
Root Beer, 12 fl.oz	165	0	41
Diet Rite, Pure Zero	0	0	0
Dr Pepper: Regular	140	0	40
Cherry Vanilla	150	0	39
Diet, all flavors	0	0	0
Fanta, all flavors	110	0	27
Fresca: Regular	3	0	0
Peach Citrus	0	0	0
Fruitopia: *See Page 153*			
GuS, average all flavors	95	0	23
Hansen's: Diet Soda	0	0	0
Natural Orange Mango, 8 fl.oz	160	0	44
Other flavors, average	150	0	44
Hawaiian Punch: Island Citrus	120	0	30
Light	15	0	3
Henry Weinhard's: Root Beer	170	0	43
Cream flavor, average	175	0	42
Hires, Root Beer	170	0	45
IBC: Root Beer	160	0	43
Cherry Limeade	170	0	44
Cream Soda; Black Cherry	180	0	48
Diet Root Beer	0	0	0

Per 12 fl.oz Unless Indicated	C	F	Cb
Icee: Coca-Cola, 12 fl.oz	100	0	27
Barq's; Minute Maid, 12 fl.oz	200	0	52
Smoothee Lemonade, 12 fl.oz	255	0	64
Jolt Cola, 12 fl.oz	150	0	39
Jones Soda: Cola	170	0	43
Other flavors, average	185	0	46
Lucozade, 500 ml	140	0	33
Manzanila Sol	160	0	43
MDX Energy Soda (Sugar Free)	0	0	0
Mello Yello, Regular	180	0	48
Minute Maid: Fruit Punch	180	0	47
Fruit Falls, 6.8 fl.oz pouch	5	0	2
Orangeade	160	0	43
Pink Lemonade	150	0	42
Soft Frozen Lemonade, 12 fl.oz	300	0	76
Light flavors	10	0	2
Fruit Juices: *See Page 154*			
Mountain Dew: Live Wire; Code Red	165	0	47
Diet flavors	0	0	0
Mug Root Beer	150	0	44
Natural Brew: Vanilla, Cream	170	0	42
Ginseng Cola, Ginger Ale	170	0	42
Root Beer	180	0	44
Nehi, Royal Crown Peach	190	0	51
Orangina: 10 fl.oz bottle	110	0	28
Pepsi: Regular/Blue/Caffeine Free	150	0	42
Diet Pepsi; Jazz	0	0	0
One, 12 fl.oz	2	0	0
Wild Cherry; Vanilla	150	0	42
Perrier, Carbonated Water	0	0	0
Pibb Xtra	145	0	39
RW Knudsen, Spritzers, average	180	0	43
RC Cola: Regular; Cherry	165	0	45
Diet Cola	0	0	0
Reed's, Ginger Brew, avg. all var.	145	0	38
7•UP: Regular	150	0	39
Cherry, Gold	150	0	39
Diet varieties, 12 fl.oz	0	0	0
7•UP Plus, 12 fl.oz	15	0	3
Safeway: Cola	160	0	44
Cherry Cola	160	0	43
Ditto Lemon Lime	165	0	41
Parker's Cream Soda	170	0	42
Parker's Root Beer	170	0	47
Diet flavors	0	0	0
Santa Cruz, Sparkling, average	135	0	32

Per 12 fl.oz Unless Indicated	C	F	Cb
Schweppes: Seltzer	0	0	0
Tonic Water; Ginger Ale, average	130	0	35
Shasta: Cream Soda	190	0	47
Cherry Cola; Doc Shasta	160	0	39
Club Soda; Diet, all flavors	0	0	0
Fruit Punch, Pineapple; Orange	200	0	50
Ginger Ale	130	0	32
Other flavors, average	175	0	45
Sierra Mist, Lemon Lime	150	0	39
Sprite: Regular	145	0	40
Tropical Remix	0	0	0
Zero	4	0	0
Squirt, Citrus Burst	150	0	40
Star Ruby (GUS): Valencia Orange	95	0	24
Other flavors	90	0	22
Stewarts: Root Beer	160	0	41
Grape	190	0	48
Key Lime	180	0	44
Sunkist: Orange	195	0	53
Diet Sunkist	0	0	0
Cherry Limeade	180	0	45
Sunny D, 12 fl.oz	180	0	44
TAB, 12 fl.oz	0	0	0
Thomas Kemper: Root Beer	140	0	34
Other flavors, average	160	0	40
Tropicana Twister, avg., 12 fl.oz	180	0	32
Vault, Zero	6	0	0
Vernor's: Ginger Ale	150	0	39
Diet, 10 fl.oz	0	0	0
Walgreens: Grape Soda, 20 fl.oz	300	0	75
Cola; Lemon Lime, 20 fl.oz	225	0	60
Red Soda; Root Beer, 20 fl.oz	225	0	60
Diet Cola	0	0	0
Welch's: Soda, 12 fl.oz	190	0	51
Sparkling	240	0	60
Wild Oats, Down to Earth	175	0	55

Powdered Soft Drink Mix

Per 8 fl.oz (Prep'd)	C	F	Cb
Capri Sun, ½ pkg	30	0	8
Cool Splashers, 8 fl.oz	60	0	16
Country Time: Lemonade	60	0	16
Other flavors, average	80	0	19
Lite	35	0	9
Crystal Light, 8 fl.oz	5	0	0
Flavoraid, ⅛ pkg	0	0	0
Kool-Aid: All flavors	60	0	16
Unsweetened, 6 fl.oz	5	0	0
Propel, ½ pkg	10	0	3
Tang, 8 fl.oz, average	40	0	10

Instant Coffee

	C	F	Cb
Powder/Granules: Regular or Decaffeinated			
1 level tsp	2	0	0.5
1 rounded tsp	4	0	1
Ground, 3 tsp	7	0	1
Brewed/Percolated, 1 cup, 8 fl.oz	4	0	1
Coffee With Milk/Cream/Creamers:			
Per Cup Coffee (8 fl.oz): Black	4	0	1
w. Whole Milk: Dash, 1 Tbsp	15	0.5	2
2 Tbsp, 1 fl.oz	25	1	2
w. 2% Milk, 2 Tbsp	20	0.5	2
w. 1% Milk, 2 Tbsp	20	0.3	3.5
w. Fat Free Milk, 2 Tbsp	15	0	3
w. Half & Half, 2 Tbsp	50	3.5	2
w. Cream (light coffee), 2 Tbsp	65	6	2
w. *Coffee Mate:* Liquid, reg., 1T.	20	1	2
Liquid Fat Free, 1 Tbsp	25	0	5
Powder, 1 heaping tsp	15	1	2
Sugar ~ Add Extra: 1 heaping tsp	25	0	6
Single portion, 1 package	25	0	6

Flavored Coffee Mixes

	C	F	Cb
Chicory: Instant Coffee, 1 tsp	5	0	1
Coffee Essence, 1 tsp	15	0	4
Caffé D'Vita: Mixes, 3 tsp	60	1.5	11
Sugar Free Mixes, 2 tsp	35	2	3
General Foods: Average, ½ oz	60	3	10
Sugar-free, average, 1 tsp	30	2.5	2
Cappuccino Coolers, ½ oz	60	0	15
Jakada *(Folgers):* Mocha Latte, 3 T.	90	2.5	15
Cappuccino, 3 tsp	80	2	16
Maxwell House: Cappuccino, 1 pkt	100	1.5	19
Van., Irish Cream, 1 envelope	90	1	20
Nescafé: Average all flavors	80	0	19

Coffee Substitute Mixes

	C	F	Cb
Roasted Cereal Beverages: (No Caffeine)			
Cafix Instant Beverage, 1 tsp	5	0	1
Kaffree Roma *(Natural Touch)* , 1 tsp	10	0	2
Postum, Instant Hot Beverage, 1 tsp	10	0	3
Revival Soy "Coffee", 1 Tbsp	0	0	1
Teeccino Caffe, 1 tsp	10	0	2

Vending Machine

	C	F	Cb
Cappuccino, 1 cup, 8 fl.oz	85	0	12

Coffee Shops/Restaurants

Per 8 fl.oz Cup (Unless Indicated)	C	F	Cb
Coffee (Regular/Percolated/Filtered)	5	0	0
Americano Drip Coffee, 1 cup	7.5	0	1
Cafe Au Lait: 1 cup, 8 fl.oz	60	3.5	5
Nonfat Milk, 1 cup, 8 fl.oz	35	0	5
Caffe Latté:			
8 fl.oz cup: w. Whole Milk	110	6	9
w. 2% Milk	100	3.5	9
w. Nonfat Milk	70	0	10
12 fl.oz: w. Whole Milk	180	9	14
w. Nonfat Milk	100	0	15
16 fl.oz: w. Whole Milk	220	11	18
w. Nonfat Milk	130	0	19
Cafe Mocha (Mochaccino): 1 cup	150	6	20
12 fl.oz	230	9	31
16 fl.oz	290	12	41
Cappuccino:			
8 fl.oz cup: w. Whole Milk	90	2.5	7
w. 2% Milk	80	3	8
w. Nonfat Milk	50	0	8
12 fl.oz: w. Whole Milk	110	6	9
w. 2% Milk	90	3.5	9
w. Nonfat Milk	60	0	9
16 fl.oz: w. Whole Milk	140	7	11
w. Nonfat Milk	80	0	12
Mocha (with cream):			
8 fl.oz: w. Whole Milk	200	11	22
w. Nonfat Milk	160	6	22
12 fl.oz: Whole Milk	290	15	33
w. Nonfat Milk	230	8	34
Iced Mocha (no cream):			
12 fl.oz: w. Whole Milk	170	6	26
w. Nonfat Milk	130	2	27
Espresso: Single (Solo)	5	0	1
Doppio (Double)	10	0	2
Espresso con Panna,			
(w. dollop whipped cream), solo	30	2.5	2
Espresso Macchiato, solo	10	0	1
Frappuccino: Tall, 12 fl.oz	180	2.5	37
Grande, 16 fl.oz	240	3	48
Frappuccino Mocha (w. Cream):			
Tall, 12 fl.oz	280	11	43
Grande, 16 fl.oz	380	15	57
Iced Latte: *Similar to Caffe Latte*			
Starbucks: *See Fast-Foods Section*			
For Complete Nutritional Data – See CalorieKing.com			

Irish & Liqueur Coffees

	C	F	Cb
Irish Coffee (no sugar)	175	10	0
Liqueur Coffee, average 1 fl.oz	100	5	7

Cocoa & Hot Chocolate

Cocoa (8 fl.oz cup): w. Whole Milk	205	8.5	22
w. Nonfat Milk	145	1	23
Tall (12 fl.oz): w. Whole Milk	280	12	26
w. Nonfat Milk	185	1	28
Hot Chocolate:			
8 fl.oz cup: w. Whole Milk	180	7	26
w. Nonfat Milk	140	2	17
Tall (12 fl.oz): w. Whole Milk	260	10	36
w. Nonfat Milk	190	2	37
Cinnabon, Mochalatta Chill, 16 oz	360	13	55

Coffee Extras

Chocolate (Cocoa) Topping, ½ tsp	5	0	1
Flavored Syrups: Regular, 2 Tbsp	80	0	20
Sugar-free, 2 Tbsp	0	0	0
Half & Half Cream, 2 Tbsp	40	3.5	1
Light Whipped Cream, 2 Tbsp	15	1.5	1
Marshmallows, miniature ½	5	0	1
Hershey's Chocolate Syrup, 2 Tbsp	200	0	48

Bottled Coffee (Chilled)

Ready-To-Drink: Per Bottle

Arizona Mocha Latte 10½ fl.oz	130	2	24

Deerfield Farms: Per 11 oz Bottle

Chai Latte, Reg./Vanilla, average	230	6	39
Mocha Cappuccino	190	3	38
Kahlúa Cappuccino Shake 15½ fl.oz	195	3	35

Main St Cafe

French Vanilla Ice Latte, 12 fl.oz	190	3	31
Nescafe, Ice Mocha Java, avg., 2 T.	80	0	19
Shock Coffee: Latte, 8 fl.oz bottle	150	2.5	28
Triple Latte, 8 fl.oz can	125	2	27
Triple Mocha, 8 fl.oz can	125	2	27

Starbucks: Per Bottle

Frappuccino: Caramel, 9.5 fl.oz	200	3	36
Coffee; Hazelnut, 9.5 fl.oz	200	3	37
Mocha: 9.5 fl.oz bottle	180	3	33
13.7 fl.oz bottle	260	4	48
Vanilla, 9.5 fl.oz	200	3	37
DoubleShot, 6.5 fl.oz can	140	6	18
Iced Coffee, 11 fl.oz can	100	1	23
Swiss Miss, Caramel Cream Hot Cocoa, 1 packet	120	2.5	22
Tully's, Bellaccino, all flav., 9.5 fl.oz	210	4	36

CAFFEINE COUNTER

Moderate caffeine intake is not harmful to healthy adults. However, frequent large amounts (over 350mq/day) may cause dependency ('caffeinism') and adversely affect health. To be safe, limit caffeine to 200mg/day. Avoid if pregnant; breast feeding; a child under 8; or have heart arrhythmias.

Caffeine (mg)

Coffee: Instant, Weak, 1 level teaspoon	30
Medium, 1 rounded teaspoon	60
Strong, 1 heaping teaspoon	100
Decaffeinated, 1 round teaspoon	2
Bags *(Folgers)*, 1 bag (6-8 fl.oz)	115
Ground, 1 Tbsp, 6g	60
Bottled (Ready-To-Drink), 9.5 fl.oz	70
Coffee Shop: Brewed, 8 fl.oz	110 - 150
Cappuccino: 1 cup, 8 fl.oz	75
Tall, 12 fl.oz	110
Large, 16 fl.oz	150
Decappuccino (decaffeinated)	5
Espresso: Regular/Solo	75
Double (Doppio) Espresso	150
Iced Coffee, 12 fl.oz	140
Latte, 1 cup, 8 fl.oz	75
Mocha, 8 fl.oz	90
Hot Chocolate, 8 fl.oz	15
Tea (Black/Green): Weak, 1 cup	20
Medium Strength, 1 cup	40
Strong, 1 cup	70
Herbal Tea	0
Iced Tea, Tall Glass/Can, 12 fl.oz	25
Soda Drinks: *Per 12 fl.oz Can*	
Coca-Cola, Pepsi (Reg./Diet)	35
Coca-Cola Blak, 8 fl.oz bottle	45
Diet Coke; TAB; RC Cola (Regular)	45
Dr. Pepper (Reg./Diet)	40
Sunkist Orange Soda; Mr PiBB	40
Jolt Cola; SunDrop	55-65
Pepsi One; Mtn Dew; Mellow Yellow; Surge	55
Energy Drinks (w. caffeine): Avg., 8 fl.oz	80
Full Throttle, 16 fl.oz can	145
Red Bull (Regular/Sugar Free), 8.3 fl.oz	80
Tilt (Anheuser-Busch), alcoholic, 16 fl.oz	70
Chocolate Bars: Milk Chocolate, 2 oz	20
Dark Chocolate, 2 oz	30
Cocoa/Hot Choc. Mix, 1 oz pkt	5
Chocolate Milk, 1 cup, 8 fl.oz	2
Choc Chip Cookies, 1 medium, 1 oz	3
Chocolate Syrup, 2 Tbsp, 1.4 oz	5

Extensive Caffeine Counter ~ www.CalorieKing.com

Quick Guide

Teas | C | F | Cb
	C	F	Cb
Regular: Bag, Loose or Instant			
Brewed, 1 cup, 8 fl.oz	2	0	0.5
(Add extra for sugar/milk)			
Herbal: Average all varieties, 1 cup	2	0	0
Bigelow: Apple Orchard, 1 cup	0	0	0
Chamomile	0	0	0
Celestial Seasonings:			
Bengal Spice; Spearmint	0	0	0
Lemon Zinger	0	0	0
Roastaroma	0	0	0
Other varieties	0	0	0
Bubble Tea, average, 12 fl.oz	175	0	41
Chai Tea: *Cafe D' Vita*, 2 Tbsp	120	3.5	21
Starbucks: *See Fast-Foods Section*			

Iced Tea | C | F | Cb
	C	F	Cb
Average All Brands			
Sweetened: 8 fl.oz	100	0	25
12 fl.oz	150	0	38
16 fl.oz	200	0	50
Unsweetened: 8 fl.oz	2	0	0

Iced Tea Mixes

Per Serving (1 Cup, Made-Up)

4C Instant	70	0	18
Carb Options, 1 cup	0	0	0
Crystal Light Sugar Free	5	0	0
Lipton: Instant	0	0	0
Instant Raspberry	80	0	19
Lemon	70	0	18
Peach/Raspb, Sugar Free	5	0	1
Nestea			
Lemonade Tea, 1⅓ Tbsp	60	0	15
Lemon flavored Iced Tea, 1⅓ Tbsp	60	0	15
Sugar Free Lemon Iced Tea, 2 tsp	5	0	2
Unsweetened Tea, 2 tsp	0	0	0
Concentrate: Green Tea, 2 Tbsp	80	0	18
Lemon Tea, 2 Tbsp	80	0	19
Raspberry, 2 Tbsp	90	0	19

> *"A woman is like a teabag. You never know her strength until she's in hot water."*
>
> ~ Eleanor Roosevelt

Bottled & Canned Teas

Per 8 fl.oz Unless Indicated

	C	F	Cb
Arizona: *Per 8 fl.oz Cup*			
Black with Ginseng	70	0	18
Green Tea(s)/Asian Plum	70	0	18
Diet Green Tea (w. Sorbitol)	5	0	2
Diet Lemon/Peach/Raspb.	0	0	0
Peach/Raspberry	70	0	18
Sweet Tea	90	0	23
Brisk: Raspberry, 12 fl.oz can	120	0	35
Diet	0	0	0
Lemon, 12 fl.oz can	120	0	33
Gold Peak, 16.9 fl.oz bottle	170	0	46
Hansen's: Natural Iced Tea, 8 fl.oz	85	0	21
Low Calorie Blueberry/Raspberry	0	0	0
Honest Tea: Green Dragon, 16 fl.oz	60	0	16
Lori's Lemon Tea	60	0	16
Lipton: *Per 16 fl.oz Bottle*			
No Lemon; Lemon	120	0	32
Peach; Raspberry	120	0	32
Diet Green Tea	0	0	0
Nantucket: Half & Half	90	0	22
Original Lemon Tea	80	0	22
Diet Lemon Tea	0	0	0
Nestea Iced Tea: Diet Lemon	2	0	0
Lemon/Peach/Raspberry, 8 fl.oz	90	0	23
Green Tea, 1 bottle, 20 fl.oz	210	0	56
Diet Green Tea	0	0	0
Oregon Chai (Concentrate): *Per ½ Cup (4 fl.oz)*			
Average all flavors	80	0	20
Sugar Free Original	0	0	0
Slightly Sweet Original	20	0	5
Pom Pomegranate Teas: *Per 13.5 fl.oz pkg*			
Black Tea	120	0	30
Hibiscus Green Tea (Light)	60	0	27
Orange Blossom Red (Light)	60	0	27
Note: Carb figures for 'Light' inlcude sugar alcohol (Erythritol) which has a lower calorie value.			
Sbarro, 16 fl.oz Bottle	180	0	48
Shasta, 8 fl.oz	80	0	20
Snapple: Reg., sweetened, avg.	100	0	26
Diet/Unsweetened	0	0	0
SoBe: Green/Lemon Tea, 8 fl.oz	100	0	25
20 fl.oz bottle	225	0	63
Ssips *(Johanna Farms)*, 8 fl.oz	100	0	24
Tazo: *Per 13.8 fl.oz Bottle*			
Berryblossom White Tea	60	0	15
Giant Peach Juiced Tea	120	0	30
Lemon ginger Iced Tea	120	0	30
Mojito Green (Diet)	0	0	0
Organic Iced Green	120	0	30
White Cranberry	140	0	35
Turkey Hill: Regular, 8 fl.oz	90	0	22
Raspberry Cooler, 8 fl.oz	110	0	28

Alcohol Guide

Excess alcohol contributes to obesity, high blood pressure and many other health problems

▶ **Health Hazards: Excessive alcohol intake** contributes to obesity, high blood pressure, stroke, heart and liver disease, some cancers, and even impotence. **Concentration and short-term memory** are reduced as well as sporting performance.

Other alcohol hazards include stomach upsets, menstrual problems, anxiety, headaches, insomnia, work absenteeism, risky behaviors, and social problems.

▶ **Alcohol contributes to obesity** through its high calories and by lessening the body's ability to burn fat. Fat storage is promoted, particularly in the belly - a health danger zone. Alcohol can also stimulate the appetite.

▶ **Alcohol is potentially more harmful while dieting.** Blood sugar levels may drop with resultant tiredness and further impairment of concentration, reflexes and driving skills - and maybe even the dieter's resolve!

LOW RISK ALCOHOL LIMITS

 WOMEN: No more than **1 drink** per day

 MEN: No more than **2 drinks** per day

(At least 2 days a week should be alcohol-free)

 1 DRINK CONTAINS 14 GRAMS ALCOHOL
- ➤ 12 fl.oz Regular Beer (5% Alc.)
- OR 14 fl.oz Light Beer (4.2% Alc.)
- OR 5 fl.oz Wine (12% Alc.)
- OR 1½ fl.oz Spirits (80 Proof)

Note: You cannot save daily drinks for one occasion. Binge drinking is particularly harmful ~ 4 drinks for males or 3 drinks for females (within 2 hours).

For some people, **safe drinking** will mean no alcohol drinks at all. Even one drink may impair driving skills, particularly if tired; and each drink after the first drink increases breast cancer risk in women by 9%.

▶ **It is advisable not to drink at all if you are:**
- pregnant, trying to conceive or breastfeeding
- taking medication or have liver or heart disease (unless approved by your doctor or pharmacist)
- planning to drive, use machinery or play sport
- studying or needing to concentrate
- a child or adolescent

Note: **Women and adolescents are more prone to** alcohol's ill-effects due to their lower body weight, smaller livers and lesser capacity to metabolize alcohol.

▶ **Ten Hints to Avoid Harmful Drinking:** *See Page 172*

HOW TO CALCULATE ALCOHOL CONTENT

Percent alcohol on label refers to alcohol volume (ml alcohol/100ml).

100ml = 3½ fl. oz

To convert to grams (weight) of alcohol, multiply the percent volume by 0.8 - since 1 ml of alcohol weighs only 0.8 grams.

EXAMPLE
12 fl.oz Can Beer
  (5% alcohol)
5% alc.volume = 5% of 12 fl.oz
    = 0.6 fl.oz
    = 18ml alcohol
    (1 fl.oz = 30ml)

Weight (18ml x 0.8) = 14.4g alc.

GOVERNMENT WARNINGS!

(1) According to the Surgeon General, women should not drink alcoholic beverages during pregnancy because of the risk of birth defects.

(2) Consumption of alcoholic beverages impairs your ability to drive a car or operate machinery, and may cause health problems.

Quick Guide

Alc ~ Alcohol (Grams)
Cb ~ Carbohydrate

Beer

Beer Contains Zero Fat

	C	Alc	Cb
Regular Beer (5% Alc. Vol.)			
7 fl.oz Glass	80	8.5	4
12 fl.oz Bottle/Can/Glass	140	14	10
16 fl.oz Bottle/Can	185	19	13
22 fl.oz Bottle	260	25	18
24 fl.oz Can	280	28	20
32 fl.oz Bottle	370	35	28
40 fl.oz Bottle	470	46	35
50 fl.oz Football	590	57	50
Light Beer (4.2% Alc. Vol.)			
7 fl.oz Glass	65	7	4
12 fl.oz Bottle/Can/Glass	110	12	7
16 fl.oz Bottle/Can	145	16	9
22 fl.oz Bottle	200	22	13
24 fl.oz Can	220	24	14
Non-Alcoholic/Near Beer			
(Less than 0.5% alcohol by volume)			
Average All Brands, 12 fl.oz	70	1	14

Beer Brands

Per 12 fl.oz Serving

Percentage alcohol listed below is by volume - not by weight.

Alc ~ Alcohol (Grams)

	C	Alc	Cb
Amber Ice (5.3% alcohol)	130	15	6
Amstel Light (3.5%)	100	10	5
Anheuser World Select (5%)	165	15	15
Anchor Steam (4.6%)	155	13	16
Arrogant Bastard Ale (7.2%)	190	20	12
Artic Ice (5.3%)	150	15	8
Artic Ice Light (3.9%)	100	11	6
Asahi Super Dry (5.2%)	150	15	11
Aspen Edge Low Carb (4.1%)	95	12	3
Augsburger Bock (4.9%)	170	14	17
Bass (5.51%)	140	16	13
Beck's (5%)	145	14	10
Beck's Light (3.8%)	105	11	6
Big Sky (4.8%)	150	14	12
Big Sky Light (4.5%)	105	13	5
Black Label (5.6%)	155	15	11
Blackhook Porter (4.9%)	160	14	14
Blatz (4.6%)	145	13	13
Blatz LA (2.3%)	75	7	6
Blatz Light (3.9%)	110	14	8
Blonde (4.3%)	140	12	10
Blue Moon: Belgian (5.4%)	170	15	14
Pumpkin Ale (5.8%)	185	16	18
Bud Dry (5%)	130	14	8

Brands (Cont)

Alc ~ Alcohol (Grams)

Per 12 fl.oz Serving

	C	Alc	Cb
Bud Light (4.2%)	110	12	7
Bud Ice (5.5%)	150	15	9
Bud Ice Light (4.2%)	110	12	7
Bud Light & Clamato (4.2%), 24 fl.oz	300	24	31
Budweiser (5%)	145	14	11
Budweiser Select (4.3%)	100	12	3
Budweiser & Clamato (5%), 24 fl.oz	370	28	41
Busch (4.6%)	135	13	10
Busch Ice (5.9%)	170	16	13
Busch Light (4.2%)	110	12	7
Carling (4.4%)	140	13	10
Carlsberg (5%)	135	13	10
Carta Blanca (4.0%)	125	11	11
Castlemaine XXXX (4.7%)	140	13	9
Cerveza Aquila (3.9%)	125	11	11
Colt 45 Malt (5.6%)	160	15	11
Coors Original (5%)	140	14	11
Coors Extra Gold (5%)	145	14	11
Coors Light (4.2%)	105	12	5
Corona Extra (4.6%)	150	13	13
Corona Light (4.1%)	105	12	5
Dos Equis Lager (5%)	130	14	9
Drop Top Amber Ale (4.8%)	165	13	15
Fosters Lager (5%)	150	14	12
George Killian's: Irish Brown (5.2%)	185	15	15
Irish Red (5%)	160	14	13
Goebel (4.1%)	130	11	12
Goebel Light (3.9%)	110	11	8
Grolsch Premium (5%)	140	14	10
Guinness Draught (4.2%)	125	12	10
Guinness Extra Stout (5.8%)	175	17	14
Hamm's (4.7%)	145	13	12
Special Light (3.9%)	110	12	7
Harp (4.5%)	150	12	13
Heineken (5%)	150	14	12
Heineken Special Dark (5.2%)	175	15	16
Heineken Premium Light (3.5%)	100	10	7
Hurricane (5.8%)	160	16	10
Icehouse (5.0%)	135	14	8
Icehouse Light (5%)	125	14	7
Jacob Best Ice (5.8%)	160	16	11
Keystone: Premium (4.4%)	110	12	5
Ice (5.9%)	145	16	7
Light (4.2%)	100	12	5
Killarney's Red Larger (5%)	200	14	23
Killain's Irish Red (4.9%)	165	14	14
King Cobra (5.9%)	170	16	12
Kirin Lager (4.9%)	145	14	11
Kirin Light (3.2%)	95	9	7
Labatt's Blue (5%)	145	14	9

Beers ◆ Ales (with Alcohol Counts)

Brands (Cont)

Alc ~ Alcohol (Grams)
Cb ~ Carbohydrate

Beer Contains Zero Fat
Per 12 fl.oz Serving

	C	Alc	Cb
Leinenkugel's: Original (4.7%)	150	13	14
Light (4.2%)	105	11	6
Lone Star: Regular (4.7%)	140	13	12
Light (3.9%)	110	11	8
Lowenbrau Dark/Special (4.9%)	160	14	15
Magic Hat #9 (4.8%)	140	14	12
Magnum Malt Liquor (5.6%)	155	16	10
Meister Brau (4.5%)	130	13	12
Memphis Brown (4.6%)	120	13	6
Michelob: Regular (5%)	155	14	13
Light (4.3%)	135	12	12
Amber Bock (5.2%)	165	15	15
Golden Draft (4.7%)	150	13	14
Golden Draft Light (4.1%)	110	11	7
Honey Larger (4.9%)	175	14	18
Michelob ULTRA (4.1%)	95	12	3
Mickey's Malt Liquor (5.6%)	160	16	11
Miller MGD (4.7%)	145	14	13
Miller MGD Light (4.2%)	110	13	7
Miller High Life (4.7%)	145	14	13
Miller High Life Light (4.2%)	110	13	7
Miller Lite (4.2%)	100	13	4
Milwaukee's Best (4.3%)	130	13	12
Milwaukee's Best Ice (5.9%)	145	16	4
Milwaukee's Best Light (4.2%)	100	13	4
Minnesota's Best (4.9%)	140	14	10
Molson Canadian (5%)	150	14	12
Molson Ice (5.6%)	160	16	12
Molson Special Dry (5%)	145	14	10
Moosehead (5%)	125	14	14
Natural Ice (5.9%)	160	17	9
Natural Light (4.2%)	95	12	3
Negra Modela (5%)	155	14	14
Newcastle Brown Ale (4.5%)	140	12	13
Northstone Amber Ale (4.9%)	150	14	8
Olde English "800" (5.9%)	160	16	11
Old Milwaukee (4.6%)	145	13	13
Light (3.9%)	110	11	8
Ice (5.9%)	180	16	15
Old Style (4.7%)	140	13	12
Old Style Light (4.2%)	115	12	7
Olympia Gold Light (2.2 %)	70	6	6
Pabst	145	13	12
Pabst Blue Ribbon (4.7%)	145	14	12

	C	Alc	Cb
Pabst Light (3.9%)	110	11	8
Pabst Extra Light (2.2%)	70	6	6
Pearl Light (2.2%)	70	6	6
Pete's Wicked Ale (5.3%)	175	15	17
Piels (4.3%)	125	12	9
Pilsner Urquell (4.4%)	155	13	16
Red Dog (5%)	150	14	14
Red Hook ESB (5.7%)	180	17	16
Red Hook India Pale Ale (4.7%)	180	13	19
Red Stripe Jamaican Ale (5.0%)	155	14	14
Rolling Rock (4.5%)	120	13	7
Sam Adams Light (4%)	130	11	10
Samuel Adams (4.6%)	170	13	18
Samuel Adams Lager (4.7%)	180	13	19
Sapporo Draft (3.9%)	135	11	14
Schaefer (4.6%)	145	13	12
Schaefer Light (3.9%)	110	11	8
Schlitz (4.6%)	145	13	12
Schlitz Light (3.9%)	110	11	8
Schmidt's (4.6%)	145	13	13
Schmidt's Light (3.9%)	110	11	8
Sheaf Stout, 5.7%	180	16	17
Sierra Nevada: Pale Ale (5.6%)	200	16	12
Big Foot (9.6%)	295	28	25
Porter (5.6%)	200	16	16
Wheat Beer (4.4%)	150	12	12
Silver Thunder (5.9%)	165	17	11
Skyy Sport (5%)	160	14	15
Sol Cerveza Especial (4%)	125	11	11
Southpaw Light (5%)	125	14	7
St Pauli Girl (5%)	135	14	9
Stella Artois, 5%, 330ml	135	14	9
Stroh's (4.6%)	145	13	13
Stroh's Light (4.0%)	130	12	10
Tecate (4.7%)	155	13	16
Tequiza (4.5%)	130	13	9
The Governator (5.2%)	150	15	11
Warsteiner Verum/Dunkel (5%)	155	14	13
Weinhard's: Pale Ale (4/6%)	150	13	13
Hefeweizen (4.9%)	155	14	12
Wheat Hook (4.8%)	150	14	12
Widmer: Hefeweizen (4.7%)	155	13	16
Zeigenbock Amber (4.4%)	145	13	13

Home-Brewed Beer: Similar to regular beers, according to alcohol content.

Alc ~ Alcohol (Grams) **Cb** ~ Carbohydrate

Non-Alcoholic Brews

Less Than 0.5% Alcohol **C** **Alc** **Cb**
Average All Brands (Busch NA, Coors NA, Kaliber, Kingsbury, O'Douls, Old Milwaukee NA, Pabst NA, Stroh's NA, Sharp's, Haake Beck, Texas Select)

	C	Alc	Cb
12 fl.oz Can/Bottle	70	1	14
O'Doul's Amber, 12 fl.oz	90	1	18

Cider

Alcoholic Cider: Average, 6% alcohol,

	C	Alc	Cb
Dry, 12 fl.oz	130	17	12
Sweet, 12 fl.oz	170	17	15
Hardcore Crisp Hard Cider (6%)	190	17	19
Hornsby's: Draft Cider (6%)	170	17	16
Hard Apple Cider (5.5%)	200	16	27
Woodchuck (5%) Amber, 12 fl.oz	200	15	21
Dark & Dry, 12 fl.oz	180	15	17
Granny Smith, 12 fl.oz	165	15	11
Wyder's: Raspb. (4%), 11.5 fl.oz	140	11	15
Peach (5%) 11.5 fl.oz	150	13	16
Pear (5%), 11.5 fl.oz	130	13	14
22 fl.oz bottle	250	25	28

Quick Guide

Table Wines
Average All Varieties (11.5% Alcohol)
Wine Contains Zero Fat

	C	Alc	Cb
4 fl.oz 1 small wine glass OR ½ large wine glass	90	11	3
6 fl.oz (¾ large wine glass)	135	16	4
8 fl.oz (1 large wine glass)	180	22	6
½ Carafe/Bottle, 375ml	290	34	10
1 Bottle, 750ml	580	68	20

Table Wines

	C	Alc	Cb
Red: Claret/Burgundy/Chianti, 4 fl.oz	80	11	2
Sparkling Reds, 4 fl.oz	90	11	3
Rose: Medium, 4 fl.oz	80	11	2
White: *Per 4 fl.oz*			
Dry (Chablis/Hock/Riesling)	75	11	2
Zinfandel Sweet (Moselle/Sauterne), 4 fl.oz	85	11	2
Sparkling, 4 fl.oz	95	11	4

Table Wines (Cont)

	C	Alc	Cb
Champagne: *Per 4 fl.oz Serving*	85	11	2
Average 1 glass, 4 fl.oz	85	11	2
w. Orange Jce (3:1 orange)	75	8	4
w. Orange Jce (1:1 orange)	65	5	7
Cold Duck, 4 fl·oz	108	11	8
Mulled Wine (Gluhwein), 4 fl.oz	180	14	20
Non-Alcoholic Wine, avg., 4 fl.oz	50	0	12
Reduced Alcohol Wine (6%):			
Average all types, 4 fl.oz	50	0	12
Sake: Rice Wine (16% alc.), 4 oz	125	15	5

Flavored Wine

Average All Brands (6% alcohol)
(Examples: Arbor Mist, Wild Vines, Boones)

	C	Alc	Cb
1 small wine glass, 4 fl.oz	80	6	11
1 large wine glass, 8 fl.oz	160	11	21
1 bottle, 750 ml (25.4 fl.oz)	510	36	67

Dessert Wines

	C	Alc	Cb
Madeira (18% alc), 2 oz	85	9	5
Marsala (18%), 2 oz	110	9	11
Port, Muscatel (18%), 2 oz	85	9	5
Sherry (18%), 2 oz			
Dry, 1 Sherry glass	65	9	0.5
Sweet/Cream, average	85	9	5
Vermouth: Dry (18%), 2 oz	65	9	0.5
Sweet (15%), 2 oz	85	7	8

Cooking Wine

Average All Brands

	C	Alc	Cb
Red/White: 2 Tbsp, 1 oz	20	3	1
1 cup, 8 fl.oz	160	22	12
Marsala, 2 Tbsp, 1 oz	35	4	2
Sherry, 2 Tbsp, 1 oz	40	4	2

COOKING WITH WINE

For alcohol to evaporate, sufficient heat and cooking time (at least 30 minutes) is required.
Red and white table wines would then contain negligible residual calories.
Sweetened wines (marsala/sherry) would contain 10 calories per 1 fl.oz.
Flambé Desserts: Only surface alcohol is burnt off, so negligible reduction in alcohol or calories.

Liquors ✦ Coolers ✦ Cocktails

Quick Guide *Alc ~ Alcohol (Grams)*

Spirits/Liquors
Includes Bourbon, Brandy, Gin, Rum, Scotch, Tequila, Vodka, Whiskey.
Note: All spirits with same proof (alcohol) have similar calories and zero fat.

Average All Brands

	C	Alc	Cb
80 Proof (40% Alcohol by Volume):			
1 fl.oz	65	9.5	0
1½ fl.oz (1 shot)	100	14	0
3 fl.oz (Double shot)	200	29	0
½ Bottle, 350 ml	810	120	0
1 Bottle, 700 ml (24 fl.oz)	1620	240	0
86 Proof (43% Alc): 1 fl.oz	70	10	0
1½ fl.oz (1 shot)	105	15	0
1 Bottle, 700 ml (24 fl.oz)	1750	250	0
100 Proof (50% Alc): 1½ fl.oz	120	18	0

Shochu (Soju) ~ Izakaya Lounges

	C	Alc	Cb
Average all types (20% alc), 2 fl.oz	65	9	0

Chu-Hai Cocktails ~ Next Page

Flavored Spirits ~ Average All Brands
Includes Malibu Rum; Captain Morgan

	C	Alc	Cb
70 Proof (35% Alc): 1½ fl.oz	105	13	1
3 fl.oz (Double shot)	210	26	3

Hard Lemon(ade) & Sodas

	C	Alc	Cb
Doc's Hard Lemon (5%), 12 fl.oz	170	14	17
Henry's Hard L'ade (5%), 12 fl.oz	285	14	46
Hooch Hard (5.2%), 330ml	215	14	32
Hooch Ice (5.7%), 330ml	230	15	32
Mike's Hard Lem. (5.2%): 11.2 fl.oz	240	13	38
16 fl.oz bottle	345	19	54
Mike's Light Lem. (4%), 11.2 fl.oz	120	10	12
Mike's Hard Iced Tea (5%), 11.2 fl.oz	195	13	27
Rick's Spiked (5.2%), 12 fl.oz	250	14	39
Twisted Tea: Half & Half (5%) 12 fl.oz	250	14	37
Hard Iced/Raspberry (5%) 12 fl.oz	220	14	30
Two Dogs (4.2%), 355ml	205	12	30

Alcoholic Energy Drinks (with Caffeine)

	C	Alc	Cb
B-to-the-E *(Anheuser-Busch)*, 10 fl.oz	150	12	17
Sparks: Per 16 fl.oz Can			
Premium Malt (6%)	345	23	47
Sparks Light (6%)	180	23	5
Sparks Plus (7%)	385	26	49
Tilt *(Anheuser-Busch)* 6.6% alc., 16 fl.oz	390	24	56

Coolers & Premix Cocktails

Ready-To-Drink
Zero Fat Unless Indicated

	C	Alc	Cb
Arbor Mist: Blenders, all flavors (12.5%), 4 fl.oz	100	11	14
Bacardi: Silver (5%), 12 fl.oz	235	14	35
Silver O³ (5%), 12 fl.oz	235	14	35
Silver Raz (5%), 12 fl.oz	235	14	35
Silver (5%), all flavors	235	14	35
Ready to Pour (1.75 liter bottle)			
Bahama Mama (10%), 4 fl.oz	130	13	16
Hurricane (12.5%), 4 fl.oz	144	12	16
Rum Island Ice Tea (12.5%), 4 fl.oz	150	14	16
Bartles & Jaymes			
Malt Based Coolers (3.9% alc): Per 12 fl.oz			
Blue Hawaiian; Melon Splash	230	11	35
Classic Original	200	11	30
Exotic Berry	210	11	33
Fuzzy Navel; Apple Passion	230	11	38
Margarita, Pina Colada	270	11	48
Strawberry Daiquiri	230	11	38
Luscious Blackberry	230	11	38
Daily's *(Ready-to-Drink):*			
Bag-In-Box Cocktails (6.9%)			
Bloody Mary, ½ cup, 4 fl.oz	70	6	6
Other flavors, 4 fl.oz	110	6	15
Frozen Pouches (5%), 10 fl.oz	280	11	44
Jack Daniels Country Cocktails (5.9%)			
Average all flavors, 6.8 fl.oz	170	10	25
Jack Daniels Hard Cola (5%) 12 oz	234	14	34
Jose Cuervo Authentic Margarita (5.9% alc)			
Margarita/Lime.Strawb. 200ml	180	10	27
Sauza Diablo (5%), 12 fl.oz	260	14	40
Seagram's Coolers (5%)			
Average all flavors	240	14	35
Skyy Blue (5%), 12 fl.oz	280	14	45
Stolichnaya Citr. (5%), 12 fl.oz	240	14	36
Smirnoff Ice (5%), 330ml	220	13	33
Black Ice (5.5%), 12 fl.oz	240	19	36
TGI Friday's: Per 3 fl.oz			
On The Rocks: Margarita (7.5%)	90	6	14
Long Island Ice Tea (15%)	130	11	14
Mudslide (10%)	200	8	18
Blenders (12.5% alc): Per 3 fl.oz			
Mudslide (12.5%)	120	8.5	12
Orange Dream (12.5%)	120	8.5	14
Strawberry Shortcake (12.5%)	115	8.5	12

Coolers & Premix Cocktails (Cont)

Ready-To-Drink

The Club Premix Cocktails (8 oz Can):
Per 4 oz Serving (½ can):

	C	Alc	Cb
Long Island Ice Tea; Manhattan	220	16	30
Margar.; Screwdriver; Vodka Martini	210	7	40
Mudslide (9g fat)	270	12	41
Pina Colada; Or. Craze; Whisk. Sour	260	10	40
Zima (5.9%), 12 fl.oz	235	15	20

Shooters
Alc ~ Alcohol (Grams)

	C	Alc	Cb
Alabama Slammer	110	14	2
Amaretto Sour	120	6	19
B52	145	14	11
Beam Me Up Scotty	145	13	13
Duck Fart	140	9	11
Jager Bomb	205	8	30
Jager Bomb (w. Sugar-Free Red Bull)	155	8	18
Jello Shot	180	14	19
Jello Shot (W. Diet Jello)	110	14	0
Kamakazie	75	8	3
Kool-Aid	160	15	14
Liquid Cocaine	135	9	9
M & M	150	11	20
Orgasm	100	12	6
Peppermint Patty	200	8	11
Stinger	170	18	12
Tequila Shot	105	14	1

Cocktail Mixers

Non Alcoholic ~ No Alcohol Added
Bacardi: *Frozen Concentrate*
(Made Up from 2 fl.oz concentrate)

	C	Alc	Cb
Margarita, 8 fl.oz	90	0	25
Pina Colada, 8 fl.oz	170	0	35
Strawberry, 8 fl.oz	120	0	35
Baja Bob's (Sugar Free),			
Cocktail/Martini Mix, 4 fl.oz	10	0	2
Daily's Pina Colada, 3 fl.oz	160	0	37
J.Cuervo Margarita, 4 fl.oz	100	0	24
Malibu Beach, all flavors, 8 fl.oz	10	0	3
Mr & Mrs T: Mai Tai, 4.5 fl.oz	140	0	33
Bloody Mary, 8 fl.oz	40	0	9
Margarita, 8 fl.oz	100	0	26
Pina Colada, 4.5 fl.oz	180	0	43
Strawberry Daiquiri, 4 fl.oz	200	0	50
Sweet 'n' Sour, 4 fl.oz	90	0	23
Sauza Margarita, 3 fl.oz	70	0	18
Skyy Cosmo, 4 fl.oz	140	0	36
TGI Fridays: Hurricane, 2.3 fl.oz	60	0	15
Long Island Ice Tea, 3.3 fl.oz	55	0	14
Mudslide, 2.3 fl.oz	120	0	24

Cocktails
Alc ~ Alcohol (Grams)

Made to Standard Recipes *(Standard Size)*
(Main Reference: The New American Bartender's Guide)
Zero Fat Unless Indicated

	C	Alc	Cb
Bacardi & Coke (w. 1½ oz Bacardi)	160	14	17
Bloody Mary (w. 1½ oz Vodka)	125	10	7
Blue Lady	220	15	7
Blushin' Russian (20g fat)	405	14	23
Bourbon & Soda (w. 2 oz Bourbon)	130	19	0
Brandy Alexander (10g fat)	300	20	15
Chi Chi, frozen, (5g fat)	215	14	17
Chu-Hais (w. 2 oz Shochu):			
On the Rocks	65	9	0
Aloha (w. 2 oz Juice)	100	9	9
Sora (Sky) Martini,			
(w. 1 oz Curacao/Plum Wine)	120	14	4
Chupa Naranjas (w. 1½ oz Tequila)	150	16	8
Cosmopolitan	215	14	12
Daiquiri (w. 2 oz Rum) avg. all types	140	19	4
Frozen Daiquiri (w. 2 oz Rum): no fruit	155	19	6
with fruit (w. 1½ oz Rum)	145	14	11
Gin Martini (w. 2 oz alcohol)	140	19	0
Grasshopper	260	17	28
Harvey Wallbanger (2 oz Alc.)	200	19	17
Highball (1½ oz Whiskey)	100	14	0
Irish Coffee (contains 10g fat)	205	14	2
Kahlua Mudslide: w.milk (3g fat)	145	11	22
w. cream (12g fat)	230	11	20
L.A. Sunrise (w. 1½ oz Vodka)	220	14	17
Lady Killer	160	14	15
Long Island Iced Tea (w. 3 oz Cola)	270	19	32
with Diet Cola (w. 3 oz Cola)	235	19	22
Mai Tai (with 2 oz Rum)	290	24	33
Manhattan	130	19	5
Margarita	180	24	7
Mint Julep (w.2½ oz Bourbon)	180	24	4
Mojito (with 2 oz Rum)	150	19	5
Moscow Mule	185	14	24
Pina Colada (contains 10g fat)	325	19	26
Red Bull & Vodka	210	14	28
with Sugar Free Red Bull	105	14	3
Screwdriver	160	14	15
Sex On The Beach	235	19	25
Spritzer (with 3 oz Wine)	65	8	2
Tequila Sunrise	200	14	25
Tom Collins (w. 2 oz Gin)	210	19	18
Vodka Soda (w. 1½ oz Vodka)	100	14	0
Vodka Tonic (w. 2 oz Vodka)	165	14	18
Whiskey Sour (w. 2 oz Whiskey)	155	19	7
White Russian (w. 10g fat)	240	19	7

Liqueurs (with Alcohol Counts)

Liqueurs/Cordials   **C**   **Alc**   **Cb**

Per 1 fl.oz

	C	Alc	Cb
Advocaat (36 Proof; 2g fat)	85	4	9
Alizé: Cognac	70	11	2
Gold/Red Passion	105	4.5	11
Amaretto (56 Proof)	110	6	17
Baileys Irish Cream (34 Proof; 5g fat)	95	4	5
Lite (30 Proof; 2g fat)	75	4	7
Benedictine (80 Proof)	90	10	5
Chambord (33 Proof)	105	5	11
Chartreuse (80 Proof)	100	10	7
Cherry Brandy (48 Proof)	80	6	9
Coffee Liqueur (53 Proof)	90	6	11
Cointreau (80 Proof)	100	10	7
Creme de Cacao (54 Proof)	100	6	15
Creme de Menthe (60 Proof)	120	7	14
Curacao (70 Proof)	95	8	6
Drambuie (80 Proof)	105	10	9
Frangelico (48 Proof)	80	6	9
Galliano (80 Proof)	100	10	8
Grand Marnier (80 Proof)	100	10	7
Kahlua (53 Proof)	90	6	11
Kirsch (80 Proof)	80	8	6
Midori (42 Proof)	80	5	11
Ouzo (80 Proof)	105	11	11
Pernod (80 Proof)	75	10	2
Sambuca (84 Proof)	100	10	7
Schnapps (80 Proof)	100	10	7
Southern Comfort (70 Proof)	80	10	3
Starbucks Coffee Liqueur (40 Proof)	80	4	13
Tia Maria (64 Proof)	90	8	9
Triple Sec (60 Proof)	80	7	4

Liqueur Coffee & Hot Drinks

Per Standard Drink

	C	Alc	Cb
Liqueur Coffee, avg. all types	200	10	10
Egg Nog	270	10	25
Hot Toddy, w. 2 oz liquor	200	19	17
Irish Coffee, w. 2 Tbsp whip. crm	80	7	4
Mulled Wine (Glühwein), 5 oz	175	14	6

Flavorings/Syrups

	C	Alc	Cb
Angostura Bitters, ¼ tsp	3	0	0
Ginger Ale, 8 fl.oz	80	0	22
Grenadine/Cassis, 2 Tbsp, 1 oz	70	0	17
Lime/Lemon Juice, 2 Tbsp, 1 oz	10	0	2
Maraschino Cherry, 1 small	8	0	2
Pure Lemon Extract (70%) avg., 1 oz	145	20	0
Sugar Syrup, 2 Tbsp, 1 oz	70	0	17
Sour Mix, 2 Tbsp, 1 oz	10	0	2
Tonic Water, 8 fl.oz	90	0	22
Vanilla Extract, (35%), avg., 1 oz	80	10	3.5

TEN HINTS TO AVOID HARMFUL DRINKING

1. **Add up the alcohol** you typically drink each day and on social occasions. How does this compare with 'low risk' amounts?

2. **Compare the alcohol content** of different drinks and select the lowest. Request half ounces of alcohol in cocktails and mixed drinks. Dilute them and keep topping off with non-alcoholic drinks.

3. **Go easy on 'Light' beers.** At 4% alcohol, on average, they are still high in alcohol compared to regular beer (5% alcohol).

4. **Try low alcohol or non-alcohol** alternatives such as fruit juices and mineral water. Take your own to parties.

5. **Before drinking alcohol,** quench your thirst with water and non-alcoholic drinks – particularly after vigorous exercise or sport.

6. **Slow the rate of drinking.** Chugging or drinking fast is the major cause of illness and death from alcohol poisoning.

7. **Avoid drinking in 'rounds'.**

8. **Have a non-alcoholic 'spacer'** between drinks (e.g. mineral water, orange juice).

9. **Don't drink on an empty stomach.** Food slows the rate of alcohol absorption.

10. **Keep track of the number of drinks** and know when to stop. Stick to a set limit.

Note: • Alcohol can be very dangerous when taken with prescription or street drugs or when you are very tired.
Extra Info: www.CalorieKing.com

"The doctor told him to cut down to just one glass a day."

Cafeteria-Style Foods

	C	F	Cb
Apple & Cinnamon, 1.23 oz	130	1.5	26
Beef Stroganoff, 5 oz	195	13	7
Beef Stroganoff w. 4 oz noodles	350	14	36
Chicken Lasagna, 1 piece	300	11	32
Chicken Chop Suey w. 4 oz rice	245	4	37
Deep Dish Burrito, 7 oz	265	13	20
Grnd Beef Casserole, 2 scoop, 6 oz	245	13	17
Italian Meat Sce for Spagh., 5 oz	150	9	9
w. 5 oz Spaghetti	350	10	49
Lasagna, 1 piece	275	11	25
Meatloaf, 3 oz	205	13	4
Ranch Beans, 2 scoops, 6 oz	350	11	45
Red Beans & Rice, 7 oz	280	9	37
Scalloped Potato/Ham, 2 scp, 6 oz	160	6	20
Stuffed Shells in Sauce (1)	105	3	17
Swedish Meatballs (3)	205	12	9
Sweet & Sour Pork/Rice, 9 oz	240	3	40
Swiss Steak w/Mushr. Gravy, 6 oz	280	11	4
Tator Tot Casserole, 2 scoops, 6 oz	260	15	20
Tenderloin Tips/Mushr. Gravy, 5 oz	210	13	3
w. 5 oz noodles	395	15	38
Tuna Noodle Casserole, 2 scp, 6 oz	180	6	17
Turkey Tetrazini, 2 scoops, 6 oz	195	7	17
Vegetable Lasagna, 1 piece	250	13	21

Croissants

	C	F	Cb
Unfilled: Medium 1½ oz	180	10	21
Filled: w. Ham (2 oz), Salad	280	14	24
w. Ham (2 oz), Cheese (2 oz)	470	30	20
w. Chick (2 oz) Cheese (2 oz)	470	30	20
w. Turkey/Ham/Chse (2 oz ea.)	580	36	20
Au Bon Pain: Ham & Cheese	340	10	46
Spinach & Cheese	250	9	32
7-Eleven: Page 246			

Bagels

	C	F	Cb
Plain: Large, 4 oz (no filling)	320	2	65
with 2 oz Cream Cheese	500	27	54
with 2 oz Lox (Smoked Salmon)	400	4	65

Also see Bagels Section: Page 104
Fast-Foods Restaurants: Page 183
Au Bon Pain: Page 187
Bruegger's: Page 193
Einstein Bros Bagels: Page 207

Sandwiches

	C	F	Cb
No Spreads Unless Indicated			
(Includes 2 Slices Bread ~ 3 oz)			
BLT (5 strips Bacon, 2 Tbsp Mayo)	600	40	46
Breaded Chicken & Salad	540	28	46
Chicken (5 oz) Salad w. Mayo.	580	30	49
Chopped Liver, Egg, Mayo.	630	25	44
Corned Beef (5 oz) w. Mustard	560	28	44
Cream Cheese w. Olives (5 large)	340	14	46
Egg Salad w. Mayonnaise	570	29	49
Egg Salad Club w. Bacon, Mayo.	780	53	49
Grilled Cheese (3 oz)	540	30	44
Ham (4 oz); Cheese (4 oz), Mayo.	910	56	44
Lobster Salad (4 oz) w. Mayo.	530	25	45
Overstuffed Tuna Salad (7 oz)	870	39	75
Philadelphia Cheese Steak S'wich	550	23	42
Reuben (6 oz Beef/Pastrami, 2 oz Cheese,			
2 Tbsp Dressing)	920	60	28
Roast Beef (4 oz) w. Mustard	460	12	45
Roast Pork (4 oz) w. Apple Sauce	500	16	55
Shrimp Salad Club w. Bacon, Mayo.	800	57	48
Sloppy Joe w. Sauce (7 oz)	600	30	45
Steak Sandwich (5 oz cooked)	680	32	41
Triple Cheese (4 oz) Melt	720	45	46
Tuna (5 oz) Salad w. Mayo.	610	30	49
Turkey Breast (5 oz) w. Mayo.	460	18	44
Turkey Breast (5 oz) w. Mustard	360	7	44
Turkey Club w. Bacon, Mayo.	830	38	31
Vegetarian w. Avocado, Cheese	820	49	72

7-Eleven: Page 246
Schlotzsky's: Page 247
Subway: Page 258

Wraps & Roll-Ups

	C	F	Cb
Average All Types			
(Meat/Chicken/Fish/Veges)			
Small size, approx. 9 oz	500	25	48
Regular, approx. 15 oz	830	40	80
Large, approx. 22 oz	1400	70	134

Fast-Foods Restaurants: Page 183
Au Bon Pain: Page 187
Sonic Drive-In: Page 252
Subway: Page 258
The Wrap: Page 263
WAWA: Page 267

Fair & Carnival Foods

Fair & Carnival Foods

	C	F	Cb
Mexican			
Burritos w. Bean/Beef, 17 oz	1100	41	104
Carne Asada, 14.5 oz	820	44	58
Fish Tacos, 1 taco, 5 oz	270	13	31
Nachos w. Cheese, 9" plate	860	59	70
Taco Chicken, 3.3 oz	210	12	16
Tamale (1), 3.5 oz	180	8	21
Taquitos, 5 oz	370	17	43
Greek			
Baklava, 2" square	245	13	32
Falafel, 11.6 oz	660	27	85
Greek Salad, 14 oz	520	48	17
Gyros, 7.5", 12 oz	680	40	55
Spanakopita, 8 oz	200	7.5	23
Italian			
Garlic Bread, ½ loaf, 10 oz	1135	40	147
Pizza Bread Pepperoni, ½ loaf, 12 oz	1115	32	151
Pizza on a Stick, 1 piece	535	28	55
Personal Pizza, 7": Cheese (1)	670	24	80
Pepperoni (1)	795	35	80
Ham & Pineapple (1)	800	31	87
Low Carb			
Beef Patty, wrapped in lettuce, 4 oz	480	33	0
Sandwiches: Per 7½" Roll			
Ham, 11 oz	645	39	47
Hot Pastrami, 9 oz	760	17	62
Roast Beef, 11 oz	620	36	46
Philadelphia Cheese Steak, 13 oz	680	36	49
Tuna, 12 oz	830	60	46
Turkey, 11 oz	665	24	65
Veggie, 11 oz	490	23	49
Oriental: Fried Egg Roll, 6 oz	400	19	44
Rice Bowl: Beef, 6" Bowl	880	13	136
Chicken, 6" Bowl	870	15	135
Hamburgers			
⅓ Pound Burger, 7.5 oz	670	41	26
Burger w. Cheese, 6 oz	550	36	25
Hot Dogs/Franks: With Bun			
Hot Dog: Regular, (1)	215	14	28
with Chili, 6 oz	450	32	32
with Chili & Cheese, 7.3 oz	500	36	31
⅓ Pound Hot Dog	550	41	31
Foot Long Hot Dog	470	26	41
Corn Dog: Regular, 4 oz	250	14	23
Jumbo, 6 oz	375	21	36
Jumbo Franks w. Bun:			
Bratwurst; Sausage; Kielbasa, avg.	800	60	28

Fair & Carnival Foods (Cont)

	C	F	Cb
Barbeque Items (Weights with Bone)	:		
Beef Stew over Rice, 2 cups	440	14	61
Chicken, 15 oz	740	24	34
Chili, 1 cup	280	11	24
Corn on the Cob, 8" (1), 16 oz	200	1	42
Pork Ribs, 18 oz	1360	68	21
Smoked Turkey Legs (1), 19 oz	1135	54	0
Potatoes & Fries			
Australian Battered Potato, 12 oz	1290	66	155
Baked Potato, 14 oz	435	0.5	100
Fries: French, 7 oz	560	24	70
Cheese Fries, 10 oz	645	38	62
Chili Fries, 10 oz	700	36	83
Chili/Cheese Fries, 13 oz	745	45	57
Curly Fries, 7 oz	620	30	78
Tasti Chips, 40 chips, 6.5 oz	780	33	117
Sweet Potato, 14 oz	405	0.5	97
Ranch Dip, 3 oz	165	14	9
Finger Foods			
Artichoke: Steamed, 6 pieces	65	0	16
Fried, 9 pieces	250	14	24
Chicken Nuggets (6)	340	17	26
Chicken Strips (4), 4.5 oz	445	21	33
Finger Steaks (2), 4 oz	400	20	26
Mushrooms, Fried, 10-12 pieces	395	26	34
Onion Rings, 3 rings	310	13	40
Onion Flower	1320	72	140
Shrimp, Fried, 10-12 pieces, 5 oz	555	30	36
Sweet Potato Strips, Fried, 4 pces	750	30	106
Zucchini, Fried, 4 slices	620	40	42
Salads/Sides			
Baked Beans, 4 oz	140	2	38
Cole Slaw, 5 oz	350	21	37
Pickle, whole (6")	30	0	8
Potato Salad, 5 oz	290	15	35
Popcorn: Plain, small, 3 oz	450	24	48
Large, 6 oz	900	48	96
Kettle Corn: Small, 5 oz	600	15	110
Large, 10 oz	1200	30	220
Cakes, Donuts, Cookies			
Funnel Cake: Plain	760	44	80
Toppings: Cinn. & Sugar, 2 tsp	30	0	8.5
Apple Cinnamon, 2 oz	85	3	36
Strawberries & Cream, 2 oz	70	0	16
Cinnamon Roll, large	730	24	114
Churros, 1½ oz	150	8	18
Donuts, Jumbo Twist, 7.5 oz	905	49	109

Fair & Carnival Foods (Cont)

Cakes, Donuts, Cookies (Cont)

	C	F	Cb
Fried Snickers, 5 oz	445	29	42
Fried Oreos, 3 cookies	300	10	33
Fried Twinkie, 1	420	34	45
Cotton Candy, 5½ oz bag	625	0	156
Red Rope Licorice, (24"), 2 oz	200	0	46
Cream Puff, 4.3 oz	500	43	22
Puff-on-a-Stick (4), 8.6 oz	995	86	44
Strawberry Crepe, 4.3 oz	280	14	36
Chocolate Dipped Straw, 1 pce	125	7	15
Fudge, 1.5 oz	200	11	25
Twinkie Dog (Sundae)	500	14	89
Key Lime Pie Bar, 6 oz	635	40	59
Cheesecake on a Stick, 6 oz	655	47	56
Cobbler, 5 oz	350	10	62
Soft Pretzel, 4.5 oz	340	2	70
Candied Apple, 7 oz	330	0.5	80

Ice Cream & Frozen Treats

	C	F	Cb
Dippin' Dots Ice Cream: Small, 4 oz	150	7	17
Medium, 8 oz	305	14	35
Large, 16 oz	600	28	70
Snow Cone, 10 oz	270	0	68
Frozen Yogurt in sugar cone, 14 oz	475	2	94
Ice Cream: Small, sugar cone, 10 oz	775	42	83
Large, sugar cone, 14 oz	935	54	96
Sherbet, 8 oz	270	4	59
Frozen Banana, choc cover, 5 oz	240	4	53

Drinks

	C	F	Cb
Lemonade, 18 fl.oz	210	0	52
Orange Julius, 20 fl.oz	490	10	96
Strawberry Julius, 20 fl.oz	430	0	98
Icee, 16 fl.oz	235	0	59
Malt, 16 fl.oz	690	33	85
Slushies, 16 fl.oz	260	0	65
Soft Frozen Lemonade, 12 fl.oz	300	0	78
Smoothies: Berry Flavors, 16 fl.oz	350	1	80

Stadium Foods

Sandwiches

	C	F	Cb
Bacon Burger, 8.3 oz	470	25	34
Cheeseburger, 8.3 oz	450	23	33
Chicken Sandwich: w. Cheese, 8.3 oz	510	29	40
no Cheese, 7.7 oz	460	25	40
w. Bacon, 8.3 oz	530	31	41
Hamburger, 7.8 oz	400	19	33
Polish Sausage Sandwich, 7 oz	565	33	46
Fries, French Fries, 6.4 oz	470	34	39
Fruit Cup, 6 oz	80	0	20

Hot Dogs

	C	F	Cb
Chili Dog, 7.7 oz	520	29	45
Hot Dog, 6.4 oz	465	21	50
Jumbo Dog, 6.4 oz	440	25	38
Kraut Dog w. Sauerkraut , 7.8 oz	490	27	41
Nachos, 40 chips w. 4 oz cheese	1100	59	132

Individual Pan Pizza (6"): Per 10 oz Pizza

	C	F	Cb
BBQ Chicken	630	24	71
Cheese	630	27	71
Pepperoni	660	30	70

Snacks

	C	F	Cb
Brownie, 2.5" x 4.5"	360	18	44
Cheese Sauce, 1.25 oz	100	8	4
Cheetos, 2.75 oz pkg	440	28	42
Chocolate Chip Cookie, 2.3 oz	280	12	40
Churros, 8", 3 oz	325	15	42
Doritos Nacho, 2.75 oz pkg	390	20	48
King Size Candy:			
Butterfinger, 3.75 oz	485	18	75
Nestle Crunch, 2.75 oz	390	21	85
Lays Chips, 2.75 oz pkg	440	28	42
Peanuts in shell, 8 oz	930	80	24
Popcorn: Small (9 cup size)	575	35	56
Large (15 cup size)	950	58	93
Red Vines, 5.5 oz box	560	0	136
Soft Pretzel: Regular, 5.5 oz	490	3.5	101
Giant, 8 oz	710	5	147
Beverages: Orange Juice, 12 fl.oz	180	0	2
Beer: Heineken, 16 fl.oz	200	0	16
Light Miller, 16 fl.oz	165	0	10
Miller Draft, 16 fl.oz	205	0	18
Jack Daniels Punch, 12 fl.oz	235	0	34
Wine, White, 9 fl.oz	190	0	6
Soda (with ½ ice), average: 20 fl.oz	160	0	40
32 fl.oz	260	0	65
Snow Cone, 18 oz (incl. 3 oz syrup)	270	0	68
Starbuck's Frappccino, 12 fl.oz	195	2.5	39

Restaurant & International Foods

Chinese & Asian Dishes

	C	F	Cb
Appetizers			
Crab Cake, 63g	105	5	0.5
Curried Meat Triangles, 1 pce	150	5	12
Dumplings: Pork, steamed, 1	40	3	4
Pork, fried, 1 dumpling	75	7	4
Vegetable, steamed, 1	25	0.5	4
Egg Rolls, mini, 3 rolls	100	3	11
Rice Paper Roll, 1	80	2	10
Spring Roll: Small, 1½ oz	100	7	10
Medium, 3 oz	200	12	20
Large, 5 oz	350	15	33
Wonton, 1 only	55	3	4
Soup: Clear, 1 bowl	30	1	4
with Noodles	100	3	12
Chicken & Corn	150	8	8
Rice: Plain, 1 cup (½ Pint), 6½ oz	240	0.5	54
2 cups (1 Pint), 13 oz	480	1	108
Fried: 1 cup, 5 oz	320	13	42
Large dish, 16 oz	1010	40	134
Noodles: Chinese Egg, ckd, 1 cup	200	3	42
Entrees & Mains: *Per Whole Dish*			
Beef Satay, 17 oz	760	50	15
Beef in Black Bean Sce, 17 oz	530	33	17
Beef with Broccoli, 16 oz	650	30	31
Chicken & Almonds, 18 oz	685	50	18
Chicken (sliced) & Broccoli	280	12	13
Chop Suey: Chicken, 20 oz	560	37	7
Pork, 20 oz	680	50	12
Chow Mein, Beef/Chicken, 24 oz	940	60	50
Crab Puff/Rangoon, 1 dumpling	80	4.5	7.5
Crispy Fried Chicken, 8 oz	485	33	12
Egg Drop Soup: w. Noodles, 1 cup	120	3	15
w/out Noodles, 1 cup	70	3	3
Egg Foo Yung w. Sauce, 1 cup	225	12	11
Lemon Chicken, 10 oz	580	32	25
Lo Mein (stir-fried)	620	29	61
Moo Shu Chicken, 2 wrapped crepes	430	16	43
Omelet, Chicken/Shrimp, 16 oz	990	82	10
Steamed Whole Fish·½ Red Snapper	500	11	1
Sweet & Sour: Fish, 20 oz	1160	58	106
Pork, 18 oz	950	50	92
Vegetable Combination, w. oil, 6 oz	250	17	19
Vegetables, Steamed (no oil), 6 oz	120	1	25
Bubble Tea, average, 12 fl oz	240	0	55
Fortune Cookie: each	25	0.5	5

Cajun & Creole

	C	F	Cb
Alligator, 4 oz cooked	160	2	0
Baked Herb Chicken, 1 serving	850	53	2
Bouillabaisse	400	15	10
Cajun Fried Turkey, 1 serving	630	25	0
Cocktail Sauce, 2 Tbsp	30	0	6
Couche-couche, ½ cup	80	0	17
Crawfish Bisque, 1 serving	500	10	10
Crawfish, cooked, 2 oz	45	0.5	0
Creole Jambalaya, 1 serving	550	30	15
Frog's Legs, steamed (2)	45	0	0
Guinea Fowl, flesh, 4 oz, ckd	160	4	0
Hogshead Cheese, ¼ cup	80	5.5	0
Jambalaya, Shrimp & Crabmeat	520	14	12
Red Beans & Rice, 1 serving	400	17	52
Roasted Quail, w. Bacon on Toast	550	25	15
Remoulade Sauce, 2 Tbsp, 1 OZ	110	11	2
Shrimp Creole, 1 serving	450	20	10
Stuffed Smothered Steak, w. 1 cup Rice	890	50	50
Turtle, cooked, 3 oz	120	3	0

Cuban

	C	F	Cb
Bl. Beans w. Rice (Moros con Cristianos)	510	22	76
Blk.-eyed Pea Fritters (Bollitos de Carita)	80	5	6
Casserole Corn Tamale	445	20	55
Chkn w. Yellow Rice (Arroz con Pollo)	925	49	87
Cuban Bread (Pan Cubano)	80	1.5	15
Donuts in Syrup (Bunuelos)	170	5	10
with Melado	100	5	10
Grilled Plantains	145	0	40
Gypsy's Arm Cake (Brazo Gitano)	260	18	42
Roast Pork S'wich (Pan con Lechon)	640	30	62
Seasoned Beef w. Olives & Raisins (Picadillo)	435	36	10
Shredded Beef (Ropa Vieja)	550	35	10
Taro Root Mash (Pure de Malanga)	315	3	69
Yuca with Citrus Garlic Dressing (Yuca con Mojo)	190	9	25

French Foods

	C	F	Cb
Blanquette d'Agneau (Lamb Stew)	800	30	17
Brioche, 1 cake	280	14	34
Bouillabaisse (Fish Stew)	400	15	10
Coq au Vin (Chicken in Wine)	800	30	16
Coquilles St. Jacques, fried, 6 lge.	300	14	2
Crème Brulée, 1 serving	460	40	21

French Foods (Cont)

	C	F	Cb
Creme Caramel (Caramel Custard)	260	10	38
Crepe Suzette, 1x6" crepe w. sauce	220	10	13
Duck a l'Orange	780	35	47
Escargots (Snails), garlic butter (6)	200	10	4
French Stick Bread, 3 slices, 2.2 oz	150	1	35
Frogs Legs, fried, 4 med. pairs	400	20	10
Lamb Noisettes, fried, 2 chops	500	40	1
Mousse au Chocolat	380	15	33
Potage Creme Crecy (Carrot Soup)	360	18	14
Salade Nicoise (Tuna/Oliv./Veg.)	450	13	14
Veal Cordon Bleu (Veal/Ham/Ch)	650	25	18
Vichyssoise (Pot./Leek Soup), 1 c.	200	9	15

Baguette & French Stick: *Page 102, 103*
Croissants: *Pages 113, 173*

German

	C	F	Cb
Bavarian Bread Dumpling, 3 small	330	10	28
Beef Goulash with Veges	520	20	46
Black Forest Cake, 1 slice	380	16	30
Bratwurst, grilled, 1 medium, 6 oz	450	37	2
Chicken: Fried, Viennese-style	530	20	28
Livers w. Apple/On., 6 oz	460	28	10
Herring, Pickled: Rollmops, 4 oz	260	16	3
with Sour Cream, 4 oz	310	20	3
Hot Sausage Curry	300	7	6
Kugelhupf Cake, 1 lge slice, 4 oz	400	23	40
Sauerbraten Pork (Pot Roast)	650	35	15
Torte: Linzer (Alm./Raspb. Jam)	430	18	58
Sacher (Choc./Apricot Jam)	260	12	23
Weiner Schnitzel, 1 medium	750	35	38

Greek

	C	F	Cb
Baklava Pastry: Small	240	13	32
Large, 3¾ oz	400	21	45
Calamari, deep fried, 1 cup	300	13	17
Chicken Kebob Plate	345	13	8
Galactobureko, 1 only			
(Filo, Custard, Pastry in Syrup)	360	15	48
Greek Chicken Salad	400	8	9
Gyros, 4 oz	380	33	6
Hummus & Pita, 4 oz	260	12	30
Kataifi, (Filo, Nut, Pastry in Syrup)	350	11	56
Moussaka, 1 serve, 8 oz	350	22	22
Soup: Argolemono (Egg Lemon Soup			
with Chicken & Rice)	85	6	5
Souvlakia (Lamb), each, 2 oz	120	6	1

Greek (Cont)

	C	F	Cb
Stuffed Tomatoes, 2 only	250	12	17
Taramasalata, 1 Tbsp, ½ oz	40	3	2
Tyropita (Filo/Egg/Cheese Pastry)	350	26	31
Tzatziki (Cucumber/Yog. Dip), 1 T.	20	1	1
Vine Leaves, stuffed, 3 rolls, 6 oz	200	5	13

See Daphne's: *See Fast-Foods Section*

Hawaiian

	C	F	Cb
Ahi Tuna, grilled (6 oz fillet), no fat	220	2	0
Chicken Long Rice, 1 cup, 7 oz	240	14	12
Gyoza, 1 only	55	2	6
Haupia (Coconut Pudd.), 1 pce (4"x 2½")	120	6	17
Hawaiian Sweet Bread, ½" sl., 2 oz	180	4.5	29
Kalua Chicken, 4 oz	280	16	0
Pork, 4 oz	350	24	0
Kim Chee (pickled cabbage), ½ c., 4 oz	20	0	5
Kulolo (Taro Pudding), 4 oz	125	5	19
Lau Lau: Chicken (1) 7 oz	280	21	3
Pork (1) 7 oz	320	26	5
Loco Moco (rice/burger/egg/gravy)	650	27	63
Lomi Salmon, ¼ cup, 4 oz	20	1	2
Malasadas (Donut), 2 oz	240	13	26
Manapua (Char Siu Pork Bun), 2.3 oz	180	8	25
Poi (mashed ckd taro), 1 c., 8½ oz	270	0.5	65
Poke, avg all types, 3 oz	90	1	0
Portuguese Sausage, 2 oz	180	15	2
Potato Salad, ½ cup, 5 oz	170	10	17
Shave Ice *(Matsumoto)*, all flavors:			
w. Icecream, 1 large	300	4	64
w. Beans, 1 large	290	0	72
Spam Musubi: w. Regular Spam	265	11	34
(4 oz rice+1.3 oz Spam/7-Eleven Hawaii)			
Homemade: w. Lite Spam (50% less fat)	220	5	34
Taro Pancake Mix, ⅓ cup (makes 2)	140	2	26
Plate Lunches:			
Chicken Katsu (9 oz) w. 2 scp Rice	1110	48	108
+ Macaroni Salad, ¾ cup	1360	68	123
or Tossed Salad + Fr. Dress. (2 T.)	1240	61	111
Hamburger (5 oz) w. 2 scoops Rice	710	24	81
Gravy + Macaroni Salad	1135	49	112
MahiMahi (7 oz) w. 2 scoops Rice	650	12	90
+ Macaroni Salad + Tartar Sce	1150	58	108
or Macaroni Salad, no Tartar Sce	935	34	108
or Tossed Salad + Fr. Dress. (3 T.)	815	27	96
or Tossed Salad, no dressing	670	12	93
Teri Beef (5 oz) w. 2 scoops Rice	790	23	94
+ Macaroni Salad, ¾ cup	1095	47	113
or Tossed Salad, no dressing	800	23	95

Restaurant & International Foods

Indian & Pakistani

	C	F	Cb
Per Serving			
(Meat dishes allow 4 oz meat/serving)			
Aloo Samosa, each	155	12	12
Alu Gosht Kari (Meat/Pot. Curry)	600	40	23
Chicken Korma	500	35	6
Chicken Pilaf (Murgh Biriyani)	700	53	50
Chicken Tikka	260	16	2
Chicken Vindaloo	400	20	8
Chapati/Roti, 7" diam. piece	60	0.5	11
Dal (Lentil Puree): 1 cup, no oil	230	1	37
1 Tbsp Tadka (oil topping)	120	13	0
Dhakla (Lentil Dish), 1" sq., 1 oz	105	5	13
Dhansak, ½ cup	105	3.5	11
Gosht Kari (Meat Curry/Tom./Pot.)	460	25	17
Lamb Pilaf	520	35	40
Lassi (Sweet or Mango), 1 cup, 8 oz	160	4	24
Masala Gosht (Beef/Tom./Gravy)	400	25	18
Mulligatawney Soup, average	300	15	8
Murgh Makhani, 1 cup	300	4	7
Naan Bread, ¼ (8" x 2"), 1 oz	75	2	11
Pappadum, 1 large/2 small	50	3	5
Pesrattu (Lentil Crepe), 9", 2.6 oz	130	5	15
Pork Vindaloo Curry	620	47	3
Rajmah (Kidney Bean Curry), 1 cup	225	5	35
Rogan Josh (Lamb/Yogurt Sce)	500	30	3
Shahi Korma (Braised Lamb)	430	28	3
Tandoori Chicken: Breast	260	13	5
Leg/Thigh portion	300	17	6

Sal Monella Restaurant

"I wonder why business is so bad these days?"

Italian Dishes

	C	F	Cb
Baked Ziti: Small	370	27	32
Regular	575	42	49
Breadstick (1), 2 oz	120	2.5	25
Broccoli Fettucine Alfredo, reg.	815	23	125
Bruschetta, 2 slices	380	17	53
Calzones, average, all types	840	34	101
Cannelloni, 1 tube, 6 oz	280	15	18
Cheese Breadstick (1), 2.4 oz	180	8	20
Cheese Ravioli w. Sauce	495	17	65
Chicken Alfredo	775	29	82
Chicken Parmigiana, 11 oz	520	22	16
Fettucine Alfredo: Small	525	15	80
Regular	775	22	119
Meat Lasagne, 16 oz	700	36	60
Meat Ravioli	725	22	102
Minestrone Soup, 1 bowl	110	2	18
Shrimp & Scallop Fettucine	595	16	81
Spaghetti w. Marinara: Small	410	6	74
Regular	600	8	111
Spaghetti w. Meatballs: Small	710	31	80
Regular	1010	42	119
Spaghetti w. Meat Sauce: Small	425	8	74
Regular	625	11	111
Vegetable Primavera	610	8	116

Pizza: *Per Slice*

Thin Crust, *(⅛ Medium, 12"):*

	C	F	Cb
Cheese, Hawaiian	200	8	21
Pepperoni	210	10	21
Sausage	280	16	22
Veggie	180	7	23

Thick/Pan Crust, *(⅛ Large, 14"):*

	C	F	Cb
Cheese, Hawaiian	350	13	40
Pepperoni	380	16	40
Veggie	330	11	41

Personal Pan Pizza, *(6"):*

	C	F	Cb
Hawaiian	600	24	70
Pepperoni	640	29	67

Desserts: Lemon Ice | 180 | 0 | 45

	C	F	Cb
Gelato: Vanilla (Milk Base), ½ cup	200	15	18
Choc. Hazelnut (Milk), ½ cup	370	29	26
Water Base, ½ cup	100	0	25
Tiramisu, 1 piece, 5 oz	400	29	30

For more listings see Fast-Foods Section.

Restaurant & International Foods

Japanese

	C	F	Cb
Sushi Rice: cooked, 1 Tbsp	25	0	5
1 cup, 5¼ oz	380	3	82
Sushi (Maki) Rolls: *Per Piece*			
Average all types (California Rolls; Crm Cheese w. Crab; Eel; Salmon; Shrimp; Tuna; Yellowtail; Vegetable)			
Small (1⅛" diam. x 1⅛" high), 0.8 oz	25	0.5	3.5
Med. (1¾" diam. x 1¾" high), 1.6 oz	50	1	7
Large (2¼" diam. x ⅞" high), 2 oz	60	1.5	9
Sushi Packs: *Per Pack*			
Average all types: 6 large pces	370	5	55
9 medium pieces	360	6	60
12 small pieces	265	3	45
Futomaki (thick roll), 6 pieces	380	5	72
Hand Roll (Cone) 4 oz	120	2	18
Inari (rice filled soybean pocket), 4 pce	420	9	73
Sushi-Nigiri (fish on rice):			
average all types, 1 piece	70	0.5	12
Sushi Plate: Assorted, 6 pieces	420	3	36
Combination (Sushi & Sushi Rolls)			
2 Sushi + 6 sm. & 3 med. rolls	400	7	72
Sashimi (Sliced Raw Seafood/Beef)			
Ika (Squid), 4 oz	105	2	0
Hamachi (Yellowtail), 4 oz	165	6	0
Maguro (Yellowfin Tuna), 4 oz	120	1	0
Niku (Beef), 5 oz	200	10	0
Saba (Mackerel), 4 oz	160	7	0
Suzuki (Sea Bass), 4 oz	110	0.5	0
Tako (Octopus), 4 oz	95	1	0
Dipping Sauces: Average, 2 Tbsp	30	0	7
Ginger Vinegar Dressing, 2 Tbsp	20	0	5
Edamame (young green soybeans):			
Steamed/Salad (in pods), 4 oz	60	3	5
Boiled beans (no pods), 4 oz	160	7	12
Katsu-don Pork w. Rice	1100	39	141
Miso Soup w. Tofu pces, 1 cup	85	3	11
Seaweed Salad, 1.5 oz	20	2	0
Sukiyaki (Beef/Tofu/Veg.), 8 oz	400	24	32
Tempura (Batter-fried Shrimp & Veges)			
3 large shrimp & veges	320	18	25
1 shrimp only	60	4	3
Teppan Yaki (Steak, Seafood & Veges)			
10 oz serving	470	30	15
Teriyaki: Beef, 4 oz serving	350	25	4
Chicken, 4 oz serving	260	9	7
Salmon, medium, 6 oz serving	270	8	3
Sake Wine (16% alc.), 3 fl oz	115	0	7
Yakatori, 1 skewer, 2½ oz	140	5	1

Kosher/Deli Foods

	C	F	Cb
Bagel/Bialy, 1 small, 2 oz	160	2	32
Beiglach (Cheese Knish)	350	17	35
Blintzes: Average, 1	120	1	25
w. Sour Crm. & Preserves	370	10	30
Borscht: (no cream), 1 cup	85	3	14
Diet/Reduced Cal., 1 cup	30	1	7
Cabbage Roll (meat/rice), 5 oz	170	6	21
Chicken Broth: 1 cup	80	8	0
with vegetables	100	8	5
with noodles	150	9	16
Lowfat, plain, 1 cup	25	1	0
Cholent, 1 med serve, 1 cup	350	16	48
Chopped Liver: 1 serve, 3 oz	110	6	5
with Egg Salad, ¼ cup	100	7	3
Farfel, dry, ½ cup	90	0.5	21
Hallah (Yeast Bread), 1 sl., 1 oz	85	2	14
Gefilte Fish Balls: Reg., medium, 2 oz	55	2	4
with jelled broth	80	2	6
Cocktail size, 1 oz	30	1	2
Sweet, medium, 2 oz	65	2	4
with jelled broth	95	2	9
Herring: Smoked, 2 oz	120	8	0
in Sour Cream, 2 oz	150	10	0
Kasha, cooked, ½ cup	100	0.5	20
Kipfel (Vanilla/Almd. Cookie), 1 pce	60	2	7
Knaidlach ~ see Matzo Balls			
Knish: Kasha/Potato, 1 only	130	4	22
Cheese, 1 only	350	17	35
Kreplach, beef, 1 piece	40	1	6
Kugel, potato/noodle, 1 serve	300	20	25
Latkes (Potato Pancake), 2 oz	200	11	22
3 Latkes w. Sour Cr./Apple Sce	750	25	95
Lochshen: Plain, 1 cup	130	2	26
Pudding, 1 cup	380	13	48
Lox (Smoked Salmon), 2 oz	65	2	0
Mandelbrot (Almond Bread),			
1 slice, ¼" thick	45	2	5
Matzo (See Page 105), 1 oz board	110	0.5	21
Matzo Balls: 2 small, or 1 large, 2"	90	3	12
Extra large ball, 3"	180	6	24
Matzo Ball Soup:			
Cup w. 2 small or 1 large ball	150	5	27
Bowl with Chicken & Noodles	325	13	34
Jerry's Deli, large bowl	560	17	56
New York Cheesecake, 4 oz	350	24	26
Pierogi, potato/cheese, 1 pce	90	4	11
Reuben S'wich w. ½ lb corned beef	920	60	28
Schmaltz (Rend'd chick. fat), 1 T.	90	10	0

Restaurant & International Foods

Korean Food

	C	F	Cb
Bibimbab (Vege & Beef on Rice), 1 cup	565	15	89
Bulgogi (Barbeque Beef), 3.5 oz	325	12	15
Galbi (Short Ribs), 16 oz	975	61	16
Gujeolpan (Pancake w. Meat & Vegetables), cup w. 1 pancake	340	11	39
Japchae (Noodle w. Vege & Meat), 1¼ cup	365	19	34
Sides:			
Kimchee (Cabbage Relish), ½ cup	30	0	6
Namool (Assorted Veges) 1 cup	125	6.5	9
Soups: Per Serving			
Muguk (Radish & Chive Soup), 6 oz	105	7	6
Samgyetang (Ginseng Chicken Soup)			
no Chicken Skin, 1 cup	520	11	60
w. Chicken Skin, 1 cup	725	35	60
Yuk Gae Jang (Spicy Beef Soup), 1¼ cup	180	13	5

Lebanese/Middle East

	C	F	Cb
Baba Ghannouj, 2 Tbsp, 1 oz (Eggplant/Sesame Dip)	70	6	2
Baklava, 1 pastry, 13/4 oz (Pastry, Nuts, Syrup)	245	18	18
Cabbage Rolls, 1 roll, 3 oz (Cabbage Leaf, Meat, Rice)	100	3	12
Cous Cous, 1 serve (Semolina, Milk, Fruit, Nuts)	400	21	43
Felafel (Chick Pea Fritter):			
Fried, 1 medium, 1 oz	60	4	4
Hummus, ¼ cup, 2.2 oz	105	3	5
Fried Kibbi, 1 piece, 3 oz (Wheat, Meat, Pinenuts)	180	8	15
Kafta, 1 skewer, 1½ oz (Ground Lamb Saus. on Skewer)	85	5	2
Kibbeh Naye, 1 cup, 9 oz (Raw Lamb, Bulgur & Spices)	450	18	28
Lebanese Omelet, 1 serving, 4 oz (Egg, Spinach, Pinenuts, Onion)	200	12	13
Pilaf, 1 cup (Rice, Onion, Rais., Apr. Spice)	400	11	60
Shawourma, 1 serve, 4 oz (Spit Roast Beef)	280	15	2
Shish Kabob, 1 stick, 2½ oz	130	7	2
Spinach Pie, 1 piece, 3½ oz	290	21	20
Sweet Almond Sanbusak, 1 pce (Pastry, Almonds, Spices)	200	15	11
Tabouli, 1 serve, 4 oz	170	14	7
Tahini Sauce, avg., 1 Tbsp	90	8	2

Mexican

	C	F	Cb
Black Bean Soup, 1 bowl	200	3	34
Bueso Fresco, ¼ cup	80	4.5	8
Burritos (Taco Bell): Bean	370	10	55
Supreme® Beef	440	18	50
Chili, plain, ¼ cup	90	6	8
Chili con Carne: w. Beans, 1 cup	310	17	15
w/out Beans, 1 cup	370	28	10
Chimichangas, Beef, 5 oz	400	19	43
Chorizo Sausage, 2 oz	265	23	0
Churros, 1½ oz	150	8	18
Corn Chips, ½ cup, 1 oz	160	10	17
Costillas Ribs, 6 oz	675	52	0
Enchilada, average	330	10	49
Fajitas, Chicken (Soft)	200	7	20
Guacamole, avg., 2 Tbsp, 1 oz	45	4	2
Horchata: Don Jose, 1 cup, 8 fl. oz	140	4	25
Cacique, 1 pint bottle, 16 fl. oz	320	7	62
Margarita (w. 1½ oz Tequila)	160	0	6
Menudo, ½ cup	55	1.5	10
Nachos: Del Taco, Regular	395	24	40
Macho Nachos	1145	63	113
Taco Bell: BellGrande®	760	43	80
Supreme®	470	26	42
Nachos: with cheese, peppers, 1 portion (6-8 nachos), 7 oz	600	33	60
with cheese, beans, ground beef, peppers, 1 portion (6-8 nachos), 9 oz	570	31	56
Nopal Cactus Salad, 1 serving	130	9	11
Papas Fritas (Fried Potatoes) (1), 6 oz	325	18	40
Piloncillo (Brown Sugar): 1 Tbsp, 13g	50	0	13
Cone, small, 3", 3 oz	325	0	81
Quesadilla, Cheese (Taco Bell)	490	28	39
Refried Beans, ¾ cup, 6 oz	160	3	26
Rice Pudding (Arroz Con Leche), 4 oz	140	3	24
Sopes (Gorditas), 2 oz	120	0	27
Taco (Taco Bell): Regular, Crispy	170	10	13
Ranchero Chicken	270	15	21
Taco Supreme®	220	14	14
Double Decker® Taco	340	14	39
Taco Salad w. Salsa	840	52	85
Taco Sauce, average, ¼ cup	15	0	3
Taco Shell, regular	50	2	8
Tamales, Beef/Chicken, avg, 4.5 oz	250	11	27
Taquitos, Beef & Cheese, 4.5 oz	330	15	36
Tostada, 1 serve	250	10	29
Tortilla, Corn, 6" diam.	70	1	14
Tortilla Chips, 1 oz	150	8	18

Extra Listings of Mexican Dishes:
- **Fast-Foods Section** (Taco Bell, Del Taco)
- **Canned Bean/Chili Products:** See Pages 71-76

Mexican (Cont)

	C	F	Cb
Breads: Bolillos, 1 roll, 3½ oz	240	4	42
Telera, 2 oz	150	1.5	19
Mexican Cornbread, 4" square	210	11	19
French Baguette, 2 oz	140	1.5	26
Cakes, Cookies, Pastries			
Banderilla (Pastry Puff), 1 shell	140	10	8
Bigotes, 7"	570	22	44
Calvos, 2½ oz	320	18	38
Capirotada (Bread Pudding), 10 oz	810	38	107
Cinnamon Cookies, 2	125	8	13
Cocadas, 1 oz	120	6	15
Cortadilo, 1 cookie, 1.9 oz	300	11	48
Concha (All Colors):			
Small (3" diam), 2½ oz	250	8	38
Medium (4" diam), 3½ oz	350	11	53
Large (5" diam), 5½ oz	550	18	84
Cream Puff with Custard, 4¼ oz	255	14	25
Cuerno, 2 oz	200	4.5	34
Cuerno Fine, 2¾ oz	330	17	40
Donus (Donuts), 4", 3½ oz	440	21	58
Elotes, 3½ oz	450	24	51
Empanadas (Average all types):			
Small, 2 oz	230	10	28
Regular, 3 oz	300	14	42
Fiesta Cookie, 2¼ oz	280	8	47
Galletas Mixtas (1), 1 oz	100	2.5	16
Guayaba, 3¼ oz	360	14	53
Jelly Rolls, 3¼ oz	240	4	46
Mantecadites (Almond Shortbread), 4½ oz	670	42	64
Mini Pound Cake, 3 oz	260	12	33
Mini Cupcakes, 1¾ oz	180	8	25
Muffins/Nino Enbuelto, large, 6 oz	465	11	48
Novcias, 2¾ oz	290	9	46
Nuez, 3¼ oz	380	17	52
Ojo De Buey, 4 oz	360	15	55
Orejas Ears, 3 oz	310	15	38
Pan Dulce (Mexican Sweet Bread), 1 bun	330	10	45
Panquecitos, 2½ oz	260	11	36
Piedras, 4 oz	470	15	76
Polvorones, 3 oz	370	18	48
Puerquitos, 5 oz	600	24	88
Rebanadas, 3½ oz	390	18	51
Roles De Canela (Cin. Roll), 4½ oz	490	15	81
Roscas, 2¾ oz	360	18	44
Semitas, 3 oz	300	10	46
Sopapillas (flaky pastry puffs), 1 pce	100	7	10
w. Honey & Cream	200	14	18
Strawberry Crème Roll (⅙), 2½ oz	240	5	45

Extra Food Listings ~ See CalorieKing.com

Polish

	C	F	Cb
Cabbage Rolls w. Sour Cr., 2 sm.	220	10	30
Chicken Casserole w. Mush., 1 cup	520	27	5
Kielbasa (Sausages, Onions, fried), 2 large	350	28	2
Meatballs in Sour Cream, 3 x 1½" balls	300	16	11
Pierogi, Fruit/Veg, 3" ball	80	2	15
Pork Goulash (Pork/Veg. Stew)	550	21	38
Pot Roast with Vegetables	630	21	28

Soul Foods

	C	F	Cb
Breakfast Sausage, fried, 2 patties	250	17	0
Brunswick Stew, 1 cup, 8.5 oz	320	14	19
Cornbread, home-made, 3 oz	200	7.5	28
Fatback, raw, ¼ oz	60	6.5	0
Ham Hock	90	6.5	2
Hog Maw	45	2.5	0
Hominy, cooked, ¾ cup	110	0.5	25
Hush Puppies, 5 pieces	260	12	35
Kale, cooked, ½ cup	20	0.5	4
Opossum	65	3	0
Oxtail	70	3.5	0
Pig Ear, ¼ ear	50	3	0
Pig Foot, ½ foot	70	4.5	0
Pig Tail, ⅓ tail	115	10	0
Poke Salad, cooked, ½ cup	16	0.5	3
Pork Brains	40	2.5	0
Pork Chitterlings, simmered, 3 oz	260	25	0
Pork Cracklings, ½ oz	80	6	0
Pork Neck Bones	65	4	0
Pork Skin, 1 cup	70	4.5	0
Pork Tongue, ⅓ tongue	75	5.5	0
Sousemeat	60	4.5	0
Succotash, ½ cup	80	1	17
Sweet Potato Pie, ⅛ of 9" pie	250	12	34
Tripe, 2 oz	55	2	0
Vienna Sausage, 2 small	90	8	1
small	45	4	0.5

Brooklyn

Restaurant & International Foods

Spanish

	C	F	Cb
Arroz Abanda (Fish with Rice)	340	8	31
Arroz Con Pollo (Rice/Chick. Sal)	500	23	50
Clams Marinara, 8 clams	330	16	22
Cochifrito (Lamb w. Lemon/Garlic)	650	25	5
Cochinillo Asado, 2 sl. (Rst Suckling Pig)	300	15	3
Cocido Madrileno (Madrid-Style Boiled Dinner)	450	27	18
Flan de Leche (Caramel Custard)	325	9	52
Fritadera de Ternera (Sauteed Veal)	450	27	2
Gazpacho, 1 bowl	60	0	15
Paella a la Valenciana (Chicken & Shellfish Rice)	900	42	70
Pollo a la Espanola (Chicken)	475	30	4
Ternera al Jerez (Veal w. Sherry)	660	29	6
Zarzuela (Fish & Shellfish Medley)	530	27	40

Thai Foods

	C	F	Cb
Appetizers: Satay Pork, 1 oz	100	4	2
Spring Roll, 1¼ oz	110	6	13
Soups: Tom Yam (Hot & Sour):			
Spicy Shrimp/Seafood, 1 cup	100	4	6
1 bowl	160	7	10
Vegetarian, 1 cup	50	0	11
Curries: Chicken w. Ginger, 1 cup	390	34	4
Thick Red Curry w. Beef, 1 cup	600	50	7
Thai Chicken Curry, 1 cup	340	23	4
Massaman Curry, 1 cup	680	57	8
Green Curry w. Pork, 1 cup	480	44	5
Pad Thai, Large serving, 18 oz	990	38	125
Fish: Steamed w. Spicy Thai Sce	450	8	46
Crispy Fried, 5 oz	290	15	9
Spicy Chicken (w. veges), stir-fry	450	22	14
Spicy Garlic Tofu w. veges, stir-fry	340	14	14
Sticky Thai Rice: Plain 1 cup, 6 oz	170	0.5	36
w. Coconut & Sesame Seeds, 1 cup	880	28	120
Stir-fried Rice Noodles, 1 c., 5½ oz	270	9	40
Stir-fried Vegetables, 1 cup	100	3	18
Salads: Green Papaya Salad	160	0	40
Spicy Prawn, 9 shrimp	170	3	15
Thai Chicken, 1 serving	330	9	17
Thai Beef Salad, 1 serving	260	9	15
Thai Noodle, 1 serving	410	13	45
Satay Chicken & Peanut Sauce:			
1 satay stick	390	24	20
Sauces: Peanut Satay, ½ cup, 4 oz	160	10	13

Vietnamese

	C	F	Cb
Banh Cuon (Steam Rice w. Pork), 1 roll	105	7	8
Bo Nuong (Beef Satay), 2 sticks	265	9	4
Bo Xao Dau Phong (Ginger Beef w.Onion, Fish Sce.)	750	30	10
Ca Chien Gung (Whole Snapper/Ging.)	600	16	6
Canh Chay (Veg./Tofu Soup)	80	3	13
Cari (Curry) Chicken, 1 cup	475	29	16
Cari (Curry) Chicken, w. Rice Noodle, cup curry & cup cooked noodles	660	29	60
Cari (Curry) Chicken, w. Steam Rice, cup curry & cup rice	650	29	55
Cuu Xao Lan (Curried Lamb, Veges in Coconut)	900	40	80
Ga Chien (Crisp Chick + Plum Sce)	900	40	105
Ga Nuong (Chicken Satay + Sce)	240	10	4
Ga Xao Rau (Marinated Chicken Braised w. Veg.)	800	26	100
Gio Lua (Lean Pork Pie), ⅛ of pie	245	12	0
Goi Cuon (Cold Spring Rolls), each	60	1	7
Rau Cai Xao Chay (Stir Fried Vege.)	400	15	65
Thit Bo Vien (Beef Balls), 6 balls	225	14	2
Thit Heo Goi Baup Cai, each (Spicy Cabbage Rolls w. Pork)	200	7	11
Soup: Per Bowl (1½ Cup)			
Bun Bo Hue (Hot & Spicy Soup)			
no Pork Feet	340	9	35
w. Pork Feet	830	45	35
Chicken & Rice Noodle Soup	400	3	35
Pho Bo (Beef Noodle Soup)	410	7	59
Pho Ga (Chicken Noodle Soup)	460	6	58
Pho Tai (Rare Beef & Noodle Soup)	440	7	73
Salad: Per ½ Cup			
Goi Du Du (Green Papaya Salad)	155	3	29
Sauce: Nuoc Cham (Fish Sauce)	5	0	1

Gourmet & Miscellaneous

	C	F	Cb
Ants Eggs/Larvae, 1 Tbsp	20	0	0
Ants, Choc. coated, 3 Tbsp	140	7	2
Bee Maggots, canned, 3 Tbsp	65	2	0
Caviar, black/red, 1 Tbsp	40	3	0
Caterpillars, canned, 2 oz	60	2	0
Frogs Legs, fried, 1 pair (large)	125	7	0
Haggis, boiled, 4 oz	350	24	22
Locusts, roasted, 1 oz	35	1	0
Silkworms, raw, 1 oz	60	2	0
Snails in garlic butter, 6 large	200	10	4
Snake, roasted, 4 oz	160	6	0

Fast-Food Chains & *Restaurants*

~ EXTRA RESTAURANTS ~ www.CalorieKing.com ~

A&W® (Aug '07)

Sandwiches & Burgers	C	F	Cb
Papa Burger	720	42	46
Double Cheeseburger	720	42	46
Bacon Cheeseburger	570	33	41
Double Bacon Cheeseburger	800	49	47
Crispy Chicken Sandwich	590	29	54
Grilled Chicken Sandwich	440	19	34
Kids Hamburger	430	22	35
Kids Cheeseburger	460	24	39

Chicken

	C	F	Cb
Chicken Strips, 3 pces	500	29	32
Hot Dogs: Plain, 3.2 oz	280	17	22
Cheese Dog, 4.4 oz	320	20	25
Coney (Chili), 4.4 oz	310	18	24
Coney (Chili) Chse Dog, 5.4 oz	350	21	27

Fries & Sides: Per Serving

	C	F	Cb
Fries: French, Regular, 4 oz	310	12	45
French, Large, 5.5 oz	430	16	62
Cheese Fries w. sauce, 6 oz	420	20	53
Chili Fries, 6 oz	400	16	51
Chili Cheese Fries, 7 oz	410	17	52
Dipping Sauces: Barbeque, 1 oz	40	0	10
Honey Mustard	100	6	12
Sweet and Sour	45	0	12
Onion Rings, 4 oz	350	20	45

Desserts

	C	F	Cb
Hot Caramel Sundae	340	9	57
Hot Fudge Sundae	350	11	54
Other Sundaes, avg.	310	8	52
Polar Swirl™: M&M; Oreo, small	720	25	107
Reese's, small	750	31	97
Soft Ice Cream Cone, regular, avg.	250	7	41

Milkshakes & Floats: Per 16 fl.oz

	C	F	Cb
Chocolate Milkshake	700	29	100
Strawberry Milkshake	670	29	90
Vanilla Milkshake	720	31	97
A&W Root Beer Float	330	4.5	70

Drinks: Per 20 fl.oz

	C	F	Cb
A&W Root Beer	270	0	72
Diet A&W Root Beer; Diet Coke	0	0	0
Coca-Cola	290	0	75
Sprite	290	0	72

Applebee's® (Aug '07)

Appetizers: Onion au Gratin Soup	C	F	Cb
Appetizers: Onion au Gratin Soup	150	8	12
Tortilla Chicken Melt	480	13	50
Veggie Patch Pizza (10") ⅛ pizza	150	9	12
Entree Meals: Includes Sides/Sauces			
Applebee's Riblets	2025	130	106
Crispy Buttermilk Shrimp	845	34	83
Crispy Orange Chicken Skillet	1710	69	209
Fiesta Lime Chicken	1285	47	136
Grilled Tilapia, w. Rice Pilaf & Mango	320	6	30
Madeira Steak Tips	910	38	82
Teriyaki Steak & Shrimp Skewers	370	7	33
Burger & Sandwiches: No Sides			
Angus Bacon Cheeseburger	940	53	58
Cowboy Burger	1150	62	89
Clubhouse Grill Sandwich	870	39	55
Tango Chicken Sandwich	460	17	44
Roll-Ups: Chicken Fajita, w. Dress.	1130	66	58
Oriental Chicken	710	25	72
Salads			
Pecan Crusted Chicken	1180	65	63
Half serving , no dressing	675	36	44
Shrimp & Spinach	570	41	14
Half serving, no dressing	220	11	10
Sizzling Fajitas: Includes 4 Tortillas			
Average all types	1900	76	174
Tortilla (8"), each, 1.6 oz	145	3	25
Teriyaki Bowls: Steak	1610	45	230
Combo Teriyaki	1440	29	224
Weight Watchers: Complete Dish			
Confetti Chicken	370	7	34
Grilled Shrimp Skewer Salad	210	2	22
Grilled Tilapia w. Mango Salsa	320	6	27
Mesquite Chicken Salad	350	4	42
Onion Soup au Gratin	150	8	10
Sizzling Chicken Skillet	360	4	43
Southwest Cobb Salad	440	8	59
Teriyaki Steak & Shrimp Skewers	370	7	33
Tango Chicken Salad	370	9	38
Tortilla Chicken Melt	480	13	50
Desserts: Per Serving			
Blue Ribbon Brownie			
w. 2 scoops Ice Cream	735	30	105
Chocolate Raspberry Layer	230	3	46
Cheesecake, Berry Lemon	230	7	34
Sizzling Apple Pie w. Ice Cream	1085	56	146
Triple Chocolate Meltdown Cake	725	31	107

*Most figures above are author calculations and not
intended for clinical use.*
For Extra Listings ~ see CalorieKing.com

Updated Nutrition Data ~ www.CalorieKing.com
Persons with Diabetes ~ See Disclaimer (Page 24)

Arby's® (Aug '07)

Breakfast: *Per Serving*

	C	F	Cb
Blueberry Muffin, 3 oz	320	12	49
Biscuit: Plain	275	15	28
Bacon, Egg & Cheese	460	28	30
Chicken	415	23	39
Sausage, Egg & Cheese	555	38	30
Croissant: Bacon & Egg	335	22	23
Ham & Cheese	275	12	22
Sausage & Egg	435	32	23
French Toastix, no Syrup, 4.3 oz	310	13	44
Sourdough S'wich. Egg & Cheese	390	12	40
Bacon, Egg & Cheese	435	16	40
Sausage, Egg & Cheese	515	27	40
Wraps: Bacon, Egg & Cheese	515	29	50
Sausage, Egg & Cheese	690	45	50

Market Fresh Salads

	C	F	Cb
Chicken Club Salad: No Dressing	485	25	31
w. Buttermilk Dressing	810	59	34
Martha's Vineyard, no Dress./Almd.	275	8	24
w. Raspb. Vinaigrette, Almonds	470	22	42
Santa Fe: no Dressing, Tortilla Strips	475	21	42
w. Dressing, Tortilla Strips	845	55	54
w. Grilled Chicken, no dressing	285	9	21

Sandwiches

	C	F	Cb
Arby's Melt	300	12	36
BBQ Bacon 'n Jack 2/For	360	16	42
Beef 'n Cheddar	445	21	44
Chicken Naturals:			
Chicken Bacon & Swiss, Crispy	625	29	52
Chicken Bacon & Swiss, Grilled	460	17	38
Chicken Fillet, Crispy	575	30	50
Chicken Fillet, Grilled	415	17	36
Cordon Bleu, Crispy	650	31	49
Cordon Bleu, Grilled	490	19	35
Southwest Chipotle, Crispy	680	37	51
Southwest Chipotle, Grilled	515	25	37
Fish Sandwich	545	25	61
French Dip & Swiss	475	18	38
Roast Beef, Regular	320	14	34
Roast Beef, Super	400	19	40
Sourdough Roast Beef Melt	355	14	40
Subs: French Dip w. Au Jus	450	12	48
Hot Ham & Swiss	500	18	45
Italian	620	33	48
Philly Beef & Swiss	670	35	46
Roast Beef	725	42	46
Turkey Sub	635	30	47

Arby's® cont... (Aug '07)

Market Fresh Sandwiches

	C	F	Cb
Chicken Salad w. Pecans	770	39	79
Roast Beef & Swiss	775	41	73
Roast Ham & Swiss	705	31	75
Roast Beef Gyro	540	29	49
Roast Turkey & Swiss	725	30	75
Roast Turkey Ranch & Bacon	835	38	75
Ultimate BLT	780	45	75
Wraps: Rst Turkey Ranch & Bacon	700	37	44
Ultimate BLT	650	44	45

Sauces & Condiments

	C	F	Cb
Dipping Sauce: BBQ, 1 oz	45	0	11
Bronco Berry, 2 oz	120	0	30
Buffalo Sauce, 2 oz	20	1	3
Cool Ranch Sour Cream, 1½ oz	160	16	2
Sauce: Arby's, ½ oz	15	0	4
Cheddar Cheese, ¾ oz	30	2	2
Chipotle Mayo, ½ oz	90	9	0
Horsey Sauce, ½ oz	60	5	3
Italian Sub, 1 oz	125	12	3
Monterey Jack Cheese, ¾ oz	25	2.5	0
Smoky Q, ½ oz	25	0	5
Sour Cream, 2 oz	120	12	2
Spicy Three Pepper, ½ oz	20	1	3
Swiss Cheese, serving, ¾ oz	30	2	1
Tangy Southwest, 2 oz	335	34	5
Dressing: Raspb. Vinaigrette, 2.2 oz	195	14	18
Buttermilk Ranch, 2.2 oz	325	34	4
Light Buttermilk Ranch, 2.2 oz	110	6	13
Santa Fe Ranch, 2.2 oz	295	31	4

Sides: Potato Cakes, 2 cakes

	C	F	Cb
Sides: Potato Cakes, 2 cakes	245	18	26
Baked Potato: Plain	270	0	63
w. Broccoli & Cheese	535	22	73
w. Butter & Sour Cream	495	24	65
w. Sour Cream	395	12	65
Deluxe	645	32	67
Fries: Curly, small, 3.7 oz	340	20	39
Homestyle, small, 4 oz	300	20	44
Chicken Tenders, 3 pieces	380	18	28
Jalapeno Bites, no Sauce, 5 bites	305	21	29
Loaded Potato Bites, no Sce, 5 bites	355	22	27
Mozzarella Sticks, no Sce, 4 sticks	425	28	38
Onion Petals, no Sauce, reg., 4 oz	330	23	35
Shakes: Vanilla, 14 fl.oz	440	13	65
Other flavors, regular, 14 fl.oz	515	13	85

Desserts

	C	F	Cb
Apple Turnover w. Icing	375	16	65
Cherry Turnover w. Icing	375	15	65

For Complete Nutritional Data ~ see CalorieKing.com

Fast - Foods & *Restaurants*

Arthur Treachers® (Aug '07)

	C	F	Cb
Meals: Per Serving			
Fish N Chips	1540	101	132
Fish Sandwich,	480	23	40
Seafood Sampler	3380	270	226
Shrimp N Chips	2050	123	225
Sides			
Cole Slaw, 5 oz	215	8.5	34
Hush Puppy (2)	275	10	42

Atlanta Bread Company®
(Aug '07)

	C	F	Cb
Bagels: Per Bagel			
Asiago Cheese	380	10	53
Cinnamon Crisp	330	2.5	68
Everything	320	3.5	60
Low-Carb Cranberry Walnut	110	3.5	16
Poppy Seed	320	5	57
Sesame	360	9	57
Other varieties, average	270	1.5	54
Sandwiches: No Cheese or Dressing			
ABC Special on French Roll	420	4.5	61
Grilled Cheese on French Bread	390	11	57
Honey Maple Ham	410	5	63
Peanut Butter & Jelly	600	14	99
Roasted Turkey Breast	430	7	61
Tangy Roast Beef	390	4	56
Veggie on Nine Grain	340	5	63
Focaccia:			
Bella Basil on Tom. & Rosemary	660	35	58
California Avocado on Tom. On.	690	40	71
Paninis: Chicken Pesto	800	35	83
Cordon Bleu	660	18	82
Cuban Pork Loin	660	19	81
Italian Vegetarian	640	16	93
Turkey Club	750	27	83
Salads: Caesar	190	10	11
Chicken Salad on Lettuce, no dr.	280	21	2
Chopstix Chicken	280	13	24
Fruit Salad, 10 oz	130	0	34
Greek Salad	200	13	13
House Salad, no dressing	50	0	11
Tuna Salad on Lettuce	360	32	4
Add Grilled Chicken, 2.5 oz	70	1.5	2
Extra Croutons, 0.5 oz	50	2	6

Atlanta Bread ® cont... (Aug '07)

	C	F	Cb
Soups: Per Serving (10 oz)			
Black Bean & Ham	250	9	40
Chicken Tortilla	190	9	20
Chunky Baked Potato	290	16	30
Classic Chicken Noodle	140	2.5	21
Cream of Broccoli	200	11	19
Creamy Tomato	130	9	10
French Onion w. Toppings	200	10	16
Garden Vegetable	100	1.5	19
Homestyle Chicken 'n Dumpling	290	18	25
New England Clam Chowder	280	16	24
Pasta Fagioli	170	6	24
Spicy Chicken Gumbo	120	2.5	16
Wisconsin Cheese	240	14	21
Breads: Per Thick Slice (2 oz)			
ABC Roll, 1 roll	260	1	54
Asiago	160	2	29
Challah	160	2.5	29
Cinnamon Raisin Loaf	150	2	28
Focaccia, round, ⅛ loaf	180	5	26
Pumpernickel	140	1.5	26
Rye; Nine Grain, avg.	155	2	28
Sourdough	140	0	29
Muffin Tops: Banana Nut	420	26	39
Blueberry	250	12	31
Chocolate Chip, 3 oz	400	19	52
Mocha	410	20	53
Pumpkin	350	13	54

For Complete Nutritional Data ~ see CalorieKing.com

Au Bon Pain® (Aug '07)

Bagels: Per Bagel	C	F	Cb
Asiago Cheese	360	8	57
Cinnamon Raisin	290	1	62
Dutch Apple	450	3.5	93
French Toast	400	7	72
Plain	280	1	57
Spreads: Plain Cream Chse, 2 oz	120	11	4
Honey Walnut	140	9	12
Veggie, 2 oz	140	12	3
Breakfast Sandwiches: Per Sandwich			
Egg on a Bagel	400	4	63
w. Bacon	480	12	63
w. Bacon & Cheese	560	18	63
w. Cheese	480	11	63
Sandwiches			
Asian Chicken Salad	430	16	50
BBQ Pulled Pork	610	18	83
Chicken & Mozzarella	680	30	58
Chicken Tarragon w. Romaine	630	29	57
Mozzarella, Tomato w. Pesto	820	43	67
Grilled Chicken w. Blue Cheese	670	29	64
Spicy Tuna on Multigrain	690	33	72
Steak w. Swiss Cheese	690	28	68
Tuna w. Cheddar & Peppers	555	18	62
Turkey w. Guacamole & Swiss	760	28	77
Wraps: Chicken Caesar	590	22	67
Fields & Feta	560	17	79
Mediterranean Wrap	570	22	80
Southwest Tuna	540	25	68
Soups: Per Medium (12 oz)			
Broccoli Cheese	315	21	22
Chicken Noodle	140	3	21
Corn Chowder	345	19	41
Garden Vegetable	75	1.5	13
Split Pea w. Ham	210	1.5	42
Vegetarian Chili	260	3	45
Breads: Average, 1.75 oz slice	130	1	27
Artisan Multigrain Bread, 1 slice	170	2	31
Bread Bowl (1)	640	3	127
Foccacia (1)	310	3.5	58
Rosemary Garlic Breadstick	200	5	33
Bread Rolls, Soft (1)	400	11	65

Au Bon Pain® cont... (Aug '07)

Yogurt & Fruit Cups: Per Serving	C	F	Cb
Yogurt & Fruit, average, 15 oz	380	4.5	75
Fruit Cup: Small, 6 oz	70	0	16
Large, 12 oz	140	0	32
Salads: Per Container			
Caesar Salad, 6 oz	210	11	16
Chef's Salad, 8⅓ oz	270	15	8
Garden Salad, Small, 4 oz	50	1	10
Gorgonzola & Walnut, 6 oz	310	27	9
Mediterranean Chicken, 15 oz	350	16	16
Thai Chicken, 11 oz	190	5	21
Tuna Garden, 11 oz	350	25	14
Turkey Medallion Cobb, 11 oz	350	20	15
Steak w. Cranb., Oranges, 11.5 oz	290	7	46
Cookies: Per Cookie			
Chocolate Chip	260	11	37
English Toffee	210	11	26
Oatmeal Raisin	230	8	37
Shortbread	310	18	34
Desserts: Apple Strudel	410	23	49
Blonde w. Nuts Brownie	570	36	57
Cherry Strudel	340	20	34
Choc Chip Brownie	420	18	63
Pecan Roll	520	28	61
Croissants: Ham & Cheese	350	18	34
Spinach & Cheese	250	14	28
Filled: Plain	260	15	28
Almond	570	38	50
Apple	230	10	31
Chocolate	330	17	42
Raspberry Cheese	330	16	41
Sweet Cheese	340	19	37
Muffins: Blueberry	510	19	76
Chocolate Chunk	590	20	83
Corn	460	16	69
Cranberry Walnut	500	24	61
Raisin Bran	410	9	74
Low-Fat: Chocolate Cake	320	2	74
Triple Berry	290	2	61
Drinks			
Hot Mocha Blast, 16 fl.oz	350	10	56
Frozen Mocha Blast, 16 fl.oz	355	10	71
Iced Cappuccino, 16 fl.oz	220	8	22
Iced Tea, 22 fl.oz	120	0	30

For Complete Nutritional Data ~ see CalorieKing.com

Fast - Foods & Restaurants

Auntie Anne's® (Aug '07)

Pretzels: With Butter	C	F	Cb
Almond	400	8	72
Cinnamon Sugar	450	9	83
Garlic	350	4.5	68
Glazin' Raisin	510	4	107
Jalapeno	310	4.5	59
Original	370	4	72
Sesame	410	12	64
Sour Cream & Onion	340	5	66
Stix, 4 sticks	245	3	48
Whole Wheat	370	4.5	72

Pretzels: Without Butter			
Almond Pretzel; Whole Wheat	350	1.5	72
Cinnamon Sugar	350	2	74
Garlic Pretzel; Sour Crm & Onion	320	1	66
Glazin' Raisin	470	0.5	104
Jalapeno	270	1	58
Original	340	1	72
Sesame	350	6	63
Stix, 4 sticks	225	1	48

Dipping Sauces			
Caramel Dip, 1.5 oz	135	3	27
Cheese Sce; Hot Salsa Chse, avg.	100	8	4
Chocolate Flavored Dip, 1¼ oz	130	4	24
Light Cream Cheese, 1¼ oz	70	6	1
Marinara Sauce, 1¼ oz	10	0	4
Sweet Dip, 1¼ oz	40	0	10
Sweet Mustard, 1¼ oz	60	1.5	8

Beverages: Per Serving			
Auntie Anne's Lemonade, 22 fl.oz	180	0	43
Dutch Ice (20 fl.oz): Kiwi-Banana	270	0	63
Blue Raspberry	230	0	55
Lemonade	450	0	110
Mocha	570	15	105
Orange Crème	400	0	92
Pina Colada; Strawberry	535	0	125
Wild Cherry	300	0	69
Dutch Smoothie: Per 20 fl.oz			
Blue Raspberry	400	14	61
Kiwi-Banana	430	14	68
Lemonade	540	14	95
Mocha	590	23	90
Orange Crème	500	14	83
Pina Colada	470	14	79
Strawberry; Wild Cherry, avg.	450	14	74

Backyard Burgers® (Aug '07)

Burgers	C	F	Cb
Back Yard Burger ⅓ lb.	470	29	38
Cheeseburger ⅓ lb	520	34	38
Bacon Cheddar	620	42	38
Barbecue Bacon	630	39	47
Black Jack	580	39	36
Chili Cheese	560	36	41
Garden Veggie Sandwich	240	6	47
Jr Burger	310	17	38
Hawaiian	550	33	44
Miz Grazi	530	34	39
Mushroom Swiss	540	36	37
Low-Carb Burger	350	27	3

Chicken Sandwiches			
Bacon Swiss	390	20	37
Barbecue	280	8	44
Blackened	290	11	39
Buffalo Ranch	540	30	51
Hawaiian Chicken	280	8	45
Honey Mustard	320	11	46
Lemon Butter Chicken	260	9	37
Savory Chicken	230	6	36
Specialities: BLT	270	16	36
Chicken Tenderloins, 3 piece	400	28	22
Chili Dog	340	20	29
Chili Cheese Dog	400	25	29
Hot Dog	310	18	27

Baked Potatoes			
Chili & Cheddar, 9 oz	330	11	48
Ranch, 7.7 oz	410	22	45
Salsa, 7.7 oz	250	5	47
Traditional/Plain, 6 oz	190	0	43

Fries			
Chili Cheese Fries, 6.7 oz	350	22	28
Seasoned Fries, regular, 3 oz	260	16	26
Waffle Fries, regular, 3 oz	240	16	23

Salads (No Dressing)			
Blackened Chicken	160	4	11
Charbroiled Chicken	140	3	11
Garden Fresh	25	0	5

Cobblers: Apple, 6 oz	430	20	61
Blackberry; Peach, 6 oz	420	20	60
Cherry, 6 oz	460	20	68

Shakes: Per 12 fl.oz			
Chocolate; Strawberry	560	26	79
Vanilla	540	26	71

For Complete Nutritional Data ~ see CalorieKing.com

Restaurants & Fast - Foods

Baja Fresh® (Aug '07)

	C	F	Cb
Burritos: No Tortilla Chips			
Baja Burrito: w. Chicken	790	38	65
w. Steak	850	46	67
Bare Burrito: w. Charbroiled Chkn	640	7	97
Vege and Cheese	580	10	101
Bean & Cheese Burrito: w. Chkn	970	35	96
w. Steak	1030	43	97
Vegetarian	840	33	96
Burrito Dos Manos: w. Chicken	760	26	94
w. Steak	795	30	95
Burrito Mexicano: w. Chicken	790	13	117
w. Steak	860	21	118
Burrito Ultimo: w. Chicken	860	36	84
w. Steak	950	44	85
Grilled Vegetarian	800	33	94
Fajitas			
Chicken w. Corn Tortillas	860	24	105
Chicken w. Flour Tortillas	1140	33	147
Nachos: w. Charbroiled Steak	2120	118	163
w. Cheese	1890	108	163
w. Chicken	2020	110	164
Quesadilla: w. Charbroiled Chkn	1330	80	84
w. Charbroiled Steak	1430	87	84
w. Cheese	1200	78	84
Vegetarian	1260	78	96
Tacos: No Tortilla Chips			
Baja Fish Taco	250	13	27
Grilled Mahi Mahi Taco	230	9	26
Baja Style Taco w. Chicken	210	5	28
w. Steak	230	8	28
w. Gulf Shrimp	200	5	28
Salads: No Dressing or Tortilla Chips			
Baja Ensalada			
w. Charbroiled Chicken	310	7	18
w. Charbroiled Shrimp	230	6	18
w. Charbroiled Steak	450	18	18
Chipotle Glaze Charbroiled Chicken	590	22	54
Tostadas: Charbroiled Chicken	1140	55	98
Charbroiled Fish	1130	55	99
Charbroiled Shrimp	1120	55	99
Charbroiled Steak	1230	63	98
Savory Pork Carnitas	1180	62	100

For Complete Nutritional Data ~ see CalorieKing.com

Baskin Robbins® (Aug '07)

	C	F	Cb
Hard Scooped Ice Cream			
Classic: Per Regular Scoop			
Chocolate	260	14	33
Chocolate Chip	270	16	28
Chocolate Chip Cookie Dough	290	15	36
Chocolate Fudge	270	15	35
French Vanilla	280	18	26
German Choc Cake	300	16	36
Gold Medal Ribbon	260	13	34
Jamoca	240	13	26
Jamoca Almond Fudge	270	15	31
Mint Choc Chip	270	16	28
Old Fashion Butter Pecan	280	18	24
Oreo Cookies 'N Cream	280	15	32
Peanut Butter 'N Chocolate	320	20	31
Pistachio Almond	290	19	25
Pralines 'N Cream	270	14	34
Reeses Peanut Butter	300	18	31
Rocky Road	290	15	36
Vanilla	260	16	26
Very Berry Strawberry	220	11	28
World Class Chocolate	270	15	33
Chocolate Roll Cake: Per Slice (4.1 oz)			
Average all flavors	290	14	36
Low-Fat Ice Cream: Espresso 'N Crm	180	4	32
No Sugar Added Ice Cream, avg.	160	2	27
Ices, Sherbets, Sorbets: Regular Scoop			
Ices, Daiquiri; Margarita	135	0	34
Sherbets, average all flavors	160	2	34
Sorbets, average all flavors	115	0	29
Signature Sundaes			
Chocolate Bliss, 10 oz	880	42	121
Peanut Butter Pie, 8 oz	850	59	68
Tiramisu, 9.6 oz	790	39	101
Low-Fat Yogurt (Hard): Regular Scoop			
Average all flavors	200	4	38
Non-Fat Yogurt (Soft Serve): Per ½ Cup			
Vanilla, 4 oz	220	0	46
Other flavors, 3 oz	180	0	34
Shakes, Smoothies, Blasts: Regular (16 fl.oz.)			
Shakes: Chocolate Ice Cream	620	30	81
Vanilla Ice Cream	690	33	85
Smoothies: Average all flavors	365	1	82
Blasts: Cappuccino w/whip cream	450	12	81
Cones: Sugar Cone	60	3	7
Cake Cone	25	0.5	4
Waffle Cone: Large	120	1.5	14
Fresh Baked	145	2	3

For Complete Nutritional Data ~ see CalorieKing.com

Ben & Jerry's®

C **F** **Cb**

Ice Cream & Frozen Yogurt ~ See Page 32
Novelty Bars ~ See Page 36

Big Apple Bagels® (Aug '07)

	C	F	Cb
***Bagels:** All types, avg., 5 oz*	**340**	**2**	68
½ bagel, 2.5 oz	**170**	**1**	34
***My Favorite Muffin:** Per Jumbo (5.8 oz)*			
Regular: Blueberry	**504**	**24**	66
Chocolate Chip	**633**	**33**	81
Cinnamon Swirl Cheesecake	**642**	**33**	84
Pumpkin Spice	**543**	**24**	78
Fat Free: Blueberry	**324**	**0**	78
Chocolate Marble	**375**	**0**	87
Cinnamon Bun	**504**	**0**	126
***Choice Bagels:** Per Bagel*			
Blueberry Cobbler	**392**	**8**	70
Cheddar Nacho	**352**	**6**	60
Cinnamon Apple Pie	**386**	**8**	68
Cinnamon Bun	**400**	**8**	70
Cinnamon Danish	**396**	**8**	72
French Toast	**372**	**4**	74
Quiche Lorraine	**354**	**8**	54
Strawberry White Chocolate	**364**	**4**	72
Swiss Melt	**368**	**8**	58
White Chocolate Swirl	**396**	**8**	70
***Cream Cheese:** Per 2 Tbsp (1 oz)*			
Plain	**90**	**9**	2
Plain Lite	**60**	**4.5**	1
Whipped: Classic Plain	**70**	**7**	1
Brown Sugar Cinnamon	**70**	**5**	5
Reduced-Fat Spring Veggie	**60**	**5**	2
Other varieties, avg	**90**	**8**	2
***Soups:** Per Cup (8 oz)*			
Boston Clam/Potato Chowder	**210**	**13**	20
Chicken Noodle; Beef Pot Roast	**110**	**4**	12
Garden Vegetable	**110**	**1**	22
Minestrone	**150**	**3**	26
Split Pea w. Ham; Hearty Vege	**95**	**2**	16

For Complete Nutritional Data ~ see CalorieKing.com

Big Boy

~ Same Menu and Data as Frish's Big Boy
Page 209

Blimpie® (Aug '07)

C **F** **Cb**

***Cold Deli Subs:** Per 6" Sub on White (w. Cheese)*			
Blimpie Best	**475**	**16**	52
Club	**440**	**12**	50
Ham & Swiss Cheese	**435**	**13**	52
Roast Beef	**450**	**13**	49
Seafood, no cheese	**350**	**8**	58
Tuna	**495**	**23**	51
Turkey	**420**	**11**	49
***Paninis:** Cuban*	**460**	**12**	50
Grilled Chicken Caesar	**560**	**26**	50
Turkey Italiano	**390**	**10**	44
***Wraps:** Chicken Caesar*	**650**	**35**	56
Zesty Italian	**680**	**33**	74
***Hot Deli Subs:** Per 6" Sub on White*			
Grilled Chicken	**375**	**9**	50
Meatball w. Cheese	**570**	**27**	55
Mexi Max	**430**	**9**	65
Steak & Onion Melt w. Cheese	**440**	**16**	49
VegiMax	**395**	**7**	60
***Salads:** Chef Salad*	**210**	**9**	9
Macaroni Salad, ⅓ container	**360**	**25**	25
Seafood Salad	**120**	**4.5**	16
Tuna Salad	**260**	**19**	6
***Dressings & Sauces:** Caesar*	**210**	**22**	2
Blimpie, 1.5 oz	**180**	**12**	24
***Soups:** Per Serving*			
Cream of Broccoli & Cheese	**190**	**12**	15
Garden Vegetable	**80**	**0.5**	14
Homestyle Chicken Noodle	**120**	**2.5**	18
Vegetable Beef	**80**	**1.5**	13
Desserts			
Cookies: Oatmeal Raisin	**190**	**8**	27
Sugar	**330**	**17**	24
Other varieties, average	**200**	**10**	26

For Complete Nutritional Data ~ see CalorieKing.com

Bob Evans® (Aug '07)

Breakfast	**C**	**F**	**Cb**
Combinations: Country Biscuit	660	45	40
Home Fries	195	7	28
Lite Sausage Breakfast	470	21	48
Pot Roast Hash Breakfast	660	39	35
Sausage Benedict	935	66	40
Farm Fresh Eggs: Eggs Benedict	420	20	35
Hardboiled (1)	60	4	1
Over Easy (1)	100	8	1
Scrambled	255	17	2
Scrambled Egg Beaters, 4.5 oz	175	12	3
Hotcake: Blueberry (1), 7.2 oz	335	9	57
Buttermilk (1), 3 oz	320	9	53
Omelets: Three Cheese	770	67	4
Farmer's Market	910	74	15
Ham & Cheddar	760	62	3
Western	780	63	8
Crepes: Raspberry (2)	1025	70	84
Plain (2)	470	36	28
Dinners: Per Serving			
Beef & Pork: Meat Loaf	280	19	9
Country Fried Steak w. Gravy	535	37	32
no Gravy	480	33	26
Slow Roasted Pork Loin, 2 pces	520	30	30
Chicken & Turkey:			
Chicken Dinner, Fried, 1 piece	325	16	14
Chicken Dinner, Grilled, 1 piece	230	13	0
Chicken Pot Pie	900	61	63
Chicken-n-Noodles	295	16	23
Slow Roasted Turkey	115	4	1
Seafood: Salmon Dinner, plain	290	13	0
Kid's Menu: Mac & Cheese	330	12	45
Mini Cheeseburgers (1)	305	19	21
Pasta	115	5	15
Plenty-O-Pancakes	500	17	79
Smiley Face Potatoes, 6 oz	515	34	48
Lunch Savors: Per Serving			
Chicken Parmesan Pasta	650	33	46
Salads: Cobb	700	46	14
Country Spinach	600	41	14
Fruit & Yogurt Plate	400	2	92
Wildfire Chkn: w. Fried Chicken	770	36	77
w. Grilled Chicken	655	32	53
Stir-Fry: Chicken	675	23	52

Bob Evans® cont... (Aug '07)

Sandwiches & Burgers	**C**	**F**	**Cb**
Burgers: Bacon Cheeseburger	715	48	32
Cheeseburger	645	41	32
Hamburger	540	32	31
Sandwiches: Big BLT	420	29	30
Fried Chicken Club	700	38	45
Grilled Chicken Club	605	35	31
Grilled Chicken, plain	400	15	30
Pot Roast	610	28	58
Turkey Bacon Melt	615	29	53
Sides			
Baked Potato Seasoned, Loaded	375	13	56
Baked Potato Seasoned, Plain	210	0	54
Broccoli Florets, 4 oz	30	0	6
Coleslaw, 4 oz	210	14	19
French Fries, 5 oz	345	14	49
Garden Side Salad, 5.3 oz	140	4	22
Garden Vegetables, 6 oz	120	7	14
Glazed Carrots, 4 oz	85	3	14
Green Beans, 6 oz	80	3	9
Mashed Potatoes, 5 oz	170	6	15
Rice Pilaf, 6 oz	130	4	20
Specialty Breads: Banana Nut, 6 oz	430	16	68
Cinnamon Swirl Roll, Frosted	575	25	79
Dinner Roll (1)	200	5	34
English Muffin (1)	130	1	25
Garlic Bread, 2 oz	220	16	16
Sourdough, 1.7 oz	135	1	25
Texas Toast, 1.8 oz	120	1	12
Beverages			
Iced Tea: Regular	5	0	1
Raspberry; Strawberry	80	0	20
Desserts, Pies, Sundaes			
Pie: Apple Dumpling Pie, 1 slice	605	28	83
Apple Dumpling A La Mode, 1 sl.	790	38	108
Apple Pie, N.S.A., 1 slice	490	30	55
Coconut Cream Pie, 1 slice	535	27	65
French Silk Pie, 1 slice	695	47	62
Oreo Cookies & Cream, 1 slice	805	45	95
Pumpkin Pie, 1 slice	545	27	69
Kids Sundae: Fudge Blast, 5 oz	270	13	36
Reese's, 5.6 oz	355	18	44

For Complete Nutritional Data ~ see CalorieKing.com

Bojangles® (Aug '07)

Cajun & Southern Style Chicken	C	F	Cb
Breast, average	280	17	11
Leg, average	265	16	11
Thigh, average	310	23	11
Wing, average	355	25	11
Sandwiches			
Cajun Filet: no Mayo	340	11	41
w. Mayonnaise	440	22	41
Grilled Filet: no Mayo	235	5	25
w. Mayonnaise	335	16	25
Snacks: Buffalo Bites	180	5	5
Chicken Supremes	335	16	26
Biscuit Sandwiches: Biscuit (plain)	245	12	29
Bacon	290	17	26
Bacon, Egg & Cheese	550	42	27
Cajun Filet	455	21	46
Country Ham	270	15	26
Egg	400	30	26
Sausage	350	23	26
Smoked Sausage	380	26	27
Steak	650	49	37
Fixins': Botato Rounds	235	11	31
Cajun Pintos	110	0	18
Corn on the Cob	140	2	34
Dirty Rice	165	6	24
Green Beans	25	0	5
Macaroni & Cheese	200	14	12
Marinated Cole Slaw	135	3	26
Potatoes, no Gravy	80	1	16
Seasoned Fries	345	16	39
Sweet Biscuits: Bo Berry	220	10	29
Cinnamon	320	18	37

For Complete Nutritional Data ~ see CalorieKing.com

Be sure to balance 'eating out' with adequate fruit and veggies.

Boston Market® (Aug '07)

Sandwiches & Burgers	C	F	Cb
Chicken Carver	700	29	68
Meatloaf Carver	940	45	96
Sirloin Dip Carver	860	37	70
Turkey Carver	530	17	55
Turkey Dip Carver	770	27	67
Salads: Per Serving (w. Dressing)			
Caesar Entree: w. Roasted Sirloin	660	51	12
w. Roasted Turkey	640	51	13
w. Rotisserie Chicken	600	48	13
Market Chopped: w. Rsd Sirloin	740	54	31
w. Roasted Turkey	720	54	32
w. Rotisserie Chicken	680	50	32
Sides: Per Serving			
Caesar Side Salad: w. Dressing	400	40	7
no Dressing	40	2	3
Cinnamon Apples, 5 oz	210	3	47
Creamed Spinach, 6.7 oz	280	23	12
Fresh Steamed Vegetables, 4.8 oz	50	2	8
Fresh Vegetable Stuffing, 4.8 oz	190	8	25
Garden Fresh Coleslaw, 3.8 oz	170	9	21
Garlic Dill New Potatoes, 5½ oz	140	3	24
Gravy, Poultry, 4 oz	15	0.5	4
Green Bean Casserole, 6 oz	60	2	9
Macaroni & Cheese, 7.8 oz	330	12	39
Mashed Potatoes (7.8 oz): no Gravy	210	9	29
w. 2 oz Poultry Gravy	235	10	32
Seasonal Fresh Fruit Salad, 5 oz	60	0	15
Sweet Corn, 6.2 oz	170	4	37
Sweet Potato Casserole, 7 oz	460	17	77
Soups: Per Serving			
Chicken Noodle, 10 oz	180	7	16
Chicken Tortilla, 8 oz	340	22	24
Desserts: Per Serving			
Apple Pie, 1 slice, 6 oz	420	20	56
Chocolate Cake, 5.1 oz	600	32	75
Choc. Chip Fudge Brownie, 5 oz	580	23	81
Cornbread, 1.6 oz	130	3.5	21
Nestle Toll House Choc. Chip Cookie (1)	370	19	49

For Complete Nutritional Data ~ see CalorieKing.com

Updated Nutrition Data ~ www.CalorieKing.com
Persons with Diabetes ~ See Disclaimer (Page 24)

Boston Pizza® (Aug '07)

	C	F	Cb
Starters: Cactus Cut Potatoes/Dip	930	64	73
Boston's Pizza Bread, no dip	510	13	83
Oven Rstd Boston's BBQ Wings	690	42	24
Soup: Baked French Onion	160	4	23
Salads: Caesar, reg., w. dressing	240	18	15
Greek, regular, w. dressing	600	57	18
Sirloin Steak w. dressing	640	48	17
Entrees: See CalorieKing.com			
Sandwiches: Boston Brute & Fries	1100	45	130
Boston Cheesesteak & Fries	1770	98	137
Chkn Santa Fe Strombli & Caesar	720	22	106
New York Steak w. Tossed Greens	510	33	12
Pizzas (Medium): Per 2 Slices			
BBQ Chicken	380	12	50
Boston Royal	420	12	54
Californian	320	4	62
Hawaiian	420	10	54
Meateor	520	20	58
Spicey Perogy	560	26	54
Ultimate Pepperoni	460	18	48
Vegetarian	360	8	54
Other Sizes: See CalorieKing.com			
Pastas (Full Order): Lasagna	680	18	90
Chicken & Mushroom Fettucini	1420	77	139
Spaghetti with Bolognese	780	9	146
Desserts: Chocolate Explosion	880	51	105
New York Cheesecake	620	33	80
For Complete Nutritional Data ~ see CalorieKing.com			

Braum's® (Aug '07)

	C	F	Cb
Cinnamon Rolls, with Icing	340	11	56
Frozen Yogurt: Per ½ Cup			
Vanilla; Peach; Strawb./Banana	120	4	17
Other flavors, average	140	5	20
Ice Cream: Per ½ Cup			
Light: Average all varieties	110	3	18
Premium: Peanut Buttercup	190	12	18
Other flavors, average	130	7	16
Pies (Baked): Average, 1 slice	400	20	50
For Complete Nutritional Data ~ see CalorieKing.com			

Buck's Pizza® (Aug '07)

	C	F	Cb
Buck's Deluxe: Med. (12"), 1 sl, ⅙	265	13	28
Large (14"), 1 slice, ⅛	270	13	29
X-Large (16"), 1 slice, ½₁₂	240	11	38
Small (9"), Whole Pizza	900	44	96
Personal (6"), Whole Pizza	400	17	69

Bruegger's Bagels® (Aug '07)

Bagels	C	F	Cb
Average all flavors, 4.3 oz	330	2	65
Softwiches (Square), avg. 4½ oz	350	3	68
Cream Cheese: Avg., 1½ oz scoop	140	13	3
Light varieties, average, 1½ oz	100	6	4
Breakfast S'wiches: Egg & Cheese	420	18	71
Egg, Cheese & Ham	460	18	73
Egg, Cheese & Sausage	640	38	72
Western Wheat Softwich	820	58	76
Bagel Sandwiches: Chicken Fajita	530	11	81
Smoked Salmon	490	10	74
Garden Veggie Softwich	380	3	76
Herby Turkey	560	14	78
Santa Fe Turkey	490	9	75
Deli Softwich: Chicken Breast	630	11	81
Chicken Salad w. Mayo	670	27	76
Ham	510	6	85
Tuna Salad w. Mayo	720	34	76
Turkey w. Mayo	550	15	74
Salads (With Dressing): Caesar	270	17	22
Chicken Caesar	370	20	23
Sesame Chicken	480	28	30
Muffins: Blueberry, 5 oz	450	19	64
Chocolate, 4½ oz	460	24	57
Cake: Lemon Pound, 3.3 oz slice	320	13	48
Cookies: Chocolate Chunk	500	22	71
Oatmeal Raisin	460	19	71
Slices: Luscious Lemon, 2.7 oz	300	16	36
Seven Layer, 4.7 o z	650	43	58
Chocolate Chunk Brownie, 2.6 oz	330	18	40
Raspberry Sammies, 2.5 oz	340	16	44
Iced Coffee: Raspb. & Cream, 20 oz	210	10	27
For Complete Menu & Data ~ see CalorieKing.com			

Burgerville® (Aug '07)

	C	F	Cb
Hamburger	300	15	29
Cheeseburger	350	19	29
Double Beef Cheeseburger	430	25	29
Half Pound Colossal	730	45	31
Colossal	520	30	30
Gardenburger	450	19	52
Turkey Club Sandwich	550	32	38
Crispy Chicken	490	19	59
Grilled Chicken	320	4.5	44
Chicken Strips, 5 pieces	320	14	26
French Fries: Regular, 5 oz	360	17	48
For Complete Menu & Data ~ see CalorieKing.com			

Burger King® (Aug '07)

Burgers & Sandwiches

	C	F	Cb
Bacon Cheeseburger	360	18	31
Bacon Double Cheeseburger	530	31	32
BK Veggie Burger (with mayo)	420	16	46
without mayonnaise	340	8	46
Cheeseburger	330	16	31
Double Cheeseburger	500	29	31
Hamburger	290	12	30
Double Hamburger	410	21	30
The Angus Steak Burger	640	33	55
Stackers: Double	610	39	32
Triple	800	54	33
Quadruple	1000	68	34

Whoppers®

	C	F	Cb
Whopper w. mayonnaise	670	39	51
without mayonnaise	510	22	51
Double Whopper w. mayonnaise	900	57	51
with Cheese, Mayo	990	64	52
without mayonnaise	740	39	51
Whopper JR w. mayonnaise	370	21	31
without mayonnaise	290	12	31
Triple Whopper	1130	74	51

Chicken & Fish

	C	F	Cb
BK Big Fish Sandwich w. tartar sce	630	30	67
Original Chicken Sandwich	660	40	52
without mayonnaise	450	17	52
Chick'N Crisp	480	31	36
without mayonnaise	320	13	36
TenderCrisp Chicken S'wich	790	44	66
TenderGrill Chkn S'wich w. mayo	510	19	49
without sauce	400	7	49
Chicken Fries: 6 pieces, no sauce	260	16	18
Chicken Tenders: 5 pieces, no sauce	215	15	13
Big Kid's Meal, 6 pces	250	15	16
Kid's Meal, 4 pieces	170	10	11
Dipping Sauces, (1 oz): Buffalo Sce	80	8	2
Honey Flavored	90	0	23
Honey Mustard	90	6	8
Ranch; Zesty Onion Ring, avg.	145	15	2
Sweet & Sour; Barbecue, avg.	40	0	11
French Fries: Small, 2.6 oz	230	13	26
Medium, 4 oz	360	20	41
Large, 5.6 oz	495	27	57
King Size, 6.8 oz	600	33	69
Ketchup, 1 packet	10	0	3
Onion Rings: Small, 1½ oz	140	7	18
Medium, 3.2 oz	310	15	37
Large, 4.8 oz	440	22	53
King Size, 5.3 oz	520	25	62
Cheesy Tots: Small, 6 pieces	215	12	20
Medium, 9 pieces	325	18	30

Burger King® cont.. (Aug '07)

Breakfast

	C	F	Cb
Biscuits: Ham, Egg & Cheese	390	22	31
Sausage, Egg & Cheese	530	37	31
Croissan'wich: Egg & Cheese	300	17	26
Bacon/Ham, Egg & Cheese, avg.	340	20	26
Sausage & Cheese	370	25	23
Sausage, Egg & Cheese	470	32	26
Double Croissan'wich:			
Bacon, Egg & Cheese	430	27	27
Sausage, Bacon & Cheese	560	39	27
Sausage, Egg & Cheese	680	51	26
Omelet Sandwich: Enormous	730	45	44
Ham	330	14	35
French Toast Sticks: 5 sticks	390	22	43
Kid's Meal (w. syrup)	660	22	102
Breakfast Syrup, 1 oz	80	0	21
Jam, Grape/Strawberry, 1 pkg	30	0	7
Hash Brown: Medium	430	28	42
Small, 3 oz	260	17	25
Cini-Minis (4), with Vanilla Icing	500	21	72
Salads: (No Dressing or Croutons)			
Garden Salad, no Chicken, 6½ oz	90	5	7
Side Garden Salad, 3½ oz	15	0	3
TenderGrill Chicken Garden Salad	240	9	8
TenderCrisp Chicken Garden Salad	410	22	26
Garlic Parmesan Croutons, ½ oz	60	2	9
Salad Dressings: Per 2 oz			
Ken's Fat-Free Ranch	60	0	15
Ken's Creamy Caesar	210	21	4
Ken's Honey Mustard	270	23	15
Ken's Light Italian	120	11	5
Ken's Ranch	190	20	2
Desserts: Dutch Apple Pie	300	13	45
Hershey's Sundae Pie	310	19	32
Drinks & Shakes: Coffee, Medium	5	0	1
Coca-Cola/Sprite/Dr Pepper (with ¼ Ice):			
Kids, 12 fl.oz	110	0	30
Small, 16 fl.oz	140	0	39
Medium, 22 fl.oz	200	0	53
Large, 32 fl.oz	290	0	79
King, 42 fl.oz	390	0	104
Icee (Coke/Minute Maid): Small	110	0	31
Medium, 11 fl.oz	140	0	40
Low-Fat Milk (1%), 8 fl.oz	100	2.5	12
Milk Shakes (Choc./Strawb.): Sm.	470	14	75
Medium	690	20	114
Large	950	29	151
Orange Juice, 8 fl.oz	140	0	33

For Complete Nutritional Data ~ see CalorieKing.com

Updated Nutrition Data ~ www.CalorieKing.com
Persons with Diabetes ~ See Disclaimer (Page 24)

California Pizza Kitchen
~ See CalorieKing.com

Captain D's Seafood® (Aug '07)

Platters: Per Platter	C	F	Cb
Fish, Shrimp & Chicken	1695	107	138
Jumbo Fish, average	1610	102	130
Super Shrimp	1380	83	122
Dinner: Per Order			
Chicken	1200	72	102
Crab	1055	60	66
Fish & Chicken	1465	93	120
Fish & Shrimp	1510	96	126
Carb Control: Fish Dinner	405	18	26
Chicken Dinner	370	17	27
Low-Cal Fare: w. Rice & Vegetables			
Baked Chicken Dinner, 1 piece	340	5	43
Baked Fish Dinner, 1 piece	375	7	42
Baked Salmon Dinner, 1 piece	540	16	54
Shrimp Scampi Dinner, 10 pieces	410	19	42
Sandwiches: Baked Chicken	185	20	48
Baked Fish	645	33	48
Desserts: Carrot Cake	390	19	50
Cheesecake	425	26	45
Chocolate Cake	300	10	49
Pecan Pie	475	26	56

Caribou Coffee® (Aug '07)

Beverages Based on 2% Milk Unless Indicated

Drinks: Per Cup (16 fl.oz)			
Smoothies: Creampop	480	23	66
Passion Green Tea	200	0.5	49
Strawberry Banana	270	0.5	65
Wildberry	235	0.5	57
Coffee Coolers: Caramel	435	11	80
Chocolate	370	12	63
Espresso; Coffee, average	230	4	46
Mint Oreo	620	26	94
Vanilla	390	13	64
Espresso: Breve	425	36	15
Campfire Mocha	560	15	97
Cappuccino	170	7	17
Espresso	10	0	2
Latte	200	8	20
Macchiato	15	0.5	2
Mocha	455	16	64
White Chocolate Mocha	520	18	70
Skinny Bou Latte: Low Cal	65	0	10
Wild: Caramel Highrise	385	14	52
Hot Apple Blast	440	11	9
Lite White Berry w. Skim	495	8	95
Mint Condition	560	17	90

Carl's Jr.® (Aug '07)

Burgers/Sandwiches	C	F	Cb
Bacon Swiss Crispy Chicken	720	35	64
Catch Fish Sandwich	660	31	75
Famous Star Hamburger	600	34	53
Charbroiled: BBQ Chicken S'wich	360	4	38
Chicken Club Sandwich	550	25	43
Santa Fe Chicken Sandwich	610	32	43
Dble Western Bacon Chseburger	970	53	71
JR. Hamburger	280	9	36
Low Carb Chicken Club S'wich	380	21	10
Sourdough Bacon Cheeseburger	680	43	43
Spicy Chicken Sandwich	560	30	59
Super Star Hamburger	810	49	54
Teriyaki Burger	660	34	61
The Six Dollar Burger	1010	68	61
Bacon Cheeseburger	1070	76	50
Double Burger	1520	111	60
Jalapeno	700	44	50
Low-Carb Burger	490	37	6
Western Bacon Burger	1140	67	84
Western Bacon Cheeseburger	710	33	71
Western Crispy Chicken	750	28	91
Potatoes: Plain, no marg.	280	0	63
Bacon & Cheese	620	29	71
Broccoli & Cheese	510	21	71
Sour Cream & Chives	410	14	65
Breakfast: Breakfast Burger	830	46	65
Bacon & Egg Burrito	570	33	37
Loaded Breakfast Burrito	820	51	52
Breakfast Bowl, Low Carb	900	73	5
Breakfast Quesadilla	390	18	38
French Toast Dip (6), no Syrup	430	18	58
Sourdough Sandwich, no meat	460	21	39
Bakery/Desserts: Chocolate Cake	300	12	48
Chocolate Chip Cookie (1)	350	18	46
Strawberry Swirl Chsecake, 3.5 oz	290	17	30
Side Orders: Chicken Stars, 9 pces	380	24	22
Chicken Breast Strips (5)	710	41	64
CrissCut Fries, 5 oz	400	24	43
French Fries, small, 3.2 oz	290	14	37
Hash Brown Nuggets, 4 oz	330	21	32
Onion Rings, 4.5 oz	460	23	56
Salads: No Dressing			
Charbroiled Chicken Salad-to-Go	260	7	17
Green Burrito Taco Chicken Salad	820	45	72
Side Salad	50	3	5

Carvel® (Aug '07)

Sundaes	C	F	Cb
Thinny-Thin: Fudge No-Fat, small	380	0	84
Strawberry No-Fat, small	290	0	63
Classic Regular: Caramel	670	34	81
Bittersweet Fudge; Hot Fudge	680	38	77
Hot Fudge	670	38	73
Strawberry	580	33	63
Novelties: Per Small			
Flying Sauces 98% Fat-Free	190	1.5	40
Parfait; Miniature Sundae No-Fat	190	0	42
Parfait; No Sugar Added	200	2.5	42
Old Fashioned Sundae No-Fat	300	0	66
No Sugar Added	360	4.5	76
Thinny-Thin Uptown Smoothies: Per Small			
Berry Times Square	300	0	73
Grand Central Cooler	250	0	63
Other varieties, average	270	0	68
Beverages: Per 16 fl.oz			
Carvelanche: Cake Mix	720	27	106
Cookies & Cream	550	30	64
Triple Fudge Cake Mix	900	41	134
Creammaccino: Classic	520	21	72
Caramel Cream	670	14	108
Mocha Fudge	690	30	94

Checkers®

~ *Same Menu & Data as Rally's Hamburgers*®
See Page 240 ~

Cheesecake Factory® (Aug '07)

10" Cheesecake: Per Slice			
P. B. Cup Fudge Ripple	930	59	93
Banana Cream	860	63	70
Brownie Sundae	970	63	96
Choc Chip Cookie Dough	1910	72	102
Dulce de Leche	1010	74	83
Kahlua Cocoa Coffee	840	55	80
Keylime Cheesecake	710	49	64
Original Cheesecake	630	45	53
Vanilla Bean Cheesecake	870	64	69
White Choc. Raspberry Truffle	900	62	80

Charley's Grilled Subs® (Aug '07)

Subs: Regular w. Dressing	C	F	Cb
BBQ Cheddar	730	28	83
Bacon 3 Cheese Steak	740	37	57
Chicken Buffalo, no cheese/dress.	680	31	62
Chicken Bacon Club	640	27	57
Chicken Cordon Bleu	650	24	61
Chicken Teriyaki, no chse/dress.	520	13	61
Italian Deli	620	29	56
Philly Cheese Steak	600	24	60
Philly Chicken, no cheese/dressing	570	20	59
Philly Ham & Swiss	600	25	58
Philly Steak Deluxe	600	24	60
Philly Veggie	600	28	65
Steak Siciliano	720	36	58
Turkey Melt, no cheese/dress.	590	22	59
Ultimate Club	660	32	54
Fresh Salads: Garden no dressing	155	9	13
Fries (Per Regular): Original	680	53	46
Cheddar & Bacon	1130	91	60
Cheddar Ranch & Bacon	1310	110	61
Ranch & Bacon	1210	102	56
Beverages: Natural Lemonade, reg.	130	0	32

Chevys Fresh Mex® (Aug '07)

Tacos: With Rice, Cheese & Tamalito	C	F	Cb
Chicken	910	41	86
Steak	970	51	87
Salmon	1090	64	70
Sea Bass	845	39	88
Fajitas: With Tamalito, no Tortillas			
Chicken	915	45	67
Shrimp	1210	85	70
Steak	1065	59	67
Homemade Beans: a la Charra	230	5	33
Refried Beans	300	15	29
Salad: With Salsa Vinaigrette Dressing			
Santa Fe Chopped	680	41	25
Tostado Fajita Chicken Salad	1230	77	63
Sides: Black Beans	210	3	33
Guacamole, 2 oz	105	10	3
Mexican Rice	210	3	39
Salsa for Chips, 5 oz	40	0	8
Sour Cream	120	12	2
Tortilla: Corn	80	1	17
El Machino	165	4	27

Corner Bakery Cafe®
For Complete Nutritional Data ~ see CalorieKing.com

Updated Nutrition Data ~ www.CalorieKing.com
Persons with Diabetes ~ See Disclaimer (Page 24)

Restaurants & Fast - Foods

Chick-fil-A® (Aug '07)

Chick-fil-A Sandwiches	C	F	Cb
Chicken Sandwich	410	16	38
Chargrilled Chicken Sandwich	270	3.5	33
Chicken Salad Sandwich	350	15	32
Cool Wraps®: Chicken Caesar	460	10	52
Chargrilled/Spicy Chicken, avg.	395	7	54
Breakfast: Plain Biscuit, 2.8 oz	260	11	38
Biscuit and Gravy	330	15	43
Biscuit: w. Bacon, Egg & Cheese	470	26	39
w. Sausage	490	32	38
Hash Browns, 3 oz	260	17	25
Chick-n-Minis, 3 count	270	11	28
Chicken Biscuit	420	19	44
Platter: Chicken	630	32	51
Bacon	550	30	44
Breakfast Burrito: Chicken	410	16	42
Sausage	450	23	39
Chicken, Egg & Cheese Bagel	500	20	49
Salads: Chick-n-Strips® Salad	400	20	21
Chargrilled Chicken Garden	180	6	9
Southwest Chargrilled Chicken	240	8	17
Salad Dressing: Per Packet (1.25 oz)			
Caesar Dressing	160	17	1
Raspberry Vinaigrette	80	2	15
Bleu Cheese; Buttermilk, avg.	150	16	1
Fat Free Honey Mustard	60	0	14
Light Italian Dressing	15	0.5	2
Spicy Dressing	140	14	2
Thousand Island	150	14	5
Strips, Nuggets: Nuggets (8-pack)	260	12	12
Chick-n-Strips® (4-count)	300	15	14
Dipping Sauces: Polynesian, 1 oz	110	6	13
Barbecue; Honey Mustard, avg.,1 oz	45	0	10
Buffalo Sce, ¾ oz	15	1.5	1
Sides: Carrot & Raisin Salad, small	170	6	28
Fresh Fruit Cups, medium, 4.4 oz	65	0	17
Coleslaw, small, 4½ oz	260	21	17
Garlic and Butter Croutons, ½ oz	70	2.5	9
Side Salad, 3.8 oz	60	3	4
Tortilla Strips, 1 pkt, ½ oz	70	3.5	9
Waffle Potato Fries, medium, 4 oz	355	17	46
Desserts: Cheesecake, 3.3 oz slice	340	21	30
Icedream® Cup, small	240	6	41
Icedream® Cone, small	160	4	28
Lemon Pie, 4 oz slice	390	13	63
Fudge Nut Brownie (1), 2.6 oz	330	15	45

Chili's® (Aug '07)

Starters: Per Order	C	F	Cb
Awesome Blossom w. Sauce	2710	203	194
¼ Whole w. Blossom Sauce	680	51	48
Boneless Buffalo Wings + Sauce	1250	89	55
Boneless Shanghai Wings	1260	71	97
Bottomless Tostada Chips w. Sce	480	36	26
Classic Nachos	1570	115	66
Fried Cheese w. Marinara Sauce	1210	89	82
Skillet Queso w. Tortilla Chips	1070	89	30
South Western Egg Rolls	810	51	59
Wings over Buffalo	1140	100	4
Guiltless Grill®: Chicken Platter	580	9	85
Chicken Sandwich	490	8	63
Burgers (No Fries): BBQ Ranch	1110	71	60
Bunless Burgers	360	25	0
Chipotle Bleu Chse Bacon Burger	1090	71	57
Ground Peppercorn	1050	68	61
Meals: Chili's Sirloin, no sides	530	41	1
Cajun Chicken Pasta w. Toast	1500	78	123
Cajun Chicken Sandwich, no Fries	820	43	66
Cheesesteak Sandwich, no Fries	1010	70	82
Chicken Caesar Pita, no Fries	650	41	31
Citrus Fire Chicken & Shrimp Fajita	720	42	34
Country Fried Steak	1890	107	148
Flame Grilled Rib Eye, no Fries	960	87	1
Grilled Baby Back Ribs	1370	82	112
Grilled Salmon w. Garlic & Herbs	700	33	53
Gr. Shrimp Alfredo Pasta w. Toast	1540	84	123
Margarita Grilled Chicken	690	14	85
Fajitas: Includes 3 Tortillas & Garnishes			
Mushroom Jack	1360	74	98
Chicken	940	30	90
Steak	1400	78	87
Salads: No Dressing Unless Indicated			
Chicken Caesar Salad w. Dressing	1010	76	39
Dinner Caesar Salad w. Dressing	520	43	27
Dinner House Salad	140	7	12
Quesadilla Explosion	980	48	81
Desserts: Choc Chip Paradise Pie	1600	78	215
Molten Choc Cake	1270	62	172

For Complete Nutritional Data ~ see CalorieKing.com

Updated Nutrition Data ~ www.CalorieKing.com
Persons with Diabetes ~ See Disclaimer (Page 24)

197

Chipotle® (Aug '07)

	C	F	Cb
Bol Salad: Per Bowl (no Rice or Tortilla)			
Burrito w. Beans: Meat & Cheese	475	22	24
Meat & Corn Salsa	475	14	45
Meat & Sour Cream or Cheese	470	23	25
Meat & Tomato Salsa	395	13	29
Fajita w. Vege: Meat & Corn Salsa	435	21	28
Meat & Sour Cream or Cheese	435	30	8.5
Meat & Tomato Salsa	355	20	12
Vegetarian: w. Guacamole			
w. Beans/Corn Salsa	420	17	52
w. Beans, Tomato Salsa	340	16	36
Burrito Bol: with Rice & Beans			
Meat & Cheese	710	29	63
Meat & Corn Salsa	710	21	85
Meat & Sour Cream or Cheese	705	30	65
Meat & Tomato Salsa	630	20	69
Vegetarian w. Guacamole:			
Rice & Beans	545	23	70
Tomato Salsa	575	23	76
Corn Salsa	655	24	92
Fajita Burrito Bol: with Rice & Beans			
Meat & Corn Salsa	1040	30	139
Meat & Sour Cream	1040	39	119
Meat & Tomato Salsa	960	29	123
Vegetables: Meat & Cheese	675	36	46
Meat & Corn Salsa	670	28	68
Meat & Sour Cream or Cheese	670	37	48
Vegetables & Meat: & Tom. Salsa	590	27	52
& Cheese or Sour Cream	1005	45	100
& Corn Salsa	1005	37	122
& Tomato Salsa	925	36	106
Taco w. 4 Crispy Shells: Per Serving			
Meat, Corn Salsa: & Cheese	705	31	57
& Sour Cream	675	32	58
Meat, Tomato Salsa: & Cheese	600	30	41
& Sour Cream	595	31	42
Vegetarian Burrito: w. Rice, Beans & Guacamole			
Black Beans	880	32	124
Corn Salsa	990	33	146
Sour Cream	985	42	126
Tomato Salsa	910	32	130

CinnaMonster® (Aug '07)

	C	F	Cb
Cinnamon Roll: Per Roll			
Caramel Pecan	840	32	120
Original	880	24	100

Chuck E. Cheese® (Aug '07)

	C	F	Cb
Appetizers: Per Serving			
Buffalo Wings (12)	660	45	3
French Fries (for s'wiches), 5 oz	240	9	37
French Fries ala Carte, 10 oz	480	17	74
Italian Bread Sticks (1)	195	8	27
Sargento Mozzarella Sticks (1)	105	6	7
Pizzas: Per Slice (Medium)			
BBQ Chicken	270	8	43
Cheese	235	7	33
Pepperoni	265	10	33
Vegetarian	235	7	36
Sandwiches: Ham & Chse, no Fries	620	28	70
Grilled Chicken Sub, no Fries	650	31	70
Italian Sub, no Fries	730	40	69
Hot Dog, no Fries	170	17	27
Hot Dog w. Cheese, no Fries	335	30	28
Desserts: Apple Pie Pizza, 1 slice	195	2	40
Birthday Cake (8"), 1 slice (⅒)	310	13	45
Cinnamon Sticks, 1 stick	200	5	33

Church's Chicken® (Aug '07)

	C	F	Cb
Fried Chicken: Per Piece			
Original: Breast	200	11	3
Leg	110	6	3
Thigh	330	23	8
Wing	300	19	7
Spicy: Breast	320	20	12
Leg	180	11	8
Thigh	480	35	20
Wing	430	27	17
Tender Strips: Original (1)	120	6	6
Spicy, 1 piece	135	7	7
Spicy Chicken Sandwich	360	18	35
Sides: Cajun Rice, regular, 3 oz	130	7	16
Cole Slaw, regular, 4.2 oz	150	10	15
Corn on the Cob, 1 ear	140	3	24
French Fries, regular, 5 oz	420	20	55
Fried Okra, regular	300	23	27
Honey Butter Biscuits (1)	250	16	26
Jalapeno Cheese Bombers, 4 oz	240	10	29
Mashed Pot. & Gravy, reg., 3.6 oz	70	2	12
Apple Pie (Fried), 3 oz	260	11	39
Sauces: Per Pkg			
BBQ; Sweet & Sour	30	0	7
Creamy Jalapeno	100	11	1
Honey Mustard	110	11	4
Purple Pepper	45	0	12
Ranch	130	13	1

Cinnabon® (Aug '07)

	C	F	Cb
Sweet Rolls: Cinnabon Bites (6)	510	19	77
Classic Cinnamon Roll (1)	815	32	117
Cinnabon Stix, 5 pieces, 85g	380	21	41
Minibon (1) 92g	340	13	49
Caramel Pecanbon (1)	1100	56	141
CinnaPretzel (1)	755	6	156
Sweet Roll Icing: Frosting Cup, 1.4 oz	180	11	20
Drinks: Mochalatta Chill, 480ml	360	13	55
For Complete Nutritional Data ~ see CalorieKing.com			

Cici's Pizza® (Aug '07)

	C	F	Cb
Buffet Pizza (12"): Per Slice (1/10)			
Alfredo; Ham & Pineapple, avg.	140	5	18
Beef; Bar-B-Que	170	6.5	19
Chse; Bacon Cheddar; Spin. Alfredo	150	5	20
Pepperoni	175	7	21
Sausage	200	7	19
Zesty Ham & Cheddar/ Pepperoni	155	6	18
Zesty Veggie	125	4.5	18

Cosi® (Aug '07)

	C	F	Cb
Pasta: Penne Marinara	930	9	180
Penne Pesto w. Chicken	1285	36	178
Penne a la Cosi	1300	37	189
Thai Chicken & Peanut Noodles	1600	28	276
Pizza: Four Cheese, 1 pizza	1280	38	185
Meatlovers, 1 pizza	1610	63	187
Spinach & Fresh Tomato, 1 pizza	1320	43	190
Sandwiches: Buffalo Blue	650	30	57
Cosi Club	700	35	59
Grilled Chicken TBM	790	43	60
Hummus & Fresh Veggies	430	8	77
Sesame Ginger Chicken	510	11	70
Smoked Ham & Brie	640	25	69
Tandoori Chicken	635	26	58
Tuna & Cheddar	955	55	55
Turkey Light	475	9	73
Melts: Bacon Turkey Cheddar	680	25	74
Grilled Chicken Parmesan	700	27	64
Salads (No Dressing): Bombay	175	3	13
Caesar	180	8	20
Chicken Caesar	340	16	21
Cobb	420	28	8
Greek	235	17	9
Mixed Greens	45	1	9
Shanghai Chicken	220	9	16
Signature	375	21	40
Regular Dressings: Per Serving (2 oz)			
Regular: Cosi Vinaigrette	355	39	2
Other varieties, average	300	30	2
For Complete Menu & Data ~ see CalorieKing.com			

Cousins Subs® (Aug '07)

7½" Subs	C	F	Cb
BLT	590	38	47
Cheese Steak	505	19	49
Chicken Breast	570	27	50
Chicken Cheddar Deluxe	670	39	51
Club	655	35	51
Double Cheese Steak	745	36	49
Garden Veggie	390	12	51
Gyro	710	41	61
Ham & Provolone	610	34	50
Hot Veggie	470	17	55
Italian Special	820	51	50
Meatball & Provolone	725	38	54
Pepperoni Melt	730	45	50
Philly Cheese Steak	530	19	55
Pizza	710	39	55
Roast Beef	610	30	50
Seafood w. Crab	640	38	60
Spicy Chicken Sedona	530	18	54
Three Cheese	685	44	50
Tuna	665	40	49
Turkey Breast	535	28	50
4" Mini Subs: (No Mayo, Cheese or Added Salt)			
BLT	300	19	24
Chicken Breast	185	1	25
Club	195	3	26
Garden Veggie	135	1	26
Ham	180	2	24
Hot Veggie	145	1	27
Roast Beef	205	3	25
Turkey Breast	175	2	26
French Fries: Small, 2.8 oz	250	13	30
Medium, 4 oz	365	19	43
Large, 5.3 oz	485	25	57
Salads: (Without Dressings)			
Chef Salad	330	14	26
Chicken Sedona	230	5	16
Garden: Salad	240	11	24
w. Chicken Breast	355	12	26
Italian	410	24	25
Seafood Salad	320	11	35
Side Salad	135	6	14
Tuna Salad	630	46	24
For Complete Menu & Data ~ see CalorieKing.com			

Updated Nutrition Data ~ www.CalorieKing.com
Persons with Diabetes ~ See Disclaimer (Page 24)

Cold Stone Creamery® (Aug '07)

	C	F	Cb
Sweet Cream Ice Cream			
Like It, average all flavors	330	20	33
Love It, average all flavors	570	31	63
Gotta Have It, average all flavors	920	50	93
Like It	240	6.5	43
Low-Fat Frozen Yogurt (Choc)			
Like It	230	1.5	48
Love It	380	3	79
Non-Fat Frozen Yogurt: Like It	230	0	48
Love It, average all flavors	380	0.5	80
Gotta Have It, average all flavors	540	1	113
Sinless Sorbet: Like It, avg.	180	0	48
Love It, avg.	300	0	80
Gotta Have It, avg.	420	0	112
Ice Cream Cake: Per Slice (⅛ of 6" Cake)			
A Cheesecake Named Desire	420	19	56
Butterfinger Bonanza	450	21	59
Chocolate Chipper	450	26	50
Midnight Delight	510	28	60
Peanut Butter Playground	490	29	54
Strawberry Passion	390	19	50
Zebra Stripes Dark	480	29	53
Waffle Cone or Bowl	160	4	29

Culver's® (Aug '07)

	C	F	Cb
Butterburgers: Cheese, Double	580	32	37
Bacon Deluxe	765	51	34
Deluxe Single	505	32	34
Deluxe, Double	685	44	34
Low-Carb	445	32	1
Favorite Sandwiches: Chkn Filet	635	30	68
Beef Pot Roast	365	16	33
Chicken Salad Sourdough	555	29	37
Grilled Chicken Breast	375	8	47
Grilled Ham & Swiss on Rye	520	26	35
Philly Ribeye Steak	515	21	46
Pork Tenderloin	705	29	87
Turkey Stacked	460	20	47
Turkey Sourdough BLT	605	33	39
Garden Fresh Salads: Chkn Caesar	360	14	15
Chicken Cashew	440	25	11
Garden Fresco Salad	225	11	25
Taco Salad	780	51	59
Side Salad	90	5	7
Fish & Chicken: With Sides			
Breaded Shrimp Dinner, 8 pieces	1250	61	148
Chicken Dinner, 2 pieces	1755	94	140
Fish n' Chips Dinner, 6 pieces	1380	83	104
North Atlantic Cod, 2 pieces	1830	116	135

Culver's® cont... (Aug '07)

	C	F	Cb
Sides			
Chili Cheddar Fries, 9.3 oz	660	34	73
French Fries, regular, 5 oz	385	17	53
Mashed Potatoes & Gravy, small	140	2	26
Onion Rings, breaded, 6.7 oz	630	36	70
Desserts: Classic Lemon Ice, 7 oz	140	0	35
Lemon Ice Smoothie, 11 oz	405	16	61
Root Beer Float, 15 oz	465	18	70
Cookie Custard Sandwich	765	38	94
Custard Dishes: 1 Scoop	305	18	30
2 Scoops	590	35	58
3 Scoops	745	44	73
Custard Cake: Turtle, 3½ oz	270	16	30
Cookies & Cream, 3½ oz	245	14	26

For Complete Nutritional Data ~ see CalorieKing.com

D'Angelo's® (Aug '07)

	C	F	Cb
Sandwiches			
Cheeseburger: Pokket	460	25	31
Sub	525	26	44
Wrap	570	25	52
Chicken Stir Fry: D'Lite Pokket	425	6	57
Sub	450	11	53
Wrap	490	9	61
Classic Veggie: D'Lite Pokket	360	7	63
Wrap	485	13	68
Grilled Chkn Breast D'Lite Pokket	390	7	52
Italian Sub	615	31	54
Number 9 Steak Sub	460	19	41
Roast Beef: D'Lite Pokket	340	5	51
Sub	320	5	48
Turkey: D'Lite Pokket	350	4	51
Sub	320	4	45
Salads: No Dressing Unless Indicated			
Caesar Salad w. Dressing	475	39	25
Chicken Stir Fry	170	3	11
Greek Salad	300	23	17
Roast Beef	130	3	10
Lobster	375	26	12
Tossed Salad	50	1	11
Turkey	160	2	10

For Extra Menu Items
and **Complete Nutritional Data**
~ See Author's Website
www.CalorieKing.com

Dairy Queen® (Aug '07)

Burgers/Sandwiches	C	F	Cb
GrillBurger: ½ lb Burger, no cheese	670	37	42
Classic, no cheese	470	23	42
Bacon Cheddar	650	37	41
Crispy Chicken Sandwich	530	29	47
DQ Homestyle: Hamburger	350	14	33
Bacon Double Cheeseburger	730	41	35
Cheeseburger	400	18	34
Double Cheeseburger	640	34	34
Ultimate Burger	780	48	33
Grilled Chicken Sandwich	350	16	49
Hot Dog, Classic	280	17	21
Chili 'n' Cheese Dog, regular	380	24	24
Entrees/Sides: On. Rings, reg., 4 oz	470	30	45
Chicken Strips, basket (4)	940	58	75
French Fries, small, 5.7 oz	425	19	58
Chicken Quesadilla, no dressing	1110	68	92

Salads: No Dressing			
Crispy Chicken Salad	420	22	30
Grilled Chicken Salad	270	11	32

Ice Cream Cones/Soft Serve			
DQ Vanilla Soft Serve, ½ cup	150	5	22
DQ Choc. Soft Serve, ½ cup	150	5	22
Chocolate Cone, medium	345	11	52
Dipped Cone, medium	480	23	60
Vanilla Cone, medium	335	10	53

Novelties: Buster Bar	480	31	45
Chocolate Dilly Bar	240	15	24
DQ Fudge Bar, No Sugar Added	50	0	13
DQ Sandwich	190	5	32
DQ Vanilla Orange Bar, NAS	60	0	17
Starkiss	80	0	21

Blizzards® & Sundaes			
Choc. Chip Cookie Dough, med.	1030	40	151
Oreo Cookie Blizzard, medium	690	26	103
Chocolate Sundae, medium	410	10	70
DQ Log Cake ⅛ cake	310	12	44
DQ Heart Cake, 1⁄10 cake	290	11	42
Reese's Peanut Butter Cup, med.	850	36	111
Royal Banana Split, medium	530	14	98
Strawberry CheeseQuake, medium	720	30	98
Drinks: Chocolate Shake, medium	765	20	110
Malts, medium, average	870	22	153
MooLatte: Cappuccino, large	700	24	105
Mocha, large	840	31	121

For Complete Nutritional Data ~ see CalorieKing.com

Daphne's® (Aug '07)

Meals: Per Plate	C	F	Cb
Chicken: Combo	530	37	9
Kabob Plate	350	10	5.5
White Meat	370	16	6
Hummus & Pita	230	12	45
Kabob Lunch w. Chicken	210	9	2
Sandwich: Gyros Pita	650	46	38
w. Chicken Breast	565	22	34

Salads			
Greek Chicken	415	18	9
Spicy Greek Chicken w. 1 oz Fire Feta	510	24	12
Soups: Avgolemono, 1 cup	100	8	7

Extras			
Fire Feta, 2 Tbsp	100	7	2
Gyros, 4 oz	380	33	6
Pita Bread, whole	190	4	33
Rice Pilaf, 6 oz	275	7.5	47
Salad Dressing, 2 Tbsp	150	16	0
Tzatziki Sauce, 1.5 oz	60	6	3

Davanni's® (Aug '07)

Hoagies: Per Half Hoagie (6") w. Mayonnaise			
Assorted	390	29	21
Cheese	385	28	21
Chicken Breast	510	31	22
Chicken Parmigana	415	19	22
Club	385	25	22
Italian Sausage	520	37	28
Meatball	465	31	31
Pastrami	440	25	22
Pizza	315	18	22
Roast Beef	370	23	21
Salami	470	36	21
Tuna	550	42	24
Turkey	355	22	22
Vegie	350	23	25
Without Cheese ~ Deduct	40	3	0
Without Mayo ~ Deduct	100	11	1
Calzones, average all varieties	750	42	65

Pizzas			
5 Meat:			
Thin, 1 slice	245	12	18
Traditional: 1 slice	300	12	30
Solo Thin	1010	62	45
The Works: Thin, 1 slice	250	13	18
Traditional: 1 slice	310	14	29
Solo Thin	735	32	70
Vegie: Thin, 1 slice	210	9	18
Traditional: 1 slice	265	10	29
Solo Thin	495	22	42

Deep Dish ~ Similar to Traditional slice

Del Taco® (Aug '07)

Breakfast	C	F	Cb
Breakfast Burrito	250	11	24
Bacon & Egg Quesadilla	450	23	40
Egg & Cheese Burrito	450	24	39
Macho Bacon & Egg Burrito	1030	60	82
Steak & Egg Burrito	580	34	41
Hash Brown Sticks (5)	250	19	20
Tacos: Big Fat Chicken Taco	340	13	38
Big Fat Steak Taco	390	19	38
Big Fat Taco	320	11	39
Chicken Del Carbon	170	5	19
Steak Taco Del Carbon	220	11	19
Taco; Soft Taco, average	160	10	13
Burritos: Combo Burrito	530	22	61
Bean & Cheese Red/Green Burrito	270	8	38
Chicken Works Burrito	520	23	57
Del Beef Burrito	550	30	42
Del Classic Chicken Burrito	560	36	41
Deluxe Combo Burrito	570	25	64
Deluxe Del Beef Burrito	590	33	45
Half Pound Red/Green Burrito, avg.	430	12	63
Macho Beef Burrito	1170	62	89
Macho Combo Burrito	1050	44	113
Spicy Chicken/Veggie Works, avg.	480	17	68
Steak Works Burrito	590	31	58
Quesadillas: Cheddar	500	27	39
Chicken Cheddar	580	31	41
Spicy Jack Chicken	570	30	40
Spicy Jack	490	26	38
Salads: Deluxe Chicken Salad	740	34	77
Deluxe Taco Salad	780	40	76
Taco Salad	350	30	10
Burgers: Cheeseburger	330	13	37
Double Del Cheeseburger	560	35	35
Del Cheeseburger	430	25	35
Nachos: Regular, 4 oz	380	24	40
Macho Nachos, 16 oz	1100	63	113
Sides: Rice Cup, 4 oz	140	2	27
Beans 'n Cheese Cup, 7.8 oz	260	3	44
Fries: Chili Cheese, 10.5 oz	670	46	51
Deluxe Chili Cheese, 12 oz	710	49	53
Medium, 7 oz	490	32	47
Macho, 10 oz	690	46	68
Shakes: Chocolate, 15 fl.oz	680	16	117
Vanilla; Strawb. avg., 15 fl.oz	545	9	97

Denny's® (Aug '07)

Breakfast	C	F	Cb
All American Slam, no toast	950	75	21
French Slam, no syrup/marg.	1180	75	74
Grand Slam Slugger w. Hash Brn	1040	55	97
Heartland Scramble, no syrup	1190	59	118
Lumberjack Slam w. Hash Brown	1140	53	108
Meat Lovers Bowl, no syrup	1230	66	109
Moons Over My Hammy	760	40	52
Original Grand Slam	740	43	56
Pancake Platter, no syrup/margarine	660	25	83
Two Egg Breakfast, no Pot. or Grits	630	46	21
Ultimate Omelette	830	62	26
Extra Breakfast Items ~ See CalorieKing.com			
Soup: Chicken Noodle, 12 oz	180	7.5	15
Vegetable Beef, 12 oz	135	4.5	18
Sandwiches (No Fries/Sauces)			
Bacon, Lettuce, Tomato	590	35	50
Boca Burger	450	10	64
Chicken Ranch Melt	890	39	84
Classic Burger, no cheese	780	45	56
Club Sandwich	550	32	39
Fish Sandwich	590	30	30
Grilled Cheese	540	30	50
Grilled Chicken, no dressing	490	13	57
Mushroom Swiss Burger	900	55	63
Philly Melt	700	32	68
Slam Burger	1080	57	115
The Super Bird Sandwich	520	25	40
Appetizers/Entrees: No Sides/Condiments			
Buffalo Chicken Strips (5)	735	42	43
Buffalo Wings (9)	975	72	11
Chicken Strips (5)	735	42	56
Country Fried Steak	645	46	30
Fish & Chips	960	54	83
Fried Shrimp Dinner	260	12	18
Grilled Chicken Dinner	280	5	4
Grilled Tilapia Dinner	530	18	33
Mini Burgers (6) w. Onion Rings	2220	136	179
Mozzarella Sticks (8)	710	41	49
Roast Turkey & Stuffing w. Gravy	510	14	66
Sampler, no condiments	1405	80	124
Smothered Cheese Fries	765	48	69
Steakhouse Strip Dinner	390	14	0
T-Bone Steak Dinner	860	65	0

Updated Nutrition Data ~ www.CalorieKing.com
Persons with Diabetes ~ See Disclaimer (Page 24)

Denny's® cont... (Aug '07)

Sides	C	F	Cb
Garlic Bread, 2 pces	170	11	15
Corn, 4 oz	110	2	23
Onion Rings, 4 oz	380	23	38
Fries: Unsalted, 5 oz	425	20	57
Seasoned, 4 oz	260	12	35
Potato: Baked, plain with skin	220	0	51
Mashed, 5 oz	170	7	23

Salads (No Dressing/Bread Unless Indicated)			
Fried Chicken Strips Salad	440	26	26
Grilled Chicken Breast Salad	260	11	10
Side Caesar with Dressing	360	26	20
Side Garden Salad, no Dressing	115	7	6
Turkey Breast	250	8	12

Dressings & Sauces			
BBQ Sauce, 1.5 oz	45	1	11
Blue Cheese, 1 oz	165	18	1
Caesar; Ranch, avg., 1 oz	135	14	1
French, regular, 1 oz	105	10	3
Honey Mustard, 1 oz	160	15	20
Italian Dressing, Fat-Free; Salsa	15	0.5	3
Sour Cream, 1.5 oz	90	9	2
Thousand Island, 1 oz	120	11	5

Desserts: Carrot Cake, 8 oz	800	45	99
Hershey's Chocolate Cake	630	33	79
Hot Fudge Brownie A La Mode	995	42	147
Pies (⅛ Whole): Apple, 7 oz	470	21	68
Cheesecake, no topping, 4 oz	580	38	51
Chocolate Peanut Butter, 6 oz	655	39	64
French Silk Pie	735	56	58
Sundaes: Banana Split	895	43	121
Single Scoop, no topping	190	14	14
Double Scoop, no topping	375	27	29
Dessert Toppings: Choc., 2 oz	135	0.5	34
Cherry, 2 oz	55	0	14
Chocolate, 2 oz	135	0.5	34
Strawberry, 2 oz	75	1	17

Drinks: Cappuccino, 8 fl.oz	100	3	28
Floats, Rootbeer/Cola, 12 fl.oz	280	10	47
Milkshake, Van/Choc., 12 fl.oz	585	26	82
Oreo Blender Blaster, 15 oz	895	46	112
Ruby Red Grapefruit Juice, 10 oz	160	0	41
Raspberry Iced Tea, 16 fl.oz	80	0	21

For Complete Nutritional Data ~ see CalorieKing.com

Dippin' Dots® (Aug '07)

Flavored Ices	C	F	Cb
All flavors, ½ cup, 3 oz	90	0	23
Frozen Yogurt: All flavors, ½ cup	100	0	21

Ice Cream: Per Serving (½ Cup)			
Average all flavors	180	9	20
Fat-Free, Fudge, No Sugar Added	90	1	18
Low-Fat, Vanilla, No Sugar Added	125	6	13
Sherbet, ½ Cup	100	1	21

Donato's® Pizza (Aug '07)

14" Traditional Pizza: Per Slice (⅛ Large)			
Chicken Vegy Medley	310	10	37
Founders Fav.; The Works, avg.	435	20	37
Hawaiian; Serious Cheese, avg.	400	18	36
Mariachi Beef/Mariachi Chkn, avg.	405	18	37
Serious Meat	460	23	39
Vegy	365	14	38
Vegy (without Cheese)	250	5	38
Salads: Tuscan Chicken, no dress.	200	8	6
Chicken Harvest, no dressing	515	32	29

Tortilla Subs			
Big Steak Hoagy w. Sauce	585	39	19
Grilled Chicken Club	575	33	22
Meatball	810	54	28
Roasted Vegy	405	26	24
Steak & Cheese	450	23	20
Big Don: Italian	720	34	67
w. Pizza Sauce	655	26	69
Sausage Italian	1000	56	68

Individual No Dough Pizza: Per Whole Pizza			
Chicken Vegy Medley	495	29	20
Classic Trio	530	37	18
Founder's Favorite	560	38	18
Hawaiian	435	26	22
Mariachi Beef	530	34	23
Mariachi Chicken	495	30	21
Pepperoni	500	35	17
Philly Cheese Steak	520	33	19
Serious Cheese	455	31	17
Serious Meat	655	46	19
Spinach	455	29	21
Vegy	420	25	23
White	390	26	15
Works	545	37	21

For Complete Nutritional Data ~ see CalorieKing.com

Domino's® Pizza (Aug '07)

Feast Pizza Classic Hand-Tossed
14" Large: *Per Slice (⅛ Pizza)*

	C	F	Cb
America's Favorite	460	23	48
Bacon Cheeseburger	490	24	46
Barbecue Feast	460	20	53
Deluxe Feast	420	19	47
ExtravaganZZa	420	20	45
Hawaiian Feast	420	17	49
MeatZZa Feast	500	26	47
Pepperoni Feast	470	24	47
Philly Cheese Steak	420	18	44
Vegi Feast	410	17	48

Feast Pizza Crunchy Thin Crust
14" Large: *Per Slice (⅛ Pizza)*

	C	F	Cb
America's Favorite	350	24	26
Bacon Cheeseburger	380	25	24
Barbecue Feast	350	21	31
Deluxe Feast	310	20	25
ExtravaganZZa	380	26	27
Hawaiian Feast	310	18	27
MeatZZa Feast	390	27	26
Pepperoni Feast	360	25	25
Philly Cheese Steak	310	19	22
Vegi Feast	300	18	26

Feast Pizza Ultimate Deep Dish
14" Large: *Per Slice (⅛ Pizza)*

	C	F	Cb
America's Favorite	490	28	46
Bacon Cheeseburger	520	29	44
Barbecue Feast	490	25	51
Deluxe Feast	450	24	45
ExtravaganZZa	520	30	47
Hawaiian Feast	450	22	47
MeatZZa Feast	530	31	46
Pepperoni Feast	500	29	45
Philly Cheese Steak	450	23	42
Vegi Feast	440	22	46

Classic Hand-Tossed
14" Large: *Per Slice (⅛ Pizza)*

	C	F	Cb
Cheese only	290	9	42
Pepperoni	340	14	42
Ham	305	9.5	42
Sausage	350	15	44
Beef	340	15	42
Ham & Pineapple	310	9.5	45
Pepperoni & Sausage	385	17	43

Domino's® Pizza cont... (Aug '07)

Crunchy Thin Crust
14" Large: *Per Slice (⅛ Pizza)*

	C	F	Cb
Cheese only	180	9.5	20
Pepperoni	230	14	20
Ham	195	10	20
Sausage	240	15	22
Beef	230	14	20
Ham & Pineapple	200	10	22
Pepperoni & Sausage	275	18	21

Ultimate Deep Dish
14" Large: *Per Slice (⅛ Pizza)*

	C	F	Cb
Cheese only	320	14	40
Pepperoni	370	19	40
Ham	335	15	40
Sausage	380	20	42
Beef	370	19	40
Ham & Pineapple	340	15	42
Pepperoni & Sausage	415	22	41

Salads: Per Serving

	C	F	Cb
Garden Fresh, ½ container	70	4	5
Grilled Chicken Caesar	100	4.5	6
Salad Dressing: Blue Cheese	230	24	2
Creamy Caesar	210	22	2
Italian	220	23	2
Lite	20	1	2
Buttermilk Ranch	220	24	2

Side Dishes: Breadsticks (1)

	C	F	Cb
Side Dishes: Breadsticks (1)	130	7	14
Chicken Kickers (1), 0.8 oz	45	1.5	3
Buffalo Wings: Barbecue (1)	230	14	6
Hot (1)	210	14	5
Cheesy Bread (1), 1.3 oz	140	7	14
Cinna Stix (1), 1.2 oz	140	7	17
Sweet Icing, 2½ oz	250	3	57
Dipping Sauce: Blue Cheese	210	22	2
Hot	120	12	3
Marinara	25	0	5
Ranch	190	21	2
Garlic Sauce	440	50	0

For Complete Nutritional Data ~ see CalorieKing.com

Updated Nutrition Data ~ www.CalorieKing.com
Persons with Diabetes ~ See Disclaimer (Page 24)

Restaurants & Fast - Foods

Don Pablos® (Aug '07)

	C	F	Cb
***Appetizers:** Per Serving*			
Beef Taquito (1), no garnish	65	3	5
Buffalo Chicken Wings (8)	1035	78	43
Chicken Flauta (1), no garnish	65	4	6
Nachos (1 order): Taco Beef	1625	113	85
Beef Fajita	1430	99	71
Chicken Fajita	1395	87	73
***Quesadillas:** Incl. Sour Cream & Guacamole*			
Cheese Quesadilla, 8 slices	1595	99	105
Mesquite Grilled Chicken, 4 slices	665	32	55
Mesquite Grilled Steak, 8 slices	1560	91	122
Portabello Mushr. & Veges, 8 slices	1505	83	136
Primo Club, 8 slices	1745	100	114
***Dips:** Per 6 oz Cup (No Chips)*			
Queso Blanco	340	27	13
Prairie Fire Bean w. Cheese	380	25	23
Spinach	315	28	8
***Burritos (No Sides):** Chicken*	880	48	70
Beef & Bean	1390	73	123
***Chimichangas:** Includes Rice & Refritos*			
Spicy Beef Chimi De Oro	1190	63	109
Chicken Chimi	815	44	71
***Rellenos:** Beef w. Sauce/Cheese*	300	17	20
Cheese w. Sauce/Cheese	395	26	19
Chicken w. Sauce/Cheese	235	11	21
***Salads** (No Dressing):* Steak Fajita	620	35	27
Chicken Fajita	565	30	28
Traditional Taco Salad, Beef	1290	80	94
***Salad Dressing:** Per 3 oz*			
Blue Cheese	450	48	3
House Vinaigrette	355	31	10
Honey Mustard	315	27	17
Low Fat French	150	4	30
Ranch	320	34	3
***Sides:** Chips & Salsa, 1 order*	340	17	43
Guacamole, 1.5 oz	50	5	2
Mexican Rice, 3 oz	105	1	21
Refritos, 5 oz	180	6	23
Salsa, 1 oz	5	0	1
Side Salad	110	7	8
Sour Cream, 1.25 oz	75	7	2
Sour Crema, 1 oz	55	5	1
Flour Tortilla , 7"	125	4	20

Extra Menu Items ~ see CalorieKing.com

Dunkin Donuts® (Aug '07)

	C	F	Cb
Donuts			
Apple/Blueberry Crumb Donut	240	10	36
Apple N' Spice Donut	200	8	29
Black Raspberry/Strawberry Donut	210	8	32
Blueberry Crumb Donut	240	10	36
Boston Kreme Donut	240	9	36
Chocolate Coconut Cake Donut	300	19	31
Chocolate Frosted Cake Donut	360	20	40
Chocolate Frosted Donut	200	9	29
Chocolate Glazed Cake Donut	290	16	33
Cinnamon Cake Donut	330	20	34
French Cruller	150	8	17
Glazed Cake Donut	350	19	41
Jelly Filled Donut	210	8	32
Kreme Filled (Choc./Vanilla)Donut	270	13	35
Lemon Glazed/Frosted Cake Donut	240	14	28
Maple/Marble Frosted Donut, avg.	210	9	29
Old Fashioned Cake Donut	300	19	28
Powdered Cake Donut	330	19	36
Strawberry Frosted; Bavarian	210	9	30
Sugar Raised Donut	170	8	22
Whole Wheat Glazed Cake Donut	310	19	32
***Muffins:** Banana Walnut*	540	25	69
Blueberry: Regular	470	17	73
Reduced Fat	400	5	78
Chocolate Chip	630	26	89
Coffee Cake Muffin	580	19	78
Corn	510	18	77
Cranberry Orange	440	17	66
Honey Raisin Bran	480	15	79
Lemon Raspberry	460	15	75
***Danishes:** Apple*	330	20	32
Cheese	340	22	30
Strawberry Cheese	320	20	31
Fancies:			
Coffee Roll: Regular	270	14	33
Chocolate Frosted	290	15	36
Donuts: Bow Tie	300	17	34
Eclair	270	11	39
Frosted Coffee Roll	290	14	36
Choc Iced Bismark	340	15	50
Fritters, Apple/Glazed, avg.	300	14	40
Cookies: Chocolate Chunk	540	23	80
Oatmeal Raisin	480	14	83
Peanut Butter Cup	590	29	73

Continued Next Page ...

Dunkin Donuts® cont... (Aug '07)

	C	F	Cb
Bagels: *Per Bagel*			
Reduced Carb w. Cheese	380	12	45
Everything	370	6	67
Onion	320	3.5	61
Sesame	380	8	64
Salt; Plain	320	2.5	62
Cream Cheese (Per Packet): Lite	120	9	5
Average of other flavors	180	17	4
Breakfast Sandwiches			
Bagel S'wich: Ham Egg & Cheese	510	16	65
Sausage Egg & Cheese	660	35	63
Biscuit S'wich: Egg & Cheese	410	25	32
Sausage Egg & Cheese	610	43	32
Croissant S'wich: Egg & Cheese	480	31	40
Sausage Egg & Cheese	690	51	40
English Muffin S'wich: Egg & Chse	280	9	34
Ham, Egg & Cheese	310	10	34
Dunkin' Deli Sandwiches			
Cravings: Chicken Bruschetta	580	25	48
Chipotle Chicken	620	26	49
Pastrami Supreme	760	42	47
Turkey Pesto	530	23	46
Deli Classics: Ham & Swiss	360	11	44
Roast Beef & Swiss	530	25	45
Tuna	550	26	49
Turkey & Cheese	510	22	45
Vegetarian	420	21	51
Favorites: Avocado & Turkey	500	22	49
Chicken Cordon Bleu	550	19	51
Steak & Cheese	510	23	45
Toasted Italian	630	34	49
Turkey & Bacon Club	510	22	44
Paninis: Meatball	480	19	56
Southwestern Chicken	420	10	57
Steak	450	12	56
Drinks: Dunkacinno, 10 fl.oz	230	10	35
Hot Chocolate, 10 fl.oz	220	8	38
Iced Coffee: 16 fl.oz	15	0	3
w. Cream, 16 fl.oz	70	6	4
w. Milk, 16 fl.oz	35	1	4
Berry Bliss; Choc-Nilla, 16 fl.oz	90	6	8
Turbo Ice, 16 fl.ox	120	7	14
Vanilla Iced Latte Lite, 16 fl.oz	80	0	3
Vanilla Chai, 10 fl.oz	230	8	40
Smoothies: All flav., Small, 16 fl.oz	360	2.5	79
Medium, 24 fl.oz	550	4	118
Coolatta: *Per 16 fl.oz*			
Coffee Coolatta®: w. Cream	350	22	40
w. Milk	210	4	42
w. 2% Milk	190	2	41
Orange Tropicana Fruit Coolatta®	370	0	92
Strawberry Fruit Coolatta®	290	0	72
Vanilla Bean Coolatta®	440	17	70

Eat 'N Park® (Aug '07)

	C	F	Cb
Breakfast			
Apple Waffles	960	44	126
Cornbeef Hash, 7.5 oz	340	23	16
Egg Beaters Breakfast	75	0	5.5
Fruit Cup	60	0.5	15
Hash Browns, 6 oz	235	12	28
Homefries, 6 oz	210	12	24
Omelette: Cheese	390	30	2.5
Ham & Cheese	465	32	3
Supreme	420	30	9
Pancake, Plain (1)	225	3	43
Burgers: American Grill	790	51	31
Bacon & Cheddar	1035	69	50
Classic Burger	815	50	40
Classic Cheeseburger	975	64	41
Mushroom & Onion	885	56	44
Superburger	705	49	38
Swiss Burger	580	32	34
Swiss, Mushroom & Onion	880	55	45
Turkey Burger	500	22	36
Sandwiches: Tuna Melt	610	41	35
Bacon Turkey Swiss	525	37	16
Chicken Bacon Deluxe	565	23	50
Chicken (Breaded)	515	19	50
Chicken Chargrill/Spicy, 4 oz	350	7	39
Chicken Fiesta, 4 oz	430	13	41
Grilled Cheese	505	36	26
Hot Roast Beef	310	6.5	33
Hot Turkey	260	5	27
PA Dutch Ham & Swiss	570	30	35
Reuben	720	49	31
Steak'n Cheese	765	50	43
Turkey Club	770	44	49
Turkey Pastrami	715	46	40
Croissants, Chicken Salad; Tuna	595	39	36
Pita: Chicken Fajita	620	19	68
Tuna	640	26	72
Turkey	445	5	67
Appetizers: Cheese Fries	880	50	93
Cheese Sticks	410	25	17
Onion Rings	210	13	19
Wings, all flavors	400	28	0.5

**For Data Updates,
Check Author's Website
www.CalorieKing.com**

Eat 'N Park® cont... (Aug '07)

	C	F	Cb
Meals: Chicken Breast, stuffed	370	17	27
Chicken Fillets (5)	530	26	28
Chicken Parmigiana: Marinara	840	33	90
Meat Sauce	900	38	86
Chicken Stir-Fry	555	25	47
Country Fried Chicken Steak	790	40	43
Rib-Eye	615	42	1
Scrod Floridian, 4 oz	120	1.5	4
Spaghetti Marinara	620	8	120
Veal Parmigiana w. Meat Sauce	820	26	107
Ziti w. Meat Balls	960	42	102
Salads & Dressings			
Buffalo Chicken Salad	605	42	42
Chicken Caesar Salad	270	9	16
Chicken Portabella Salad	320	11	23
Garden Salad	100	3	16
Spinach & Chicken	375	17	9
Taco Salad	805	41	70
Dressings: Bleu Cheese, 2 Tbsp	90	7	7
French Fat Free	70	0	17
Italian Fat Free	10	0	3
House, 2 Tbsp	115	11	2.5
Thousand Island , 2 Tbsp	95	10	3
Desserts: Cheesecake, Plain	505	36	40
Banana Fudge Sensation	975	44	147
Grilled Sticky A La Mode	730	39	81
Ice Cream, 2 scoops	285	16	33
Pies: Apple (NAS)	340	10	61
Peach (NAS)	300	10	50
Chocolate Pudding (Sugar Free)	90	2.5	13
Strawberry Shortcake	685	26	114

Edo Japan® (Aug '07)

Meals: Per Regular Serving	C	F	Cb
Beef Yakisoba	575	26	54
Chicken & Beef	560	17	68
Chicken Yakisoba	430	6	52
Curry Chicken	395	5	87
Ginger Pork	520	10	71
Grilled Vegetables	325	1	71
Hawaiian Chicken	500	7.5	71
Seafood Grill	495	8	73
Sukiyaki Beef	635	26	68
Teriyaki Chicken	490	7.5	68
Teriyaki Shrimp	465	6	72

Einstein Bros®/Noahs® (Aug '07)

	C	F	Cb
Bagels: Average, 4.2 oz	350	1	75
Chocolate Chip Bagel, 4 oz	370	3	76
Egg Bagel	340	3	69
Sesame Dip'd	380	5	75
Cream Cheese Shmear: Plain, 2 T.	70	7	1
Plain Reduced Fat, 2 Tbsp	60	5	2
Smoked Salmon, 2 Tbsp	65	6	2
Flavors, average, 2 Tbsp	70	5	2
Spreads: Fruit, 2 Tbsp	75	0	19
Honey Butter, 1 Tbsp	90	8	4
Peanut Butter, 2 Tbsp	190	15	8
Breakfast Sandwiches			
Lox & Bagel Sandwich	660	27	79
Spicy Elmo Egg Sandwich	650	35	50
Bagel Omelet Sandwiches:			
Black Forest Ham & Swiss	660	21	76
Cheddar	590	20	74
Santa Fe	720	28	78
Smoked Bacon & Cheddar	680	26	75
Turkey Sausage & Cheddar	660	23	74
Grilled Panini Omelet Sandwiches:			
Spinach & Bacon	930	49	72
Steak & Egg Ranchero	690	27	67
Sandwiches			
Grilled Panini: Cheese Steak	690	29	69
Country Cheese	540	20	49
Italian Chicken	690	27	68
Signature: Club Mex on Challah	730	38	60
Einstein Club on Grilled White	670	29	54
Tasty Turkey on Asiago Bagel	600	18	81
Veg Out on Sesame Bagel	500	13	82
Salads: Asiago Chicken Caesar	740	54	25
Bros Bistro	810	69	37
Chicken Chipotle	630	40	38
Soups: Per Bowl (14 oz)			
Broccoli Sharp Cheddar	380	23	43
Crab Chowder	520	38	30
Chicken Noodle	160	7	13
Cookies: Chocolate Chip	520	24	68
Trail Mix	480	19	70
Coffee: Cafe Latte, 12 fl.oz	140	5	13
Cappuccino, 12 fl.oz	90	3.5	9

Fast - Foods & *Restaurants*

El Pollo Loco® (Aug '07)

	C	F	Cb
Flame-Grilled Chicken			
Chicken Breast w. Skin	225	9	0
Leg	80	4	0
Thigh	215	14	0
Wing	90	5	0
Burritos			
Classic: BRC	390	10	61
Classic Chicken	500	14	63
Grilled Signature: Twice Grilled	770	37	58
Ultimate Grilled	620	20	80
Bowls: Caesar	495	25	46
Chicken Tostada w. Shell	805	40	77
Original Pollo	500	4	84
Ultimate Pollo	820	25	90
Loco Favorites			
Cheese Quesadilla	420	23	35
Chicken Nachos	1060	55	98
Chicken Quesadilla	565	27	53
Chicken Taquitos w. Salsa	250	14	23
Taco Al Carbon	155	5	17
Salads: Per Serving (no Dressing)			
Pollo Caesar	205	9	16
Loco	60	3	7
Tostada w. Shell	625	30	71
Tostada Salad no Shell	245	5	41
Side Dishes: Per Individual Serving			
Cole Slaw, 5 oz	205	16	12
Corn Cobbette, 3 oz	40	0	10
French Fries, 5.5 oz	445	19	61
Fresh Vegetables, 4 oz	70	4	6
Garden Salad, 4.8 oz	120	11	9
Pinto Beans, 6 oz	155	4	24
Spanish Rice, 4 oz	160	1	33
Tortilla Chips, small, 2 oz	395	21	50
Tortillas: 6" Corn (3) 3 oz	210	3	42
6½" Flour (3), 3 oz	330	12	48
Condiments			
Dressings: Light Cilantro	70	5	6
Creamy Cilantro	220	23	2
Guacamole, 1.7 oz	75	6	6
Jalapeno Hot Sauce, 0.3 oz pkg	5	0	1
Sour Cream	105	10	2
Salsa: Avocado	30	2	2
Chipotle; House	5	0	1
Pico de Gallo	10	0	2
Desserts: Churro (2)	415	25	43
Caramel Flan, 5.5 oz	305	12	46
Soft Serve, Regular, 5 oz	300	8	48

For Complete Nutritional Data ~ see CalorieKing.com

Fatburger® (Aug '07)

	C	F	Cb
Burgers: Baby Fat	300	15	24
Bacon & Egg Sandwich	440	27	31
Chicken Sandwich	360	13	32
Chili Dog	510	26	45
Fatburger	520	29	32
Fatburger w. Cheese	590	35	39
Kingburger	820	41	64
Kingburger w. Cheese	890	47	64
Turkey Burger	550	31	38
Shakes (17 fl.oz): Vanilla	820	34	116
Chocolate, Strawberry, average	910	40	124
Fries & Sides: Chili Cup, 7.6 oz	270	15	13
Fat Fries, 8 oz	550	26	72
Skinny Fries, 5.5 oz	490	20	71
Onion Rings, 5.5 oz	510	29	57

For Complete Nutritional Data ~ see CalorieKing.com

Fazoli's® Italian Food (Aug '07)

	C	F	Cb
Classic Pasta Bowl: Per Serving			
Classic Sampler Platter	810	25	110
Classic Ziti w. Meat Sauce, regular	700	22	95
Classic Ziti w. Meat Sauce, small	480	15	65
Ravioli w. Marinara Sauce	500	15	71
Ravioli w. Meat Sauce	550	20	71
Six Layer Lasagna	630	23	75
Six Layer Lasagna w. Broccoli	690	28	79
Spaghetti w. Marinara Sauce, reg.	670	4	132
Ultimate Sampler Platter	980	29	134
Oven-Baked Pasta: Per Serving			
Baked Chicken Parmesan	960	33	117
Baked Spaghetti	680	22	90
Baked Spaghetti w. Meatballs	940	40	100
Twice Baked Lasagna	800	36	78
Twice Baked Ziti	830	37	76
Paninis: Four Cheese & Tomato	500	21	51
Grilled Chicken	440	8	53
Smoked Turkey	610	28	52
Pizzas: Per Serving			
Double Slice, Cheese	500	20	57
Double Slice, Pepperoni	560	25	57
Mega Slice, Cheese	750	30	85
Mega Slice, Pepperoni	840	38	85

Updated Nutrition Data ~ www.CalorieKing.com
Persons with Diabetes ~ See Disclaimer (Page 24)

Fazoli's® cont... (Aug '07)

Submarinos (7")

	C	F	Cb
Club	820	31	95
Ham n' Swiss	760	25	95
Original	1180	67	94

Salads: Dressing Not Included

	C	F	Cb
Garden Side Salad	25	0	4
Caesar Side Salad	40	2	4
Chicken Caesar Salad	200	7	14
Chicken and Pasta Caesar Salad	440	15	41
Grilled Chicken Salad	100	2	6
Italian Market Salad	620	41	32
Pasta Side Salad	320	12	41

Salad Dressing: Italian Dressing

	C	F	Cb
Italian Dressing	160	14	7
Fat Free Honey Mustard	60	0	15
Caesar Dressing	230	25	1
Honey French	220	18	14
Thousand Island	210	20	6
Ranch Dressing	220	24	2
Lite Ranch Dressing	120	12	2

Breadsticks, Soup, Meatballs

	C	F	Cb
Breadstick (1), dry	100	1.5	20
Minestrone Soup, small bowl	90	2	19

Desserts

	C	F	Cb
Chocolate Chunk Cookie	510	26	68
Cheesecake: Original	290	22	17
Turtle	450	28	43
Freezi's, average all flavors	380	3.5	92

Kids Meals: Lasagna

	C	F	Cb
Lasagna	260	13	21
Fettuccine Alfredo	290	5	50
Cheese Ravioli w. Meat Sauce	300	8	42
Pizza: Cheese	270	11	31
Pepperoni	310	14	31
Spaghetti: w. Meatballs	350	7	55
w. Marinara or Meat Sauce, avg.	270	2	53

For Complete Nutritional Data ~ see CalorieKing.com

Fox's Pizza Den® (Aug '07)

12" Pizzas: Per Slice (⅛ Pizza)

	C	F	Cb
Cheese	155	5	21
Pepperoni	180	7	21

16" Pizzas: Per Slice (1⁄10 pizza)

	C	F	Cb
Cheese	220	7	30
Pepperoni	250	9	30

Firehouse Subs® (Aug '07)

Subs: Per Medium

	C	F	Cb
Chicken Salad	760	46	63
Engine Company	385	7	56
Engineer	380	14	61
Ham Sub	430	7	62
Hero Sub	460	12	61
Hook & Ladder	400	10	60
Italian Sub	660	31	60
NY Steamer	520	20	56
Roast Beef	400	8	56
Tuna Salad	610	28	62
Turkey Sub	370	4	58
Veggie Sub	370	11	60

Freshens® (Aug '07)

Frozen Yogurt: Per Serving

	C	F	Cb
Soft Serve Yogurt, 1 oz	25	0.5	5

Ice Creams

	C	F	Cb
Hand Dipped Ice Cream, ½ cup	150	12	21

Smoothies: Per Container (21 fl.oz)

	C	F	Cb
All That Razz	360	0	79
Berry Breeze	305	0	77
Blueberry Bay	375	0	81
Caribbean Craze	290	0	73
Fitness Fuel	520	5	81
Jamaican Jammer	355	0	78
Mango Beach	90	0	48
Maui Mango	290	0	74
Mystic Mango	355	3	82
Orange: Shooter	335	3	77
Sunrise	355	3	81
Peach: Passion	150	0	32
Sunset	270	0	60
Peachy Pineapple	325	0	69
Pina Collider	430	4	88
Pineapple Paradise	330	4	77
Raspberry Royale	270	0	67
Strawberry: Oasis	80	0	49
Shooter	245	0	64
Squeeze	315	0	68
Sunrise	155	0	35

Snacks: Per Serving (3 oz)

	C	F	Cb
Pretzel Logic: Gourmet Bites	115	9	4
Gourmet Pretzels, ½ pretzel	255	3	49

Fast - Foods & *Restaurants*

Frisch's Big Boy® (Aug '07)

	C	F	Cb
***Breakfast: HealthSmart,** Egg Beaters,*			
Plain Omelette	310	8.5	38
Scrambled	310	8.5	38
Vegetarian Omelette	340	8.5	45
***Health Smart Meals:** Tossed Salad*	45	0.5	6
Grilled Chicken Breast	325	10	22
Lemon Baked Cod	490	4.5	72
Spaghetti Marinara	420	6.5	76
Vegetable Stir-Fry	610	3.5	134
***Sandwiches:** Big Boy*	600	26	35
Brawny Lad	420	21	30
Buddie Boy	760	34	80
Fish Sandwich	690	48	41
Small Hamburger	445	30	30
Super Big Boy	830	66	35
Swiss Miss	635	44	28
***Sides:** Chili*	315	18	19
French Fries	360	19	45
Onion Rings	580	41	45
Tartare Sauce	370	40	1
Trio Salad	620	46	18
***Soups:** HealthSmart Cabbage Soup*	50	0.5	9
***Beverages:** HealthSmart Shake*	160	0	33

Gold Star Chili® (Aug '07)

Meals
	C	F	Cb
Bowls: Low Carb Coney, 10.4 oz	570	47	7
Veggie Chili, 9 oz	160	2	29
Coney	285	14	30
Cheese Coney, 5.6 oz	345	18	31
Chili, 8 oz	215	12	8
Chili Cheese Nachos, 8½ oz	410	25	30
Chili Cheese Sandwich	290	12	30
Chili Sandwich	210	5	32
Regular 2-Way	420	11	58
Bean	490	12	71
Onion	435	11	62
Onion Bean	505	12	75
Regular 3-Way	650	30	59
Regular 4-Way	665	30	63
Regular 5-Way	735	30	76
Super 5-Way	1140	51	109
Tex Mex, 8 oz	210	9	17
***Sides:** Fries, 5 oz*	365	19	44
Garlic Bread: Without Cheese, 2 oz	215	13	19
w. Cheese, 2½ oz	270	18	19
Side Salad	70	5	2

Gino's East® (Aug '07)

	C	F	Cb
***Deep Dish Pizza:** Medium 11" ~ Per Slice (⅙ Pizza)*			
Cheese	410	11	58
Crumbled Sausage	420	21	38
Pepperoni	450	15	57
Spinach	410	11	59
***Deep Dish Pizza:** Small 6" ~ Per Whole Pizza*			
Cheese	720	16	116
Crumbled Sausage	800	22	116
Pepperoni	780	20	116

Golden Corral® (Aug '07)

Meals
	C	F	Cb
Bourbon Street Chicken, 3.5 oz	210	11	5
Fish Fillet Cajun Style, 2 pces	210	10	18
Fresh Fried Chkn, Leg or Thigh (1)	250	19	2
Meatloaf, 3.5 oz	190	10	10
Sirloin Steak, Buffet, 3 oz	220	13	0
Steakburgers, Lunch, 6 oz	860	55	0
Turkey Breast w. Wing, 2 oz	70	3	1
Whitefish Cajun, 3 oz	110	7	0
***Sides:** Baked Potato, plain (1)*	110	0	25
Glazed Sesame Carrots	260	16	27
Macaroni Salad, ½ cup	190	8	26

Godfather's™ Pizza (Aug '07)

	C	F	Cb
***Golden Pizza:** Per Slice*			
Cheese: Medium, ⅛ pizza	220	8	26
Large, 1/10 pizza	250	9	28
Combo: Medium, ⅛ pizza	290	13	28
Large, slice, 1/10 pizza	330	15	30
Original Pizza			
Cheese: Mini, ¼ pizza	150	4	20
Medium, ⅛ pizza	260	7	34
Jumbo, 1/10 pizza	430	13	53
Combo: Mini, ¼ pizza	210	8	22
Medium, ⅛ pizza	350	14	37
Jumbo, 1/10 pizza	580	24	57
Thin Pizza			
Cheese: Medium, ⅛ pizza	180	8	16
Large, 1/10 pizza	220	10	19
Combo: Medium, ⅛ pizza	250	13	18
Large, 1/10 pizza	290	16	21
Sides			
Breadstick (1)	80	2	14
Cheesestick, 1 piece, ⅙ whole	130	3.5	18
Choc. Chip Cookie, slice, ⅛ whole	195	8	30
Potato Wedges, 4 oz	190	9	24

Updated Nutrition Data ~ www.CalorieKing.com
Persons with Diabetes ~ See Disclaimer (Page 24)

(The) Great American Bagel Co® (Aug '07) Ⓒ Ⓕ Ⓒb

	C	F	Cb
Bagels: Plain	390	1.5	85
4-Grain Honey; Cinn. Raisin	420	1.5	88
Apple/Blueberry Crumb, average	570	8	106
Banana Nut; Cheddar Herb, avg.	410	5	82
Blueberry; Onion; Strawberry	380	1	83
Cheddar Salsa	430	11	83
Cheese Twist	740	20	107
Chocolate Chip	390	4	75
Cinnamon Sugar; Egg	390	2	83
Cranb. Nut; P'nut Butter Choc Chip	400	6	72
Jalapeno Cheddar	330	4.5	58
Pumpernickel; Pumpkin, average	330	1.5	72
Pumpkin Chocolate Chip	350	3.5	67
Spinach Herb	300	1	60
Stuffed Pepperoni	500	12	74
Stuffed Spinach	720	22	98
Sun-Dried Tomato Basil	390	1.5	75
Other varieties, average	370	2	75

Green Burrito (Aug '07)

Burritos: Bean & Cheese	760	36	87
Grilled Chicken	1030	52	91
Meat Bean & Cheese: Chicken	660	28	67
Ground Beef	820	43	71
Steak	700	31	68
The Green Burrito w. Steak	920	34	117
Sides: Chips, 2 oz	300	15	75
Chips & Cheese, 5 oz	690	40	133
Guacamole, 1.4 oz	50	3	6
Green Sauce w. Jack & Cheese	400	27	43
Make Any Entree a Plate			
Beans Rice & Tortilla Chips	440	17	85
Pinto Beans & Cheese	330	16	43
Rice, 5 oz	220	3.5	43
Sour Cream, 1.4 oz	50	3.5	3
Specialties: Enchiladas w. Cheese	420	26	31
Super Nachos: Chicken; Steak	1020	56	165
Ground Beef	1170	70	167
Taco Salad: Chicken	790	45	68
Ground Beef	950	59	71
Steak	830	47	68
Taquitos: Chicken, 2 taquitos	160	8	18
Chicken, 5 taquitos	370	17	42
Tacos: Fish, 6 oz	290	14	34
Hard: Chicken; Steak	200	11	14
Ground Beef	300	19	16
Soft: Chicken	200	8	19
Ground Beef	270	14	20

(The) Great Steak & Potato Company® (Aug '07)

Sandwiches	C	F	Cb
Cheeseburger, Kids	350	19	20
Chicken Philly	715	34	64
Chicken Teriyaki	760	34	74
Ham Delight	675	31	63
Ham Explosion	530	15	63
Phillyburger	615	41	23
Super Steak	710	34	60
Turkey Philly	640	28	60
Veggie Delight	700	38	62
Sides: Per Serving			
Bacon, 2 slices	85	4	1
Chicken Nuggets, Kids, 2.8 oz	185	10	11
Fries: Kids, 11.5 oz	850	44	128
Small, 13.9 oz	1065	55	142
Regular, 15.6 oz	1195	62	159
Large, 27.5 oz	2105	109	281
Potato Skins, 7 oz	755	57	54
Potato, Plain, 10.5 oz	215	0	45
Meat: Per Serving (Sides Not Included)			
Chicken, 5 oz	125	1	1
Gyro, 4 oz	280	29	14
Ham, 4 oz	165	6	2
Salami, 2 oz	145	11	1
Steak, 4 oz	140	6	0
Turkey, 4 oz	155	1	0
Salad: Chef Salad	300	12	9
Tossed Salad	40	0	8
Side Salad	20	0	4
Vegetables: Broccoli, 3 oz	25	0	4
Other vegetables, avg., 1 serving	10	0	2
Salad Dressings: Per Serving			
Low-Cal Mayo, ½ oz	40	4	1
Mayonnaise, ½ oz	100	11	0
Sauces: Cheese, 2 oz	80	5	0
Teriyaki Glaze, 1.2 oz	45	0	10
Tzatziki, 1 oz	90	9	1
Bun: Regular Bun, 3.5 oz	290	3	55
Large Bun, 5 oz	380	4	72
Pita, 3 oz	165	1	33
Drinks: Medium, 16 fl.oz			
Lemonade	210	0	56
Mountain Dew	240	0	59
Pepsi; Sierra Mist	210	0	54

Fast - Foods & *Restaurants*

Haagen-Dazs® (Aug '07)

Ice Cream: Per ½ Cup

	C	F	Cb
Baileys Irish Cream	270	17	23
Banana Split	280	16	31
Butter Pecan	310	23	21
Cherry Vanilla	240	15	23
Chocolate	270	18	22
Chocolate Chip Cookie Dough	310	20	29
Chocolate Peanut Butter	360	24	27
Coffee; Cookies & cream	270	18	23
Macadamia Brittle	300	20	25
Mango	250	14	28
Mint Chip	300	19	26
Pistachio	290	20	22
Strawberry	250	16	23
Triple Chocolate	330	21	31
Vanilla	270	18	21
White Chocolate Raspberry Truffle	310	18	32

Extra Flavors ~ See CalorieKing.com

Light Ice Cream: Dutch Chocolate

	C	F	Cb
Dutch Chocolate	190	5	33
Pineapple Coconut	210	4.5	37
Other varieties, average	220	7	33
Sorbet: Chocolate, Low-Fat	130	0.5	28
Coconut	160	16	25
Zesty Lemon	110	0	28
Fat-Free: Mango	120	0	37
Orchard Peach	130	0	33
Raspberry	120	0	30
Strawberry	120	0	30
Tropical	150	0	38

Frozen Yogurt: Per ½ Cup

	C	F	Cb
Chocolate Fudge Brownie	200	2.5	35
Coffee; Vanilla; avg.	200	4.5	31
Strawberry Fat Free	140	0	31
Strawberry Banana	160	2	32
Vanilla Raspberry Swirl	170	2.5	32
Wildberry	180	2	34
Low-Fat: Coffee; Vanilla	200	4.5	31
Dulce de Leche	190	2.5	35

Ice Cream Bars ~ See Page 37

Hardee's® (Aug '07)

Breakfast

	C	F	Cb
Big Country Platter: Bacon	980	56	90
Chicken	1140	61	105
Country Steak	1150	68	98
Biscuit: Egg	450	29	35
Bacon, Egg & Cheese	560	38	37
Country Ham	440	26	36
Breakfast Sandwiches: Frisco	420	20	37
Smoked Sausage	710	54	30
Loaded Breakfast Burrito	780	51	38
Loaded Omelet	270	21	2
Low Carb Breakfast Bowl	620	50	6
Sunrise Croissant with Ham	430	26	28

Hardee's® cont... (Aug '07)

Sandwiches: (Lunch/Dinner)

	C	F	Cb
Chicken Sandwiches: Spicy Chkn	470	26	46
Big Chicken Filet	850	42	76
Buffalo Chicken	780	36	74
Charbroiled BBQ Chicken	415	5	58
Charbroiled Chicken Club	560	30	33
Hot Ham N Cheese	420	18	39
Big Hot Ham N Cheese	520	24	40
Regular Roast Beef Sandwich	330	16	29
Big Roast Beef Sandwich	470	23	38
Cheeseburger ⅓ lb	680	39	52
Double Cheeseburger ¼ lb	510	26	38
Hamburger	310	12	36
Double Hamburger ¼lb	420	19	37
Fish Supreme Sandwich	500	27	38
Hot Dog	420	30	22
Six Dollar Burger ½ lb	1060	72	60
Thickburger: Original, ⅓ lb	850	57	54
Double Thickburger, ⅔ lb	1240	90	55
Grilled Sourdough, ½ lb	1080	82	42
Bacon Cheese, ⅓ lb	910	63	50
Double Bacon Cheese,⅔ lb	1300	96	51
Mushroom N Swiss, ⅓ lb	720	42	48
Monster, ⅔ lb	1410	107	47
Low Carb, ⅓ lb	420	32	5
Kids Meals: Hamburger w. Kids Fries	560	24	67
Cheeseburger w. Kids Fries	600	27	68
2 Chicken Strips w. Kids Fries	500	25	50
Fried Chicken: Breast portion	370	15	29
Leg portion	170	7	15
Thigh portion	330	15	30
Wing portion	200	8	23
Sides: Chili Cheese Fries	850	48	76
Crispy Curls: Small, 4 oz	340	17	43
Medium, 4.7 oz	410	20	52
Chicken Strips (3), 5 oz	380	21	27
Chicken Strips (5), 8.5 oz	630	34	45
Coleslaw, small, 4 oz	170	10	20
French Fries: Kids, 2.8 oz	250	12	32
Small, 4.4 oz	390	19	51
Medium, 5.9 oz	520	24	67
Large, 6.7 oz	610	28	78
Mashed Potato & Gravy, small	90	2	17
Dessert: Apple Turnover	290	15	36
Chocolate Chip Cookie	290	11	44
Shakes: Average all flavors, 16 fl.oz	700	33	86
Malts: Average all flavors, 16 fl.oz	780	35	91

Extra Menu Items ~ see CalorieKing.com

Restaurants & Fast - Foods

Harvey's® (Aug '07)

Sandwiches & Burgers	C	F	Cb
Angus Burger	390	17	34
Angus Burger w. Cheese	440	21	35
Angus Patty, By Itself, 1 patty	215	15	4
Cheeseburger	440	23	35
Hamburger	380	18	35
Grilled Chicken Sandwich	340	6	52
VeggieBurger	315	9	39
Patty: Original, By Itself, 1 patty	210	16	4
VeggieBurger, By Itself, 1 patty	150	7	7
Sides			
French Fries: Large, 5.3 oz	400	17	58
Regular, 4.2 oz	320	14	47
Value, 3.1 oz	240	10	35
Gravy, 3.2 oz	35	1	5
Onion Rings: Large, 4.3 oz	420	21	52
Regular, 2.8 oz	280	14	35
Poutine	640	33	67
Salads: Dressing Not Included			
Garden Salad	40	0	8
Entree. Chicken Salad	140	1.5	16
Garden Salad	70	0.5	16
Salad Dressings			
Creamy Caesar	140	14	2
Creamy Garlic Peppercorn Ranch	140	14	2
Fat-Free Honey Dijon	50	0	12
Light Italian	60	4	6
Sauces			
Barbecue Sauce	50	0	12
Ketchup	10	0	2
Light Mayonnaise, ½ oz	45	5	1
Spicy Buffalo, 1 oz	50	3.5	1
Dipping: Barbecue	90	0	21
Honey Mustard	160	12	13
Plum	125	0	33
Sweet n' Sour	80	0.5	17
Breakfast: Bacon, 3 Strips	40	2	0
Extra Egg (1)	90	6	0
Homefries	300	19	29
Sandwich: Breakfast Club	440	22	33
Breakfast Club Deluxe	480	24	33
Sausage (1)	130	9	3
Toast: White, 2 slices	180	2	35
Whole Wheat, 2 slices	170	2	32
Chicken: Chicken Strips, 3 pieces	310	16	24
Patty, Grilled, By Itself, 1 patty	170	4	1
Hot Dogs: Regular: w. Bun	320	14	34
Regular, By Itself	160	12	3

Hogi Yogi® (Aug '07)

Frozen Yogurt: Per ½ Cup	C	F	Cb
Chocolate Base, 2.5 oz	80	0	17
Vanilla (No Sugar Added): Base, 2.6 oz	100	0	22
Regular Sandwiches: Club	340	5	47
BBQ Chicken	360	4.5	59
Roast Beef	300	4.5	46
Smokey Turkey	320	3	46
Turkey	290	3	57
Vegetarian	240	2.5	45
Smoothies: Per 24 oz			
Berry Blast	310	0	70
Fruit Safari	370	3.5	84
Jungle Mist	430	4	101
Peach Treat	430	0	105
Pina Collision	450	4.5	105
Pure Passion	430	4	99
Ragin Rasberry	370	3.5	84
Strawberry Kist	420	0.5	98

Hot Dog on a Stick® (Aug '07)

Menu Items	C	F	Cb
Hot Dog on a Bun	470	26	41
Hot Dog on a Stick	250	14	23
Veggie Dog	180	3	24
American Cheese on a Stick	240	13	22
Pepper Jack Cheese on a Stick	240	13	21
French Fries, 7 oz	700	37	83
Lemonade (12 fl.oz): Original	135	0	34
Cherry/Lime, average	170	0	42
Sugar Free Lemonade	10	0	2

Hot Stuff Pizza® (Aug '07)

	C	F	Cb
Pizza: Per Slice (⅛ Medium or ¹⁄₁₀ Large)			
Beef	320	12	34
Canadian Bacon	320	11	25
Cheese	350	12	25
Double Pepperoni	390	18	37
Garden Style	300	11	34
Italian Sausage	340	15	37
Masterpiece Supreme	330	14	34
Pepperoni	350	14	37
Pork Sausage	340	15	33
Western Omelet	320	15	30

Hungry Howie's Pizza® (Aug '07)

	C	F	Cb
Pizzas: Per Slice (Cheese Only)			
Small, ⅛ pizza	160	3.5	20
Medium, ⅛ pizza	190	5.5	23
Large, ⅒ pizza	210	5	25
X-Large, ⅛ pizza	395	9.5	42
Calzone Subs: Pizza, ½ sub	690	34	67
Deluxe Italian, ½ sub	505	18	61
Sides: Chicken Tenders, 2 pieces	140	4.5	11
Howie Wings, 5 wings	180	13	0
Toppings: Per Slice (For Medium or Large Pizza)			
Anchovies	55	3	0
Bacon	40	0.5	0.5
Banana Peppers	10	0	1.5
Beef; Pepperoni; Sausage	30	2	0.5
Black Olives; Green Olives	10	0.5	0.5
Green Peppers; Mushroom	0	0	0.5
Ham	5	0.5	0
Onions	5	1	0.5
Pineapple	5	0.5	1.5

I Can't Believe It's Yogurt® (Aug '07)

	C	F	Cb
Original Frozen Yogurt: Per Serving (4 oz)			
Chocolate; Vanilla	140	8	17
Strawberry	150	7	19
Low-Fat Frozen Yogurt: Per Bar (5.5 oz)			
Chocolate	120	2.5	23
Smoothies: Per Serving (8.5 oz)			
Ana-Bana-Berry	80	0	21
Might Berry	130	0.5	30
Raspberry Rush	110	0.5	26
Strawbapple; Strawberry Skinny	60	0	16
Strawberry Banana	130	0.5	30

In-N-Out Burger® (Aug '07)

	C	F	Cb
Burgers: Hamburger w. Onion	390	19	39
w. Mustard/Ketchup, no Spread	310	10	41
Protein Style, no Bun	240	17	11
Cheeseburger w. Onion	480	27	39
w. Mustard/Ketchup, no Spread	400	18	41
Protein Style, no Bun	330	25	11
Double Double® (2 patty/2 sl. chse)	670	41	39
w. Mustard/Ketchup, no Spread	590	32	41
Protein Style, no Bun	520	39	11
French Fries, 4.4 oz	400	18	54
Drinks: Milk, 10 fl.oz	180	6	18
Coca-Cola®; Dr. Pepper, 16 fl.oz	200	0	54
Lemonade, 16 fl.oz	180	0	40
Root Beer; Seven-Up® 16 fl.oz	220	0	54
Shakes, average all flavors, 15 fl.oz	690	36	83

For Complete Nutritional Data ~ see CalorieKing.com

IHOP® (Aug '07)

	C	F	Cb
Pancakes: (Syrup/Butter extra)			
Buttermilk (1), 1.7 oz	110	3	17
Short Stack, 3	330	9	51
Full Stack, 5	550	15	85
Country Griddle Cakes (1), 2 oz	120	3.5	19
Harvest Grain 'N Nut (1) 2¼ oz	180	9	20
Crepe-Style, 2 oz	120	6	14
Syrup: 1 Tbsp	50	0	12
Whipped Butter, 1 Tbsp	80	9	0
Waffles (Plain): Regular (1), 3 oz	310	15	37
Belgian, Regular (1), 4 oz	390	19	48
Breakfast: Per Serving			
Classic Combos: Cntry Fried Steak/Eggs	1530	105	73
Fruity Country Griddle Cakes Combo	960	56	83
Harvest Grain 'N Nut Combo	1035	65	80
T-Bone Steak & Eggs	1310	86	63
Signature, Rooty Tooty Fresh & Fruity, average all flavors	855	45	84
Omlette Feast			
Colorado Omelette: No pancakes	790	68	5
with 3 buttermilk pancakes	1205	83	66
The Big Steak Omelette: No pancakes	910	72	14
with 3 buttermilk pancakes	1325	87	75
Burgers			
Sourdough Bacon Burger Melt:			
Burger Only	690	41	37
with French Fries	1265	74	104
with Onion Rings	1230	88	64
with Salad & 2½ T. Reg. Dress.	870	56	47
Entrees: Old Fashioned Pot Roast	765	48	30
with Mashed Potatoes	965	53	65
Salad: Southwestern Chicken Fajita,			
with Tortilla Shell	1110	85	48
no Tortilla Shell	890	67	35

Jack's® (Aug '07)

	C	F	Cb
Sandwiches: Big Bacon Burger	700	42	45
Big Jack Burger	500	27	40
Chicken Fillet Sandwich	640	31	69
Double Big Jack Cheese Burger	930	60	43
Double Cheeseburger	590	33	37
Grilled Chicken	410	15	44
Hamburger	270	8	35
Sides: Brown Gravy, 1 oz	10	0	2
Coleslaw, 4 oz	210	16	17
Green Beans, 4 oz	25	0	5
Mashed Potatoes, 4 oz	70	0.5	15

For Complete Nutritional Data ~ see CalorieKing.com

Jack in the Box® (Aug '07)

Breakfast	**C**	**F**	**Cb**
Biscuit: Bacon, Egg & Cheese	430	25	34
Sausage	440	29	32
Sausage, Egg & Cheese	740	55	35
Spicy Chicken	460	22	44
Breakfast Jack: Regular	290	12	29
w. Sausage	450	28	29
Sourdough	420	24	31
Ultimate	570	27	49
Croissant: Sausage	580	39	37
Supreme	450	25	36
Extreme Sausage Sandwich	670	48	31
Hash Browns (1), 2 oz	150	10	13
Meaty Burrito,No Salsa	480	29	29
Sandwiches & Burgers			
Bacon Bacon Cheeseburger	840	56	51
Bacon Ultimate Cheeseburger	1090	77	53
Junior Bacon Cheeseburger	430	25	30
Ultimate Cheeseburger	1010	71	53
Hamburger	310	14	30
Hamburger w. Cheese	350	17	31
Deluxe Hamburger: No Cheese	370	21	31
w. Cheese	460	28	33
Jumbo Jack: Regular	600	35	51
w. Cheese	690	42	54
Sourdough Jack	710	51	36
Chicken & Fish			
Bacon Chicken Sandwich	440	24	39
Chicken Breast Strips (4)	500	25	36
Chicken Fajita Pita, no salsa	300	10	31
Chicken Sandwich	400	21	38
Ciabatta: Bruschetta Chicken	640	24	67
Grilled Chicken Chipotle	690	28	65
Fish & Chips, medium, 8.8 oz	660	35	67
Jack's Spicy Chicken Sandwich	620	31	61
w. Cheese	700	37	62
Sourdough Grilled Chicken Club	530	28	34
Southwest Chicken Pita, no salsa	230	3.5	34
Tacos & Snacks			
Bacon Cheddar Potato Wedges	720	48	52
Beef Taco (1), regular	160	8	15
Egg Rolls (3)	390	18	45
Monster Beef Taco (1)	240	14	20
Stuffed Jalapenos (3)	225	13	22

Jack in the Box® cont... (Aug '07)

Fries & Rings	**C**	**F**	**Cb**
Natural Cut Fries: Medium, 5.9 oz	450	23	54
Kids portion, 2.8 oz	210	10	28
Seasoned Curly Fries, med., 4.4 oz	405	23	44
Onion Rings (8), 4.2 oz	500	30	51
Salads: No Dressing or Condiments			
Asian Chicken	160	1.5	5
Chicken Club	320	16	4
Side Salad	50	3	2
Southwest Chicken	365	14	8
Sauces & Dressings			
Dipping Sauce: Barbecue, 1 oz	45	0	11
Buttermilk House, 1 oz	130	13	3
Frank's Red Hot Buffalo, 1 oz	10	0	2
Sweet & Sour, 1 oz	45	0	11
Tartar, 1½ oz	210	22	2
Sauce: Mayo-Onion, ½ oz	90	10	1
Soy, 0.3 oz	5	0	1
Taco, 0.3 oz	0	0	0
Condiments			
Cheese: American/Swiss, 1 slice	45	3.5	1
Provolone, 1 slice	70	6	0
Ketchup	10	0	2
Mustard	5	0	1
Salsa	5	0	1
Sour Cream	60	5	2
Desserts			
Cheesecake, 3.6 oz	310	16	34
Double Fudge Cake, 3 oz	310	11	49
Ice Cream Shakes: Per Regular			
Chocolate Ice Cream	885	42	114
Oreo Cookie Ice Cream	935	49	108
Strawberry Ice Cream	875	41	111
Vanilla Ice Cream	785	43	84

For Complete Nutritional Data ~ see CalorieKing.com

Jamba Juice® (Aug '07)

Juices: Per Original	**C**	**F**	**Cb**
Carrot	150	1	34
Lemonade	450	0	112
Orange Banana	350	1.5	84
Orange Carrot	240	1.5	56
Orange	330	1.5	77
Vibrant C	380	1	92
Shots: Average all, 4 fl.oz	70	0	14
Wheatgrass, 1 fl.oz	10	0	1
Yogurt Blend:			
Bright Eyed & Blueberry	380	1	76
Sunrise Strawberry	400	1	83
Smoothies: Per Original			
Aloha Pineapple	500	1.5	117
Banana Berry	450	1	106
Berry Lime Sublime	460	2	106
Caribbean Passion	440	2	102
Chocolate Moo'd	680	8	138
Citrus Squeeze	470	2	110
Coldbuster	430	2.5	100
Grape Escape	300	0	74
Mango A Go-Go	470	2	110
Mega Mango	330	1	80
Orange A Peel	440	1.5	102
Orange Berry Blitz	410	2.5	94
Orange Dream Machine	540	2.5	111
Peach Pleasure	460	2	108
Peanut Butter Moo'd	840	21	139
Peenya Kowlada	690	5	152
Protein Berry Pizzazz	440	1.5	92
Raspberry Rainbow	300	1	73
Razzmatazz	480	2	112
Strawberry Whirl	310	0.5	76
Strawberries Wild	450	0.5	105
Energy: Acai Supercharger	420	5	86
Matcha Green Tea Blast	440	0.5	97
Light Smoothies:			
Berry Fulfilling	260	1	57
Mango Mantra	280	1	64
Strawberry Nirvana	250	0.5	55
Tropical Awakening	270	1	62
Baked Goods			
Pretzels: Apple Cinnamon	410	5	78
Savory: Cheddar Jalapeno Twist	250	5	41
Pizza Protein Stick	230	6	33
Sweet: Blueberry Cinnamon Swirl	320	6	55
Honey Berry Bran	320	12	48

Jimmy John's® (Aug '07)

Giant Club Sandwiches	**C**	**F**	**Cb**
Beach Club	795	37	76
Billy Club	865	40	77
Bootlegger Club	720	27	74
Club Lulu	760	33	74
Club Tuna	725	29	79
Country Club	840	38	75
Gourmet Smoked Ham Club	850	40	76
Gourmet Veggie Club	855	46	77
Hunter's Club	855	38	75
Italian Night Club	975	52	77
Low-Fat Sandwiches: Turkey Tom	555	26	54
Turkey Breast	405	0.5	70
Plain Slims: Figures based on French Bread			
Double Provolone	590	20	72
Ham & Cheese	540	12	72
Roast Beef	420	1.5	70
Salami, Capicola, Cheese	625	21	72
Tuna Salad	580	19	74
Turkey Breast	405	1	70
Subs: Figures based on 8" French Bread, Mayo, Cheese, Sce			
Big John	565	27	54
JJBLT	635	34	54
Pepe	685	37	55
The J.J. Gargantuan	1010	55	60
Totally Tuna	510	20	58
Turkey Tom	555	26	54
Vegetarian	640	36	57
Vito	580	25	56
Low-Carb Unwiches: Includes Mayo, Cheese & Sauce			
Hunters Club	520	38	8.5
The J.J. Gargantuan	770	55	11
Sides: Jimmy Chips, average 1 oz	160	8	18
Cookies, average	420	18	63

*Zero trans fat . . . but
still high in total fat!*

Restaurants & Fast - Foods

Johnny Rockets® (Aug '07)

Original Hamburgers	C	F	Cb
Hamburger #12	880	57	58
Chili Size	1255	84	67
Original Burger	790	50	57
Patty Melt	785	48	48
Rocket Double	1190	79	58
Rocket Single	830	52	57
Route 66	910	63	53
Smoke House	970	60	60
St Louis	990	68	53
Streamliner	420	11	60
Turkey Single	730	42	56
Sandwiches: Chicken Club	1070	39	126
Egg Salad	690	49	41
Grilled Chicken Breast	630	33	52
Grilled Cheese	540	30	40
Grilled Ham & Cheese	515	24	40
Tuna Melt	755	45	40
Tuna Salad	710	46	41
Other Favorites			
Chicken Club Salad:			
with Chicken Tenders	650	40	46
with Grilled Chicken Breast	530	33	23
Chicken Tenders	520	22	47
Chili Dog	815	55	46
Garden Salad	250	20	5
Hot Dog	420	23	38
Extras: Bacon, 0.7 oz	100	7	0
Extra Patty, 3 oz	270	20	1
Chili, 2½ oz	170	15	3
Grilled Onions or Mushrooms, 1 oz	20	2	2
Starters			
American Fries, 8 oz	530	23	77
Half Fries & Half Rings, 9.3 oz	720	36	92
Cheese Fries, 10 oz	760	42	78
Chili Bowl, 10 oz	870	69	24
Chili Fries	1085	67	91
Onion Rings, 6.8 oz	500	34	22
Rocket Wings, regular order	540	20	33
Desserts: Apple Pie	930	59	88
Hot Fudge Sundae	830	47	93
A la mode, 8 oz	520	32	52
Drinks (Medium): Rootbeer	170	0	49
Coke; Sprite	170	0	43
Lemonade	170	0	49
Float	420	26	42
Shakes: Chocolate, 20 oz	1100	60	120
Strawberry, 20 oz	810	48	82
Vanilla, 20 oz	1120	60	130
Extra for Malt, ½ oz	60	2	10

Kenny Rogers Roasters® (Aug '07)

Chicken	C	F	Cb
½ Chicken, No Skin or Wing	315	10	1
with Skin	515	28	2
¼ Dark Meat, No Skin	170	7	1
with Skin	270	17	1
¼ White Meat, No Skin or Wing	145	2	1
with Skin, serving	245	11	1
Grilled Breast Platter	990	52	100
Tenders (3)	510	37	24
Tenders Platter	1315	79	119
Pies: Chicken Pot Pie	710	33	78
Pitas: BBQ Chicken	400	7	51
Chicken Caesar	605	35	34
Roasted Chicken	685	35	42
Turkey: Sliced Breast	160	2	0
Salads (No Dressing): Side Salad	25	0	5
Chicken Caesar	285	9	18
Pasta	230	12	28
Roasted Chicken	290	10	19
Sour Cream & Dill Pasta	230	16	20
Tomato Cucumber	125	2	10
Sandwiches			
Chicken Tender	695	46	45
Chicken Tender Pita	610	38	45
Grilled Chicken	525	29	32
Turkey	385	12	30
Side Dishes: Cinnamon Apples	200	5	41
Cole Slaw	225	16	18
Cornbread Stuffing	325	19	34
Corn Cob	70	0.5	14
Corn Muffin	165	6	25
Sweet Corn Niblets	115	0.5	28
Creamy Parmesan Spinach	120	6	10
Honey Baked Beans	150	1	32
Italian Green Beans	115	8	10
Macaroni & Cheese	200	6	24
Potatoes: Baked Sweet	265	0	62
Garlic Parsley	260	12	37
Potato Salad	390	27	34
Real Mashed	295	14	39
Rice Pilaf	175	5	43
Steamed Vegetables	50	0	8
Zucchini & Squash Santa Fe	70	5	8
Soups: Chicken Noodle, 1 bowl	90	2	12
Chicken Noodle, 1 cup	55	1	7

KFC® (Aug '07)

	C	F	Cb
Chicken: Extra Crispy™			
Breast, 5.7 oz	440	27	15
Drumstick, 2.1 oz	160	10	6
Thigh, 4 oz	370	28	12
Whole Wing, 1.8 oz	170	11	6
Original Recipe®: Breast, 5.7 oz	360	21	7
Breast, no skin or breading, 4 oz	140	2	1
Drumstick, 2 oz	130	8	2
Thigh, 4.4 oz	330	24	8
Whole Wing, 1.6 oz	130	8	4
Crispy Strips, 3 pieces	350	19	16
Popcorn Chicken: Kids, 3 oz	290	19	16
Individual, 4 oz	400	26	22
Large, 5.6 oz	550	35	30
Wings: Hot Wings (5)	350	24	14
Honey BBQ Wings (5)	390	24	23
Honey BBQ Wings, Boneless (5)	450	20	41
Famous Bowls: Potato w. Gravy, 19 oz	740	35	80
Rice w. Gravy, 13 oz	620	28	67
Sandwiches: Honey BBQ	280	4	40
Double Crunch	470	23	38
Crispy Twister	550	28	49
Oven Roasted Twister w. Sauce	420	17	40
Tender Roast: w. Sauce	380	13	29
without Sauce	300	5	28
KFC Snacker: Regular	290	13	29
Fish: w. Sauce	330	15	31
without Sauce	290	12	29
Honey BBQ	210	3	32
Ultimate Cheese	280	11	30
Chicken Pot Pie, 15 oz	770	40	70
Salads: (No Dressing or Croutons)			
Crispy BLT/Caesar Salad, average	350	18	17
Roasted BLT/Caesar Salad, average	220	7	8
Parm. Garlic Croutons, ½ oz pouch	60	3	8
Dressings: Creamy Parm. Caesar	260	26	4
Original Ranch, 2 oz	200	20	3
Fat-Free, 1½ oz	35	0	8
Golden Italian Light, 1½ oz	45	2.5	6
Sides: Baked Beans, 4.8 oz	220	1	45
Biscuit, 2 oz	220	11	24
Coleslaw, 4.6 oz	180	10	22
Corn on the Cob (3") 2.9 oz	70	1.5	13
Green Beans, 4 oz	50	1.5	7
Macaroni & Cheese, 4.8 oz	180	8	18
Mashed Potatoes: w. Gravy, 4.8 oz	140	5	20
Potato Salad, 4.5 oz	180	9	22
Potato Wedges, small, 3.6 oz	260	13	33
Desserts: Apple Pie Mini's, 3	330	16	44
Double Choc. Chip Cake, 2.7 oz	330	16	41
Lil' Bucket™: Choc. Cream, 4 oz	280	13	38

Koo♦Koo♦Roo® (Aug '07)

	C	F	Cb
Rotisserie Chicken			
Leg & Thigh, 4.8 oz	300	18	1
Breast & Wing, 6.5 oz	355	16	1
Half Rotisserie Chicken, 11.3 oz	655	34	2
Original Skinless Flame Broiled Chicken™			
3 Piece Original Dark, 5 oz	320	16	5
Original Breast, 4.1 oz	190	5.5	0
Roasted Turkey: Breast, sliced, 4 oz	180	8	0
Hand-Carved Turkey Sandwich	600	32	31
Traditional Turkey Dinner	690	29	67
Turkey Pot Pie	885	44	83
Salads: Per Regular (No Dressing)			
BBQ Chicken Salad	365	14	22
Chicken Caesar Salad	285	11	12
Chinese Chicken Salad	550	28	39
Koo Koo Roo House Salad	115	4	16
Chicken Bowls (No Sce): Chargrilled	570	18	57
Southwest	570	18	66
Tostada: With Shell & Dressing	1130	77	69
Without Shell or Dressing	530	22	45
Dressings/Sauces			
BBQ Vinaigrette, 2 oz	100	4	14
Caesar Dressing, 1½ oz	235	26	1.5
Chinese Salad Dressing, 3 oz	325	26	26
Chipotle Sauce, 1 oz	130	14	0.5
Cilantro Ranch Dressing, 2 oz	200	21	2
Cranberry Sauce, 1 oz	45	0	11
Curried Mustard Sauce, 3 oz	630	69	3
Soup: Chicken Noodle, 5 oz	70	3	5
Ten Vegetable, 5 oz	95	2	16
Sandwiches: BBQ Chicken w. Sce	560	11	71
Original Chicken Breast w. Dressing	660	28	62
Chicken Caesar w. Dressing	780	35	62
Wrap: Caesar Chicken w. Dressing	755	39	60
Burritos: Original Chicken	710	28	71
California Chicken	810	41	60
Sides: Baked French Fries, 5 oz	250	7.5	42
Baked Yams, 6 oz	200	0	47
Black Beans, 6 oz	125	2.5	22
Buffalo Wings (no sauce), 6 wings	605	27	42
Creamed Spinach, 5 oz	100	6.5	10
Lahvash (flatbread), each	60	0.5	12
Mashed Potatoes, 6.5 oz	185	5	32
Macaroni & Cheese, 6 oz	340	16	32
Roasted Garlic Potatoes, 5 oz	135	4.5	21
For Complete Nutritional Data ~ see CalorieKing.com			

Kilwin's® ~ *see CalorieKing.com*

Kohr Bros® ~ *see CalorieKing.com*

Kolache® ~ *see CalorieKing.com*

Updated Nutrition Data ~ www.CalorieKing.com
Persons with Diabetes ~ See Disclaimer (Page 24)

Krispy Kreme® (Aug '07)

Doughnuts	C	F	Cb
Apple Fritter	380	21	46
Caramel Kreme Crunch	380	21	46
Chocolate Iced Glazed Cruller	290	15	37
Chocolate Iced Cake	270	14	36
Chocolate Iced Custard Filled	300	17	35
Chocolate Iced Glazed	250	12	33
Chocolate Iced Kreme Filled	350	20	38
Chocolate Iced with Sprinkles	260	12	38
Cinnamon Apple Filled	290	16	32
Cinnamon Bun	260	16	28
Cinnamon Twist	240	15	23
Dulce de Leche	290	18	30
Glazed Blueberry Cake	330	17	43
Glazed Chocolate Cake	300	15	41
Glazed Cinnamon	210	12	24
Glazed Cruller	240	14	26
Glazed Kreme Filled	340	20	38
Glazed Lemon Filled	290	16	35
Glazed Raspberry Filled	300	16	38
Glazed Sour Cream	340	18	42
Key Lime Pie	320	17	40
Maple Iced Glazed	240	12	32
New York Cheesecake	320	19	35
Original Glazed	200	12	22
Powdered Cake	280	14	37
Powdered Strawberry Filled	290	16	33
Sugar Doughnut	200	12	21
Traditional Cake Doughnut	230	13	25
Whole Wheat Glazed	180	11	19
Doughnut Holes: Orig. Glazed (5)	200	11	25
Glazed Cake, Regular/Chocolate (4)	210	11	28

Chiller Beverages: *No Cream Topping*

Fruity Chillers, *No Cream Topping:*

	C	F	Cb
Average all flavors,12 fl.oz	180	0	43
20 fl.oz	300	0	73

Kremey Chillers, *Includes Whipped Cream Topping:*

	C	F	Cb
Orange & Kreme: 12 fl.oz	585	24	90
20 fl.oz	985	40	152
Lemon Sherbert: 12 fl.oz	590	24	93
20 fl.oz	995	40	157
Choc./Latte/Mocha, avg. 12 fl.oz	630	25	102
20 fl.oz	1065	43	172

For Complete Nutritional Data ~ see CalorieKing.com

Krystal® (Aug '07)

Burgers/Sandwiches	C	F	Cb
B.A. Burger	470	27	39
w. Cheese	530	32	40
BA Double Bacon Burger	800	53	41
Krystal Burger	160	7	17
Krystal Chik	240	11	24
Bacon Cheese Krystal	190	10	16
Cheese Krystal	180	9	17
Double Krystal	260	13	24
Double Cheese Krystal	310	16	26
Chili Cheese Pup	210	12	17
Corn Pup	260	19	19
Plain Pup	170	9	15
Sampler Combo (Krystal, Chik, Chili Cheese Pup, Fries, 24 oz drink)	1320	50	171

French Fries	C	F	Cb
Regular, 4.2 oz	470	20	53
Chili Cheese Fries, 7.3 oz	540	28	59

Sides	C	F	Cb
Krystal Chili	200	7	22
Chik'n Bites, Small, 4 oz	310	19	16
Chik'n Bites & Salad	290	20	12
Kryspers	190	13	17

Breakfast Items	C	F	Cb
Krystal Sunriser Sandwich	240	14	14
Biscuit: Bacon, Egg & Cheese	390	23	33
Chik Biscuit	360	15	40
Plain Biscuit	270	13	33
Sausage Biscuit	480	33	33
Biscuit & Gravy	280	14	34
Country Breakfast	660	42	46
Scrambler, 11 oz	440	26	33
4-Carb Scrambler: Bacon	370	29	4
Sausage	600	51	3

Desserts: Apple Turnover, fried	220	10	31
Lemon Icebox Pie	260	9	41

Drinks: *Per Small Serving (16 fl.oz w. ¼ ice)*

	C	F	Cb
Coca-Cola Classic	160	0	40
Coca-Cola Classic, frozen	145	0	36
Diet Coke	0	0	0
Sprite	155	0	39

For Complete Nutritional Data ~ see CalorieKing.com

For Data Updates, Check Author's Website www.CalorieKing.com

219

La Rosa's Pizzeria® (Aug '07)

Pan Crust Medium Pizza: Per Slice	C	F	Cb
Blanca, ⅒ pizza	350	22	28
Cheese	300	16	30
Deluxe/Pepperoni Topper, avg.	370	21	31
Meat Topper	400	23	30
Veggie Topper	320	16	32

Traditional Crust Medium Pizza: Per Slice			
Blanca, ⅒ pizza	260	16	17
Cheese	200	10	19
Deluxe/Pepperoni Topper, avg.	280	16	20
Meat Topper	300	18	20
Veggie Topper	220	11	21

Stuffed Pizza Pie: Per Slice			
Cheese	340	14	40
Meat	790	53	44
Veggie	395	18	43

Calzones: Per Calzone (No Dipping Sauce)			
3 Meat & 3 Cheese	1080	55	102
3 Veggie & 3 Cheese	860	34	105
Cheese	840	34	101
Cheese & Pepperoni	960	45	101
Philly Cheese Steak	870	39	90

Hoagy: No Cheese/Dressing/Sauce/Chips			
Baked Buddy, 8.7 oz	665	28	62
Baked Royal, 9 oz	600	22	62
Meatball, 11.7 oz	690	26	77
Original Steak, 11.3 oz	730	35	65
Philly Steak, 9.3 oz	620	25	64

Lite & Low Fat Menu			
Grilled Chicken Hoagy, low fat	520	9	56
Grilled Chicken Salad, low fat	380	10	40
Lite Deluxe Pizza, Medium, 1 slice	190	6	27
Minestrone Soup, 12 oz bowl	130	2	22

Pasta Dinner: No Sides			
Cheese Ravioli	660	26	80
Lasagna w. Meat Sauce	735	38	61
Meat Ravioli	620	22	102
Spaghetti: w. Meat Sauce	700	18	104
w. Meatballs	870	28	119
w. Traditional Sauce	640	12	113

Chicken Wings: (12)			
BBQ Wings (12)	1255	77	48
Special Recipe Wings (12)	1260	87	21
Spicy Hot Wings (12)	1250	85	26

For Complete Nutritional Data ~ see CalorieKing.com

La Salsa Fresh Mexican Grill® (Aug '07)

Appetizers: Tortilla Chips, serving	C	F	Cb
Tortilla Chips, serving	900	42	108
Chips, Guacamole & Salsa	1180	68	125
Nachos w. Chicken, no Beans	1515	86	128
Nachos w. Steak, no Beans	1530	90	127

Burritos: Chips and Salsa Not Included			
Baja Fish	920	56	67
Bean & Cheese: w. Black Beans	635	20	87
w. Chicken/Carnitas, avg.	590	23	57
w. Steak, no beans	605	27	56
California Veggie: w. Beans, avg.	750	32	96
no Beans	660	31	80
California: w. Beans, avg.	750	32	96
w. Carnitas, no Beans	765	35	81
w. Chicken, no Beans	795	35	82
w. Steak, no Beans	810	39	81
Fire-Rstd Bowl: w. Steak, no Beans	665	38	65
w. Carnitas/Chkn, avg., no Beans	650	34	66
Grande: w. Steak, no Beans	810	41	81
w. Carnitas/Chkn, avg., no Beans	795	37	82
Los Cabos Shrimp, no Chips & Salsa	785	40	88
Original Gourmet: w. Steak	665	32	62
w. Carnitas/Chicken, avg.	650	28	63
Overstuffed Grilled Burrito:			
w. Chicken	950	46	63
w. Steak	980	53	62
Sonora Fish, no Chips & Salsa	630	25	63
The No Rice No Beans: w. Carnitas	780	40	69
w. Chicken	810	40	70
w. Steak	825	44	69
Three Pepper Fajita: w. Carnitas	820	39	86
w. Chicken	850	39	87
w. Shrimp	785	37	86
w. Steak	865	43	86

Meal Platters: Beans, Chips and Salsa Not Included			
Carnitas Guadalajara Taco	445	20	56
Cheese Enchilada	665	38	62
Enchilada: w. Carnitas	645	29	63
w. Chicken	685	29	65
w. Steak	705	34	67
Taquitos & Quesadilla: w. Chicken	2160	120	174
w. Steak	2170	124	173
Three Pepper Fajita: w. Carnitas	1220	38	208
w. Chicken	1485	46	212
w. Steak	1515	53	210
Two Soft Tacos: w. Carnitas	550	22	77
w. Chicken	570	22	78
w. Steak	580	24	77

La Salsa Fresh® cont... (Aug '07)

	C	F	Cb
Quesadillas: No Chips/Salsa			
Classic Quesadilla: w. Carnitas	995	61	61
w. Chicken	1025	61	62
w. Steak	1040	65	61
Grande: w. Carnitas, no Beans	1085	63	79
w. Chicken, no Beans	1115	63	80
w. Steak, no Beans	1130	67	79
Stuffed Fajita: w. Steak	955	60	55
w. Carnitas/Chicken, avg.	940	57	56
Salads: Chips and Salsa Not Included			
Chile Lime Salad: w. Carnitas	645	46	49
w. Chicken	775	50	51
w. Steak	790	54	50
Chipotle Shrimp Salad	800	56	52
Taco Salad: w. Steak, no Beans	885	47	88
w. Carnitas/Chkn, avg., no Beans	870	43	89
Sides: Chips & Salsa	200	10	25
Black Beans: with Cheese	200	3	33
no Cheese	180	1	33
Pinto Beans: with Cheese	175	3	28
no Cheese	155	1	28
Rice: with Cotija Cheese	120	5	22
no Cotija Cheese	100	3	22
Tacos: Chips and Salsa Not Included			
Baja Fish Taco	450	26	42
Baja Style Shrimp Taco	370	26	29
Carnitas Guadalajara Taco	320	17	30
La Salsa: w. Steak Taco	275	12	28
w. Carnitas/Chicken, avg.	265	10	29
Sonora Fish Taco	235	11	19
Taquitos (3)	1910	109	162

LaMar's® (Aug '07)

	C	F	Cb
Bars: Caramel Iced, Unfilled	430	18	59
Chocolate Iced: Unfilled	540	22	81
Bavarian Cream Filled	600	22	96
Chocolate/White Fluff Filled	810	35	120
Bizmarks: Bavarian Cream	620	22	101
Blueberry/Lemon Filled, avg.	530	21	80
Cherry Filled	550	19	88
Donuts: Apple Spice Cake	340	17	44
Bluberry Cake	350	17	44
Chocolate Iced Cake	330	18	37
Old Fashioned Sour Cream	420	18	60
Ray's Chocolate Glazed	290	11	44
Ray's Original Glazed	220	10	31
White Iced Cake	320	17	38
Other Items: Apple Fritter	650	26	91
German Chocolate Knot	480	27	54
Cinnamon Roll	690	25	106
Cinnamon Twist	770	26	120
Raisin Nut Cinnamon Roll	850	27	137

Little Caesar® (Aug '07)

	C	F	Cb
Pizza: Per Slice			
12" Round: Cheese, ⅛ pizza	180	6	23
Pepperoni, ⅛ pizza	210	7.5	23
12" Thin Crust: Cheese, ⅛ pizza	140	7	13
Pepperoni, ⅛ pizza	170	8.5	13
14" Round: Cheese, ⅒ pizza	200	6.5	25
Meatsa, ⅒ pizza	280	13	26
Pepperoni, ⅒ pizza	230	8	25
Supreme, ⅒ pizza	270	10	31
Veggie, ⅒ pizza	240	7.5	32
14" Thin Crust: Cheese, ⅒ pizza	160	7.5	14
Pepperoni, ⅒ pizza	180	14	14
16" Round: Cheese, 1/12 pizza	220	7	27
Pepperoni, 1/12 pizza	240	8.5	27
18" Round: Cheese, 1/14 pizza	230	7	30
Pepperoni, 1/14 pizza	260	9	30
Large Deep Dish: Cheese, ⅛ pizza	320	12	37
Pepperoni, ⅛ pizza	350	14	38
Medium Deep Dish: Cheese, ⅛ pizza	320	12	37
Extras			
Baby Pan! Pan!, 1 piece, 5.1 oz	360	16	34
Chicken Wings (1)	70	5	0
Crazy Bread: 1 stick	90	2.5	15
Cinnamon, 2 sticks	100	2	19
Crazy Sauce, 4 oz	45	0	9
Italian Cheese Bread, 1 piece	130	6	13
Deli Sandwiches			
Ham & Cheese	640	29	66
Italian	800	44	66
Veggie	600	27	67
Side Salads: Per Individual Container			
Antipasto	140	7.5	6
Caesar	90	3	12
Greek	120	6.5	11
Tossed	100	3	15
Salad Dressings: Per Serving			
Caesar	230	25	1
Greek	270	29	0
Italian	220	23	2
Ranch	230	24	2
Fat-Free: Italian	25	0	5

For Complete Nutritional Data ~ see CalorieKing.com

Lone Star Steakhouse® (Aug '07)

Meals	**C**	**F**	**Cb**
Grilled Chicken, 6 oz	185	2.5	0
Grilled Pork Chops (2) 16 oz	1430	100	0
Mesquite Grilled Steaks:			
Cajun Ribeye, 16 oz	1250	101	0
Chopped Steak, 12 oz	900	71	0
Delmonico, 11 oz	860	69	0
Five Star Filet, 9 oz	740	60	0
New York Strip, 14 oz	1035	80	0
San Antonio Sirloin, 12 oz	770	55	0
T-Bone, 20 oz	1540	124	0
Texas Ribeye, 14 oz	1090	88	0
Baby Back Ribs, 12 oz	970	80	0
Shrimp Dinner, 3.5 oz	105	1.5	1
Slow Roasted Prime Rib, 16 oz	1250	101	0
Sweet Bourbon Salmon, 6 oz	240	11	0
Texas Teasers Ribs, 6 oz	485	40	0
Sides: Per Serving			
Baked Potato	665	18	114
Baked Sweet Potato	635	8	137
Lone Star Chili, 6 fl.oz	230	15	8
Sauteed Mushrooms	115	9	6
Sauteed Onions	100	7	8
Steamed Vegetables	70	1	14
Texas Rice	80	2	12
Soups			
Black Bean, 6 fl.oz	190	4	31
Desserts			
Homemade Cobbler	240	8	43

Long John Silver's® (Aug '07)

Sandwiches: Ultimate Fish	530	28	49
Fish Sandwich	470	23	48
Chicken Sandwich	360	15	40
Sides: Cheese Sticks (3)	140	8	12
Fries: Small, 3 oz	230	10	33
Large, 5 oz	385	17	55
Coleslaw, 4 oz	200	15	15
Corn Cobbette, no butter	90	3	14
Crumblies, 1 oz	170	12	14
Hushpuppies (1)	60	2.5	9
Rice, 4 oz	180	3.5	34
Soup: Clam Chowder, 1 bowl	170	8	19
Chicken: Battered Plank, 1 piece	140	8	9
Seafood: Battered Fish, 1 piece	260	16	17
Battered Shrimp, 1 piece	45	3	3
Clam Strips, 3 oz	240	13	22
Desserts: Per Serving			
Chocolate Cream Pie	310	22	34
Pecan Pie	370	15	55
Pineapple Cream Pie	290	13	39

For Complete Nutritional Data ~ see CalorieKing.com

Luby's® (Aug '07)

Entrees: (Without Sides)	**C**	**F**	**Cb**
Blackened Chicken Breast	350	15	5
Blackened Tilapia	270	11	5
Carved Ham	300	11	6
Chicken Piccata	420	25	13
Grilled Chicken Breast w. skin, 8 oz	415	23	1
Grilled Chicken Breast no skin, 8 oz	335	16	1
Lemon Basil Salmon	355	20	1
Pan Grilled Fillet	330	12	19
Roasted Chicken, ½, no skin	460	23	0
Roasted Turkey, no skin, no Gravy	280	3	0
Sides			
Bread Rolls: White	130	3	23
Whole Wheat	170	5	23
Black-eyed Peas	220	5	33
Blue Lake Green Beans	85	5	9
Broccoli	80	4	9
Cabbage	70	5	6
Carrots	95	4	15
Cauliflower, Peas & Carrots	65	4	7
Corn	190	5	38
Fresh Green Beans	90	5	10
Grapefruit	45	0	12
Holiday Rice	165	3	30
Jell-O	100	0	24
Mixed Melons	70	0	20
Pineapple	50	0	12
Pinto Beans	190	5	28
Roasted Mixed Vegetables	135	8	16
Spinach	65	4	5
Salads: Marinated Cucumbers	115	8	13
Grilled Chicken Caesar w. Dressing	790	50	23
Grilled Chicken Caesar, no Dressing	550	26	23
Mediterranean Vegetables	140	10	1
Mixed Field Greens, no Dressing	35	0	7
Spinach Salad, no Dressing	50	2	5
Spring Mix, no dressing	35	0	7
Dressings: Per Tablespoon (½ fl.oz)			
Blue Cheese	90	9	0
Caesar	75	8	0
French	80	7	5
Greek	30	3	0
Honey Mustard; Italian	75	7	4
Ranch	55	6	1
Thousand Island	50	5	2
Soups: Chicken Noodle, 1 bowl	235	9	21

For Complete Nutritional Data ~ see CalorieKing.com

Restaurants & Fast - Foods

McDonald's® (Aug '07)

Burgers/Sandwiches

	C	F	Cb
Big Mac	540	29	45
Big N'Tasty	460	24	37
Big N'Tasty w. Cheese	510	28	38
Cheeseburger	300	12	33
Double Cheeseburge	440	23	34
Filet-O-Fish Sandwich	380	18	38
Hamburger	250	9	31
McChicken	360	16	40
McRib Burger	490	25	44
McVeggie Burger	350	8	47
McVeggie Burger w. Cheese	400	12	49
Quarter Pounder:	410	19	37
w. Cheese	510	26	40
Double w. Cheese	740	42	40
Chicken Fajita	220	8	26
Deli Sandwiches: Trio	410	7	61
Turkey BLT Toasted	500	15	61
Grilled Chicken Flatbread Sandwich	520	23	55
New York Reuben: w. Corned Beef	560	23	58
w. Turkey	540	19	60

Premium Chicken Sandwiches:

	C	F	Cb
Crispy Chicken Classic	500	17	61
Crispy Chicken Club	660	28	63
Crispy Chicken Ranch BLT	600	23	64
Grilled Chicken Classic	420	10	51
Grilled Chicken Club	570	21	52
Grilled Chicken Ranch BLT	520	16	53

Snack Wrap

	C	F	Cb
Chipotle BBQ: w. Grilled Chicken	270	10	26
w. Crispy Chicken	330	16	33
Honey Mustard: w. Grilled Chicken	260	9	27
w. Crispy Chicken	320	15	34
Ranch: w. Grilled Chicken	270	10	26
w. Crispy Chicken	330	16	32

Extra Value Meals

	C	F	Cb
Large Fries & Large Soda, add	880	30	156

French Fries

	C	F	Cb
Small, 2.6 oz	250	13	30
Medium, 4 oz	380	20	47
Large, 6 oz	570	30	70

McDonald's® cont... (Aug '07)

Chicken McNuggets®/Sauces

	C	F	Cb
Chicken McNuggets: 4 pieces	170	10	10
6 pieces	250	15	15
10 pieces	420	24	26
Sauce: Barbecue, 1 oz pkg	50	0	12
Honey, ½ oz pkg	50	0	12
Hot Mustard, 1 oz pkg	60	2.5	9
Sweet 'N Sour, 1 oz pkg	50	0	12

Chicken Selects® Breast Strips

	C	F	Cb
Strips: 3 pieces	380	20	28
5 pieces	630	33	46
Sauces (1.5 oz pkg): Creamy Ranch	200	22	2
Spicy Buffalo	70	7	1
Tangy Honey Mustard	70	2.5	13
Chipotle Barbecue	70	0	18

Breakfast Menu

	C	F	Cb
Biscuit: Regular, 25 oz	250	11	32
Large, 3.2 oz	320	16	39
Bacon Egg & Cheese, large	520	30	43
Bacon Egg & Cheese, regular	450	25	36
Sausage w. Egg, large	570	37	42
Sausage w. Egg, regular	500	32	35
Breakfast Steak	120	8	0
Big Breakfast, regular	720	46	49
Deluxe Breakfast, regular	1070	55	109
English Muffin, 2 oz	140	1.5	27
Grape/Strawberry Jam	35	0	9
Hash Browns (1), 1.9 oz	140	8	15
Hotcakes: Plain (3)	350	9	60
w. Margarine (2 pats), no Syrup	430	18	60
w. Margarine (2 pats) & Syrup (1)	610	18	105
McGriddles: Bacon, Egg & Chse	460	21	48
Sausage	420	22	44
Sausage, Egg & Cheese	560	32	48
McMuffin: Egg	300	12	30
Sausage	370	22	29
Sausage w. Egg	450	27	30
Sausage, 1.4 oz patty	170	15	1
Sausage Breakfast Burrito	300	16	26
Scrambled Eggs (2)	170	11	1
Warm Cinnamon Roll: Regular	440	19	60

Breakfast Value Meal (Extras)

	C	F	Cb
If Hash Browns & Coffee (black/no sugar,) add	140	8	15
If Hash Browns & Orange Juice, add	280	8	48

Salads/Desserts/Drinks ~ Next Page ...

McDonald's® cont... (Aug '07)

Salads: (No Dressing)	C	F	Cb
Asian Salad: w. Crispy Chicken	380	17	33
w. Grilled Chicken	300	10	23
Bacon Ranch Salad: No Chicken	140	7	10
w. Crispy Chicken	350	16	23
w. Grilled Chicken	260	9	12
Caesar Salad: No Chicken	90	4	9
w. Crispy Chicken	300	13	22
w. Grilled Chicken	220	6	12
South West Salad: w. Crispy Chicken	400	16	41
w. Grilled Chicken	320	9	30
Fruit & Walnut, Snack Size	210	8	31
Side Salad, 3.1 oz	20	0	4
Butter Garlic Croutons, ½ oz	60	1.5	10
Salad Dressings: Per Package			
Newman's Own: Ranch Dressing	170	15	9
Creamy Caesar Dressing	190	18	4
Low-Fat: Balsamic Vinaigrette	40	3	4
Family Recipe Italian	60	2.5	8
Sesame Ginger Dressing	90	2.5	15
Soups: Broccoli Cheese	180	9	19
Chicken Noodle	100	0	16
Vegetable Beef	120	1	20
Desserts/Cookies/Shakes/Sundaes			
Apple Dippers w. Caramel Dip	105	0.5	23
Apple Dippers, 1 pkg	35	0	8
Caramel Dip, 0.7 oz	70	0.5	15
Baked Apple Pie, 2.7oz	270	12	36
Cookies: Oatmeal Raisin (1)	150	6	22
Chocolate Chip Cookie (1)	160	7	22
Sugar Cookie (1)	150	6	21
McDonaldland® Cookies: 2 oz	250	8	42
Chocolate Chip Cookies, 2 oz	270	11	39
Fruit 'n Yogurt Parfait: Regular	160	2	31
without Granola	130	2	25
Ice Cream: Kiddie Cone, 1 oz	45	1	8
Vanilla Reduced Fat Cone, 3.2 oz	150	3.5	24
Van. Red'd-Fat Ice Cream only, 3 oz	130	3.5	20
McFlurry™: M&M®, 12 fl.oz cup	620	20	96
Oreo®, 12 fl.oz cup	560	16	88
Swamp Sludge: 12 fl.oz cup	510	16	80
16 fl.oz cup	710	23	110
Sundaes: Hot Caramel Sundae	340	8	60
Hot Fudge Sundae	330	10	54
Strawberry Sundae	280	6	49
Peanuts (for Sundaes)	45	3.5	2
Triple Thick Shakes, average all flavors:			
12 fl.oz cup	430	10	75
16 fl.oz cup	570	13	101
21 fl.oz cup	760	18	134
32 fl.oz cup	1150	27	201

McDonald's® cont... (Aug '07)

	C	F	Cb
Drinks: 1% Low Fat Milk, 8 fl.oz	100	2.5	12
Coffee (black), 16 fl.oz	0	0	0
Half & Half Creamer, 1 pkg	20	2	0
Sugar Packet (1)	15	0	4
Cappuccino: *Per 12 fl.oz*			
French Vanilla	215	6	38
Original; Swiss Mocha	205	4	39
White Choc. Raspberry	225	9	34
Coca-Cola or Sprite (No Ice):			
Childs, 12 fl.oz cup	110	0	33
Small, 16 fl.oz cup	150	0	43
Medium, 21 fl.oz cup	210	0	58
Large, 32 fl.oz cup	310	0	86
Diet Coke	0	0	0
Hi-C Orange Drink (No Ice):			
Child, 12 fl.oz cup	120	0	32
Small, 16 fl.oz cup	160	0	44
Medium, 21 fl.oz cup	240	0	64
Large, 32 fl.oz cup	350	0	94
Iced Coffee, average all flavors:			
Small, 16 fl.oz	130	5	21
Medium, 24 fl.oz	190	8	29
Large, 32 fl.oz	270	11	4
Iced Tea	0	0	0
Orange Juice: 12 fl.oz cup	190	0	44
16 fl.oz cup	250	0	57
Powerade Mountain Blast (with ⅓ Ice):			
Child, 12 fl.oz	70	0	22
Small, 16 fl.oz	100	0	27
Medium, 21 fl.oz	150	0	38
Large, 32 fl.oz	220	0	58
Whipped Hot Chocolate, 12 fl.oz	195	1	43

For Updates & Complete Nutritional Data
~ see CalorieKing.com

Restaurants & Fast - Foods

Manhattan Bagel® (Aug '07)

Bagel (East Coast): Per Bagel (4 oz)

	C	F	Cb
Blueberry	360	1	80
Cheddar Cheese	340	1	72
Chocolate Chip	370	3	75
Cinnamon Raisin	340	1	76
Cranberry Orange	340	1	75
Egg, 4 oz	330	1.5	72
Jalapeno Cheddar; Marble Rye	330	1	72
Lower Carb 9-Grain	210	3.5	28
Oat Goodness	350	3	73
Plain, 4 oz	330	1	72
Pumpernickel; Rye	340	1	73
Spinach	330	1	72
Sundried Tomato	330	1	72
Whole Wheat	320	1	71
Cream Cheese: Reduced Fat, 2 Tbsp	60	5	1

For Complete Nutritional Data ~ see CalorieKing.com

Max & Erma's® (Aug '07)

Appetizers

	C	F	Cb
Black Bean Roll-Ups	575	10	95
Entrees: Blue Cheese NY Strip	1340	107	9
Caribbean Chicken (lunch)	535	20	60
Salads: No Breadstick			
Hula Bowl w. Dressing	575	7	79
Half Hula Bowl w. Dressing	365	4	57
Baby Greens Salad, no dressing	120	11	6
Shrimp Stack Salad	320	12	33
Sandwiches & Hamburgers			
Burger Stack w. Broccoli	1105	81	6.5
Chicken Stack w. Broccoli	825	51	6.5
Sides			
Buttered Broccoli, 3.5 oz	105	9	4.5
Fruit Salad, 4.5 oz	55	0	16
Garlic Breadstick (1)	155	6	21
Hearty Beef Chili Soup	390	15	39
Beverages: Fruit Smoothie	125	0.5	28
Dressings: Per 2 Tablespoons (1 fl.oz)			
Bleu Cheese	200	21	0.5
Italian	110	12	1
Ranch	120	12	0.5
Fat Free: French	125	0	31
Honey Mustard	60	0	14
Low-Fat Tex Mex Dressing	25	0	2.5

For Complete Nutritional Data ~ see CalorieKing.com

Mazzio's® (Aug '07)

Appetizers: Per Serving

	C	F	Cb
Breadsticks, no sauce, ¼ order	150	3	26
Cheese Dippers, no sce, ⅓ order	405	18	47
Cinnamon Sticks, no sce, ¼ order	625	36	70
BBQ Chicken Wings, no sce, ⅓ order	190	12	7
Nachos: Beef w. Jalapenos, ½ order	485	34	20
Cheddar w. Jalapenos, ½ order	425	30	19
Calzones: Per Slice (⅒ Whole)			
Ham & Cheddar, no Sauce	245	7.5	32
Pepperoni	260	10	32
Pastas: Without Garlic Toast			
Fettuccine Alfredo	1060	56	106
Spaghetti w. Marinara Sce	640	8	120
Lasagna: w. Meat Sauce	950	52	64
w. Marinara Sauce	705	30	73
w. Alfredo Sauce	1265	94	55
Sandwiches			
Focaccia: Chicken, Bacon & Swiss	1020	70	49
Ham & Cheddar	745	47	47
Mazzio's Sub	770	50	45
Turkey & Swiss	720	38	46
Tuscan Smash	645	34	45
Hoagie: Chicken, Bacon & Swiss	1360	73	120
Ham & Cheddar	1090	50	119
Mazzio's Sub	1110	52	117
Turkey & Swiss	1060	41	118
Tuscan Smash	985	36	117
Pizzas: Per Slice (⅛ Medium Pizza)			
Cheese: Original Crust	235	9	30
Thin Crust	180	9	18
Chicken Club: Original Crust	260	9	31
Thin Crust	205	9	19
Mazzio's Works: Original Crust	310	14	31
Thin Crust	255	14	20
Meatbuster: Original Crust	285	13	30
Thin Crust	235	13	19
Mexican: Original Crust	315	14	35
Thin Crust	260	14	23
Pepperoni: Original Crust	255	11	30
Thin Crust	200	11	18
Sausage: Original Crust	275	12	30
Thin Crust	225	13	19
Supremebuster: Original Crust	260	10	31
Thin Crust	205	11	18
Veggie: Original Crust	230	8	31
Thin Crust	180	8	20
Sides: Garlic Toast, 1 pce, 1.4 oz	160	10	15
Kosher Pickle Spear, 1 oz	5	0	1
Potato Chips, 1 oz	150	10	15

For Complete Nutritional Data ~ see CalorieKing.com

Mimi's Cafe® (Aug '07)

Breakfast	C	F	Cb
Hot off the Griddle, French Toast	305	13	40
Hot off the Griddle, Pancakes	955	35	139
Three Egg Omelette w. Sides, Low-Fat	480	5	69
Two Egg Breakfasts w. Sides	385	25	26
Carb Conscious Specialties			
Mimi's Breakfast	680	22	21
Chicken & Vegetable Platter	780	43	24
Fresh Salmon w. Steamed Veges	460	28	8
Half Pound Cheeseburger in Lettuce	730	41	13
Mediterranean Omelette w. Tomato	545	35	25
Petite Chopped Cobb Salad, no Dr.	605	51	13
Top Sirloin Steak w. Steamed Veges	580	27	7
Two "AA" Large Eggs w. Tom./Saus.	415	32	5
Sandwiches			
Classic Beef Dip	520	15	43
Fresh Roasted Turkey Breast: Reg.	530	27	28
Low-Fat, ½ sandwich	335	9	42
Ham & Cheddar Grill	1210	77	74

For Complete Nutritional Data ~ see CalorieKing.com

Miami Subs® (Aug '07)

Burgers	C	F	Cb
Deluxe Burger	785	59	31
Deluxe Cheeseburger	860	65	32
Deluxe Bacon Cheeseburger	920	69	32
Platters: Chicken Breast	745	41	57
Gyros	1420	93	81
10 Wings w. Fries & Blue Cheese	1020	67	50
Salads: Caesar w. Dressing	460	34	26
Chicken Caesar w. Dressing	610	39	28
Chicken Club	490	25	23
Garden	310	18	21
Greek	285	15	24
Side Greek w. Dressing	80	5	4
Cheesesteaks (6"): Original	410	11	45
Classic	420	11	47
Chicken Philly Classic	550	27	46
Works	530	22	51
Pitas: Gyros	660	39	46
Chicken	390	13	33
Subs(6"): Ham & Cheese	450	18	79
Italian Deli	515	24	49
Meatball	490	22	49
Tuna	470	18	44
Turkey	485	18	67
Sides: Mozzarella Sticks	755	56	34
Onion Rings	870	68	55
Spicy Fries: Regular	530	39	39
Large	1040	72	85

Mr. Goodcents® (Aug '07)

	C	F	Cb
Cold Sub: *Per Half Sandwich on Wheat Bread*			
Centsable Sub	495	20	57
Cheese Mix	570	26	57
Ham & Cheese	420	10	62
Italian Sub	620	34	57
Mr. Goodcents Original	480	28	29
Oven Roasted Chicken Breast	355	6	54
Penny Club	365	7	56
Pepperoni & Cheese	750	54	32
Roast Beef	370	7	54
Hot Sub: *Per Half Sandwich on Wheat Bread (w. Cheese)*			
Chicken Bacon Ranch	580	31	28
Chicken Parmesan	525	15	61
Meatball	715	33	65
Pasta: Chicken Parmesan	695	12	100
Red Sauce on Mostaccioli	520	4	100

Mr. Hero® (Aug '07)

	C	F	Cb
Sandwiches: *Per 7" Sub*			
Hot Subs: Grilled Chkn Philly	440	14	48
Cheesesteak: Grilled Steak Philly	450	14	48
Hot Buttered Deluxe	565	33	48
Cold Subs: Classic Italian	585	36	49
Tuna & Cheese	665	47	47
Turkey & Cheese	455	20	46
Ultimate Italian	610	33	51
Meatball	620	32	53
Romanburger	715	47	49
Round: Bacon Cheeseburger	350	23	23
Chicken	420	22	23
Fish	410	23	31
Tuna	430	33	22
Pasta: Breadsticks w. Sauce, 5 oz	290	9	47
Spaghetti Dinner, 16.8 oz	610	8	110
Spaghetti w. Meatballs, 19.8 oz	845	26	116
Salads: Garden Salad	35	0.5	7
Grilled Chicken	225	10	7
Seafood Crab	450	37	17
Side Salad	30	0.5	6
Tuna Salad	740	69	8
Dressings: Buttermilk, 2 oz	290	29	6
Creamy Italian, 2 oz	190	17	11
Croutons, ½ oz	60	2	9
Fat-Free: French ; Ranch	70	0	18
Side Orders: Onion Rings, 6 oz	565	32	64
Cheddar Cheese Sauce, 1.5 oz	60	4.5	5
Potato Waffers, 3.7 oz	335	17	42
Desserts: Cheesecake, plain, 3.5 oz	350	26	26
Cheesecake w. Cherries, 4.7 oz	385	26	35

Restaurants & Fast - Foods

Mrs Fields Cookies® (Aug '07)

	C	F	Cb
Brownies: Per Brownie (2.6 oz)			
Butterscotch Blondie	350	14	52
Double Fudge	360	20	45
Pecan Fudge	360	20	46
Special Walnut Fudge & Blondie	350	16	43
Toffee Fudge	360	19	47
Walnut Fudge	360	20	45
Cakes			
Blueberry, 3 oz slice	270	12	36
Carrot Cake, 3 oz slice	280	13	37
Chocolate, 3 oz piece	350	21	35
Chocolate Chip, 3 oz piece	350	17	45
Cinnamon Sugar Pecan, 2.1 oz slice	270	14	32
Lemon Bundt, 2.1 oz slice	300	14	40
Raspberry, 3 oz piece	270	12	36
Raspberry Chocolate Chip, 2.1 oz	260	12	36
Cookies			
Bite Size Nibblers: Cinn. Sugar (3)	170	8	22
Debra's Special (3)	170	7	23
Peanut Butter (3)	180	10	20
Semi-Sweet Chocolate (3)	170	8	24
Triple Chocolate (3)	170	9	23
White Chunk Macadamia (3)	180	9	23
Butter Cookie (1)	200	8	29
Coconut & Macadamia (1)	280	13	39
Cut Out Cookie (1)	400	19	56
Debra's Special (1)	200	9	25
Peanut Butter (1)	210	12	24
Semi-Sweet Chocolate (1)	210	10	29
w. Walnuts (1)	220	11	29
Triple Chocolate (1)	210	11	28
White Chunk Macadamia (1)	230	12	27
Muffins: Blueberry (1), ¾ oz	70	3	10
Chocolate Chip (1), ¾ oz	80	4	11
Mandarin Orange (1), ¾ oz	80	3	9
Raspberry (1), ¾ oz	70	3	10

For Complete Nutritional Data ~ see CalorieKing.com

My Favorite Muffin®

~ Same Menu & Data as
Big Apple Bagel (See Page 189) ~

Nathan's Famous® (Aug '07)

	C	F	Cb
Burgers			
¼ lb Burger	535	30	42
¼ lb Burger w. Cheese	850	61	45
Bacon Cheeseburger	705	44	43
Super Burger	865	61	42
Cheesesteaks: Chicken	565	19	62
Original	740	43	50
Supreme	785	43	61
Fish Sandwich	465	20	41
Hot Dogs: Nathan's Famous (1)	310	20	22
Sides			
French Fries: Regular, 9.6 oz	545	37	46
Large, 13.4 oz	760	52	65
Super, 21 oz	1190	82	101
Nuggets (6), 3.5 oz	350	27	20
Onion Rings, 5.6 oz	560	44	36

For Complete Nutritional Data ~ see CalorieKing.com

Noodles & Company® (Aug '07)

	C	F	Cb
Classics			
Buttered Noodles & Parm.	1010	36	134
Chicken Noodle Soup	290	9	37
Mushroom Stroganoff	1000	45	116
Pad Thai	720	9	147
Pesto Cavatappi	760	30	89
Tomato Marinara	560	13	87
Wisconsin Mac & Cheese	970	44	99
Noodle-Less: Chicken Rustica	530	26	11
Mediterranean Mixed Grill	190	2	43
Shrimp Curry Saute	190	6	20
Sweet Chili Chicken	470	14	29
Specialties: Bangkok Curry	400	10	71
Indonesian Peanut Saute	820	21	128
Japanese Pan Noodle, no oil	620	1.5	128
Pasta Fresca	660	19	93
Penne Rosa	670	32	70
Thai Curry Soup	360	15	49
Whole Grain Tuscan Fettuccine	500	17	70
Salads			
Caesar Salad w. Dressing	440	35	28
Chinese Chop Salad	340	21	37
Market Salad w. Fat Free Dressing	190	2	43
The Med Salad	360	16	40
Spicy Peanut Noodle Salad	480	9	83
Spicy Thai Caesar Salad	220	19	11
Sides: Potstickers (3)	330	17	34
Cucumber Tomato Salad	100	0	21

Ninety Nine (Aug '07)

	C	**F**	**Cb**
Appetizers			
All Star Sampler, ¼ platter	450	29	23
Boneless Wings & Skins Sampler, ¼	360	21	18
Outrageous Potato Skins, ¼ platter	300	23	13
Toasted Ravioli	210	12	16
Desserts			
Apple Fortune	870	39	123
Little Midnight Fudge Hero	430	23	54
Low Carb Cheesecake	380	29	35
Strawberry Shortcake	590	25	88
Towering Midnight Oreo Fudge Cake	860	47	109
Sandwiches: *No Sides*			
BBQ Pulled Pork Sandwich	710	34	52
Buffalo Chicken Sandwich	1120	60	87
Cajun Mushroom Steakburger	1210	81	64
Philly Steakburger	860	47	53
Tuscan Steakburger	1110	75	54
Veggie Burger	790	37	71
Salads			
Boneless Buffalo Wing Salad	980	60	71
w/o dressing or bread	540	25	42
Calypso Coconut Shrimp Salad	1000	65	90
Tropical Chicken Salad	850	41	71
Wild Bleu Chicken & Spinach Salad	1270	82	67
Meals			
Cape Cod Seafood Trio, no pot./vege	670	40	20
Captain's Combo Platter	2320	143	166
Grilled Chicken Fajitas	1400	58	118
Grilled Double BBQ Turkey Tips	1620	65	138
no sides	610	3	42
Shrimp Scampi	1270	55	143
Smothered Sirloin Tips, no vege	810	40	9
Teriyaki Chicken, w. Rice, no vege	750	16	66
Sides			
Double Bleu Iceberg Wedge	450	41	9
Garlic Redskin Mashed Potatoes	300	14	42
Honey Butter Biscuit w. honey butter	300	14	38
Honey Butter, ¼ oz	35	3	3
Onion Rings, garnish	360	24	32
Rice Side Dish, 8.5 oz	340	8	60
Cole Slaw, 7 oz	320	26	20
French Fries, 8 oz. raw weight	550	35	48
Rustic Bread w. Garlic Sauce	140	3	27
Soup: *Per Cup*			
Seafood Chowder, no topping	390	20	31

O'Charley's® (Aug '07)

	C	**F**	**Cb**
Appetizers: *Per Serving*			
Chicken Quesadilla Dip	990	59	53
Chicken O'Tenders w. Buffalo Sce (6)	810	53	31
Chips & Salsa	520	18	82
Fried Cheese Wedges (7)	880	60	55
Spinach & Artichoke Dip	940	51	107
Brunch: *Per Order (w. Brunch Potatoes & Toast)*			
Cajun Chicken Omelette	870	63	13
Spanish Omelette	1180	80	66
Ultimate Omelette	1180	79	68
Strawberry Waffle	1290	50	196
Chicken: *Per Order*			
Chicken Parmesan w. Vegetables	860	42	70
Chkn Tenders Dinner, w. Sauce	850	57	34
Chicken Teriyaki on Rice	500	6	57
Grilled Chicken Dinner	460	13	26
Salad: *No Dressing*			
Black & Bleu Caesar	920	65	21
O'Charley's Caesar Salad	490	30	13
Cajun Chicken	740	49	17
California Chicken	560	26	42
Southern Fried Chicken	720	41	34
Sandwiches: *No Fries*			
Bacon & Cheese Trio Chicken	800	40	53
Buffalo Kickin', no dressing	980	58	72
French Dip	650	23	70
Grilled Chicken Flatbread, no sides	770	28	83
Grilled Chicken Sandwich	610	27	52
Three Cheese Bacon Burger	1050	63	51
Seafood:			
Coconut Shrimp w. Sauce, no sides	650	26	88
Sides: *Baked Potato, plain*	420	24	52
Cole Slaw	250	19	19
French Fries, Adult	300	18	30
Rice Pilaf	200	5	31
Smashed Potatoes	370	12	47
Vegetable Medley	180	14	13
Steak & Ribs: *Per Serving (No Sides or Fries)*			
Steak Tips Monterey, 1 order	1000	64	47
Choice Sirloin, 5 oz	260	14	0
Filet Mignon, 9 oz	500	30	0
Flame Grilled Sirloin: 7 oz	430	28	0
10 oz	580	35	0
Prime Rib: 10 oz	1020	79	3
16 oz	1630	127	4
Full Rack of Ribs	1480	96	76
Ribeye Steak, 12 oz	810	55	0

Updated Nutrition Data ~ www.CalorieKing.com
Persons with Diabetes ~ See Disclaimer (Page 24)

$\mathcal{R}estaurants$ & Fast - Foods

Old Country Buffet® (Aug '07)

	C	F	Cb
Entrees: BBQ Beef Ribs, 5 oz	300	23	7
BBQ Smoked Sausage, 1 T., 2.8 oz	140	10	9
Breakfast Quiche, 1 Tbsp., 3.7 oz	220	15	12
Carved: Beef Brisket, 3 oz	200	11	1
Ham, 3 oz	140	9	0
Peppered Pork Loin, 3 oz	160	8	0
Roast Beef, 3 oz	230	15	0
Roast Turkey, 3 oz	170	8	0
Salmon Filet, 3 oz	190	12	0
Chicken Wings: Hot, Drummies (1)	35	2	0
Hot, Wing (1)	25	1.5	0
Teriyaki, Drummie (1)	50	2.5	2
Teriyaki, Wing (1)	50	2.5	2
Chicken Hand Breaded Fried:			
Breast, 5 oz	310	16	3
Drumstick (1), 1.4 oz	90	6	2
Thigh (1), 3.1 oz	210	14	4
Chicken, Traditional Baked: Breast	280	12	0
Drumstick (1), 1.4 oz	90	6	0
Thigh (1), 3.2 oz	160	11	0
Fish: Patties, 1 piece, 2.6 oz	160	9	13
Fried, 1 piece, 1.3 oz	80	3.5	9
Shrimp, fried, 6 shrimp, 1.9 oz	110	5	11
Smoked Saus. & Sauerkraut, 1 link	190	17	2
Spanish Rice, 1 Tbsp., 3 oz	140	9	9
Salads: Per Spoon Unless Indicated			
California Coleslaw, 3.5 oz	90	0.5	22
Macaroni Vegetable Salad, 3.5 oz	230	15	20
Marinated Vegetables, 3.5 oz	60	3.5	6
Seven Layer Salad, 2.6 oz	180	17	4
Tossed Green Salad, 1 cup, 1.6 oz	5	0	1
Sides: Baked Potato (1), 6.3 oz	160	0	39
Hashed Browns, 2.8 oz	110	6	13
Soups: Chili Bean, 4 fl.oz ladle	100	3.5	9
Corn Chowder, 4 fl.oz ladle	140	8	15
Navy Bean Soup, 4 fl.oz ladle	50	0	10
Desserts			
Cheesecake, plain, 1 piece, 2.8 oz	220	10	29
Chocolate Decadence Cake, 1 piece	200	9	27
Cookie, Sugar Free Ranger (1)	100	5	11
Hot Fudge Sundae Cake, 3 oz	160	3.5	32
Pumpkin Pie, 4.2 oz	270	9	31
Pudding: Chocolate, 1 Tbsp, 3 oz	150	7	19
Reduced Sugar/Calorie, 3 oz	70	1	14
Vanilla, 1 Tbsp (3 oz), 86g	140	6	19
Soft Serve Ice Cream, avg., 4 oz	140	4.5	24

Olive Garden® (Aug '07)

	C	F	Cb
Appetizers			
Bruschetta	440	21	57
Sicilian Scampi (4)	460	31	16
Stuffed Mushrooms (2)	385	31	12
Entrees (Includes Vegetables):			
Lunch: Lasagna Classico (4"x4½")	860	47	54
Eggplant Parmigiana	900	39	78
Fettuccine Alfredo	850	58	70
Sausage & Peppers Rustica	885	51	71
Dinner: Pork Fillettino	1010	58	116
Chicken Castellina	895	46	78
Manicotti Formaggio	800	38	57
Mixed Grill, 21.4 oz	840	43	65
Stuffed Chicken Marsala	1315	87	72
Garden Fare Selections (Lower Fat)			
Lunch: Capellini Pomodora, 13 oz	410	9	52
Chicken Giardino, 15.5 oz	410	12	40
Linguine alla Marinara, 10.6 oz	340	6	48
Shrimp Primavera, 19 oz	485	12	65
Dinner: Chicken Giardino, 21.5 oz	560	15	59
Capellini Pomodora, 21 oz	645	14	84
Linguine alla Marinara, 17 oz	550	8	79
Shrimp Primavera, 26 oz	705	24	84
Extras: Minestrone Soup, 6 fl.oz	160	1	30
Breadstick, plain, 1 stick	140	1.5	26
Dressing (Low Fat): Italian	37	2	4
Parmesan Peppercorn, 2 fl.oz	45	2	5

(The) Old Spaghetti Factory® (Aug '07)

	C	F	Cb
Lunch Entrees: Fettuccine Alfredo	1130	83	71
Chicken Parmigiana, 19 oz	840	34	84
Garlic Cheese Bread Starter, 13½ oz	1220	85	105
Lasagna, 13 oz	520	27	29
Manicotti, 11½ oz	510	21	55
Pot Pourri, 10 oz	480	22	54
Spinach & Cheese Ravioli, 11 oz	480	15	59
Spinach Tortellini w. Alfredo, 12 oz	930	56	82
Spaghetti: w. Clam Sauce, 10 oz	460	19	56
w. Meatballs, 13.5 oz	610	24	62
w. Meat Sauce & Mizithra, 9.2 oz	450	19	53
w. Mizithra/Mushr./Tom. Sauce	450	19	52
w. Rich Meat Sauce, 10 oz	310	3.5	55
w. Sausage & Meat Sce, 13.7 oz	620	29	57
w. Tomato & Meat Sauce, 10 oz	300	3.5	56

On the Border® (Aug '07)

	C	**F**	**Cb**
Salads: With Dressing Unless Indicated			
Chicken Chopped Salad, w. dressing	1330	89	54
Chicken Fiesta, Blackened	1150	75	54
Chicken Fiesta, Grilled	1140	74	52
Grande Taco Salad, Beef, no dress.	1450	102	78
House Salad, no dressing	170	10	15
Sizzling Beef Fajita, no dressing	910	65	24
Sizzling Chicken Fajita, no dressing	760	48	23
Dressings: Per Serving (2 fl.oz)			
Chipotle Honey Mustard	310	29	11
Jalapeno Ranch	180	19	3
Ranch Dressing	220	23	2
Smoked Jalapeno Vinaigrette	230	22	8
Sweet Pepper Vinaigrette	270	25	10
Fat-Free, Balsamic Vinaigrette	50	0	5
Low-Fat, Ranch	110	6	11
Soups: Chicken Tortilla, 1 bowl	350	22	24

For Complete Nutritional Data ~ see CalorieKing.com

Orange Julius® (Aug '07)

	C	**F**	**Cb**
Original (Orange, Strawberry):			
Small, average, 16 fl.oz	220	0	55
Medium, average, 20 fl.oz	275	0.5	68
Large, average, 32 fl.oz	450	1	109
Classic Smoothy® Drinks: Per 16 fl.oz			
Bananarilla; Tripleberry, average	300	7	56
Cool Cappuccino	390	10	69
Pina Colada; Tripleberry, average	360	7	70
Strawberry Banana	400	7	77
20 fl.oz Size ~ Add 25% to above figures			
32 fl.oz Size ~ Double the above figures			
Premium Smoothy: Per 20 fl.oz			
Banana Chill	550	10	134
Berry Lively; Blackberry Toner, avg.	450	1	100
Blackberry Storm	630	8	130
Blueberration	350	1.5	90
Cocoa Latte Swirl	640	9	122
Orange Swirl	490	10	96
Raspberry Crush	330	2	83
Strawb. Treasure; Raspb. Creme	540	8	103
Strawberry Xtreme	410	0.5	87
Tart 'N' Berry	450	1	102
Tropi-Colada	560	8	110
Wild Blue Twist	490	0.5	115
Add Banana, 1 medium	110	0.5	27
Nutrifiers: Avg. all types, ¼ oz	15	0	4

Outback Steakhouse® (Aug '07)

	C	**F**	**Cb**
Aussie-Tizers			
Aussie Chse Fries (28 oz), w. dress.	2900	182	240
Bloomin Onion (23 oz), w. dressing	2210	134	241
Gold Coast Coconut Shrimp, w. Sce	690	30	97
Grilled Shrimp on the Barbie w. Sce	660	42	32
Kookaburra Wings w. Sauce (10)	1160	75	65
Lobster-Crab Cakes w. Sauce (2)	840	72	33
Steaks: Meat Only ~ Add Extra for Sides			
Ayers Rock Strip (New York Strip) 12 oz	850	66	0
Outback Special, 12 oz Sirloin	780	55	0
Prime Minister's Prime Ribs:			
8 oz cut	450	38	0
12 oz cut	675	57	0
16 oz cut	905	77	0
Rockhampton Rib-Eye, 14 oz	730	40	0
The Melbourne, P/house, 20 oz	1365	110	0
Lean meat only	700	37	0
Victoria's "Center Cut Filet": *With ¼" Fat*			
Tenderloin, 7 oz	490	37	0
Tenderloin, 9 oz	630	48	0
Victoria's "Crowned Filet": *No Sides*			
Tenderloin (7 oz) w. Horseradish	840	64	21
Tenderloin (7 oz) w. Bleu Chse	1110	86	22
Tenderloin (9 oz), w. Horseradish	1005	79	22
Tenderloin (9 oz), w. Bleu Chse	1270	101	22
Meals: Hearts of Gold Chicken	870	55	22
Hearts of Gold Tilapia	640	31	23
Alice Springs Chicken	1080	60	23
Salad: Queensland w. Dressing	1100	88	45
Queensland Salad, no Dressing	705	47	37
Sides: Aussie Chips, 7½ oz, w. Ketchup	725	32	100
Fresh Veggies	80	1	14
Grilled Onions, 7.5 oz	180	11	19
Jacket Potato, Plain, 9 oz	270	0	63
Jacket Potato, w. Butter/Cheese	400	14	63
Mushrooms, Sauteed, 8 oz	150	11	12
Desserts: Cheesecake Olivia	700	38	79
Choc. Thunder from Down Under	1220	78	134

Most figures above are author calculations and not intended for clinical use.

For Extra Listings ~ see CalorieKing.com

Panda Express® (Aug '07)

Meals	C	F	Cb
Chicken: Black Pepper, 5½ oz	200	12	11
Orange Chicken, 5½ oz	500	27	42
w. Mushrooms, 5½ oz	130	6	8
Chicken Kung Pao Cashew, 5½ oz	200	9	12
BBQ Pork, 5½ oz	400	23	15
Beef & Broccoli, 5½ oz	150	7	11
Sweet & Sour Pork, 5½ oz	400	23	15
Mixed Veges, 5½ oz	90	7	8
Fried Tofu w. Veges, 5½ oz	120	8	10
Rice & Noodles: Per Order (8 oz)			
Chow Mein	390	12	59
Fried Rice	450	14	67
Steamed Rice	380	2.5	81
Appetizers: Chkn Egg Roll (1), 3 oz	170	8	17
Chicken Potsticker, 6 pces	440	25	49
Veggie Spring Roll (1)	80	3.5	11

Panera Bread® (Aug '07)

Bagels: Blueberry	330	1	69
Dutch Apple & Raisin	370	3	78
Plain	290	1	61
Spreads: Plain Cream Cheese, 2 oz	200	19	2
Reduced Fat, average, 2 oz	140	13	2
Salad: Asian Sesame Chkn w. Dr.	450	22	31
Caesar w. Dressing	440	32	25
Classic Cafe w. Dressing	400	37	18
Greek w. Dressing	520	48	17
Grilled Chicken Caesar w. Dressing	560	34	26
Sandwiches: Asiago Roast Beef	700	32	56
Bacon Turkey Bravo	750	26	83
Chicken Salad on Whole Grain	580	25	71
Italian Combo	1110	56	91
Mediterranean Veggie	590	13	100
Sierra Turkey	960	53	80
Smoked Ham & Swiss on Rye	680	34	52
Smoked Turkey Brst on Sourdough	430	14	44
Smokehouse Turkey Panini	700	23	73
Tuna Salad on Honey Wheat	720	44	51
Turkey Artichoke Panini	840	38	85
Tuscan Chicken	740	30	79
Soup (8 oz): Boston Clam Chowder	300	11	19
Broccoli Cheddar	230	16	13
Chicken Noodle, Low Fat	100	2	15
Cream of Chicken & Wild Rice	200	12	19
French Onion, no Cheese/Croutons	80	3	12
Vegetarian: Black Bean	160	1	31
Garden Vegetable	90	0.5	17
Muffins: Banana Nut Muffie	230	11	31
Chocolate Chip Muffie	240	10	36
Pumpkin Muffie	310	7	49
Low Fat Tripleberry Muffin	270	2.5	57
For Extra Listings ~ see CalorieKing.com			

Papa Gino's® (Aug '07)

Appetizers: Per Serving	C	F	Cb
BBQ Chicken Tender, small, 4.1 oz	260	9	28
Buffalo Chkn Tenders, small, 4.2 oz	200	7	12
Cheese Breadsticks, small, 7.2 oz	535	24	58
Cheese Garlic Bread, large, 3.8 oz	220	5	36
Cinnamon Sticks, small, 3.6 oz	310	10	50
French Fries, small, 6.3 oz	330	19	38
Mozzarella Sticks, small, 5 oz	350	15	35
Pastas: Entree Size			
Papa Platter, Penne/Spagh., plain	1005	34	136
Ravioli	445	20	49
Spaghetti & Meatballs	895	30	123
Spaghetti Chicken Parmigiana	1080	41	128
Pizzas: Per Slice			
Large Thin Crust: BBQ Chicken	275	6	38
Buffalo Chicken	240	6	32
Cheese	225	6	32
Chicken Pepper	285	9	33
Garlic Chicken	290	11	35
Meat Combo	325	14	33
PapaRoni	325	15	33
Pepperoni	270	10	32
Super Veggie	245	7	35
Works	300	12	34
Subs: Per Small Sub			
BLT	685	31	72
Italian	905	48	69
Meatball	730	33	76
Meatball Parmesan	830	36	76
Seafood Salad	680	34	69
Steak & Cheese	695	30	68
Steak	600	23	65
Super Steak	740	30	78
Tuna	735	38	67
Turkey	445	2	72
Salads			
Buffalo Chicken Tender	320	15	32
Caesar	190	8	20
Chicken Bacon Cheddar	480	21	26
Chicken Tender	280	10	30
Garden	175	6	27
Italian Chopped	575	50	12
Side: Caesar	70	3	7
Garden	65	2	10
Dressings: Bleu Cheese, 1.1 oz	150	15	3
Caesar, 3 oz	395	43	0
Ranch, 3 oz	285	31	3
Honey Dijon, Fat-Free	60	0	13

Papa John's® (Aug '07)

	C	F	Cb
Original Crust (14"): *Per Slice (⅛ Whole)*			
All the Meats w. Beef	350	16	38
BBQ Chicken & Bacon	340	11	44
Cheese	300	11	39
Garden Fresh	280	9	40
Hawaiian BBQ Chicken	340	11	46
Pepperoni	310	13	38
Sausage	330	15	37
Spinach Alfredo/Chicken	290	11	37
The Works	330	11	39
Thin Crust (14"): *Per Slice (⅛ Pizza)*			
BBQ Chicken & Bacon	290	14	29
Cheese	240	13	22
Garden Fresh	210	11	23
Grilled Chicken Alfredo	240	13	20
Grilled Chicken Club	270	14	25
Hawaiian BBQ Chicken	290	14	31
Pepperoni	260	15	23
Sausage	280	17	23
Spicy Italian	320	14	24
Spinach Alfredo/Chicken	230	13	21
The Works	280	14	23
Side Orders: *Bread Stick (1), 2 oz*	140	2	26
Cheese Sticks, 2 sticks	370	16	42
Papa's Chickenstrips, 2 strips	160	8	10
Cinna Swirl Pie, ½ pie, 3.7 oz	390	14	53
Sauce: Garlic, 1 oz	150	17	0
Honey Mustard, 1 oz	150	15	5
Pizza, 1 oz	20	0	3

Papa Murphy's® (Aug '07)

	C	F	Cb
Pizzas: *Per Slice (Family Size)*			
Deeper Dish, Traditional, ⅛ pizza	440	24	34
Gourmet: Chicken Garlic, 1/12 pizza	320	14	30
Classic Italian, 1/12 pizza	350	18	30
Veggie, 1/12 pizza	300	13	31
Papa's: BBQ Chicken, 1/12 pizza	335	13	37
Cheese, 1/12 pizza	260	10	29
All Meat; Cowboy, 1/12 pizza, avg.	350	17	30
Hawaiian, 1/12 pizza	285	11	33
Murphy's Combo, 1/12 pizza	355	18	31
Pepperoni, 1/12 pizza	310	15	29
Specialty; Perfect, 1/12 pizza, avg.	310	14	31
Rancher, 1/12 pizza	325	15	30
Veggie Combo, 1/12 pizza	285	12	32
Continued Next Page ...			

Papa Murphy's® cont... (Aug '07)

	C	F	Cb
Pizzas: *Per Slice (Family Size)*			
Stuffed: Big Murphy, 1/16 pizza	360	16	40
Other varieties, 1/16 pizza	370	16	39
Thin Crust deLITEs: Cheese, 1/10	140	6.5	13
Hawaiian, 1/10 pizza	150	6.5	15
Meat, 1/10 pizza	190	10	13
Pepperoni, 1/10 pizza	165	9	13
Veggie, 1/10 pizza	150	8	13
Salads: Club, no Dressing	315	19	18
Garden, no Dressing	160	11	10
Italian, no dressing	220	16	9

Pei Wei Asian Diner (Aug '07)

	C	F	Cb
Appetizers: *Per Serving*			
Crab Wontons (4)	190	13	9
Crispy Potstickers (4)	130	7	10
Edamame, ½ dish	155	8	12
Minced Chicken w. Lettuce Wraps	250	4	31
Spring Rolls (2)	90	5	11
Meals: *Per ½ Dish/Bowl*			
Dan Dan Noodle, Chicken	390	7	54
Fried Rice: Beef	580	21	56
Chicken	470	11	56
Japanese Udon Noodles: Beef	600	26	57
Chicken	490	16	57
Lo Mein Noodles: Chicken	460	11	61
Beef	570	21	61
Pad Thai: Beef	670	30	63
Chicken	560	20	61
Soba Miso Bowls: Shrimp	360	6	51
Beef	530	18	53
Chicken	420	8	53
Teriyaki Bowl w. Brown Rice: Beef	580	17	66
Chicken	460	7	64
Teriyaki Bowl w. White Rice: Beef	560	16	62
Chicken	440	6	60
Salads: *Per ½ Dish (no Dressing)*			
Asian Chopped Chicken	200	8	10
Spicy Chicken	210	2.5	23
Salad Dressings: *Per Serving*			
Lime Vinaigrette, 2 oz	230	20	13
Sesame Ginger, 2 oz	70	16	5
Sauces: Lettuce Wrap, 2 oz	70	4.5	2
Sweet Chile, 2 oz	140	0	34
Thai Peanut, 2 oz	170	11	15
Sides: *Per ½ Dish*			
Noodles: Egg	210	2.5	39
Rice	130	0	32
Udon	100	0	20
Rice: Brown	170	1.5	37
White	200	0	44
Soups: Hot & Sour, 1 bowl	500	28	37
Wonton, 1 bowl	260	4.5	49

$\mathcal{R}estaurants$ & Fast - Foods

Penn Station® (Aug '07)

Subs (6")	C	F	Cb
Artichoke: w. mayo	360	18	37
No mayo	260	7	37
Cheese Bread	250	5.5	42
Chicken Salad	360	15	41
Chicken Teriyaki	435	13	48
Grilled Vegetarian	245	4	46
Ham Dagwood, no cheese	260	6.5	35
Philadelphia Cheesesteak	500	25	45
Philadelphia Cheesesteak, no mayo	395	14	45
Reuben	500	21	40
Reuben, no 1000 Island Dressing	390	12	37
Tuna Salad	365	15	41
Turkey Dagwood	420	18	36
Turkey Dagwood, no Cheese/Mayo	240	4	34

Pepe's Mexican® (Aug '07)

Burritos:	C	F	Cb
Beef & Bean	510	24	52
Beef & Bean Suizo	640	34	55
Chicken & Bean	480	21	51
Chicken & Bean Suizo	610	31	54
Pork & Bean	470	19	51
Pork & Bean Suizo	600	29	54
Flauta: Beef, plain	160	9	10
Beef w. cheese & sauce	190	12	11
Chicken, plain	190	10	16
Chicken w. cheese & sauce	230	13	17
Taco Salad: (Includes Taco Shell)			
Beef w. 4 oz salsa	550	26	52
Chicken w. 4 oz salsa	520	23	51
Pork w. 4 oz salsa	500	20	52
Without Taco Shell, deduct	210	7	32
Tacos: Beef Crisp	210	11	16
Beef Soft Corn	250	10	28
Beef Soft Flour	250	11	24
Chicken Crisp	190	9	15
Chicken Soft Corn	230	8	27
Chicken Soft Flour	230	9	23
Pork Crisp	170	6	16
Pork Soft Corn	220	6	27
Pork Soft Flour	220	7	24
Tostada			
Beef & Bean	380	23	26
Beef & Bean Suiza	440	29	26
Chicken & Bean	360	21	21
Chicken & Bean Suiza	410	26	25
Pork & Bean	350	20	26
Pork & Bean Suiza	410	25	26

Perkin's® Family Restaurant (Aug '07)

Entrees	C	F	Cb
Chicken Dinner	620	13	60
Fish Dinner	470	7	60
Fruit Cup	50	0.5	12
'Lite & Healthy'	105	2	15
Omelettes: Country Club	930	79	6
Deli Ham & Cheese	960	79	8
'Everything' Omelette	695	54	9
Granny's Country Omelette	940	82	5
w. 9 oz Hash Browns	1245	90	57
Salads: Chef's, Mini	215	11	7
Muffins: Banana	650	33	78
Blueberry; Pumpkin	550	26	78
Bran Muffin	550	16	94
Carrot	455	26	55
Chocolate Chips	620	26	81
Cranberry Nut	585	29	75
Lemon Poppyseed	685	33	88
Oat Bran	455	15	68
Peaches & Cream; Apple, avg.	520	23	72
Raspberry & Cream	585	26	81
Pancakes: Buttermilk (1), no syrup	140	4.5	20
Short Stack (3), no syrup	425	14	60
Regular Stack (5), no syrup	705	24	100
Pies (Per Slice): Apple Pie, ⅛ pie	375	15	56
Wildberry, ⅙ pie	390	16	66
Bundt Cake, w. Icing (sugar free)	385	17	70

For Complete Nutritional Data ~ See CalorieKing.com

Petro's® (Aug '07)

Petro: Per Serving	C	F	Cb
Chicken: small	465	24	43
medium	665	36	59
large	970	52	88
Lite: small	380	12	48
medium	530	16	66
large	785	24	99
Original: small	515	30	43
medium	735	43	58
large	1075	63	87
Pasta Lite: small	335	2.5	52
medium	495	3.5	79
large	680	4.5	107
Pasta: small	405	16	45
medium	625	26	67
large	850	36	91
Veggie: small	525	28	52
medium	745	41	70
large	1090	60	105

Petro's® cont... (Aug '07)

Chili: Per Serving (Medium Container)	C	F	Cb
Chicken	275	4	43
Original	370	14	42
Veggie	385	11	48
Baked Potato: #1 Lite (1)	365	0.5	74
#2 Butter Sour Cream (1)	480	18	74
#3 Loaded (1)	680	33	78
#4 Loaded w. Chili (1)	780	37	90
#5 Broccoli 3 Cheese (1)	655	30	77
Hot Dogs			
Chili	315	17	28
Chili & Cheese	345	19	29
Loaded	350	19	30
Plain	265	14	22
Slaw	350	16	23
Tostitos Chips: Per Serving			
Loaded Ultimate Nachos	880	51	79
Tostitos Chips: Queso	500	27	60
Ransalsa	560	35	61
Salsa	415	18	62
Salads			
Garden, small	45	0.5	8
Petro, Original	570	36	42
Petrol, Grilled Chicken	740	41	42

For Complete Nutritional Data ~ see CalorieKing.com

Peter Piper® Pizza (Aug '07)

Cheese Pizza: Per Slice	C	F	Cb
Hand-Tossed Crust (14"), ⅛ pizza	290	9	38
Hand-Tossed Crust (16"), 1⁄12 pizza	260	8	33
Healthy Dining: Orig. Crust, 1 slice	300	6	38
Ultra Thin Crust, slice	130	4	15
Original Crust (14"), ⅛ pizza	300	9	37
Original Crust (16"), 1⁄12 pizza	260	8	32
Pan Crust (14"), ⅛ pizza	290	9	38
Pan Crust (16"), 1⁄12 pizza	290	8	38
Thin Crust (14"), 1⁄12 pizza	150	5	14
Thin Crust (16"), 1⁄16 pizza	140	5	13
Pepperoni Pizza: Per Slice			
Hand-Tossed Crust (14"), ⅛ pizza	290	10	37
Hand-Tossed Crust (16"), 1⁄12 pizza	260	8	33
Original Crust (14"), ⅛ pizza	300	10	36
Original Crust (16"), 1⁄12 pizza	260	8	32
Pan Crust (14"), ⅛ pizza	330	10	44
Pan Crust (16"), 1⁄12 pizza	280	9	37
Thin Crust (14"), 1⁄12 pizza, 48g	150	6	13
Thin Crust (16"), 1⁄16 pizza, 47g	140	6	13
Appetizers: Breadsticks (2)	250	10	36
Chicken Strips, 2 pieces	300	9	26
Garlic Cheese Bread, 2 slices	310	14	37
Wings, 2 pieces	110	8	0

For Complete Nutritional Data ~ see CalorieKing.com

P F Chang's® (Aug '07)

Appetizers: Per Whole Dish	C	F	Cb
Crab Wontons w. Plum Sauce	530	26	52
Harvest Spring Rolls (4)	350	15	46
Lettuce Wraps: Chicken	510	12	68
Vegetarian	420	4.5	70
Peking Dumplings: Pan-Fried	430	24	31
Steamed	390	19	31
Seared Ahi Tuna w. Mustard	310	11	21
Shrimp Dumplings: Pan-Fried	330	13	26
Steamed w. Ginger Sauce	290	9	26
Spare Ribs: w. Barbecue Sauce	1280	79	47
Northern Style	730	55	6
Vegetable Dumplings: Pan-Fried	370	12	53
Steamed	330	8	53
Desserts: Banana Spring Rolls	815	37	130
Great Wall of Chocolate	2240	89	376
New York Style Cheesecake	950	55	88
Meals: Per Whole Dish			
Beef: A La Sichuan	1180	64	56
Mongolian	1180	73	29
Orange Peel	1580	85	115
Chicken: w. Black Bean Sauce	700	25	33
Chang's Spicy	930	37	88
Ginger & Broccoli	660	26	45
Kung Pao, regular	1240	80	58
Mu Shu	720	38	50
Orange Peel	1150	47	127
Philip's Better Lemon	1060	42	113
Spicy Ground w. Eggplant	810	40	73
Sweet & Sour	770	20	107
Duck, Cantonese Roasted	900	54	63
Lamb, Wok Seared	1080	80	29
Seafood: Cantonese Scallops	400	16	26
Cantonese Shrimp	330	12	21
Chang's Lemon Scallops	950	27	100
Crispy Honey Shrimp	1380	64	147
Hot Fish	1340	71	111
Kung Pao Scallops	1130	56	66
Kung Pao Shrimp	980	58	58
Lemon Pepper Shrimp	710	36	59
Oolong Marinated Sea Bass	520	12	40
Orange Peel Shrimp	1020	41	118
Salt & Pepper Prawns w. Sauce	850	50	53
Sichuan From The Sea: Calamari	1000	39	110
Scallops	1030	35	98
Shrimp	730	37	55
Wild Alaskan Salmon Lemon Pepper	700	36	36
Traditions Lunch: Beef w. Broc.	900	54	28
Almond Cashew Chicken	670	28	47
Crispy Honey Chicken	1000	38	111
Lo Mein Beef	1530	112	74

P F Chang's® cont... (Aug '07)

Meals (Cont): Per Whole Dish	C	F	Cb
Traditions Lunch: Lo Mein Chkn	1510	104	95
Moo Goo Gai Pan	660	34	32
Shrimp w. Lobster Sauce	410	21	18
Vegetarian Plate: Buddha's Feast	430	6	80
Coconut Curry Vegetables	690	46	48
Garlic Snap Peas	210	10	23
Ma Po Tofu	540	19	51
Shanghai Cucumbers	120	6	8
Sichuan Asparagus	200	6	34
Sichuan Green Beans	610	40	48
Spinach Stir-Fried w. Garlic	140	6	16
Stir-Fried Eggplant	600	34	64
Soups: Hot & Sour, 1 bowl	650	15	86
Pin Rice Noodle, 1 bowl	740	30	91
Wonton, 1 bowl	350	10	44

For Complete Nutritional Data ~ see CalorieKing.com

Philly Connection® (Aug '07)

Sandwiches: Regular Serving	C	F	Cb
Cheesesteak: Hoagie	490	23	42
Mushroom	460	19	43
Pizza Steak	470	19	44
Steak	350	11	40
The Original	460	20	41
The Works	490	19	52
Hoagie: Chicken	430	19	42
Chicken Parmesan	440	14	45
Chicken Works	440	14	54
Italian	500	26	40
Tuna	580	35	39
Turkey	420	20	41
Veggie Delite	410	16	55
Philly Lite: Chicken Hoagie	290	3.5	42
Chicken Parmesan	330	6	44
Chicken Works	330	5	54
Grilled Chicken	290	3.5	42
Turkey Hoagie	280	4	41
Veggie Hoagie	260	2.5	54
Specialty: Cheese Chicken	400	12	43
Meatball Parmesan	590	33	46
Sides			
Chicken Tenders, 9.5 oz	600	28	44
Salads			
Cheesesteak	330	18	15
Chicken Tenders	360	15	33
Grilled Chicken Salad	150	2	15
Grilled Chicken Caesar	190	5	13
Philly Lite: Garden	40	0.5	15
Grilled Chicken	150	2	15
Turkey	130	2.5	11
Tuna	290	18	9
Turkey	130	2.5	11
Veggie Delite	230	10	27

Piccadilly Cafeteria® (Aug '07)

Meals: No Sides Included	C	F	Cb
Beef: Chopped Steak Fried, 4.5 oz	415	33	6
Roast Leg, small, 4 oz	350	22	2
Steak: Filet Mignon, 6 oz	340	20	1
New York Strip, 10 oz	875	71	1
Ribeye, 10 oz	1040	91	2
Chicken: Breast, Mesquite Smoked	210	8	1
Baked Cajun, Boneless Breast	430	27	9
Fish: Catfish Cajun Baked	405	28	6
Catfish Filet Stuffed	550	40	9
Tilapia Baked	210	11	10
Trout Almondine Baked, large	490	22	11
Trout Cajun Baked	520	27	7
Trout Filets Baked	465	19	10
Pork Loin: Bone in Roast, 5 oz	375	13	10
Shrimp, Fried	460	19	34
Turkey Breast, Carved, 5.5 oz	265	10	5
Salads			
Caesar Salad, 3 oz	145	11	7
Chef's Salad, Small, 6 oz	145	9	4
Italian Coleslaw, 3.7 oz	165	16	5
Louisianne Bowl	45	3	2
Mexican	60	3	8
Piccadilly Bowl	25	0	6
Shrimp Remoulade	515	28	33
Dressings			
Au Jus, 3 fl.oz	5	0	1
Blue Cheese, 2 Tbsp	160	18	1
Cheese Sauce, 2 fl.oz	35	1	5
French, 2 Tbsp	130	13	5
Italian, 2 Tbsp	160	17	1
Ranch, 2 Tbsp	150	17	1
Ranch Fat-Free, 2 Tbsp	35	0	7
Thousand Island, 2 Tbsp	170	18	2
Soups: Per 9.5 oz (No Rice)			
Gumbo: Chicken	100	2	11
& Sausage	225	15	10
Extras			
Broccoli w. Cheese Sauce	105	7	9
Cabbage: Buttered, Steamed	70	5	6
Bacon Seasoned	105	8	6
Cauliflower, Buttered	90	6	8
Fried Okra	240	13	26
Greens: Collard Mustard & Turnip	135	10	3
Turnip w. Diced Turnips, 3.2 oz	150	12	4

Pizza Hut® (Aug '07)

C F Cb

Fit 'N Delicious Pizzas: *Per Slice (⅛ Medium Pizza)*

	C	F	Cb
Diced Chkn, Red Onion, Peppers	170	5	23
Diced Chkn, Mushroom, Jalapeno	170	5	22
Ham, Red Onion, Mushroom	160	4.5	23
Ham, Pineapple, Diced Red Tomato	160	4.5	23
Peppers, Red Onion, Diced Tom.	150	4	23
Tomato, Mushroom, Jalapeno	150	4	22

Pan Pizza: *Per Slice (⅛ Medium Pizza)*

	C	F	Cb
Cheese	270	13	27
Chicken Supreme	270	12	28
Italian Sausage & Onion	300	15	28
Meat Lover's	370	22	28
Pepperoni	280	14	27
Pepperoni Lover's	330	18	28
Sausage Lover's	320	17	28
Super Supreme	330	17	29
Supreme	310	16	28
Veggie Lover's	250	11	28

Personal Pan Pizza: *Per Pizza*

	C	F	Cb
Cheese	620	26	69
Italian Sausage & Onion	690	33	71
Pepperoni	640	29	67
Supreme	710	34	70
Super Supreme	720	39	71
Veggie Lover's	560	22	70

Thin 'n Crispy: *Per Slice (⅛ Medium Pizza)*

	C	F	Cb
Cheese; Chicken Supreme, avg.	200	8	21
Italian Sausage & Onion	230	11	23
Meat Lover's	310	18	22
Pepperoni	210	10	21
Pepperoni Lover's	260	14	21
Sausage Lover's	240	13	21
Supreme	230	11	22
Super Supreme	260	13	23
Veggie Lover's	180	7	23

Hand Tossed: *Per Slice (⅛ Medium Pizza)*

	C	F	Cb
Cheese; Chicken Supreme, avg.	230	10	25
Italian Sausage & Onion	260	12	26
Meat Lover's	340	19	25
Pepperoni	240	11	24
Pepperoni Lover's	290	15	25
Sausage Lover's	280	14	25
Super Supreme	290	14	26
Supreme	270	13	26
Veggie Lover's	210	8	26

Pizza Hut® cont... (Aug '07)

C F Cb

Stuffed Crust: *Per Slice (⅙ Large Pizza)*

	C	F	Cb
Cheese	360	16	37
Chicken Supreme	370	15	39
Italian Sausage & Onion	410	20	39
Meat Lover's	520	39	28
Pepperoni	390	19	37
Pepperoni Lover's	430	21	38
Super Supreme	430	21	40
Supreme	420	21	39
Veggie Lover's	340	14	38

The Full House XL: *Per Slice*

	C	F	Cb
Cheese Only	280	12	30
Chicken Supreme	270	10	31
Meat Lover's	370	20	31
Pepperoni	280	13	30
Pepperoni Lover's	270	11	30
Quartered Ham	260	10	32
Super Supreme	330	16	32
Supreme	310	14	31
Veggie Lover's	260	10	31

P'zone Pizza: *Per ½ Pizza*

	C	F	Cb
Classic	610	21	71
Meat Lover's	680	28	70
Pepperoni	610	22	69

Dessert Pizza: Apple Dessert

	C	F	Cb
	260	5	52
Cherry Dessert Pizza	260	4.5	47

Pasta: *Per Serving*

	C	F	Cb
Cavatini Pasta	420	15	55
Cavatini Supreme Pasta	460	18	56
Spaghetti: w. Marinara	490	8	90
w. Meat Sauce	640	20	92
Meatballs	630	19	92

Sides: Breadsticks, 1.3 oz

	C	F	Cb
	150	6	20
Buffalo Wings, Hot (1)	60	3.5	1
Buffalo Wings, Mild (1)	55	3.5	1
Ranch Dipping Cup, 1½ oz	210	23	3
Garlic Bread, 1 piece	160	10	14

Pizza Pizza® (Canada) (Aug '07)

Pizza: Per Slice (⅛ Classic Medium)	C	F	Cb
Bacon Dble Cheeseburger	220	7	29
Big Bacon Bonanza	220	7	29
Canadian Eh!	230	7	30
Cheese	200	5	29
Classic Super	210	6	30
Garden Veggie	190	4.5	30
New York Style Pepperoni	230	8	29
Pepperoni & Mushroom	210	6	30
Pepperoni	210	6	29
Sicilian	240	9	30
Spicy BBQ Chicken	200	4.5	30
Tropical Hawaiian	220	7	30

Small Pizza: Per Slice
Deduct 10% fewer calories/fat/carbs from figures for medium pizza

Large Pizza: Per Slice
Add 10% more calories/fat/carbs from figures for medium pizza

	C	F	Cb
Classic Slice: Big Bacon, 1 slice	710	26	88
Other varieties, average, 1 sl.	640	19	88
Signature Slice: Bacon Chkn, 1 sl.	830	39	88
Other varieties, avg., 1 slice	620	22	85
Oven Toasted Sandwiches			
Italian Deli Classic	680	32	48
Meatball	520	23	52
Mediterranean Veggie	560	27	57
Mesquite BBQ Chicken	500	11	62
Philly Cheese Steak	530	14	61
Stuffed S'wich: Classic Super	340	11	45
Mediterranean Veggie	390	15	49
Tropical Hawaiian	360	12	47
Chicken			
Bites, 3 pieces	230	11	14
Crispy Wings, 6 wings	720	46	22
Crunchers, 6 pieces	315	22	29
Lightly Breaded Wings, 6 wings	660	40	36
Strips, 3 pieces	310	16	22
Fries: Regular, 5 oz	410	20	55
Garlic Stix: Regular (3)	665	39	68
Four Cheese (3) w. 1 oz cheese	760	47	68
Garlic Bread: Regular, 5 pieces	760	42	79
with Cheese, 4 pieces	800	49	63
Drinks			
Lipton's Brisk, 12 fl.oz	120	0	31
Mug Root Beer, 12 fl.oz	160	0	41
Orange Crush, 12 fl.oz	180	0	48
7-UP, 12 fl.oz	160	0	43

Pizza Ranch® (Aug '07)

Pizzas, 12": Per Slice (⅛ Pizza)	C	F	Cb
Original: BBQ Beef	220	8	28
BBQ Chicken	210	6	27
Bacon Cheeseburger	220	9	26
Beef; Canadian Bacon, avg.	210	7	25
California Chicken	250	12	26
Cheese; Chicken Broccoli, avg.	220	8	26
Garlic Cheese	230	11	25
Italian Sausage; Pepperoni	220	9	25
Prairie; Sweet Swine, avg.	210	7	26
Roundup; Tabasco Pepperoni	230	10	26
Stampede	250	10	27
Texan	240	9	31
Skillet: BBQ Beef	230	8	30
BBQ Chicken	220	6	29
Bacon Cheeseburger	230	9	28
Beef; Canadian Bacon, avg.	220	7	27
Bronco; California Chicken, avg.	270	12	28
Cheese; Chicken Broccoli, avg.	230	8	28
Garlic Cheese	240	11	27
Italian Sausage; Pepperoni, avg.	230	9	27
Prairie; Sweet Swine	220	7	28
Roundup; Tabasco Pepperoni	240	10	28
Stampede	260	11	29
Texan	250	9	33
Thin: BBQ Beef	170	7	17
BBQ Chicken	150	6	16
Bacon Cheeseburger	170	8	15
Beef; Canadian Bacon, avg.	150	7	14
California Chicken; Bronco, avg.	200	11	15
Cheese; Chicken Broccoli, avg.	160	8	14
Garlic Cheese	170	10	14
Italian Sausage; Pepperoni, avg.	160	8	14
Prairie; Sweet Swine, avg.	150	7	15
Roundup; Tabasco Pepperoni	180	9	15
Stampede	190	10	16
Texan	190	9	20
Broasted Chicken: Breast, 1 pce	440	23	4
Leg, 1 piece	190	12	2
Thigh, 1 piece	370	26	4
Wing, 1 piece	190	13	2
Sides: Potato Wedges (1)	60	0	13

For Complete Nutritional Data ~ see CalorieKing.com

Planet Smoothie® (Aug '07)   C F Cb

Cool Blended Smoothies
Per 22 fl.oz Unless Otherwise Stated

	C	F	Cb
Captain Kid, 12 fl oz	195	1.5	47
PBJ	560	17	97
Shag-a-delic	430	1	104
The Last Mango	355	3.5	82
Twig & Berries	300	0.5	74
Vinnie del Rocco	385	3.5	92

Energy Smoothies: *Per 22 fl.oz*

Berry Bada-Bing	360	0.5	88
Chocolate Elvis	520	9	109
Frozen Goat	360	1	85
Grape Ape	305	0.5	78
Road Runner	280	0.5	72
Spazz	265	0.5	68

Workout Smoothies: *Per 22 fl.oz*

Big Bang	350	0.5	80
Chocolate Chimp	400	1	94
Merlin's Pineapple LB	415	1.5	57
Strawberry LB	485	1.5	78

Pollo Tropical® (Aug '07)

Chicken

Boneless Chicken Breast, 2 pieces	240	3	0
Quarter Chicken: Dark Meat w. skin	290	18	0
no skin	190	10	0
White Meat w. skin	325	16	0
no skin	205	6	0
TropiChop: Vegetarian	580	13	109
Chicken w. Rice & Black Bean	565	10	95
Chicken w. Yellow Rice & Veges	340	5	50
Grilled Chicken Deluxe	410	6	51
Pork w. Rice & Black Beans	715	23	97
Pork w. Yellow Rice & Vegetables	480	18	52
Ropa Vieja (shredded beef)	620	17	98
Salad, Chicken Caesar w. dressing	670	41	13
Sandwiches: Chicken Caesar	880	34	71
Grilled Chicken	825	25	84
Roast Pork	770	26	83
Sides: Corn Combo, 4 oz	120	4	19
Boiled Yucca, Combo, 7.5 oz	190	0	51
Fried Yucca, Combo, 6 oz	500	24	69
Macaroni & Cheese, Combo, 4.9 oz	190	11	17
Sweet Plantains, Combo, 5 oz	300	7.5	62
Yellow Rice w. Veggies, Combo, 5 oz	165	2.5	31

For Complete Nutritional Data ~ see CalorieKing.com

Popeye's® (Aug '07)   C F Cb

	C	F	Cb
Chicken: Chkn Breast, Mild/Spicy	360	22	8
Chicken Leg, Mild/Spicy	110	7	3
Chicken Thigh, Mild/Spicy, avg.	280	20	7
Chicken Wing, Mild/Spicy, avg.	150	10	5
Sides: Biscuit, 2.1 oz	240	13	26
Cajun Rice, regular, 4.1 oz	170	6	22
Cinnamon Apple Turnover, 3 oz	250	12	34
Coleslaw, regular, 5 oz	260	23	14
Corn on the Cob (1), 7.8 oz	190	2	37
French Fries, 3 oz	310	17	35
Mashed Potatoes: no Gravy, reg.	100	3	17
w. Gravy, regular, 5 oz	120	4	18
Red Beans & Rice, regular, 6 oz	320	19	31

Port of Subs® (Aug '07)   C F Cb

Light Submarine: *Per 5" Sub (Five Grams of Fat or Less)*

	C	F	Cb
#2 Ham Turkey	330	5	46
#5 Smoked Ham Turkey	320	5	46
#6 Vegetarian, no Cheese	240	2	44
#7 Roast Beef	315	4	43
#8 Turkey	315	4	47
#9 Peppered Pastrami	295	4	44
#10 Roasted Chicken Breast	305	3	44
#14 Smoked Ham	300	4	44
#18 Roast Beef Turkey	315	4	45

Cold Submarine Sandwiches: *Per 5" Sub (No Mayo.)*

#1 Ham Salami Capicolla & Pepperoni w. Provolone	530	26	45
#2 Ham & Turkey w. Provolone	435	15	46
#3 Salami & Turkey w. Provolone	465	20	46
#4 Ham & Salami w. Provolone	470	21	45
#5 Smkd Ham & Turkey w. Cheddar	430	15	47
#6 Vegetarian w. Avocado & Olives	600	33	49
#7 Roast Beef w. Provolone,	420	14	43
#8 Turkey w. Provolone	420	14	47
#9 Peppered Pastrami w. Swiss	440	17	44
#10 Rstd Chicken Brst w. Provolone	410	13	45
#11 Ham w. American	380	20	45
#12 Salami w. Provolone	480	25	45
#13 Combination of Cheeses	510	26	44
#14 Smoked Ham w. Swiss	445	17	45
#15 Salami & Pepperoni w. Prov.	510	27	45
#16 BLT Sandwich	520	30	43
#17 Tuna no Cheese	420	18	45
#18 Rst Beef & Turkey w. Provolone	420	14	45

Updated Nutrition Data ~ www.CalorieKing.com
Persons with Diabetes ~ See Disclaimer (Page 24)

Port of Subs® cont... (Aug '07)

Hot Subs: Per 8" Sub	C	F	Cb
Grilled Chicken	565	11	68
Hot Pastrami	760	17	62
Meatball	655	25	76
Tortilla Wrap: *Per Wrap (12" Tortilla)*			
Chicken Caesar	630	34	35
Hot Grilled Chkn & Smokey Cheddar	485	18	35
Turkey & Bacon Ranch	590	38	34
Tortilla (1)	200	7	27
Sauces & Dressings: *Per 2 Tablespoons*			
Mayo & Mustard Mix	110	12	0
Mayonnaise	130	14	0
Mustard	0	0	0
Soups: *Medium Bowl (6 oz)*			
Campbell's: Boston Clam Chowder	105	4	13
Broccoli Cheese	120	6	13
Minestrone	55	1	8
Roasted Chicken Noodle	85	2	9

Pret A Manger® (Aug '07)

Bakery: Blondie Cake	310	17	34
Banana Loaf Cake	420	24	48
Brownie Slice	390	20	51
Carrot Loaf Cake	460	29	47
Pecan Pie	510	27	63
Raspberry Bar	420	20	60
Salads: *Per Pack*			
Chef Salad & Greens	400	24	12
Cobb & Greens	460	25	47
Fresh Mozzarella, Tomato & Greens	380	31	17
Grilled Chicken & Citrus	300	13	20
Chicken Avocado	580	23	62
Tuna Salad	430	19	43
Sushi: Deluxe Sushi, 4 rolls, 9 oz	365	3.5	65
Salmon Nigiri, 7 pce, 6 oz	245	3.5	43
Sandwiches			
Bacon Lettuce & Tomato S'wich	550	21	51
Chicken & Avocado Sandwich	580	23	62
Chicken & Bacon Sandwich	520	15	59
Chicken & Mozzarella Baguette	580	19	72
Chicken Coronation	620	27	78
Ham & Swiss Baguette	620	16	66
New York Brunch Sandwich	590	18	53
Rst Beef Arugula & Parm. Baguette	670	21	63
Turkey Club Sandwich	530	21	59
Wraps: Avocado Salad	460	30	36
Just Made Mozzarella	630	32	43
Murray's Turkey Club	480	13	39

For Complete Menu ~ See CalorieKing.com

Pretzelmaker® (Aug '07)

Pretzels	C	F	Cb
Bites: Small, 5.3 oz	450	11	80
Medium, 7½ oz	640	16	112
Large, ½ order, 5.8 oz	255	7.5	44
Cinnamon Sugar, 3.8 oz	330	4	65
Original: Pretzel (1) 4.2 oz	310	4	59
Butter Flavor & Salt (1) 4.6 oz	370	5	71
Caramel Crunch (1) 4.2 oz	300	4	58
Cinnamon (1) 3.8 oz	330	4	65
Garlic (1) 4.2 oz	310	4	60
Iced Cinnamon Swirl (1) 3.8 oz	330	4	65
Parmesan (1) 4 oz	310	3.5	60
Pretzel Dog (1) 5½ oz	480	29	38
Ranch (1), 4.2 oz	320	4.5	60
Sauces: *Per Container*			
Caramel, 2 oz	140	0	35
Cheddar Cheese, 1½ oz	70	5	6
Cream Cheese/Icing, 2 oz	200	20	2
Honey Mustard, 1½ oz	80	0	20
Ketchup, 2 packets, 0.6 oz	20	0	4
Mustard, 2 packets, 0.3 oz	10	0	1
Nachos Cheese, 1½ oz	80	5	7
Pizza Sauce, 1½ oz	20	0.5	6
Beverages			
Smoothies (20 fl.oz): Coffee	640	21	107
Mocha	620	20	106
Peach; Raspberry	650	20	117
Strawberry Banana	650	20	115
Fat Free: Peach; Raspberry	480	0	130

Pretzel Time® (Aug '07)

Pretzels			
Bites: Plain, small, 5.3 oz	450	11	80
Medium, 7½ oz	640	16	112
Large, ½ order, 5.8 oz	255	7.5	44
Caramel Nut (1), 4.5 oz	390	7	74
Cinnamon Sugar (1), 4.3 oz	370	8	68
Italian Parmesan (1), 4.2 oz	360	9	61
Plain (1), 3.8 oz	290	2	61
Ranch (1), 4.2 oz	240	7	63

Continued Next Page...

Updated Nutrition Data ~ www.CalorieKing.com
Persons with Diabetes ~ See Disclaimer (Page 24)

Pretzel Time® cont... (Aug '07)

Sauces & Dressings: Per Container	C	F	Cb
Caramel Sauce	140	0	35
Cream Cheese Icing	180	9	22
Cheddar/ Nacho Cheese Sauce	80	5	4
Cream Cheese Sauce	200	20	4
Ketchup	20	0	4
Mustard	10	0	1
Pizza Sauce	20	.5	6

Quizno's Subs® (Aug '07)

Signature Subs: No Dressing	C	F	Cb
Classic Italian Sub: Small, 9 oz	645	30	60
Regular, 11½ oz	730	33	69
Large, 19½ oz	1200	58	102
Honey Mustard Chkn w. bacon, large	1355	40	137
Philly Cheese Steak, large, 10½ oz	720	16	92
Steakhouse Sub (6"), 6½ oz	510	21	52
The Traditional (8") 16 oz	800	24	94
Turkey Ranch Swiss (8")	690	18	89
Low-Fat Subs (Small): Turkey Lite	335	6	52
Honey Bourbon Chicken	360	6	45
Sierra Smoked Turkey w. Sauce	350	6	53
Flatbread Sandwiches: No Dressing			
Antipasto	760	40	62
Classic Cobb	515	13	62
Chicken Caesar	560	12	62
Roasted Chicken	660	23	62
Flatbread Chopped Salads: No Dressing			
Classic Cobb	530	16	57
Chicken	745	33	57
Chicken Caesar	640	22	57
Antipasto	905	54	61
Dressings: Beef Au Jus, 4½ oz	25	0.5	3
Caesar Dressing	295	32	2
Honey Mustard, 2 oz	140	6	22
Italian Vinaigrette, 1 oz	130	14	3
Ranch Dressing, 2 oz	285	30	3
Toasted Gourmet Bread Bowls			
Country French Chicken	830	31	96
Southwest Chicken	850	33	96
Signature Steak 'N Chili	885	34	101

Rally's Hamburgers® (Aug '07)

Burgers/Sandwiches	C	F	Cb
Rallyburger	435	22	35
with Cheese	490	27	35
Big Buford	745	48	35
Chicken Fillet Sandwich	400	15	43
Chili w. Cheese & Onion: 7 oz	360	22	20
13 oz size	670	41	37
Super Barbecue Bacon	595	31	49
Super Double Cheeseburger	760	48	37
French Fries: Regular	210	11	26
Large	320	16	39
X-Large	425	21	52
Shakes: Vanilla, small	320	11	49
Other flavors, small	410	12	73

Ranch 1® (Aug '07)

	C	F	Cb
Salads: Gourmet Greens	220	7	31
Chicken on Gourmet Greens	350	11	31
Zesty Caesar Salad	180	3	31
Zesty Chicken Caesar Salad	280	6	31
Sandwiches: American Rancher	390	10	51
Club Sandwich	470	16	53
Grilled Chicken Philly	450	14	53
Ranch Classic	370	5	53
Spicy Grilled Chicken	420	11	58
Side Kicks: Fruit Cup, 8.3 oz	90	0.5	18
Ranch Fries, regular, 4.5 oz	350	14	51
Specialties: Chicken Tenders	370	15	7
Baked Potato: w. Broccoli	510	0.5	117
w. Cheese	790	25	118
w. Chicken	610	4	114
Grilled Chkn & Vegetable Platter	790	7	129
Grilled Chicken Fajita	330	16	25
Grilled Chicken Hot Pasta	580	10	86

Note: Figures are only estimates
For extra listings and data ~ See CalorieKing.com

Updated Nutrition Data ~ www.CalorieKing.com
Persons with Diabetes ~ See Disclaimer (Page 24)

Restaurants & Fast - Foods

Red Lobster® (Aug '07)

Lighthouse Menu

	C	F	Cb
Fresh Fish: *Per Serving*			
Broiled Flounder, lunch portion	240	5	0
Atlantic Salmon, full portion	580	33	0
Atlantic Salmon, half portion	260	12	0
Broiled Flounder, dinner portion	240	5	0
Rainbow Trout, full portion	510	25	6
Rainbow Trout, half portion	275	14	2
Tilapia, full portion	345	10	0
Tilapia, half portion	185	6	0
Meals: *Per Serving*			
Grilled Chicken Breast	315	8	0
Signature Shellfish: *Per Serving*			
Garlic Chili Jumbo Shrimp	140	3	1
Garlic Grilled Jumbo Shrimp	140	3	1
Chilled Jumbo Shrimp Cocktail	140	1	2
Live Maine Lobster, 1¼lb	145	1	2
Lobster Chops	320	8.5	4
North Pacific King Crab Legs	490	9	0
Rock Lobster Tail	260	3	0
Snow Crab Legs	260	4.5	0
Sides: *Per Serving*			
100% Pure Melted Butter, 1 oz	190	21	0
Baked Potato w. Pico de Gallo	185	2	37
Baked Potato, no topping	180	2	36
Cheddar Bay Biscuit (1)	160	9	17
Cocktail Sauce, large	85	2	17
Garden Salad, no dressing	50	2	9
Jumbo Shrimp Cocktail	140	2	1
King Crab Legs	165	3	0
Lemon Wedge (1)	5	0	1
Petite Shrimp Topping	30	1	1
Red Wine Vinaigrette Dressing	50	3	5
Seasonal Vegetables w. butter	145	11	9
Seasoned Broccoli	55	0	10
Snow Crab Legs	130	2	0
Wild Rice Pilaf	205	5	36

For Complete Nutritional Data ~ see CalorieKing.com

Rita's® (Aug '07)

	C	F	Cb
Italian Ice: Kids, 7.5 oz	165	0	43
Regular, 12 oz	265	0	69
Large, 19 oz	415	0	109
Quart, 32 oz	705	0	185
Cream Ice: Kids, 7.5 oz	195	2	44
Regular, 12 oz	310	4	70
Large, 19 oz	495	6	109
Quart, 32 oz	830	11	187
Custard: Kids, 5 oz	285	15	32
Regular, 6.75 oz	385	21	43
Large, 9.75 oz	555	30	62
Gelati w. Custard: Vanilla, Reg., 10 oz	365	13	59
Vanilla, large, 17 oz	560	17	102
Chocolate, regular, 10 oz	350	11	60
Chocolate, large, 17 oz	535	14	101
Misto w. Custard: Van., reg., 15 oz	420	7	90
Vanilla, large, 23 oz	620	10	135
Chocolate, regular, 15 oz	410	7	90
Chocolate, large, 23 oz	605	9	135
Sugar Free: *(w. Sorbitol)*			
Ice: Kids, 7.5 oz	65	0	24
Regular, 12 oz	100	0	39
Gelati w. Van. Custard, reg., 10 oz	300	13	45
Misto w. Van. Custard, reg., 15 oz	245	8	57

For Complete Nutritional Data ~ see CalorieKing.com

Robeks (Aug '07)

Smoothies: *Per 12 fl.oz*	C	F	Cb
Acai Energizer	167	1	36
Big Wednesday	172	1	40
Cardio Cooler	215	1	44
Citrus Stinger	194	1	40
Cranberry Quest	173	0	40
Dr. Robeks	181	1	40
Green Tea Sensation	222	1	42
Guava Lava	180	1	42
Hummingbird	185	1	44
Mahalo Mango	174	1	42
Malibu Peach	153	0	36
Outrageous Raspberry	174	1	39
Passionfruit Cove	168	1	38
Pomegranate Passion	196	0	48
Pomegranate Power	211	0	50
Raspberry Romance	172	1	42
Robeks Rejuvenator	193	1	43
Robeks MuscleMax	202	1	38
Strawnana Berry	179	0	44
Venice Burner	231	1	46
Zen Berry	190	1	45

Fast - Foods & *Restaurants*

Rocky Rococo® (Aug '07)

	C	F	Cb
Pastas: *Per Serving*			
Can't Decide, 14 oz	465	9	77
Fettuccine w. Alfredo Sauce:			
Regular, 14 oz	460	14	66
Light, 7 oz	230	7	33
Spaghetti with Meat Sauce: Reg.	500	7	87
Light, 7 oz	250	3	44
Spaghetti w. Meatballs: Reg., 15 oz	630	16	89
Light, 7.5 oz	315	8	45
Spaghetti w. Tomato Sauce: Reg.	470	4	87
Light, 7 oz	235	2	44
Pizzas: *Per Regular Slice*			
Cheese	380	9	54
Garden	390	10	56
Pepperoni	425	13	54
Sausage	495	19	54
Sausage Mushroom	500	19	55
Sides			
Breadsticks: w. Marinara Sce (6)	420	7	72
w. Jalapeno Cheese Sauce (6)	530	18	72
Wheat Muffin (1)	200	4	38

Roly Poly® (Aug '07)

	C	F	Cb
Sandwiches: *Per ½ Sandwich (Wheat Bread)*			
Baked Ham & Roast Pork:			
BarBQ Pork Melt	300	10	26
Italian Classic	330	12	28
Key West Cuban Mix	300	9	27
Peachtree Melt	330	11	28
Porky's Nightmare	310	12	26
Chicken: Basil Cashew Chicken	290	11	27
Catalina Chicken Salad	305	12	26
Chicken Caesar	310	12	28
Chicken Cordon Bleu	305	11	27
Chicken Fajita	280	8	27
Chicken Popper	245	7	29
Cobb Salad	320	14	28
Delhi Chicken	320	12	32
Hickory Chicken	335	11	27
Oriental Chicken	260	6	31
Santa Fe Chicken	270	9	27
Seafood: Popeye's Tuna	310	4.5	30
Classic Tuna Melt	335	18	26
Texas Tuna Melt	310	13	26
Thai Hot Tuna	330	13	27
Tuna Luau	325	15	29

Round Table® Pizza (Aug '07)

	C	F	Cb
Large Pizza (14"): *Per Slice (⅛ Whole)*			
Cheese: Pan Crust	300	9	38
Skinny Crust	190	8	18
Chkn & Garlic Gourmet: Pan Crust	330	11	39
Skinny Crust	210	9	19
Chicken Smokehouse: Pan Crust	350	12	39
Skinny Crust	230	10	20
Gourmet Veggie: Pan Crust	320	11	40
Skinny Crust	200	9	19
Guinevere's Garden Delight: Pan Cr.	300	8	39
Skinny Crust	180	7	20
Hawaiian: Pan Crust	310	8	40
Skinny Crust	190	7	20
Italian Garlic Supreme: Pan Crust	360	15	39
Skinny Crust	240	13	18
King Arthur Supreme: Pan Crust	340	12	39
Skinny Crust	240	12	19
Maui Zaui w. Polynesian Sce: Pan	340	11	43
Skinny Crust	220	9	22
Maui Zaui w. Zesty Red Sce: Pan Cr.	330	11	40
Skinny Crust	220	9	20
Montague's All Meat Marvel: Pan	360	14	38
Skinny Crust	260	14	18
Pepperoni: Pan Crust	320	11	38
Skinny Crust	210	10	18
Smokehouse Combo: Pan Crust	370	14	40
Skinny Crust	250	13	20
Ulti-Meat Premium All-Meat: Pan	390	16	38
Skinny Crust	270	15	18
Wombo Combo: Pan Crust	360	14	39
Skinny Crust	240	12	19
Sandwiches			
Chicken Club	760	34	67
Ham Club	810	37	76
RT Pizza Sandwich	690	34	65
RT Veggie Sandwich	680	29	79
Turkey Club	800	37	75
Sides			
Buffalo Wings, 6 pieces	420	28	2
Garlic Bread, 4.7 oz	470	21	59
Garlic Bread with Cheese, 6.7 oz	630	33	59
Honey BBQ Wings, 6 pieces	390	25	8

For Complete Nutritional Data ~ see CalorieKing.com

Updated Nutrition Data ~ www.CalorieKing.com
Persons with Diabetes ~ See Disclaimer (Page 24)

Roy Rogers® (Aug '07)

Breakfast Itrems	C	F	Cb
Big Country Breakfast: w. Bacon	740	43	61
w. Sausage	920	60	61
w. Ham	710	39	67
Burgers			
Hamburger	260	9	33
Cheeseburger	300	13	34
¼ lb Hamburger	430	18	41
¼ lb Cheeseburger	470	22	42
Sourdough Grilled Chicken	500	21	46
Sandwiches: Roast Beef	260	4	30
Chicken Fillet	500	24	49
Grilled Chicken	340	11	32
Fries: Regular	350	15	49
Large	430	18	59
Desserts: Hot Fudge Sundae	320	10	50

Rubio's Fresh Mexican Grill® (Aug '07)

Burritos	C	F	Cb
Baja Gourmet Seafood, Fish	740	40	70
Baja Grill: Carne Asada	680	32	58
Carnitas	630	29	59
Chicken	630	24	58
Bean & Cheese Burrito	820	36	88
Especial: Carne Asada	940	37	117
Carnitas	890	33	118
Chicken	890	29	117
Fish Burrito	740	40	70
Grilled Mesquite Shrimp Burrito	710	31	77
HealthMex Chicken Burrito	530	10	77
Mahi Mahi Burrito	720	36	56
Tacos			
Carne Asada w. Corn Tortilla	250	10	23
Carnitas w. Corn Tortilla	230	9	34
Chicken w. Corn Tortilla	300	15	24
Fish, Especial w. Corn Tortilla	370	22	29
Fish, Original w. Corn Tortilla	300	16	27
HealthMex: Chicken	170	3	23
Mahi Mahi	180	3	22
Mahi Mahi w. Corn Tortilla	310	16	23
Street Taco: Carne Asada	130	6	10
Carnitas	110	5	11
Chicken	110	3.5	10
Taquitos, Chicken (3)	290	11	34
Quesadillas			
Carne Asada Quesadilla	990	61	58
Cheese Quesadilla	830	52	56
Chicken Quesadilla	950	54	58
Shrimp Quesadilla	920	56	58

Rubio's cont... (Aug '07)

Wrapsaladas: No Dressing	C	F	Cb
Chipotle Ranch: Carnitas	730	32	85
Chicken	730	27	83
Mahi	750	29	81
Shrimp	720	30	85
Steak	780	35	83
Baja Caesar: Carnitas	600	23	73
Chicken	600	17	72
Mahi	590	17	70
Shrimp	600	20	74
Steak	650	26	72
Salads			
Baja Caesar Salad	500	37	16
Chicken Chopped Salad	570	33	35
Chicken Fiesta Salad	480	33	12
Chipotle Ranch Salad	750	51	42
HealthMex Chicken Salad	260	2	34
Dressings: Serrano Grape, 1.3 oz	40	0	1
Meals			
Grilled Grande Bowl: Carne Asada	730	40	60
Chicken	690	33	60
Mahi Mahi	710	35	58
Shrimp	670	35	61
Nachos: Grande	1270	78	111
Carne Asada	1420	87	113
Chicken	1380	80	113
Three Taco Combos: w. Chips & Beans			
Carne Asada	1060	44	116
Carnitas	1010	41	118
Chicken	1220	59	117
Fish Especial	1420	78	134
Fish	1220	62	128
Burrito Combos: w. Chips & Beans			
Baja Grill Carne Asada	990	44	104
Baja Grill Carnitas	940	42	106
Baja Grill Chicken	940	36	105
Fish	1050	52	116
Sides			
Cheese, 1 oz	100	8	1
Sour Cream, 1 oz	60	6	1
Black Beans, 7 oz	170	2	28
Carne Asada, 3 oz	160	8	2
Carnitas, 3 oz	120	6	3
Chicken, 3 oz	120	2	2
Chips, 1½ oz	210	11	28
Chips, side order, 3 oz	430	22	56
Churro, 1½ oz	170	8	22
Guacamole, 7.7 oz	340	22	16
Original & Pinto Beans, 9.3 oz	420	18	50
Pinto Beans, 7 oz	190	3	37
Rice: 2 oz	80	1	16
Side order, 4 oz	160	1.5	33

For Complete Nutritional Data ~ see CalorieKing.com

Ruby Tuesday® (Aug '07)

Appetisers: Per Serving	C	F	Cb
Asian Dumplings	110	5	12
Avocado Quesadilla	170	13	13
Chicken Quesadilla	225	14	12
Classic Sampler	340	19	27
Fire Wings	220	16	3
Grand Sampler	325	19	19
Jumbo Lump Crab Cake	110	8	4
Point Reyes Blue Cheese Chips	510	37	31
Southwestern Spring Rolls	180	10	16
Thai Phoon Shrimp	195	13	12
Wisconsin Cheddar Fries	300	17	27
Steaks: No Sides			
Peppercorn Mushroom Sirloin	605	36	16
Point Reyes Prime Sirloin	760	45	0
Premium Aged Prime Sirloin	545	30	0
Rib Eye	590	35	6
Sirloin & Crab Cake	475	22	15
Top Sirloin, 9 oz	255	6	2
Premium Baby Back Ribs:			
Classic BBQ, Half Rack	495	32	14
Memphis Dry Rub, Half Rack	535	40	3
Chicken: No Sides			
Bistro Barbecue Chicken	660	33	16
Chicken & Broccoli Quiche	735	58	24
Chicken Bella	625	36	14
Chicken Fresco	465	23	7
Chicken Oscar	470	22	4
Gourmet Chicken Pot Pie	1460	115	43
Parmesan Chicken Penne	1655	96	126
Seafood: No Sides			
Asian Glazed Salmon	425	27	7
Creole Catch	310	16	0
Jumbo Lump Crab Cake	890	48	70
Lemon Grilled Salmon	460	32	1
Louisiana Fried Shrimp	425	17	40
New Orleans Seafood	495	31	2
Parmesan Shrimp Penne	1220	64	108
Salmon Oscar	540	37	4
Handcrafted Burgers: No Sides			
Alpine Swiss Burger	1375	98	66
Avocado Chicken Burger	865	51	52
Avocado Turkey Burger	1035	63	56
Bacon Cheeseburger	1195	85	52
Bella Turkey Burger	1145	71	62
Bison Bacon Cheeseburger	1070	71	53
Bison Burger	890	57	53
Buffalo Chicken Burger	1040	71	67
Chicken BLT Burger	980	63	64
Classic Cheeseburger	1105	78	52
Hickory Chicken Burger	865	47	62

Ruby Tuesday® cont... (Aug '07)

Handcrafted Burgers (Cont)	C	F	Cb
Point Reyes Blue Cheese Burger	1280	93	52
Ruby's Classic Burger	1015	71	52
Smokehouse Burger	1390	96	77
Turkey Burger	810	45	53
Veggie Burger	955	52	75
Premium Burgers: Gr. Salmon BLT	1150	77	51
Jumbo Lump Crab Burger	755	45	63
Triple Prime Burger	885	56	53
Triple Prime Cheddar Burger	1065	70	53
Rubi Minis: Ruby Minis (4)	1310	90	74
Turkey Minis (2)	520	33	33
Salads			
Club House Salad	895	60	38
Carolina Chicken Salad	1020	72	45
Grilled Salmon Salad	590	35	21
Dressings, Sauces: Per 1 oz Serving			
Asian Barbecue Sauce	60	3	7
Avocado Ranch	60	5	3
Balsamic Vinaigrette Dressing	35	2	4
Barbecue Sauce	50	0	13
Blue Cheese Dressing	175	19	3
Caesar Dressing	100	10	2
Lemon Butter; Parmesan Cream Sce	95	9	1
Marinara Sauce	20	1	2
Parmesan Cream Sauce	95	9	2
Peanut Sauce	65	3	8
Ranch Dressing	100	11	1
Light Ranch Dressing	55	5	1
Salsa	10	0	3
Sweet & Spicy Chili Sauce	170	17	2
Sides			
Tomato & Mozzarella Salad	110	7	7
Tossed Caesar Salad	175	15	7
Sauteed Baby Portabella Mushr.	175	14	9
White Cheddar Mashed Potatoes	275	16	24
Baked Potato:			
w. Butter & Sour Cream	460	19	62
w. Cheese & Bacon	615	32	63
Brown Rice Pilaf, w. Cheese & Tom.	220	6	35
Fresh Hot Fries	360	13	57
Desserts			
Double Chocolate Cake	980	48	124
Gourmet Cookie & Ice Cream	620	29	84
Blondie	675	31	93
Chocolate Tallcake	605	21	94
Fresh Strawberries & Ice Cream	840	40	103

For Complete Menu ~ see CalorieKing.com

Updated Nutrition Data ~ www.CalorieKing.com
Persons with Diabetes ~ See Disclaimer (Page 24)

Restaurants & Fast - Foods

Runza® (Aug '07)

Sandwiches	C	F	Cb
Original Overstuffed Sandwich	495	17	65
Cheese Overstuffed Sandwich	555	21	66
BBQ Chicken Sandwich, grilled	390	9	46
Fish Sandwich	490	24	50
Polish Dog	425	26	30
Smothered Chicken, grilled	380	10	41
Special Deluxe Chicken, crispy	485	19	51
Burgers			
Junior: Cheeseburger	325	17	28
Cheeseburger Runza	305	14	30
Swiss Mushroom	380	21	26
Legendary: ¼ lb Cheeseburger	430	21	32
½ lb Double Cheeseburger	640	32	37
¼ lb Bacon Cheeseburger	515	29	36
¼ lb Legend Supreme	765	37	62
¼ lb Swiss Cheese Mushroom	450	25	36
Sides			
French Fries: Small, 3.1 oz	280	15	31
Medium	410	23	46
Large	625	35	70
Frings, 6.3 oz	540	28	64
Onion Rings: Medium, 4 oz	370	20	41
Large, 6.5 oz	590	32	66
Onion Ring Dip, 2.1 oz	90	6	4
Salads: *No Dressing*			
Tossed Salad w. Crispy Chicken	435	27	29
Tossed Salad w. Grilled Chicken	275	13	13
Dressing: Ranch, 2.4 oz	300	32	5
Reduced Calorie Ranch, 2.5 oz	170	11	17
Lite Italian, 2.6 oz	85	5	10
Raspberry Vinaigrette	25	0	6
Soups: *Per Bowl*			
Boston Clam Chowder	320	23	33
Broccoli Cheese	360	27	35
Cauliflower Cheese	335	26	32
Chicken Noodle	170	5	21
Homemade Chili	310	10	26
Potato w. Bacon	305	20	40
Vegetable Cheese	330	22	28
Wisconsin Cheese	425	35	36
Kids-Size: Mini Corn Dogs (5)	275	17	25
Chicken Strips (2)	185	10	11
Desserts & Drinks			
Chocolate Chip Cookie (1)	310	16	34
Vanilla Shake, regular, 12 fl.oz	465	16	69
Oreo Shake, regular, 12 fl.oz	605	24	84
Pepsi Slushie, medium, 18 fl.oz	225	0	60

Ryan's® Family Steakhouse (Aug '07)

Main Courses: Sides Not Included	C	F	Cb
BBQ Beef, 6 oz	225	12	9
BBQ Chicken, ¼, 5 oz	230	15	5
Carved Turkey Breast, 6 oz	280	12	0
Chkn Fried Beef Steak (1), no gravy	180	9	16
Chkn Fried Beef Steak (1), w. gravy	220	11	24
Chicken Pot Pie, 8 oz	350	16	48
Grilled Chicken Breast, plain, 6 oz	280	18	0
Grilled Pork Chop: Plain, 1 chop	240	14	1
BBQ; Teriyaki, avg , 1 chop	160	8	8
Grilled Salmon, 7 oz entree	240	9	0
Grilled Sliced Sausage: BBQ Sce, 6 oz	555	48	8
in Peppers and Onions, 4 oz	450	42	6.5
Grilled Teriyaki Chicken Thighs, 6 oz	215	6	6
Macaroni and Cheese, 8 oz	350	16	40
Meat Lasagne, 8 oz	370	16	30
Meat Loaf, 4 oz	220	12	9
Mexican Casserole, 8 oz	415	16	46
Pizza: Cheese, 1 slice, 3½ oz	200	10	11
Pepperoni, 1 slice, 3½ oz	230	13	10
Rotisserie Chicken, ¼, 5 oz	250	15	0
Salisbury Steak w. gravy, 1 patty	200	11	11
Sirloin Steak: 8 oz	485	33	0
10½ oz	640	44	0
16 oz	970	67	0
Sirloin Tips, 5.5 oz	330	23	0
Stuffed Alaskan Pollock Fillet, 6 oz	360	30	18
Taco Beef, 4 oz	180	10	8
Vegetable Lasagne, 8 oz	355	16	30
White Turkey w. gravy, 6 oz	140	3	6.5
Sides: Baked Potato, plain, 8 oz	250	0	57
Bowtie Pasta and Veges, 8 oz	210	0	38
Chicken Salad, Low-Fat, 8 oz	245	4	24
Coleslaw, 4 oz	180	12	12
Corn Cobbet (1) 4 oz	90	6	11
Garlic Mashed Potatoes, 4 oz	120	4	18
Glazed Baby Carrots w. Sauce, 4 oz	125	8	12
Low Carb Grilled Veges, 8 oz	40	0	8
Marinated 7-Bean Salad, 6 oz	300	0	66
Pinto Beans, 4 oz	105	2	16
Potato Salad, 6 oz	280	12	33
Sweet Pot. w. M'mallows, 4 oz	240	18	16
Yellow Squash w. Onions, 4 oz	50	2	7
Desserts: Cheesecake, plain, 1 sl.	190	15	11
Ice Cream Cone (flat bottom)	20	0	4
Key Lime Pie, 1 slice	410	17	58
Lemon Creme Cake, 1 slice	170	15	9
Cookies: Oatmeal Raisin (1)	110	3.5	18
Sugar Cookie (1)	120	5	18

7-Eleven® (Aug '07)

Breakfast Sandwiches	C	F	Cb
Big Bite Breakfast Sandwich	430	27	29
Croissant: w. Bacon, Egg & Chse	400	33	34
w. Ham, Egg & Chse	390	22	34
Engl. Muffin w. Saus., Egg, Chse	450	24	37
Sausage, Egg & Cheese Biscuit	500	31	34
Sausage, Egg & Twister Roll	430	27	29
Hot Dogs (Big Bite)			
¼ Pound Hot Dog, no bun	360	34	6
⅓ Pound Hot Dog, no bun	480	45	3
Spicy Bite, 1 link, 4 oz	425	38	2
Bacon Cheeseburger Bite, no bun	270	12	1
Reynoldos Jumbo Burritos (10 oz)			
Beef & Bean; Beef & Potato	590	20	82
Red Hot Burrito	640	20	88
Green Burrito	710	26	93
Sandwiches (7-Eleven)			
Black Forest Ham	380	6	59
Chicken Salad, 7.3 oz	500	28	44
Chicken w. Ancho Lime Spread	500	26	47
Classic Chicken Caesar, 8.3 oz	590	27	45
Classic Sub on Roll, 7.6 oz	380	6	44
Combo Sub w. Turkey, 5.5 oz	270	7	33
Ham & Swiss, 4.9 oz	330	11	39
Hearty Ham, 8.3 oz	570	30	48
Pastrami & Swiss on Wheat	480	21	48
Smoked Turkey w. Chse/Mayo	550	27	46
Turkey & Ham on Tom. Basil Brd	490	23	42
Turkey & Ham on White Bread	350	6	53
Tuna Salad, 7.5 oz	540	27	45
Bakery Stix™ Treats: Per Stick (3.5 oz)			
Grilled Cheese	270	11	30
Ham & Cheese	280	12	32
Pepperoni & Cheese	340	18	30
Sushi: California Rolls, 3 pieces	155	2	39
Imperial Rolls, 3 pieces	210	11	22
Salads			
Tuna Macaroni Salad, 8 oz	270	8	29
Reser's Coleslaw, 3½ oz	130	7	17
Reser's Macaroni Salad, 3½ oz	220	15	20
Reser's Potato Salad, 3½ oz	200	10	19
Go-Go Taquitos			
Beef Taco & Cheese, 3 oz (1)	250	11	30
Fiesta Chicken, 3 oz (1)	220	12	23
Jalapeno & Cream cheese, 3 oz	240	13	27
Monterey Jack Chkn, 3 oz (1)	280	14	30
Go-Go French Toast Sticks, 3 oz	270	16	23

7-Eleven® cont... (Aug '07)

Donuts & Muffins (World Ovens)	C	F	Cb
Donuts: Blueberry Cake (1)	330	22	31
Chocolate Iced (1)	250	11	35
Glazed (1)	250	16	24
Jelly (1)	420	16	66
Sour Cream Donut (1)	450	19	65
Muffins: Banana Nut, 7 oz	660	26	97
Blueberry, 5.6 oz	310	8	54
Brownies: Original, 5 oz	570	28	83
Peanut Butter Cup Brownie, 4.4 oz	560	20	55
Walnut Brownie, 5 oz	600	31	78
Fountain Drinks (Figures Assume ⅓ Ice)			
Coca-Cola/Pepsi/Dr.Pepper/7Up:			
Gulp, 20 oz	195	0	51
Big Gulp, 32 oz	310	0	82
Super Gulp, 44 oz	430	0	112
Double Gulp, 64 oz	625	0	163
Diet Coke/Diet Pepsi, 16 oz	1	0	0
Slurpees: Average All Flavors,			
12 oz size	95	0	24
22 oz size	175	0	44
28 oz size	220	0	56
40 oz size	315	0	80
Crystal Light, 12 fl.oz	45	0	9
Hawaiian Punch; Dr Pepper, avg.,			
12 oz size	180	0	48
22 oz size	330	0	88
28 oz size	420	0	112
40 oz size	600	0	160
Cafe Select Coffee: 12 fl.oz	8	0	2
16 fl.oz size	10	0	2
20 fl.oz size	14	0	3
24 fl.oz size	16	0	4
Hot Drinks: Hot Chocolate, 8 fl.oz	180	3	36
French Vanilla Cappuccino, 8 fl.oz	160	6	26

Updated Nutrition Data ~ www.CalorieKing.com
Persons with Diabetes ~ See Disclaimer (Page 24)

Sammy's®
Woodfired Pizza (Aug '07)

Healthy Dining Meals	C	F	Cb
Pasta: Grilled Vegetable Penne	620	21	84
Tomato Angel Hair Pasta	700	18	115
Individual Salad: Chinese Chicken	450	12	47
Chopped Chicken	425	11	30
Oak Roasted Salmon on Ponzu	470	19	21
Fresh Tomato Basil Soup	110	5	10
Roast Chicken Pesto Wrap	480	20	22
Vegetarian Pizza, ½ pizza	885	21	130

Samurai Sam's® (Aug '07)

Bowls: Per Regular Bowl (w ith White Rice)	C	F	Cb
Low-Carb Bowl	230	4	16
Spicy Beef'n Broccoli	620	13	97
Sweet & Sour Dark Chicken	610	10	96
Sweet & Sour White Chicken	580	4.5	96
Teriyaki Dark Chicken & Steak	540	9	83
Teriyaki Dark Chicken	540	10	79
Teriyaki Steak	530	8	86
Teriyaki Veggie	370	0.5	80
Teriyaki White Chicken & Steak	520	6	83
Salads: Oriental Chicken	220	4	9
Sesame Garden Toss	490	13	57
Sides: Grilled Chicken Egg Roll, 3 oz	150	7	17
Oriental Salad Dressing, 1 oz	70	2	12
Teriyaki Sauce, 1 oz	40	0	9
Wraps: with White Rice			
Teriyaki Dark Chicken	670	16	95
Teriyaki Steak	650	14	101
Teriyaki Veggie	510	8	94
Teriyaki White Chicken & Steak	650	13	98

Sbarro's® (Aug '07)

Entrees	C	F	Cb
Baked Ziti w. Sauce	700	41	43
Chicken Parmigiana	520	22	16
Meat Lasagna	650	37	36
Spaghetti w. Sauce	820	28	120
Pizza: Per Slice (Thin Crust)			
Cheese	460	13	60
Pepperoni	730	37	61
Sausage	670	31	60
Supreme	630	27	63
Stuffed Pizza: Per Slice			
Spinach & Broccoli	790	34	89
Pepperoni	960	42	89

Schlotzsky's® (Aug '07)

Oven-Toasted Sandwiches: Per Medium Sandwich	C	F	Cb
Angus, Beef & Provolone	755	29	80
Angus, Corned Beef Reuben	920	41	78
Angus, Corned Beef	580	13	77
Angus, Pastrami Reuben	920	40	78
Angus, Pastrami & Swiss	905	36	82
Angus, Roast, Beef & Cheese	785	33	73
BLT	545	18	74
Chicken & Pesto	565	14	72
Chicken Breast	510	6	77
Chipotle Chicken	540	12	72
Chipotle Grilled Chicken	580	13	76
Dijon Chicken	575	11	79
Dijon Grilled Chicken	615	12	83
Fresh Tomato & Pesto	555	19	73
Grilled Chicken & Pesto	650	22	74
Grilled Chicken Breast	545	7	80
Homestyle Tuna	595	20	73
Mediterranean Tuna	535	11	76
Santa Fe Chicken	620	15	76
Santa Fe Grilled Chicken	655	16	80
Smoked Turkey Breast	500	7	76
Smoked Turkey Reuben	890	37	83
Texas Schlotzsky's	755	31	73
Turkey & Guacamole	550	12	80
Turkey Bacon Club	770	29	76
Original Style: The Original	770	34	76
Cheese	770	34	76
Deluxe	955	46	78
Ham & Cheese	730	27	78
Turkey	815	33	78
Panini: Classic Swiss & Tomato	625	26	63
Grilled Chicken Romano	540	15	61
Italiano	735	32	67
Mozzarella & Portobello	485	15	63
Smoked Ham Crostini	645	23	67
Smoked Turkey & Guacamole	580	21	67
Wraps: Asian Chicken	390	4	70
Feta & Portobello	500	32	46
Grilled Chicken & Guacamole	550	29	49
Homestyle Tuna	365	13	46
Mediterranean Tuna	325	7	48
Parmesan Chicken Caesar	515	26	47
Bread/Buns: Dark Rye, medium	330	2	68
Jalapeno Cheese, medium	340	4	63
Sourdough, medium	330	2	67
Wheat, medium	340	3	67

Continued Next Page ...

Updated Nutrition Data ~ www.CalorieKing.com
Persons with Diabetes ~ See Disclaimer (Page 24)

Schlotzsky's® cont... (Aug '07)

8" Pizzas: Per Pizza

	C	F	Cb
BBQ Chicken & Jalapeno	685	16	98
Baby Spinach Salad	470	8	83
Bacon, Tomato & Portobello	615	22	76
Combination Special	640	25	76
Double Cheese	600	21	74
Fresh Tomato & Pesto	560	19	73
Grilled Chicken & Pesto	650	22	74
Mediterranean	560	20	74
Pepperoni & Double Cheese	685	30	74
Smoked Turkey & Jalapeno	640	19	78
Thai Chicken	700	22	85
Vegetarian Special	540	17	74

Salads: without Dressing/Croutons Unless Indicated

	C	F	Cb
Baby Spinach & Feta	195	15	10
Caesar Salad	100	5	10
Chicken Salad	290	15	12
Fruit Salad	100	0	25
Garden Salad	50	1	12
Greek Salad	135	8	13
Grilled Chicken Caesar w. Croutons	220	8	12
Ham & Turkey Chef Salad	250	13	14
Pasta Salad	70	3	12
Potato Salad	240	13	29
Side Salad	25	1	7
Turkey Chef Salad	295	15	15

Soups: Per Cup

	C	F	Cb
Boston Clam Chowder	215	11	23
Broccoli Cheese	185	12	13
Chicken Tortilla	150	6	13
Hearty Vegetable Beef	110	5	12
Old Fashioned Chicken Noodle	90	2	11
Potato w. Bacon	180	9	26
Timberline Chili	230	8	26
Vegetarian Vegetable	85	1	19
Wisconsin Cheese	305	22	24

Kid's Meals: without Cookie or Drink

	C	F	Cb
Cheese Pizza	480	13	73
Cheese Sandwich	395	15	48
Ham & Cheese Sandwich	425	16	49
Pepperoni Pizza	520	17	73

Desserts

	C	F	Cb
Brownie	415	24	47
Carrot Cake	715	42	80
Cheesecake	350	23	30
Cookies: Chocolate Chip	160	7	24
Fudge Chocolate Chip	165	8	22
Oatmeal Raisin	150	5	24
Sugar	155	7	22
White Choc Macadamia	170	8	22

Second Cup® ~ *see CalorieKing.com*

Shakey's® (Aug '07)

Pizzas (12"): Per Slice (1/10 Pizza)

	C	F	Cb
Cheese only:			
Thin Crust	135	5	13
Thick Crust	170	5	22
Homestyle Pan	305	14	31
Onion/Olives/Mushrooms:			
Thin Crust	125	5	14
Thick Crust	160	4	22
Homestyle Pan	320	15	32
Sausage Pepperoni:			
Thin Crust	165	8	13
Thick Crust	205	8	22
Homestyle Pan	375	20	31
Sausage Mushroom			
Thin Crust	140	6	13
Thick Crust	180	6	22
Homestyle Pan	340	17	31
Pepperoni:			
Thin Crust	150	7	13
Thick Crust	185	6	22
Homestyle Pan	345	15	31
Shakey's Special:			
Thin Crust	170	9	13
Thick Crust	210	8	22
Homestyle Pan	385	21	32

Other Items

	C	F	Cb
3-Piece Chicken & Potato	945	56	51
5-Piece Fried Chicken & Potato	1700	90	130
Hot Ham & Cheese Sandwich	550	21	56
Potato Wedges, 15 pieces	950	36	120
Shakey's Super Hot Hero	810	44	67
Spagh. w. Meat Sce/Garlic Bread	940	33	134

Sheetz® (Aug '07)

Coffeez™: Per 16 fl.oz

	C	F	Cb
Hot Chocolate, medium	250	4	52

Cupo'ccino®: Per Medium (16 fl.oz)

	C	F	Cb
Cupo'ccino: Almond Amaretto	275	8	52
Fat-Free French Vanilla	140	0	34

M.T.O Cold Subs: Per 6" Sub (No Cheese Unless Indicated)

	C	F	Cb
BLT Sub	405	13	53
Cheese	255	1	51
Chicken Salad	505	22	60
Club	375	4	56
Deli	370	10	54
Ham	330	3	54
Italian	450	12	53
Roast Beef,	295	3	52
Tuna Salad	470	17	60
Turkey	310	3	53

Updated Nutrition Data ~ www.CalorieKing.com
Persons with Diabetes ~ See Disclaimer (Page 24)

Sheetz® cont... (Aug '07)

M.T.O® Hot Subs: *Per 6" Sub*

	C	F	Cb
Chicken	375	5	51
Meatball w. Marinara Sauce	395	12	55
Pepperoni	455	19	51
Steak	445	11	52

M.T.O Deli Bagel: *No Cheese Unless Indicated*

	C	F	Cb
Chicken Salad	490	23	57
Deli	355	11	51
Ham & Cheese	125	1	15
Italian	430	13	50
Roast Beef	310	4	48
Tuna Salad	455	18	57
Turkey	290	4	50

M.T.O Hot Dogz: *No Cheese*

	C	F	Cb
Deli Dogz,	610	32	53
Hot Dogz	265	15	24

M.T.O Nachos: *Per Serving, No Topping*

	C	F	Cb
Nachos Bueno w. Nacho cheese	505	23	65

M.T.O Salads: *No Dressing Unless Indicated*

	C	F	Cb
Chef Salad	145	3	12
Crispy Chicken	270	8	30
Garden Salad	25	0	7
Grilled Chicken	145	4	7
Grilled Chicken Caesar w. Dressing	405	27	19
Steak Salad	215	10	8
Taco Salad	255	10	38

M.T.O Breakfast: *Includes Cheese*

	C	F	Cb
Shmagels: Bacon & Egg	575	28	53
Egg	425	16	51
Ham & Egg	490	17	54
Shmiscuits: Bacon & Egg	595	37	40
Egg	445	28	38
Ham & Egg	510	26	41
Sausage & Egg	620	42	38
Shmuffins: Bacon & Egg	465	27	30
Egg	315	15	28
Ham & Egg	380	16	31
Sausage & Egg	490	32	28
Steak & Egg	505	25	29

Sides

	C	F	Cb
Fryz: Bag, 3.2 oz	160	6.5	23
Cup, 5.1 oz	260	11	37
Cheese, 14.3 oz	650	30	81
Smokehouse, 15.3 oz	975	52	103

Shoney's® (Aug '07)

Breakfast

	C	F	Cb
All Star Breakfast, no extras	190	15	1.5
Deluxe Pancake Platter	1610	32	299
Half Stack Pancake Platter	930	14	187
Big Eater Steak Brkfast, no extras	630	41	1.5
Country Fried Steak Breakfast	990	66	49
Sunrise Breakfast	975	60	88
Sausage Biscuit (1)	540	34	42

Burgers

	C	F	Cb
All-American: Burger	690	32	44
Bacon Cheeseburger	890	49	44
Mushroom Swiss Burger	970	57	49
Famous Patty Melt	945	60	40
Half-O-Pound Burger	1350	53	130

Sandwiches

	C	F	Cb
Blackened Chicken	885	21	122
Charbroiled Chicken	895	22	122
Chicken Parmesan Sandwich	750	30	80
Corned Beef Reuben	795	53	37
Fish Sandwich	830	16	126
Fried Chicken Sandwich	560	14	77
Original Slim Jim Sandwich	1005	33	123
Raymond's French Dip	500	14	53
Turkey Club/Whole Wheat	945	52	47
Ultimate Grilled Cheese S'wich	895	46	77

Steaks

	C	F	Cb
BBQ Ribs	1520	78	124
Choice Sirloin, 6 oz	1225	51	127
Half-O-Pound w. Grilled Onions	1335	52	133
Half-O-Pound w. Grilled Mushr.	1320	52	127
Ribeye, 8 oz	1480	75	127
Southwest Half-O-Pound	1305	70	83
T-Bone, 12 oz	1810	100	127

Surf & Turf:

	C	F	Cb
Ribeye & 5 Fried Shrimp	1640	82	138
Ribeye & 6 Grilled Shrimp	1590	81	128
Sirloin & 5 Fried Shrimp	1380	58	138
Sirloin & 6 Grilled Shrimp	1330	57	128
T-Bone & 5 Fried Shrimp	1970	107	138
T-Bone & 6 Grilled Shrimp	1920	105	128

Rib Combos, w. Fries:

	C	F	Cb
¼ Rack & BBQ Chicken	1230	54	103
¼ Rack & Tenderloins	1370	70	120
¼ Rack & Fried Shrimp	1145	50	113
¼ Rack & Grilled Shrimp	1125	52	103

Continued Next Page ...

Shoney's® cont... (Aug '07)

Blue Plate Specials

	C	F	Cb
Cajun Whitefish	480	10	56
Baked Whitefish	510	8.5	58
Grandma's Meatloaf w. Glaze	1090	46	93
Grandma's Meatloaf w. Gravy	1090	48	87
Original Country Fried Steak	1150	62	103
Grilled Liver & Onions	710	22	79
Ham Steak Dinner (no veges)	665	25	60
Roast Beef Platter (no veges)	880	30	96

Pasta: Per Serving

	C	F	Cb
Chicken Alfredo	1705	78	170
Italian Feast	1435	45	204
Pasta Ya-Ya	1850	81	176
Shrimp Alfredo	1780	85	171

Seafood: Fish 'n' Shrimp

	C	F	Cb
Fish 'n' Shrimp	1100	39	129
Fried Fish Platter	1050	38	123
Grilled Cod/Salmon Lite, avg.	200	4	0
Grilled Salmon	750	19	95
Grilled Shrimp	720	20	96
Grilled Shrimp Lite	320	8	30
Shrimper's Feast	1030	39	128
Shrimp Stir Fry	875	19	131

Chicken: Chicken Stir Fry

	C	F	Cb
Chicken Stir Fry	1200	35	172
Charbroiled Blackened Chicken	830	26	100
Charbroiled Chicken Breast	800	23	99
Fried Chicken Tenderloins	1160	60	121
Monterey Chicken	910	40	83
Smothered Chicken	890	34	90

Junior Meals: Fish 'N Chips

	C	F	Cb
Fish 'N Chips	310	11	29
Chicken Dinner	190	10	12

Sides: Baked Potato, Plain

	C	F	Cb
Baked Potato, Plain	350	6	67
French Fries, 4 oz	215	10	25
Onion Rings, 1 order (7 rings)	500	15	83

Desserts, Ice Cream, Sundaes

	C	F	Cb
Apple Pie: a la Mode	1205	53	174
w. NutraSweet	455	18	64
Cheesecake, 1 slice, 4 oz	365	25	23
Hot Fudge Sundae	600	30	75
Original Strawberry Pie, 1 slice	330	17	45
Ultimate Hot Fudge Cake	875	37	126
Cherry/Peach Pie w. Nutrasweet	480	20	68
Caramel Sundae	620	27	83
Chocolate Milk Shake	1080	51	141
Strawberry Sundae	610	27	85
Walnut Brownie a la Mode	575	34	60

Sizzler® (Aug '07)

Hot Entrees: (No Sides)

	C	F	Cb
Hamburger	625	33	36
Dakota Ranch Steak: 6 oz	315	20	0
8 oz	420	27	0
9½ oz	500	32	0
Hibachi Chicken Breast, w. Pineapple	195	3	13
Lemon-Herb Chicken Breast	140	3	0
Malibu Chicken Patty, each	310	19	11
Salmon	250	12	0
Santa Fe Chicken Breast	150	3	0
Shrimp: Broiled	150	6	0
Fried, 4 only	225	2	35
Mini	150	1	24
Shrimp Scampi	145	3	0
Swordfish	315	14	0

Low Carb Grill Menu

	C	F	Cb
Grilled Salmon w. Broccoli	405	19	14
Hibachi Chicken w. Broccoli	295	6	15
Petite Sizzler Steak w. Broccoli	520	26	11

Hot Bar

	C	F	Cb
Broccoli Chse Soup, 4 oz	140	9	10
Chicken Noodle Soup, 4 oz	30	1	4
Chicken Wings, 1 oz	75	4	4
Clam Chowder, 4 oz	120	6	11
Focaccia Bread, 2 pces	110	7	9
Meatballs, 4 balls	155	11	5
Minestrone Soup, 4 oz	35	0	7
Pasta: Fettucine, 2 oz	80	1	15
Spaghetti, 2 oz	80	0	16
Potato Skins, 2 oz	160	8	22
Refried Beans, ¼ cup	60	1	11
Saltine Crackers, 2 crackers	25	1	4
Taco Filling, 2 oz	105	5	3
Taco Shells, each	50	2	7

Dessert Bar: Chocolate Syrup, 1 oz

	C	F	Cb
Chocolate Syrup, 1 oz	90	0	21
Choc/Vanilla Soft Serve, 4 oz	135	4	24
Strawberry Topping, 1 oz	70	0	18
Whipped Topping, 1 Tbsp	10	1	1

Salads & Toppings

Prepared Salads: *Per 2 oz*

	C	F	Cb
Carrot & Raisin	130	10	10
Chinese Chicken; Teriyaki Beef	55	2	6
Mediterranean Minted Fruit	30	0	7
Mexican Fiesta	55	1	10
Old Fashioned Potato	85	5	10
Red Herb Potato	120	9	9
Seafood	55	3	4
Seafood Louis Pasta	65	2	9
Spicy Jicama	15	0	4
Tuna Pasta	135	10	6

Updated Nutrition Data ~ www.CalorieKing.com
Persons with Diabetes ~ See Disclaimer (Page 24)

Restaurants & Fast - Foods

Sizzler® cont... (Aug '07)

Sides	C	F	Cb
Baked Potato, plain	220	0	50
Cottage Cheese, 2 oz	50	1	2
Eggs, 1 oz	45	3	0
Garbanzo Beans, ¼ cup	65	1	11
Kidney Beans, ¼ cup	50	0	10
Olives, 1 oz	60	6	1
Peaches, ¼ cup	35	0	9
Peas, ¼ cup	30	0	6
Real Bacon Bits, 1 Thsp	30	2	2
Turkey Ham, 1 oz	60	5	0
Dressings: Per 2 Tbsp (1 oz)			
Blue Cheese	110	12	1
Honey Mustard	160	16	4
Italian, Lite	15	0	2
Japanese Rice Vinegar, Fat Free	10	0	2
Parmesan Italian	100	10	2
Ranch	120	12	2
Ranch, Reduced-Calorie	90	8	4
Thousand Island	145	15	3

Skyline Chili® (Aug '07)

Burritos	C	F	Cb
All Chili, burrito	560	30	37
All Chili Deluxe, burrito	650	35	45
Salads: Without Dressing			
Buffalo Chicken Salad	150	7	7
Classic Chicken Salad	150	7	8
Garden Salad	80	5	6
Greek Chicken Salad	170	8	9
Greek Salad	60	3.5	5
Southwestern Chkn w. Tortilla Chips	760	44	66
Meals: Per Regular Serving			
Coney w. Cheese	340	22	17
Coney, no Cheese	220	12	17
Black Bean & Rice, 3-Way	800	40	74
Black Bean & Rice, 4-Way	810	40	77
Black Bean & Rice, 5-Way	880	40	89
Black Bean & Rice, Spaghetti	490	12	79
Bowls: Chili	270	16	6
Chili Bean	270	12	17
Chili Cheese	440	30	6
Coney	870	69	9
Loaded Chili	580	40	18
Vegetarian Black Beans & Rice	320	9	46

Skyline Chili® cont... (Aug '07)

Meals (Cont): Per Regular Serving	C	F	Cb
Chili Spaghetti: Regular	450	18	43
w. Bean & Onion	530	17	64
w. Bean	520	17	61
w. Onion	470	17	51
Steamed Potatoes: Plain	310	0	72
Cheddar	740	41	72
Chili	440	8	74
Sour Cream	570	27	72
Wraps			
Buffalo Chicken	520	21	55
Classic Chicken	510	21	55
Greek Chicken	510	21	54
Southwest Chicken	670	30	85
Sides: Cheese	230	19	1
Chili	130	8	3
Crackers	100	3	20
French Fries	630	33	79

Smoothie King® (Aug '07)

Berry Smoothies: Per 20 oz	C	F	Cb
Blackberry Dream	345	0.5	86
Blueberry Heaven	260	1	58
Cranberry Supreme	575	0.5	139
Raspberry Sunrise	335	1	85
Strawberry Kiwi Breeze	300	0	77
Low-Fat Fruit Smoothies: Per 20 oz (No Turbinado)			
Angel Food	230	0.5	56
Cranberry Cooler	440	0	109
Grape Expectations	250	0.5	94
Mangofest	320	0	78
Youth Fountain	165	0.5	42
High Protein Smoothies: Per 20 oz			
Almond Mocha	300	13	22
Banana	305	11	33
Chocolate	300	13	22
Lemon	390	13	41
Pineapple	380	13	41

Continued Next Page ...

Updated Nutrition Data ~ www.CalorieKing.com
Persons with Diabetes ~ See Disclaimer (Page 24)

Smoothie King® cont... (Aug '07)

	C	F	Cb
Heart Smart Smoothies: *Per 20 oz*			
Power Punch Plus	400	2	90
Super Punch Plus	515	0.5	18
The Activator: Chocolate	320	1.5	70
Strawberry	480	1.5	107
Vanilla	335	1.5	71
Sorbet Smoothies: *Per 21.6 oz*			
Banana Berry Treat	330	1	81
Berry Punch	350	0	88
Fruit Fusion	390	1	91
Island Impact	325	0	81
Kids Kups			
Berry Interesting	150	0	37
Choc-A-Laka	210	2	44

Snappy Tomato (Aug '07)

	C	F	Cb
Large Pizzas: *Per Slice (⅛ Pizza)*			
Buffalo Grilled Chicken	250	8	32
Cheese Pizza	220	7	30
Hawaiian Pizza	370	18	33
Meat Topper Pizza	430	23	31
Pepperoni Pizza	340	17	31
Ranch Pizza	370	21	31
Snapperoni Pizza	390	22	31
Supreme Pizza	340	17	32
Veggie Pizza	240	8	33
Sides			
Chicken Snappers, 2 pieces, 82g	150	5	12
Grilled Chicken Breast Hoagie, 87g	110	4.5	3
Hoagie Bun, 140.6g	380	6	68
Hoagie Patty (1),113g	290	22	5
Snappy Wings, 3 pieces, 74g	160	11	0

Sonic Drive-In® (Aug '07)

	C	F	Cb
Burgers			
Sonic Burger w. Mayonnaise	630	37	53
Sonic Burger w. Mustard	540	25	52
Cheeseburger w. Mayonnaise	700	42	55
Cheeseburger w. Mustard	600	31	54
Bacon Burger	770	47	55
SuperSonic Cheeseburger: w. Mayo	970	63	56
w. Mustard	870	52	55
Jr. Burger	320	16	29
Jr. Cheeseburger	380	21	30
Sandwiches/Coneys/Wraps			
Coney: Extra-Long Cheese (1)	600	33	54
Corn Dog (1)	250	15	23
Sandwiches: Breaded Chicken	670	33	66
Grilled Chicken	330	11	32
Toaster Sandwiches: Chicken Club	690	35	64
Bacon Cheeseburger	690	37	58
Wraps: Chicken Strip	480	20	56
Fritos Chili Cheese	670	38	66
Grilled Chicken	380	11	44
Chicken			
Chicken Strip Dinner	920	43	97
Jumbo Popcorn Chicken:			
Snack, no Sauce, 4 oz	370	21	27
Large, no Sauce, 6 oz	560	32	41
Popcorn Chicken Sauces: BBQ	45	0	11
Honey Mustard	90	7	7
Ranch	150	16	1
Fresh Tastes Salads: *No Dressing*			
Grilled Chicken	310	14	19
Jumbo Popcorn Chicken	490	28	39
Santa Fe Grilled Chicken	370	15	29
Salad Dressings: *Per Serving (2 oz)*			
Golden Italian Fat-Free	50	0	13
Honey Mustard	240	21	14
Original Ranch	260	28	0
Original Ranch Light	120	7	14
Sides			
French Fries: Plain, regular, 2.6 oz	210	10	28
w. Cheese, regular, 3.3 oz	280	15	29
w. Chili & Cheese, regular, 4.3 oz	300	18	31
Mozzarella Sticks (5), no Sauce	410	21	35
Onion Rings, regular, 5½ oz	500	28	55
Tater Tots: Plain, regular, 3 oz	220	14	23
w. Cheese, regular, 3.6 oz	290	19	25
w. Chili & Cheese, regular, 4.6 oz	310	21	26

Updated Nutrition Data ~ www.CalorieKing.com
Persons with Diabetes ~ See Disclaimer (Page 24)

Sonic Drive-In® cont... (Aug '07)

Breakfast

	C	F	Cb
Burritos: Bacon Egg & Cheese	470	27	35
Ham Egg & Cheese	440	21	35
Sausage Egg & Cheese	470	30	38
SuperSonic	550	35	47
French Toast Sticks: w. Syrup (4)	580	26	80
no Syrup (4)	500	26	59

Breakfast Sandwiches

	C	F	Cb
Bistro: Bacon Egg & Cheese	470	27	35
Ham Egg & Cheese	430	21	35
Sausage Egg & Cheese	560	37	35
Toaster: Bacon Egg & Cheese	540	30	46
Ham Egg & Cheese	500	23	46
Sausage Egg & Cheese	630	39	46

Desserts (Frozen Favorites): Per Regular

	C	F	Cb
Banana Split	450	12	82
Vanilla Cone	180	6	30
Vanilla Dish	240	9	36
Cream Pie Shakes: Banana	685	21	117
Chocolate	770	20	136
Coconut	680	22	112
Strawberry	730	20	128
CreamSlush: Lemon-Berry; Strawb., avg.	455	13	81
Other varieties, average	440	13	77
Floats: Diet Coke; Diet Dr Pepper	235	8.5	9
Coca-Cola	305	8.5	5
Malts/Shakes: Chocolate	645	19	108
Banana; Vanilla, avg.	560	20	86
Pineapple; Strawberry, avg	600	19	98
Sonic Blast: Butterfinger	685	31	91
M&M's; Oreo	670	21	99
Reese's Peanut Butter Cups	630	21	99
Single Topping Sundaes: Chocolate	410	13	67
Hot Fudge	440	18	63
Pineapple; Strawberry	380	13	60

Drinks: Barq's Root Beer, 24 fl.oz

	C	F	Cb
Drinks: Barq's Root Beer, 24 fl.oz	310	0	112
Cranberry Juice, regular	175	0	46
Limeade Cranberry, medium	200	0	53
Fruit Smoothie: Strawberry, reg.	460	0	113
Strawberry-Banana, regular	440	0	108
Tropical, regular	500	0	124

For Complete Nutritional Data ~ see CalorieKing.com

Souper Salad® (Aug '07)

Soups: Per Serving (5 oz)

	C	F	Cb
Adobe Rice & Chicken	100	5	10
Black Bean	80	2	20
Cherokee Joe's Cornbread	70	1.5	13
Chicken Noodle	80	3	9
Chicken Tortilla	60	2	7
Holiday Harvest	90	6	5
Mama Mia Chicken; Zucchini Chkn	80	3	9
Minestrone	70	1	13
Mr. B's Hot & Sour Chicken	60	1.5	8
Red French Onion, no Crouton	40	1	6
Seafood Bisque	120	8	8
Pasta Tortellini	100	3.5	14
Seafood Bisque	120	8	8
Spicy Meatballs w. Rice	100	4.5	10
Vegetable Lentil	70	0	16
Vegetarian Vegetable	50	0.5	11

Bread

	C	F	Cb
Blueberry Bread, piece	150	2.5	29
Cheese Drop Biscuit	70	3	8
Cornbread	170	4.5	30
Garlic Breadstick, piece	130	4.5	18
Gingerbread, piece	180	6	30

For Complete Nutritional Data ~ see CalorieKing.com

Souplantation® (Aug '07)

Soups: Per Cup

	C	F	Cb
Low Fat: Chicken Tortilla	100	3	5
Classical Minestrone	120	2	20
Vegetable Medley	90	1	14
Regular Soup: Per Cup			
Chesapeake Corn Chowder	280	16	30
Cream of Mushroom	290	21	15
Irish Potato Leek	260	16	23
Manhattan Clam Chowder	130	4	16
Minestrone w. Italian Sausage	210	11	14
Navy Bean w. Ham	340	10	30
Vegetarian Harvest	190	8	23
Chili: Low-Fat Kettle House, 1 cup	230	3	26
Breads: Sourdough	150	0.5	27
Buttermilk Cornbread, 1 pce	140	2	27
Focaccia: Garlic Asiago	140	5	19
Tomatillo	140	6	16

Fresh Tossed Salads: Per Cup

	C	F	Cb
Antipasto Salad; BBQ, average	140	10	6
Caesar Salad Asiago	190	14	10
Won Ton Chicken Happiness	150	8	12

Continued Next Page ...

253

Fast - Foods & *Restaurants*

Souplantation® cont... (Aug '07)

	C	**F**	**Cb**
Prepared Salads: *Per ½ Cup*			
Aunt Doris' Red Pepper Slaw	70	0	18
Baja Bean & Cilantro	180	3	29
BBQ Potato	160	8	20
Carrot Raisin	90	3	17
Dijon Potato w. Garlic Dill Vinegar	150	12	9
Greek Couscous w. Feta Cheese	170	9	19
Oriental Ginger Slaw w. Krab	70	3	9
Southern Dill Potato	120	3	20
Thai Noodle w. Peanut Sauce	170	8	17
Zesty Tortellini	190	15	18
Dressing & Croutons: *Per 2 Tbsp*			
Balsamic Vinaigrette	180	19	1
Blue Cheese Dressing	140	14	3
Italian Dressing, creamy	120	13	1
Fat Free	20	0	5
Honey Mustard Dressing	150	13	8
Fat Free	45	0	10
Ranch Dressing	130	13	1
Fat Free	50	0	2
Thousand Island Dressing	110	11	3
Croutons, Garlic Parmesan, 5 pces	40	3	2
Hot Tossed Pastas: *Per Cup*			
Bruschetta	260	4	41
Creamy Bruschetta	360	16	43
Garden Vegetable: w. Meatballs	270	7	42
w. Italian Sausage	300	10	42
Italian Vegetable Beef	270	6	43
Vegetarian Marinara w. Basil	260	4	44
Muffins: Chocolate Brownie	170	8	20
Georgia Peach Poppyseed	150	6	20
Tangy Lemon	140	4	24
Wildly Blue Blueberry, small	140	5	22
Fruit Medley Bran	80	0.5	17
Desserts			
Apple Cobbler, ½ Cup	350	10	64
Apple Medley (fat-free), ½ cup	70	0	18
Banana Royale (fat-free), ½ cup	80	0	20
Chocolate Chip Cookie, small	70	3	10
Chocolate Lava Cake, ½ cup	295	8	55
Jello, flavored, ½ cup	85	0	20
Rice Pudding, ½ cup	110	2	20
Vanilla Pudding, ½ cup	140	4	24
Chocolate Syrup, 2 Tbsp	70	0	18
Granola Topping, 2 Tbsp	110	4	16
Soft Serve: Chocolate, ½ cup	95	0	21
Vanilla Soft Serve (reduced fat)	140	4	22

For Complete Nutritional Data ~ see CalorieKing.com

Southern Tsunami® (Aug '07)

	C	**F**	**Cb**
Sushi: *Per Pack*			
California Roll, 12 pieces	360	6	66
California Roll & Inari, 9 pieces	505	11	87
California Roll Plus	495	10	88
Cream Cheese Roll w. Salmon (12)	515	20	59
Crunchy Shrimp Roll, 12 pieces	510	21	64
Dragon Roll, 12 pieces	505	18	66
Eel Roll (Freshwater Eel), 12 pieces	495	16	65
Eel Roll (Sea Eel), 12 pieces	435	12	66
Futomaki	505	6	96
Inari, 4 pieces	420	9	73
Inari & Maki	560	9	102
M&M Roll: Shrimp & Avocado (16)	330	5	59
Tuna & Cucumber, 16 pieces	305	1	57
Nigiri: Cuttlefish, 1 piece	40	0	8.5
Egg Cake, 1 piece	75	1	13
Fish Roe, 1 piece	60	0.5	9
Fresh Salmon, 1 piece	70	1	9
Fresh Water Eel, 1 piece	110	5	11
Octopus, 1 piece	55	1	9
Sea Eel, 1 piece	90	3	11
Shrimp, 1 piece	45	0	8
Smoked Salmon, 1 piece	70	1	9
Tilapia, 1 piece	50	0.5	9
Tuna, 1 piece	60	0	8
Yellowtail, 1 piece	55	0.5	8
Ocean Crab Roll, 12 pieces	390	7	60
Orange Roll, 12 pieces	385	5	67
Rainbow Roll, 12 pieces	490	9	66
Snack Pack: Cucumber, 16 pieces	265	0	57
Imitation Crab & Cucumber (16)	290	1	61
Spicy Roll: Salmon, 12 pieces	485	16	59
Shrimp, 12 pieces	395	11	57
Tuna, 12 pieces	450	11	57
Tempura Roll, 12 pieces	530	11	82
Tofu Roll, 12 pieces	320	3	62
Tsunami Roll, 12 pieces	470	13	71
Vegetable Combo: 12 pieces	350	7	60
24 pieces	445	4	92
Combinations: Fullmoon, 12 pcs	425	13	64
Marina Plate, 6 pcs	380	8	52
Meteor Special, 14 pieces	385	3	69
Seaside, Tuna & Salmon, 16 pcs	360	3	58
Seaside, Tuna, Salmon, Shrimp, Eel	355	4	59
Shoreline, 12 pieces	480	8	78
Stardust, 16 pieces	540	12	94

Spaghetti Warehouse® (Aug '07)

Lunch	C	F	Cb
Minestrone Soup	80	1.5	12
Grilled Chicken Marinara	530	8	65
Seafood Marinara	385	5	65
Spaghetti: w. Tomato Sauce	425	5	82
w. Marinara Sauce #12	440	5	84
Spicy Marinara Sce Spaghetti	280	4	52
Vegetable Primavera	340	4	65
Dinner			
Minestrone, 1 bowl	110	2	18
Grilled Chicken Marinara	640	10	85
Grilled Halibut Dinner	880	14	106
Grilled Marinated Chicken Breast	910	17	116
Marinara Sauce #12	520	6	99
Seafood Marinara	520	8	86
Spaghetti w. Tomato Sauce	525	6	101
Spicy Marinara Sce Spaghetti	330	6	60
Vegetable Primavera	610	8	116

*This Triple Decker (Carnegie Deli, New York)
contains up to 3 lb meat and 8 oz cheese
~ approx. 4000 calories and 300 grams fat.
Note: Only half the sandwich is shown
– the other half is hidden behind!
Carnegie's challenge: Eat one Triple Decker
. . . get the second one free!*

Starbuck's® (Aug '07)

Figures Based on Grande (16 fl.oz)
Without Whip Unless Indicated

Classic Favorites	C	F	Cb
Apple Juice	240	0	60
Apple Juice, Steamed	230	0	58
Brewed Coffee			
Caffe Misto: w. Whole Milk	130	7	10
w. Nonfat Milk	70	0	10
w. Soy Milk	95	3	13
Espresso Hot			
Caffe Americano	20	0	3
Caffe Latte: w. Whole Milk	230	12	18
w. Nonfat Milk	135	0	20
w. Soy Milk	175	5	24
Caffe Mocha: w. Whole Milk	305	12	41
w. Nonfat Milk	225	2.5	42
w. Soy Milk	255	6.5	46
Cappuccino: w. Whole Milk	145	7	1
w. Nonfat Milk	90	0	13
w. Soy Milk	110	3	15
Caramel Macchiato: w. Whole Milk	270	10	34
w. Nonfat Milk	190	1	35
w. Soy Milk	225	5	38
Con Panna: 1 doppio, 2 fl.oz	35	2.5	3
1 solo, 1 fl.oz	20	1.5	1.5
Dulce de Leche Latte: w. Whole Milk	390	10	63
w. Nonfat Milk	310	0	64
w. Soy Milk	345	4	67
Espresso: 1 doppio, 2 fl.oz	10	0	2
1 solo, 1 fl.oz	5	0	1
Macchiato, w. Whole Milk: 1 doppio	15	0	2
1 solo, 1 fl.oz	10	0	1
White Choc. Mocha: w. Whole Milk	440	16	61
w. Nonfat Milk	360	5.5	62
w. Soy Milk	390	9.5	66
Espresso Iced			
Caffe Americano	15	0	2.5
Caffe Latte: w. Whole Milk	140	6.5	11
w. Nonfat Milk	85	0	13
w. Soy Milk	115	3	15
Caffe Mocha: w. Whole Milk	205	7.5	34
w. Nonfat Milk	165	2.5	35
w. Soy Milk	195	4.5	37
Dulce de Leche Latte: w. Whole Milk	300	5.5	56
w. Nonfat Milk	260	0	57
w. Soy Milk	280	2.5	59
White Choc. Mocha: w. Whole Milk	345	11	54
w. Nonfat Milk	305	6	55
w. Soy Milk	325	8	57
Espresso: 1 doppio, 2 fl.oz	10	0	2
1 solo, 1 fl.oz	5	0	1

Continued Next Page ...

Starbuck's® cont... (Aug '07)

Figures Based on Grande (16 fl.oz)
Without Whip Unless Indicated

	C	**F**	**Cb**
Frappuccino Blended Coffee			
Caffe Vanilla	295	3	63
Caramel	255	3.5	51
Cinnamon Dolce	245	3	51
Coffee	225	3	45
Dulce de Leche	280	3	59
Espresso	195	2.5	38
Java Chip	325	7.5	61
Mocha	255	3.5	52
White Chocolate Mocha	295	4.5	57
Frappuccino Blended Creme			
Double Chocolate Chip	365	7.5	69
Dulce de Leche	365	2	76
Strawberries & Creme	415	2	89
Tazo Chai	315	2	64
Tazo Green Tea	360	2.5	74
Vanilla Bean	325	2.5	67
White Chocolate	420	6	79
Frappuccino Light Blended Coffee			
Caffe Vanilla	185	0.5	39
Caramel	145	1	29
Coffee	120	0.5	23
Dulce de Leche	165	0.5	35
Espresso	100	0.5	19
Java Chip	200	4.5	37
Mocha	140	1.5	29
White Chocolate Mocha	185	2.5	35
Frappuccino Light Blended Creme			
Orange Creme	125	0	29
Raspberry Chocolate	195	1.5	44
Tazo Iced Tea Shaken			
Black Tea	85	0	21
Green Tea	85	0	21
Or. Passion Tea & Lemonade	75	0	19
Passion Tea & Lemonade	125	0	33
Frappuccino Juice Blend			
Pomegranate	215	0	52
Tangerine	155	0	37
Drink Extras			
Flavored Syrup: 1 pump, 0.35 oz	20	0	5
Sugar-Free, 1 pump, 0.35 oz	0	0	0
Mocha Syrup, 1 pump, 0.6 oz	25	0.5	6
Topping: Caramel, 0.53 oz	15	0.5	2
Chocolate, 1 serving, 0.14 oz	5	0	1
Sprinkles, 1 serving	0	0	0.5
Whipped Cream Topping:			
Cold Beverage, 1 venti, 1.2 oz	110	11	3
Hot Beverage, 1 venti, 0.78 oz	70	7	2

Starbuck's® cont... (Aug '07)

Note: Baked items below are approximate only, and
vary between regions

	C	**F**	**Cb**
Apple Fritter, Top Pot	480	22	64
Bagels: Cinnamon Raisin	310	2	65
Plain	310	1	62
Bars: Crispy Marshmallow Square	370	10	71
Toffee Almond	450	20	61
Oat: Cranberry	440	17	69
Organic Blueberries	380	16	55
Bread, Roasted Red Pepper Bialy	290	7	44
Brownies, Espresso	340	19	40
Cakes: Marble Pound	370	27	55
Old-Fashioned Crumb	500	23	68
Coffee Cakes: Banana Walnut	470	27	63
Reduced-Fat: Blueberry	310	10	58
Banana Chocolate Chip	390	8	76
Banana Dulche	360	7	72
Cinnamon Swirl	300	8	59
Orange Creme	320	8	56
Cookies: Chocolate Chip	400	21	53
Chocolate Truffle	390	24	50
Oatmeal Raisin	350	12	56
Croissants: Butter	300	15	36
Pain Au Chocolat	450	24	50
Cupcakes: Vanilla	330	16	44
Chocolate Chocolate	350	19	44
Danish, Cheese	370	18	42
Doughnut, Old Fashioned	450	21	59
Empanada, Mango Pineapple	330	17	40
Loaves: Banana Walnut	410	17	60
Cinnamon Sour Cream	460	22	61
Lemon	430	21	59
Raspberry Swirl	350	11	61
Zucchini Walnut	460	22	50
Muffins: Banana Bran	400	14	68
Blueberry	430	16	65
Lemon Cream Cheese	460	22	60
Low-Fat Blueberry Apricot	360	5	74
Mini: Bran	150	5	26
Zucchini Walnut	380	24	39
Roll, Cinnamon	470	16	76
Sandie, Dulce de Leche	150	8	18
Scones: Blueberry	400	18	55
Cherry Almond Multigrain	430	20	56
Cranberry Orange	420	16	66
Maple Oat Nu	440	21	57
Raspberry Thumbprint	370	16	51
Twist, Cinnamon	480	21	68

Ice Cream & Ice Cream Bars ~ See Page 35, 38
For Bottled Drinks ~ See Page 164

Updated Nutrition Data ~ www.CalorieKing.com
Persons with Diabetes ~ See Disclaimer (Page 24)

Restaurants & Fast - Foods

Steak Escape® (Aug '07)

	C	F	Cb
Small Sandwiches (7"): *No Cheese or Condiments*			
Chicken Philly	410	6	60
Chicken Portion	120	4	0
Classic Italian	470	11	60
Meatball Sub	630	26	69
Philly Cheesesteak	420	6	60
Ragin Cajun Chicken	410	5	58
Steak Portion	130	5	0
Turkey Club	380	2	62
Wild West BBQ	455	6	60
Large Sandwiches (12"): *No Cheese or Condiments*			
Chicken Philly	640	10	84
Chicken Portion	240	8	0
Classic Italian	760	22	85
Meatball Sub	1120	52	102
Philly Cheesesteak	660	12	84
Ragin Cajun Chicken	630	10	80
Steak Portion	260	10	0
Turkey Club	580	3	88
Wild West BBQ	730	12	84
Fresh Salads: *No Cheese or Condiments*			
Side Salad	40	0.5	8
Grilled Salad: w. Chicken	175	5	11
w. Ham	130	2	8
w. Steak	185	6	11
w. Turkey	130	2	8
Smashed Potatoes: Plain, 14 oz	245	0	53
w. Chicken	385	4	56
w. Ham	340	2	59
w. Steak	395	5	56
w. Turkey	340	2	59
Loaded: Bacon & Cheddar	635	26	91
Ranch & Bacon	690	34	87
Fresh Cut Fries: *Per Serving*			
Small, 6 oz	500	26	67
Medium, 7.9 oz	650	34	87
Large, 11.3 oz	920	48	123
Loaded: Bacon & Cheddar	905	44	88
Ranch & Bacon	1045	71	84
Condiments			
Mayonnaise, 1 oz	100	11	0
BBQ Sauce, 1 oz	40	0	9
Cheddar Cheese, 1 oz	115	8	1

For Complete Nutritional Data ~ see CalorieKing.com

Steak 'n Shake® (Aug '07)

	C	F	Cb
Meals			
All-American Melt Sandwich	1230	97	54
Chicken Fingers, no fries	615	46	22
Chili 3-Way	660	36	63
Chili 5-Way	1035	67	66
Chili Deluxe, 6 oz cup	515	38	17
Fish Fillet Sandwich w. Cheese	825	58	54
Frisco Melt Sandwich	1175	93	44
Grilled Cheese & Bacon Sandwich	790	61	41
Grilled Chicken Breast Sandwich	470	26	34
Original Dbl Steakburger w. Cheese	580	38	29
Original Single w. Cheese	400	23	29
Philadelphia Sandwich	850	53	63
Triple Steakburger	690	47	29
Turkey Melt Sandwich	950	70	47
Fries: French, reg., 5 oz	475	23	62
French, large, 7.25 oz	685	34	90
Cheddar Cheese, reg., 5 oz	580	31	68
Salads: Beef Taco Salad w. dress.	940	59	76
Chicken Chef Salad no dressing	465	32	10
Fried Chicken Salad w. dress.	1050	81	48
Soups: Chicken Gumbo, 6 fl.oz cup	85	3	10
Chicken Noodle, 6 fl.oz cup	70	2	8.5
Cream of Broccoli, 6 fl.oz cup	135	8	11
Vegetable Beef, 6 fl.oz cup	115	7	10
Breakfast: Bacon 'n Egg (1) Works	625	47	36
Biscuits, Gravy 'n Hash Browns	1585	99	154
Buttermilk Pancakes (2)	160	2.5	31
Country Scrambler	1030	78	51
Cinnamon Swirl French Tst, 3 sl.	265	7	44
One Egg, cooked w. Margarine	140	13	1
Silver Dollar Hash Browns	370	25	35
Steak 'n Eggs Breakfast	1015	80	36
Sandwich on Bagel: Egg & Chse	565	19	76
Egg, Cheese & Bacon	675	29	77
Desserts: Apple Cobbler	505	22	76
Hot Fudge Brownie	490	23	69
Hot Fudge Sundae	515	27	64
Outrageous Parfait, no cream	770	40	95
Pumpkin Pie, (⅛) w. topping	395	14	61
Beverages: Root Beer Float	555	22	87
Hot Chocolate, 7 fl.oz, no topping	140	3.5	27
Orange Freeze, regular	615	19	101
Shake: Chocolate, no Cream reg.	685	22	110
Banana; Vanilla, regular	670	21	106

Subway® (Aug '07)

6" Sandwiches (6g Fat or Less)   **C** **F** **Cb**

Figures based on wheat bread and toppings: lettuce, tomato, onion, green peppers, olives and pickles. Cheese, oil or mayo not included.

	C	F	Cb
Ham	290	5	47
Oven Roasted Chicken Breast	310	5	48
Roast Beef	290	5	45
Subway Club	320	6	47
Sweet Onion Chicken Teriyaki	370	5	59
Turkey Breast	280	4.5	46
Turkey Breast & Ham	290	5	47
Veggie Delite	230	3	44

Other 6" Sandwiches

Figures based on wheat bread plus lettuce, tomato, onion, green peppers, olives and cheese.

	C	F	Cb
Chicken & Bacon Ranch	580	30	47
Cold Cut Combo	410	17	47
Italian BMT	450	21	47
Meatball Marinara	560	24	63
Spicy Italian	480	25	45
Steak & Cheese	400	12	48
Subway Melt	380	12	48
Tuna	530	31	44

Mini Subs (4")

	C	F	Cb
Ham	180	3	30
Roast Beef	190	3.5	30
Tuna, with cheese	320	18	30
Turkey Breast	190	3	30

Mini Wraps: Subway Club

	C	F	Cb
Subway Club	310	8	40
Sweet Onion Chicken Teriyaki	360	9	52
Veggie Delite	210	5	37
Other Varieties, average	280	7	39

Double Meat Subs (6")

	C	F	Cb
Ham	350	7	50
Chicken Bacon Ranch w. Cheese	710	35	48
Cold Cut Combo w. Cheese	550	28	49
Italian BMT w. Cheese	630	35	49
Meatball Marinara w. Cheese	860	42	82
Oven Roasted Chicken	400	8	51
Roast Beef	360	7	46
Steak & Cheese	540	18	52
Subway Club	420	8	50
Subway Melt w. Cheese	490	17	51
Sweet Onion Chicken Teriyaki	480	7	65
Turkey Breast	330	5	48
Turkey Breast & Ham	360	7	50

Pizza (8")

	C	F	Cb
Cheese	680	22	96
Cheese & Veggies	740	25	100
Pepperoni	790	32	96
Sausage	830	30	97

Subway® cont... (Aug '07)

Breakfast Sandwiches   **C** **F** **Cb**

	C	F	Cb
6" Sub: Cheese	400	17	43
Chipotle Steak & Cheese	580	31	48
Double Bacon & Cheese	500	25	44
Honey Mustard Ham & Cheese	460	19	51
Western with Cheese	440	18	45
Breakfast Wraps: Cheese	390	19	37
Chipotle Steak & Cheese	570	33	41
Double Bacon & Cheese	480	27	38
Honey Mustard Ham & Cheese	450	21	45
Western w. Cheese	420	20	39

Sandwich Fillings (on 6" Sub or Salad)

	C	F	Cb
Cheese Slices, ½ oz	45	3.5	1
Cucumber, Lettuce, Pickles, Peppers	5	0	1
Tomato (3 slices), Onion, Olives	5	0	2
Meats: Bacon, 2 strips	45	3.5	0
Ham, 2 oz	60	2	3
Italian BMT Meats, 2¼ oz	180	14	2
Meatballs, 7 oz	300	18	19
Roast Beef, 2 oz	70	2	1
Subway Club Meats, 3 oz	100	3	3
Tuna, 2½ oz	260	24	0
Turkey Breast, 2 oz	50	1	2

Sauces & Dressings:

	C	F	Cb
Chipotle Southwest, 1¼ Tbsp	95	10	1
Honey Mustard, fat-free, 1¼ Tbsp	30	0	7
Mayonnaise: Reg., 1 Tbsp, ½ oz	110	12	0
Light, 1 Tbsp, ½ oz	50	5	1
Mustard, Yellow or Brown, 2 tsp	5	0	1
Olive Oil Blend, 1 teaspoon	45	5	0
Ranch Dressing, 1¼ Tbsp	120	13	1
Red Wine Vinaigrette, 1¼ Tbsp	30	0	6
Sweet Onion Sauce, 1¼ tbsp	40	0	9
Vinegar, 1 teaspoon	0	0	0

Salads (6g Fat or Less)

Includes lettuce, tomato, onions, green peppers, olives, carrot, cucumber. Dressing and croutons are not included in data.

	C	F	Cb
Ham	120	3	14
Oven Roasted Chicken Breast	140	2.5	11
Roast Beef	120	3	12
Subway Club	150	4	14
Sweet Onion Chicken Teriyaki	210	3	26
Turkey Breast	110	2.5	13
Turkey Breast & Ham	120	3	14
Veggie Delight	60	1	11

Salad Dressings: *Per Package (2 oz)*

	C	F	Cb
Fat-Free Varieties	35	0	7
Ranch	320	35	3

Subway® cont... (Aug '07)

	C	F	Cb
Soups: *Per Cup (10 oz)*			
Chicken & Dumpling	170	5	23
Chili Con Carne	290	8	35
Cream of Broccoli	160	7	18
Cream of Potato w. Bacon	240	13	26
Golden Broccoli & Cheese	200	12	17
Minestrone	80	1	15
New England Style Clam Chowder	150	5	20
Roasted Chicken Noodle	80	2	11
Spanish Style Chicken w. Rice	110	2	17
Wild Rice w. Chicken	210	11	21
Breads: Wrap	190	4.5	33
6" Hearty Italian; Parmesan Oregano	220	3	41
6" Honey Oat	250	3.5	48
6" Italian Herbs & Chse; Monterey	250	5	40
6" Italian White	200	2	38
6" Wheat	200	2.5	40
Cookies & Desserts			
Cookies: Oatmeal Raisin (1)	200	8	30
Peanut Butter (1)	220	12	26
Sugar (1)	220	12	28
Chocolate varieties, avg. (1)	220	10	30
White Chip Macadamia Nut	220	11	29
Apple Pie, 2½ oz	250	10	37
Apple Slices, 1 package, 2.5 oz	35	0	9
Raisins, 1 package, 1½ oz	140	0	33
Fruizle Express: *Per Small Cup*			
Berry Lishus	110	0	28
Berry Lishus w. Banana	140	0	35
Peach Pizzazz	100	0	26
Pineapple Delight	130	0	33
Pineapple Delight w. Banana	160	0	40
Sunrise Refresher	120	0	29

For Complete Nutritional Data ~ see CalorieKing.com

Jared Fogle lost over 200 lbs with low-fat Subway® Sandwiches and lots of walking·

Sub Station® (Aug '07)

	C	F	Cb
Sandwiches			
Per ½ Sub (Incl. Oil, Vinegar, Salad)			
Ham & Cheese	580	36	48
Ham, Turkey & Cheese	605	37	49
Turkey & Cheese	600	37	48
Roast Beef & Cheese	630	40	44
Ham, Salami, Pepperoni, Cappicola, Bologna, Turkey & Cheese	825	57	43

Sweet Tomatoes®

~ Same Menu & Data as Souplantation (See Page 253) ~

Swiss Chalet® (Aug '07)

	C	F	Cb
Burgers: Includes Garnishes			
Bacon Cheese Burger	870	46	45
Hamburger	730	49	44
Veggie Burger	430	13	51
Rotisserie Chicken: Meat Only			
Double Leg w. Skin	630	38	4
Half Chicken, w. Skin	610	31	5
Quarter Chicken: Leg, no Skin	230	11	1
Leg meat w. Skin	310	19	2
Breast meat, no Skin	210	7	0
Breast meat w. Skin	300	11	3
Chicken Pot Pie, 1 pie	640	33	52
Appetizers			
Baked Garlic Cheese Loaf, 9 oz	730	31	83
Chalet Chicken Wings, 8 wings	1030	59	38
Chicken Fingers, 4 strips	420	21	32
Perogies w. Cajun Sauce, 6.5 oz	420	10	69
Soup: Chalet Chicken, 1 cup	160	4	17
Side Salads: Greek	220	18	9
Caesar Salad	360	32	15
Meals:			
From The Grill: No Flatbread			
BBQ Ribs: Regular Cut	630	38	4
Large Cut BBQ Ribs	1270	77	9
Feature Cut BBQ Ribs	420	26	3
Entree Salad: w. Chicken	410	25	13
Vegetable	270	21	14
Grilled Chicken Breast	130	1.5	41
Lighter Favorites: Includes Salad & Vegetables			
Quarter Chicken Breast Dinner	360	11	14
Santa Fe Grilled Chicken Salad	300	4	35
Spinach Chicken Salad, no dress.	370	10	19
Vegetables Stir-Fry, no rice	270	2.5	54
w. Grilled Chkn Breast, no rice	400	4	55

Fast - Foods & *Restaurants*

Swiss Chalet®cont... (Aug '07)

Sides

	C	F	Cb
Baked Potato	220	0	48
Flatbread, 1.6 oz	120	1.5	23
Butter, ½ oz	100	11	0
Coleslaw Ramekin	70	4	6
Corn Chips, 1 oz	140	7	6
French Fries, 6 oz	470	25	56
Gravy, 4 oz	40	1	7
Mashed Potatoes	120	5	21
Mushrooms, 6 oz	220	16	11
Rice Pilaf	280	3.5	57
Sour Cream & Chives, 1½ oz	70	5	3

Sandwiches: No Sides

Chicken Club Wrap	570	20	51
Chicken on Kaiser, white meat	440	8	31
Grilled Santa Fe Chicken	380	4	49
Messy Chicken, white meat	490	12	40

Salad Dressings: Light Italian, ½ oz

Salad Dressings: Light Italian, ½ oz	35	2	3
1000 Isle Dressing, ½ oz	55	4	2
Famous Chalet Sauce, 4 oz	30	1	5
French Dressing, ½ oz	65	6	2
Light Mayonnaise, ½ oz	45	5	1
Balsamic Vinaigrette, ½ oz	70	7	2

Dipping Sauce: Blue Cheese, ½ oz

Dipping Sauce: Blue Cheese, ½ oz	50	5	2
Cajun Sauce, 2 oz	100	9	3
Salsa, 1½ oz	20	0	4
Tangy Plum Sauce, 1 oz	50	0	13

Desserts: Apple Blossom

Desserts: Apple Blossom	490	25	62
Apple Pie	330	14	49
Carrot Cake	700	45	70
Chocolate Eruption Cheesecake	820	55	72
Coconut Cream	310	16	39
Colossal Caramel Fudge Chsecake	700	39	78
Cranberry, Raspberry Yogurt	120	2	23
Lemon Meringue Pie	280	9	47
Pecan Pie	530	28	63
Swiss Alps Choc Layer Cake	590	39	55

Ice Cream: Butter Pecan

Ice Cream: Butter Pecan	150	7	15
Chocolate	115	5	17
Vanilla	125	6	16
Sauce: Butterscotch	100	0	26
Chocolate	80	0	21
Strawberry	40	0	9

For Complete Nutritional Data ~ see CalorieKing.com

Taco Bell® (Aug '07)

Burritos

	C	F	Cb
7-Layer Burrito	490	18	65
Bean Burrito	350	9	54
Burrito Supreme Beef, avg	420	17	51
Chili Cheese Burrito	270	8	39
Fiesta Burrito Beef	370	13	49
Fiesta Burrito Chicken; Steak, avg.	330	8	48
Grilled Stuft Beef	680	30	76
Grilled Stuft Chicken; Steak, avg.	640	23	73

Tacos: Taco, regular/Crunchy

Tacos: Taco, regular/Crunchy	170	10	13
Taco Supreme	210	13	15
Double Decker Taco Supreme	370	17	40
Soft Taco Beef	200	9	21
Soft Taco Ranchero Chicken	270	14	21
Soft Taco Supreme Beef	250	13	23

Big Bell Value Menu: Per Serving

Burrito, ½ lb Cheesy Bean & Rice	470	20	58
Burrito, ½ lb Beef & Potato	530	23	66
Burrito, ½ lb Beef Combo	440	18	51
Burrito, Spicy Chicken	400	17	48
Caramel Apple Empanada	290	14	37
Cheesy Fiesta Potato	290	17	29
Double Decker Taco	320	13	38
Taco, Grande Soft	430	20	43
Taco, Spicy Chicken Soft	170	6	20

Gorditas: Gordita Baja Beef

Gorditas: Gordita Baja Beef	340	19	29
Gordita Baja Chicken; Steak	320	16	29
Gordita Supreme Beef	310	16	29
Gordita Supreme Chicken; Steak	290	12	28
Gordita Nacho Cheese Beef	300	14	31
Gordita Nacho Cheese Chkn; Steak	280	11	29

Chalupas: Chalupa Baja Beef

Chalupas: Chalupa Baja Beef	410	27	30
Chalupa Baja Chicken; Steak	390	23	29
Chalupa Supreme Beef	410	27	30
Chalupa Supreme Chicken	360	20	29
Chalupa Supreme Steak	360	21	29
Chalupa Nacho Cheese Beef	370	22	32
Chalupa Nacho Cheese Chkn; Steak	350	18	30

Fresco Style (Less Than 10g Fat)

Burritos: Bean	330	7	54
Fiesta Chicken	330	8	48
Supreme Chicken/Steak	330	8	49
Enchiritos: Beef	260	8	34
Chicken	240	5	32
Steak	230	6	32
Gordita Baja: Beef	250	10	29
Chicken; Steak, average	230	7	29
Tacos: Regular/Crunchy, average	150	8	13
Soft Taco Beef	180	7	21
Soft Beef Chicken/Steak	160	5	20
Tostada	200	6	27

Taco Bell® cont... (Aug '07)

	C	F	Cb
Nachos and Sides: Nachos, 3.5 oz	320	20	32
Nachos Supreme	460	26	42
Nachos BellGrande	790	44	79
Pintos 'n Cheese, 4.5 oz	180	7	20
Mexican Rice, 4.6 oz	200	9	26
Cinnamon Twists, 1.25 oz	160	5	27
Specialities			
Border Bowl: Zesty Chicken	730	40	69
w/out Dressing	490	16	64
Southwest Steak	690	28	79
Crunshwrap Supreme	560	24	70
Enchirito: Beef	380	18	35
Chicken; Steak, avg.	350	16	33
Express Taco Salad with Chips	630	34	58
Fiesta Taco Salad with Shell	860	46	82
without Shell	490	25	43
MexiMelt	290	16	23
Mexican Pizza, 7½ oz	540	31	47
Quesadilla: Chicken	540	30	40
Steak	490	28	39
Tostada	250	10	29
For Complete Nutritional Data ~ see CalorieKing.com			

Taco Cabana® (Aug '07)

Grilled Chicken: Per Serving			
¼ Chicken White, 5 oz	295	14	1
No Skin, 4 oz	170	3	0
¼ Chicken Dark, 4.5 oz	300	18	0.5
No Skin, 3.5 oz	170	7	1
Fajitas: Beef, 4 oz	245	12	4
Chicken White, 4 oz	190	6	3
Chicken Dark, 4 oz	235	11	2
Sides: Black Beans, 4 oz	110	0.5	21
Borracho Beans, 4 oz	110	2.5	17
Chips, 2 oz	290	14	36
Guacamole, 1 oz; Sour Cream, 1 oz	50	4	2
Queso, 3 oz	185	12	7
Refried Beans, 4 oz	170	6	21
Salsa, all types, 1 oz	10	0	2
Spanish Rice, 4 oz	180	5	30
Tortillas: 6" Flour	130	3.5	22
6" Table Corn	60	1	11
Tortilla Soup: Small, 8.5 oz	250	8.5	21
Large, 19 oz	375	13	32
Tacos: Bean & Cheese	290	12	35
Black Bean	215	5	37
Carne Guisada	200	8	20
Crispy Beef	150	7	13
Soft Chicken	220	9	21

Taco Cabana® cont...

	C	F	Cb
Burritos			
Bean & Cheese	710	27	85
Beef/Chicken, average	660	25	75
Black Bean	560	11	95
Breakfast Tacos: Barbacoa	310	15	2
Chorizo & Egg	250	12	22

Taco John's® (Aug '07)

	C	F	Cb
Burritos: Bean Burrito	380	10	53
Bean Burrito, no Cheese	320	7	53
Beefy Burrito	430	20	41
Chicken & Potato Burrito	460	20	54
Combination Burrito	400	15	47
Crunchy Chicken & Potato Burrito	590	30	62
Meat & Potato	490	20	55
Super Burrito	450	20	49
Grilled Burrito: Steak	600	35	46
Beef; Chicken, avg.	590	30	48
Tacos: Bravo	340	15	39
Crispy Taco	180	10	13
Softshell Taco	220	10	21
Softshell Taco, Steak	190	10	19
Softshell Taco, Chicken	190	5	19
Taco Burger w. Cheese	280	10	28
Regional Menu Items			
Burrito: Ranch Beef	420	22	41
Ranch Chicken	390	18	40
Smothered	505	21	55
Chili Enchilada	315	16	24
Mexi Rolls w. Nacho Cheese (6)	470	21	47
Potato Oles, Chili Cheese	610	36	59
Specialties: Cheese Quesadilla	480	30	39
Chicken Taco Salad, no Dressing	540	30	44
Chicken Festiva Salad, no Dressing	400	25	24
Potato Oles Bravo	530	35	50
Potato Oles Super	1060	70	91
Super Nachos	830	50	73
Super Nachos Chicken	780	45	62
Taco Salad, no Dressing	580	30	46
Sides: Mexican Rice	250	5	45
Nachos	380	20	38
Potato Oles, medium	620	35	67
Refried Beans	395	15	50
Desserts: Apple Grande	240	10	41
Choco Taco	385	20	48
Churro	235	11	31
For Complete Nutritional Data ~ see CalorieKing.com			

Taco Mayo® (Aug '07)

Burritos	C	F	Cb
Bean	495	16	71
Beef	490	23	41
Chicken Supreme	405	16	39
Combo	495	20	56
Super Burrito	540	24	58
Quesadillas			
Cheese	590	35	45
Chicken	670	37	46
Fajita Chicken	700	39	47
Fajita Steak	725	41	47
Tacos			
Crispy Taco	160	10	10
Soft: Beef Taco	230	11	17
Chicken Taco	185	6	16
Tostada	295	13	37
Tostada Melt	525	32	35
Salads			
Acapulco Chicken Salad	760	55	39
Taco Salad	705	38	57
Taco Chicken Salad	440	23	30
Taco Steak Salad	445	25	30
Sides			
Mexicali Rice	160	1	36

Target Food Court (Aug '07)

	C	F	Cb
Breakfast: Pancakes (3) + Syrup	490	4	104
Breakfast Sandwich w. Bacon	380	20	29
Cinnamon Swirl French Toast, 2 slices	230	5	36
Pretzels (Cinnabon): Cinnamon, 5¾ oz	550	9	105
Mega Cinnamon, 6½ oz	650	15	115
Salted Pretzel, 5½ oz	435	3.5	89
Meals: Bowl of Chili, 9 oz cup	300	10	32
Chicken Breast Sandwich, 4 oz	280	9	31
Chicken Tenders, 5 strips, 3 oz	280	19	14
Hot Dog Meal: w. Chips & Soda	570	22	84
w. Apple Sauce & Soda	520	12	93
Hot Dog: Plain, 3½oz	260	12	28
All Beef Meat, 5 oz	350	20	38
Cheddar, 4 oz	310	16	30
Macaroni & Cheese: 8 oz	340	13	41
w. Apple Sauce & Soda Meal	600	13	106
w. Chips & Soda, Meal	650	23	97
Mini Pizza (6"), 5½ oz	360	14	42
Nachos w. Cheese, 40 chips, 4 oz	1100	59	132
Spaghetti O's Meal: w. Chips & Soda	490	11	93
w. Apple Sauce & Soda	440	1	102

For Complete Nutritional Data ~ see CalorieKing.com

Taco Time® (Aug '07)

Burritos	C	F	Cb
Beef, Bean & Cheese	615	23	66
Big Juan Beef Burrito	640	25	71
Big Juan Chicken Burrito	620	24	69
Casita Burrito, Beef	645	31	54
Chicken & Black Bean	400	18	45
Chicken BLT	580	39	38
Crisp Burrito: Bean	425	18	53
Meat	550	30	39
Chicken	420	25	32
Soft Bean Burrito	380	10	58
Soft Meat Burrito	490	21	48
Veggie Burrito	490	16	70
Tacos			
Crisp Taco	295	17	16
½ lb Chicken Soft Taco	385	16	41
½ lb Soft Taco	510	23	46
Soft Taco	315	15	23
Super Soft Taco	510	23	50
Specialties			
Cheddar Fries, Medium, 7 oz	505	35	40
Cheddar Melt	205	11	17
Mexi Fries®, Medium, 6 oz	390	25	40
Mexi-Rice, 4 oz	160	2	30
Nachos: Regular, 10.5 oz	680	38	61
Deluxe, 15.25 oz	1050	57	91
Stuffed Fries, Medium, 6.2 oz	640	44	50
Refritos, 7 oz	325	10	44
Taco Cheeseburger	635	36	48
Salads: Per Serving			
Chicken Fiesta, 12 oz	390	19	35
Chicken Taco	370	21	27
Taco Salad, regular	480	28	30
Tostada Salad	630	33	48
Sauces & Dressings: Per 1 oz			
Green Sauce	10	0	2
Original Hot Sauce	10	0	2
Salsa Fresca	65	0	16
1000 Island Dressing	120	12	3
Desserts: Cinnamon Crustos	375	15	47
Fruit Filled Empanadas	250	9	37

For Complete Nutritional Data ~ see CalorieKing.com

Tacone® (Aug '07)

Gourmet Wrapped Sandwiches	C	F	Cb
Campfire, ½ wrap	340	12	41
Malibu Melt, ½ wrap	360	17	25
Pilgrim, ½ wrap	260	14	21
Thai Cone, ½ wrap	300	9	35

For Complete Nutritional Data ~ see CalorieKing.com

Restaurants & Fast - Foods

TCBY® (Aug '07)

	C	F	Cb
Soft Serve Frozen Yogurt: Average all Flavors			
96% Fat-Free: Kids Cup	110	2	18
Junior Cup	200	4	33
Small Cup	290	6	47
Regular Cup	370	8	60
Large Cup	450	10	74
Non-Fat: Junior Cup	160	0	33
Small Cup	220	0	46
Regular Cup	290	0	60
Large Cup	350	0	73
No Sugar Added/Non-Fat: Small	190	0	41
Regular Cup	240	0	53
Large Cup	290	0	65
Low-Carb Lovers: Small	170	10	25
Regular	300	18	45
Large Cup	360	22	56
Waffle Cones: Kids	70	1	15
Regular	110	2	22
Hand Scooped Frozen Yogurt: Average all Flavors			
Kids Cup	90	3	14
Junior Cup	140	5	22
Small Cup	180	6	28
Regular Cup	280	10	44
Large Cup	370	13	58
No Added Sugar, Vanilla:			
Small Cup	100	1	24
Regular Cup	160	1	38
Large Cup	210	1.5	50
Fruithead Smoothies: Per 20 fl.oz Cup			
A Lotta Colada: no Yogurt	380	12	69
w. Yogurt	550	17	99
Berry Slim: no Yogurt	300	0	75
w. Yogurt	410	3	95
Healthy Balance: no Yogurt	300	0	75
w. Yogurt	410	3	95
Holy-Cal: no Yogurt	360	0	94
w. Yogurt	470	3	114
Peachy Lean: no Yogurt	360	0	96
w. Yogurt	470	3	116
Raspberry DeLITE: no Yogurt	240	0	59
w. Yogurt	360	3	85
Raspberry Revitalizer: no Yogurt	300	0	79
w. Yogurt	370	3	84
Tropical Replenisher: no Yogurt	240	0	61
w. Yogurt	370	3	87
Workout Whey: no Yogurt	340	0	92
w. Yogurt	460	3	112

TCBY® cont... (Aug '07)

	C	F	Cb
Sorbet: Average all Flavors			
Kids Cup	80	0	19
Junior Cup	150	0	35
Small Cup	200	0	49
Regular Cup	260	0	63
Large Cup	320	0	17
Frappe Chillers: Per 16 fl.oz Cup			
Caramel de Leche	240	9	32
Coffee	190	7	25
French Vanilla	200	9	23
Frozen Hot chocolate	230	9	32
Mocha	240	9	31

Teriyaki Stix® (Aug '07)

	C	F	Cb
Bowls: Beef Bowl	620	7	102
Chicken Bowl; Hot & Spicy	730	15	101
Chicken Curry	680	17	92
Teriyaki Chicken Salad	360	13	26
Teriyaki Special	740	13	111
Veggie Bowl	440	1	99
Yakisoba	360	4.5	56

The Taco Maker® (Aug '07)

	C	F	Cb
Burritos			
Bean	295	9	43
Beef	445	16	44
Chicken	375	12	44
Crisp Bean; Crisp Beef, avg.	420	27	30
Enchiladas: Beef	375	20	22
Cheese	595	38	25
Chicken	320	13	21
Nachos: Cheese	605	35	49
Chips 'n Beans	290	16	32
Macho Nacho w. Beef	815	50	57
Macho Nacho w. Guacamole	845	55	62
Salad: Chicken Fiesta	625	35	38
Taco	685	42	39
Tacos: Crisp	185	9	16
Crisp Super	310	15	24
Soft	180	6.5	20
Soft Super	390	15	43
Tater Gem Fries, Regular	485	30	48

Tim Hortons® (Aug '07)

Sandwiches

	C	F	Cb
Tim's Own: Chicken Salad	380	9	55
Garden Vegetable w. Dressing	400	14	57
Ham & Swiss w. Tim's Own Dress.	440	12	56
Turkey Bacon Club w. Mustard	440	8	63
Turkey Breast w. Tim's Own Dress.	390	5	59

Soup: Per Bowl (10 oz)

Beef Stew	235	8	25
Chili	300	16	18
Cream of Broccoli	190	5	31
Creamy Field Mushroom	170	7	25
Hearty Vegetable	70	0	14
Minestrone	120	3	24
Tim's Own, Chicken Noodle	120	2	18
Tomato Florentine	95	2	18
Turkey Rice	120	1.5	21

Cookies

Chocolate Chip	150	7	21
M&M w. Chocolate Chips	160	7	22
Oatmeal Raisin	150	6	22
Peanut Butter	160	9	18
Peanut Butter Chocolate Chunk	170	10	19

Donuts: Per Donut

Cake: Chocolate Glazed	260	10	39
Old Fashion Plain	260	19	20
Sour Cream Plain	270	17	27
Filled: Blueberry	230	8	36
Boston Cream	250	9	38
Canadian Maple	260	9	41
Strawberry	230	8	36
Honey Cruller	320	19	37
Yeast: Apple Fritter	300	11	49
Other varieties, avg.	210	8	30

Baked Goods: Per Serving

Croissant: Butter	340	18	38
Cheese	370	20	37
Tea Biscuit: Plain, 3 oz	250	9	35
Raisin, 3 oz	290	10	45
Cinnamon Roll: Frosted	470	25	57
Glazed	420	23	50
Danish: Cherry Cheese	330	13	46
Chocolate	430	24	51
Maple Pecan	380	20	46

Bagels: Plain

Plain	260	1.5	52
Blueberry Cinnamon Raisin	270	1	55
Everything	280	2	53
Onion	260	1.5	53
Sundried Tomato	310	3.5	59

Tim Hortons® Cont... (Aug '07)

Muffins: Per Muffin

	C	F	Cb
Blueberry Bran	340	10	56
Cranberry Fruit	360	11	60
Chocolate Chip Plain	430	14	71
Fruit Explosion	350	10	61
Raisin Bran	380	9	67
Strawberry Sensation	370	11	62
Wheat Carrot	400	19	55
Low-Fat varieties	290	2.5	62

Timbits, Low-Fat

Cake: Chocolate Glazed	70	2.5	10
Old Fashion Plain	70	5	5
Filled, all varieties	60	2	10
Yeast: Apple Fritter	50	1.5	9
Honey Dip	60	5	9

Desserts

Yogurt: Strawberry w. Berries	150	2.5	28
Creamy Vanilla w. Berries	160	2.5	32

Beverages: Per Serving

Cafe Mocha, 10 fl.oz	170	7	27
Cappuccino: Eng. Toffee, 10 fl.oz	220	6	40
French Vanilla, 10 fl.oz	240	7	39
Iced w. 2% Milk, 12 fl.oz	300	15	41
Coffee w. sugar/cream, 10 fl.oz	75	3.5	9
Hot Chocolate, 10 fl.oz	240	6	45
Iced Tea, 12 fl.oz	50	1	10

T.J. Cinnamons® (Aug '07)

Bakery

Chocolate Twist, 2½ oz	250	12	34
Cinnachips			
50/50 blend of Pecan Chips, 10 oz	1130	50	157
Cinnamon Twist, 1 roll, 2½ oz	260	14	33
T.J. Icing, 1 oz	120	5	18
Original Roll: no icing, 5.3 oz	510	10	73
w. Cream Cheese Icing	650	17	95
Pecan Sticky Bun, 1 bun, 6½ oz	690	22	91

Beverages: Per Serving (12 fl.oz)

Coffee	0	0	0
Mocha Chill: no Whipped Cream	260	4	46
w. Whipped Cream	310	7	49

For Extra Menu Items + Full Nutritional Data
~ See Author's Website
www.CalorieKing.com

Updated Nutrition Data ~ www.CalorieKing.com
Persons with Diabetes ~ See Disclaimer (Page 24)

Restaurants & Fast - Foods

Togo's Eatery® (Aug '07)

Sandwiches: Regular 6" Roll

	C	**F**	**Cb**
Albacore Tuna	450	10	69
Avocado & Cucumber	590	26	79
Avocado & Turkey	670	27	78
Black Forest Ham & Cheese	630	24	67
Cheese Sandwich	660	30	70
Chunky Chicken & Almond Salad	750	43	64
Cold Roast Beef	680	22	68
Egg Salad & Cheese	650	28	69
Hummus	790	31	104
Salami & Cheese	760	37	70
The Italian	740	37	68
Turkey & Bacon Club	600	21	65
Turkey & Cheese	600	18	71
Turkey Ham & Cheese	600	19	70
Turkey Roast Beef & Cheese	670	23	70
BBQ Beef	530	13	64
California Roasted Chicken	620	15	68
French Onion Dip	640	16	66
Hot Pastrami	810	42	72
Meatballs in Zesty Tomato Sauce	690	23	80
Pastrami Reubin	650	25	68
Roast Beef	680	22	68
Savory BBQ Chicken	520	6	79
Sicilian Chicken	670	22	73

Large Size: Add 50% to Regular Size

Topz® (Aug '07)

Sandwiches & Burgers

½ lb Black Angus Burger: w. sauce	735	40	40
no sauce	670	34	37
¼ lb Black Angus Chili Burger	490	21	42
¼ lb Black Angus Burger: w. sauce	505	25	40
no sauce	445	19	37
Gardenburger	355	12	46
Grilled Chicken Breast Burger	395	10	39
Turkey Burger	450	19	40
Sandwiches: Classic Grilled Cheese	415	18	47
Ginger Grilled Ahi	385	11	37
Grilled Cheese & Tomato	420	18	48

Sides

Aero Fries, 5.6 oz	380	14	58
Aero Onion Rings, 5.8 oz	300	11	46
Chili Cheese Fries 10.6 oz	590	27	66
Signature Chili, 10.2 oz	330	17	17

Tropical Smoothie Cafe (Aug '07)

Sandwiches	**C**	**F**	**Cb**
American Albacore	725	30	86
Cheese BLT	715	37	72
Chicken Caesar	625	25	66
Chipolte Chicken	660	27	71
Club Sandwich	705	26	77
Ham & Cheese	605	19	78
Roast Beef	680	30	63
The Italian	750	39	71
Turkey Bacon Ranch	670	23	69
Tuscan Turkey	440	13	67
Wraps: Breakfast Wrap (Bacon)	535	23	55
Breakfast Wraps (Ham)	525	18	57
Buffalo Chicken	565	21	61
Cool Tuna Wrap	645	27	71
King Caesar	555	27	55
Sesame Chicken	755	24	103
Totally Turkey	655	27	58
Veggie Veggie	615	26	72
Western Wrap	535	18	59

Salads: No Cheese or Dressing

Chef Salad	170	2	12
Garden Classic Salad	60	0.5	10
Sesame Chicken Salad	415	10	54
Thai Chicken Salad	355	4	54

Low Fat Smoothies (with Turbinado)

Blimey Limey; Cool Breeze, avg.	410	0	102
Blue Lagoon	330	1	80
Hawaiian Breeze	360	0	88
Island Fever; Orange Passion, avg.	455	0.5	111
Rockin Raspberry	515	0.5	125
Strawberry Beach	450	0	109
Sunrise Sunset	390	0.5	96
Fat Buster	375	0.5	91
Health Nut	620	10	104
Lean Machine; Paradise Point, avg.	475	0.5	115
Muscle Blaster	595	3	119
Peanut Paradise	810	22	119

Dessert Smoothies (with Turbinado)

Beach Bum, avg. all flavors	570	5.5	126
Chocolate Chiller	555	7	118
Coconut Royale	730	11	155
Mocha Madness	645	12	127
Peanut Butter Cup	840	24	142

With Splenda, deduct 200 calories & 50g carbs

Tubby's® (Aug '07)

Subs: Per Regular Sandwich

		C	F	Cb
Burger Subs: Big Tub	670	56	55
Burger Special	900	59	59
Cheeseburger	910	60	59
Pizza Burger	930	47	62
Taco Burger	825	47	67
Deli Style Subs: Ham & Cheese	570	30	54
Club Sub	700	41	53
Tubby's Famous	665	39	55
Turkey & Cheese	600	32	51
Turkey Club Sub	680	38	52
Specialty Subs: BLT	635	42	50
Cold Veggie	460	14	66
Italian Sausage	730	45	56
Tuna Salad	415	18	47
Veggie Stir Fry	650	27	90
Chicken Subs: Per Regular Sandwich			
Chicken & Broccoli	550	23	56
Chicken & Cheddar	545	23	54
Chicken Club Sub	705	41	53
Chicken Fajita Sub	445	12	57
Grilled Chicken	345	5	52
Steak Subs: Per Regular Sandwich			
Mushroom Steak	835	26	52
Pepper Steak	710	46	52
Pizza Steak	985	57	85
Steak & Cheese	825	56	51
Steak Special	745	46	58

Una Mas® (Aug '07)

Burritos

		C	F	Cb
Bean & Cheese	925	44	85
Fresca	580	12	99
Gallito Griller	1025	57	62
Grilled Fajita Burrito: Chicken	765	31	87
Steak	850	36	88
Pineapple Thai	660	19	87
San Lucas Fish, Baja Style	425	26	34
San Lucas Fish, Cabo Style	320	19	26
Tacos: Chicken Taco	250	7.5	33
Crispy Chicken Taco Plate	330	17	30
Steak Taco	280	9	33
Veggie Taco	235	6.5	37
Nachos, 1 serving, 24 oz	1850	102	188
Quesadillas			
Monterey Chicken	960	57	61
Monterey Steak	1040	61	61

Uno Chicago Grill® (Aug '07)

Entrees

		C	F	Cb
Veggie Burger, no sides	500	11	71
Chicken Parmesan, no sides	940	21	140
Chicken Spinoccoli	1550	80	117
Flatbread Pizza: Individual			
Four Cheese	1570	56	93
Spinach, Mushroom & Gorgonzola	930	40	93
Soup: French Onion Bowl, 13 oz	230	12	19
Veggie Bowl, 12 oz	110	1.5	25
Salads: House, no dressing	120	1	25
Caesar w. dressing	430	35	21
Greek Salad, w. dressing	430	40	17
Honey Crisp Chicken w. dressing	760	38	65

For Complete Nutritional Data ~ see CalorieKing.com

Wahoo's Fish Taco® (Aug '07)

Bowls

		C	F	Cb
Carne Asada, Steak	760	22	90
Chicken, Skinless Breast	750	18	90
Fish of the Day	705	16	90
Classic Burrito (A la Carte)			
Fish, average	455	14	51
Chicken, average	545	17	50
Carne Asada	515	20	49
Carnitas	595	26	49
Shrimp	470	14	51
Veggie	600	14	98
Mushroom	415	14	57
Tacos: Carne Asada, Steak	195	7	18
Carnitas, Pork	230	10	18
Chicken, Skinless Breast	210	6	18
Fish of the Day	175	4	19
Veggie	200	4	33
Sides: Beans	445	2	80
Rice	475	6	94
Salads: Chips Not Included			
Carne Asada, Steak	555	33	13
Chicken, average	560	28	15
Fish, average	420	23	15

For Complete Nutritional Data ~ see CalorieKing.com

Restaurants & Fast - Foods

WAWA® (Aug '07)

Breakfast & Baked Goods

	C	F	Cb
Bagel: Plain	285	1	61
w. Butter	505	23	64
w. Cream Cheese	430	13	67
Bagel Melts: Ham & Cheese	495	13	67
Pepperoni & Cheese	750	38	67
Pork Roll & Cheese	580	23	68
Breakfast Bowls: *Per Bowl*			
Creamed Chipped Beef on a Bisc.	475	25	54
Sausage Gravy on a Biscuit	515	29	53
Croissant, Regular, 2 oz	190	9	24
Hash Brown (1), 1.7 oz	90	5	10
Muffins: Banana Walnut, 6 oz	605	36	71
Blueberry, 6.2 oz	620	34	76
Chocolate Chip, 4 oz	680	36	83
Corn, 6 oz	650	31	83
Sizzli Bagels: Bacon Egg & Chse	460	19	53
Sausage Egg & Cheese	560	29	54
Sizzli Biscuits: Bacon Egg & Chse	535	34	45
Sausage Egg & Cheese	640	44	46
Sizzli Muffins: Bacon Egg & Chse	360	20	29
Sausage, Egg & Cheese	460	29	30

Hot Sandwiches: *No Cheese Unless Indicated*

	C	F	Cb
Chicken Breaded Club w. Cheese	710	36	56
Chicken Caesar w. Cheese	455	12	49
Roasted Pork Kaiser	395	15	38
Classics: Roasted Pork w. Cheese	760	33	66
Meatball w. Cheese	1005	55	81
Roast Beef w. Cheese	645	21	67

Cold Sandwiches: *No Cheese Unless Indicated*

	C	F	Cb
Chicken	465	6	64
Ham	265	6	28
Italian w. Pesto & Rstd Peppers	725	32	67
Roast Beef	400	7	35
Roast Beef Classic	595	10	62
Roast Beef on White	330	6	26
Turkey Carolina Honey Smoked	235	4	32
Turkey on White	415	6	67
Seafood Salad	455	22	53
Tuna Salad	575	36	45
Veggie	330	3	62

WAWA® cont... (Aug '07)

	C	F	Cb
Cold Shortis: American	435	18	40
BLT; Cheese, average	495	28	37
Chicken Salad	505	28	42
Egg Salad w. Cheese	630	41	43
Turkey	295	5	43
Hot Shortis: Chicken Steak	315	7	36
Meatball w. Cheese	640	37	49
Roast Beef w. Cheese	400	14	40
Wraps: Buffalo Blue Chicken	260	4	37
Roast Beef & Pepper Jack	410	16	38
Roasted Chicken Caesar	295	5	39
Smoked Turkey Supreme	305	10	42
Turkey Bacon & Colby Jack	440	22	35
Hot Dogs: ¼ lb Beef Frank	385	28	23
All Beef Hot Dog	250	15	22
Big Bacon Cheese Dog	710	50	39
Hot Sausage	310	20	21
Kielbasa	290	17	21
Bowls: *Per Bowl*			
Chili, 15 oz	535	13	86
Roast Beef, 12 oz	465	27	39
Meatballs, 11 oz	565	20	76
Roasted Pork, 12 oz	545	35	38
Sides: *Per Medium*			
Beef Stew, 11 oz	265	12	22
Chili, 11 oz	220	8	28
Homestyle Chkn & Noodles, 11 oz	325	16	25
Macaroni & Beef, 11 oz	335	12	41
Macaroni & Cheese, 11 oz	460	22	50
Mashed Potatoes, 11 oz	470	31	47
Meatballs in a Cup, 4 oz	365	27	14
Soups: *Per Medium (11 oz)*			
Boston Clam Chowder	295	15	26
Chicken Corn Chowder	360	24	29
Cream of Broccoli	255	16	21
Vegetable Beef & Barley	150	5	19
Drinks: Cappuccino, 12 fl.oz	175	7	27
French Vanilla Cappuccino, 12 fl.oz	220	7	30
Low-Fat Cappuccino, 12 fl.oz	240	1	52
Mocha Alert, 12 fl.oz	195	7	34

Wendy's® (Aug '07)

Sandwiches	C	F	Cb
Baconator Burger	830	51	35
Jr Bacon Cheeseburger	370	18	34
¼ lb Double Stack	420	20	34
¼ lb Deluxe Double Stack	470	24	35
¼ lb Single Burger	430	20	37
Chicken Temptations: Ultimate	320	7	36
Spicy Chicken Fillet	440	16	46
Homestyle Fillet	430	16	48
French Fries: Small, 4 oz	330	16	43
Medium, 5 oz	415	20	54
Large, 6.5 oz	540	26	69
Kids, 2.5 oz	210	10	27
Chicken: Crispy Nuggets, 5 pce	230	15	12
Sauce: Barbecue Honey	45	0	10
Spicy Hawaiian	70	0	17
Garden Sensations Salads			
Caesar Side Salad, no dress./topping	80	4.5	6
Caesar Chicken: no dress./topping	180	6	8
w. Dressing/Croutons	530	32	34
Chicken BLT Salad: no dress./topping	330	18	11
w. Croutons/Dressing	650	44	30
Cranberry Pecan Chicken: no dress.	260	6	30
w. Berry Balsamic Vinaigrette	350	10	42
Mandarin Chicken: no dress./topping	170	2.5	16
w. Dressing/Nuts/Noodles	520	25	49
Side Salad, no Dressing	35	0	8
Southwest Taco: no dress./topping	430	22	30
w. Chips/Sour Cream/Dressing	680	39	49
Kids Meal: Hamburger only	280	9	34
Cheeseburger only	320	12	34
Crispy Nuggets, 4 pces, no sauce	185	12	10
Baked Potatoes: Plain, 10 oz	270	0	61
Bacon & Cheese	440	12	75
Broccoli & Cheese	330	2	66
Sour Cream & Chives	320	4	63
Plain w. Buttery Spread	320	6	61
Sides: Chili, small, 8 oz	220	6	24
Chili, large, 12 oz	330	9	35
Cheddar Cheese, shredded, 2 Tbsp	70	6	1
Hot Chili Seasoning, 1 pkg	5	0	2
Mandarin Orange Cup, 5 oz	80	0	19
Saltine Crackers (2)	25	0.5	4
Yogurt w. Granola Cup, 5.7 oz	250	6	42
Chocolate Chip Cookie, 2 oz	270	12	37
Frosty: Original Chocolate, 4 oz	170	4	29

For Complete Nutritional Data ~ see CalorieKing.com

Western Sizzlin® (Aug '07)

Steaks (Meat Only, Raw Wts)	C	F	Cb
New York Strip, 14 oz	900	60	0
Ribeye, 10 oz	520	28	0
Sirloin: 8 oz Steak	540	33	0
16 oz Steak	1080	66	0
T-Bone, 20 oz	1230	99	0
Baked Potato, plain, 8 oz	245	0	58

Wienerschnitzel® (Aug '07)

Breakfast	C	F	Cb
Biscuit: w. Bacon	330	17	35
Egg & Bacon	390	21	36
Egg, Bacon & Cheese	440	25	36
Egg, Sausage & Cheese	540	34	40
Burrito: Egg, Bacon & Cheese	490	25	39
Chili Cheese	470	21	43
Country Breakfast, 10.1 oz	640	40	47
French Toast Sticks	490	29	49
Hash Browns, 2.8 oz	290	25	14
Platter w. Bacon	600	40	40
Burgers: Chili Cheeseburger	350	13	32
Deluxe Cheeseburger	450	23	33
Deluxe Hamburger	400	19	33
Double Chili Cheeseburger	560	24	35
Fries: Regular, 4.6 oz	340	25	28
Large, 6.4 oz	470	34	39
Chili Cheese, 8.1 oz	540	38	39
Hot Dogs: Chili Dog	290	13	31
Chili Cheese Dog	340	17	31
Deluxe; Kraut; Mustard; Relish, avg.	270	12	30
All Beef: Chili Dog	380	21	33
Chili Cheese Dog	430	25	33
Other varieties, avg.	365	20	31
Turkey: Chili Dog	270	11	31
Chili Cheese Dog	320	15	31
Other varieties, average	250	10	28
For Pretzel Bun add extra	145	3	26
Sandwiches: Bacon Ranch Chkn	430	21	37
Italian Sausage	350	17	29
Pastrami	580	35	38
Polish Sausage	490	29	39
Sides: Onion Straws, 3.4 oz	430	35	25
Ranch Dressing, 1.2 oz	120	12	2
Desserts: Freezee, average	630	25	100
Banana Split	820	24	149
Chocolate Dipped Cone, 6 oz	490	29	57
Plain Cone, 6 oz	300	11	49

Whataburger® (Aug '07)

Burgers/Sandwiches	C	F	Cb
Justaburger	310	16	30
Whataburger: Burger	620	32	61
No Bun	265	19	8
w. Bacon & Cheese	775	44	62
w. Bacon & Cheese, no bun	425	31	9
w. Cheese, no bun	355	26	9
Whataburger Jr.	320	16	32
Double Meat Whataburger	850	49	61
Triple Meat Whataburger	1070	67	61
Grilled Chicken: Sandwich	460	18	45
no bun	250	12	13
Honey BBQ Chicken Strip S'wich	1110	60	102
Whatacatch Sandwich	490	30	42
Whatachick'n Sandwich	510	19	59
Sides:			
French Fries: Small, 3 oz	260	13	31
Medium, 4½ oz	400	20	47
Large, 6 oz	530	27	63
Onion Rings: Medium, 4.3 oz	420	27	37
sLarge, 6.4 oz	630	40	55
Chicken & Salads			
Chicken Strips (2)	390	25	23
Chicken Strips Salad	580	39	35
w. Cheddar Cheese, no Bacon	600	39	32
Garden Salad	60	0	12
w. Cheddar Cheese, no Bacon	220	15	11
Grilled Chicken Salad	230	7	19
w. Cheddar Cheese, no Bacon	400	22	19
Dressings: Per 2 oz Package			
Buttermilk Ranch	310	33	3
Caesar	190	19	3
Thousand Island	150	13	10
Reduced-Fat Ranch	230	22	6
Low-Fat Vinaigrette	40	1.5	5
Shakes			
Chocolate; Strawb. Med., 27 fl.oz	1075	30	186
Small, 17 fl.oz	670	19	116
Vanilla, Medium, 27 fl.oz	965	29	152
Small, 17 fl.oz	605	18	95
Breakfast			
Cinnamon Roll, roll, 128g	400	7	80
Hash Brown Sticks (4), 65g	200	12	20
Texas Toast, 1 slice	180	8	25

Whataburger® cont... (Aug '07)

Breakfast (Cont)	C	F	Cb
Biscuit: Plain	300	17	32
w. Bacon	350	20	32
w. Gravy	510	35	49
w. Sausage	540	38	32
Honey Butter Chicken	600	38	51
Biscuit Sandwich: w. Egg & Chse	460	29	33
w. Bacon, Egg & Cheese	510	32	33
w. Sausage, Egg & Cheese	700	50	33
Breakfast On A Bun: w. Bacon	400	22	29
w. Sausage	590	40	29
Breakfast Platter (Biscuit/Eggs/Hash Brown):			
w. Bacon	740	45	53
w. Sausage	930	63	53
Pancakes: Plain (3)	580	8	112
w. Bacon	630	12	112
w. Sausage	820	29	112
Taquito: w. Bacon & Egg	380	21	27
w. Bacon, Egg & Cheese	430	25	27
w. Potato & Egg	430	23	37
w. Potato, Egg & Cheese	480	27	37
w. Sausage & Egg	410	24	27
w. Sausage, Egg & Cheese	460	28	27
Desserts: Hot Apple Pie	230	11	29
Chocolate Chunk Cookie	230	11	33
White Choc. Macadamia Cookie	250	14	30

Winchell's® (Aug '07)

Baked Products	C	F	Cb
Croissant	260	17	28
Cake Donuts: Chocolate Iced	230	15	28
Traditional Cake	215	14	26
Yeast Raised Donuts: Per Donut			
Chocolate Bar	240	16	29
Chocolate Round/Twist	240	16	29
Glazed Round/Twist	230	15	27

White Castle® (Aug '07)

Beverages: Per Medium (20 oz) Unless Indicated	C	F	Cb
Barq's Red Cream Soda	250	0	70
Coca-Cola, Classic/Cherry, avg.	230	0	61
Hot Chocolate, medium, 12 fl.oz	140	4	26
Iced Tea	170	0	46
Icee, all varieties	145	0	42
Orange Juice, 6 fl.oz	80	0	20
Choc./Strawberry Shake, avg.	400	4	82

White Castle® Cont... (Aug '07)

Sandwiches & Burgers

	C	F	Cb
Bacon Cheeseburger	200	12	13
Cheeseburger	160	9	13
Chicken Supreme	230	10	22
Double Bacon Cheeseburger	360	23	19
Double Cheeseburger	290	18	19
Double Jalapeno Cheeseburger	320	20	20
Double White Castle	250	14	19
Fish w. Cheese Sandwich	180	8	18
Jalapeno Cheeseburger	170	10	13
Chicken Breast w. Cheese Sandwich	210	8	21
Chicken Ring Sandwich w. Cheese	190	10	17
Surf & Turf Sandwich	390	22	27
White Castle Burger	140	7	13

Sides:

	C	F	Cb
Chicken Rings, 6 rings	340	23	15
Clam Strips, 4 oz	250	22	5
Fish Nibblers, 14 pieces	280	16	21
French Fries, 3.8 oz	310	15	39
Mozzarella Cheese Sticks, 3 sticks	250	14	22
Onion Rings, 13 rings	750	39	91

Sauces:

	C	F	Cb
Cheese Sauce, 1½ oz	130	10	6
Honey Mustard Fat-Free, 1 oz	50	0	13
Horseradish Mustard, 5.5g pkg	5	0	0
Marinara Sauce, 1 oz	15	0	3
Nacho Cheese Sauce, 1.6 oz	50	4	3
White Castle Zesty Zing, 1 oz	120	11	4

Yoshinoya® (Aug '07)

Bowls

	C	F	Cb
Beef Bowl: Regular	840	30	109
Large	1160	41	153
Chicken Bowl: Regular	760	15	125
Large	1110	22	180
Combo Bowl: Regular	750	19	117
Large	1220	36	171
Shrimp & Beef Bowl, Regular	1280	44	184
Kids Meal Bowl	340	11	48
Vegetable Beef Bowl: Regular	770	23	114
Large	1090	32	163
Vegetable Bowl: Regular	530	3.5	116
Large	780	5	169

Side Orders:

	C	F	Cb
Beef	370	28	6
Chicken & Vegetables	300	12	21
Rice	460	2.5	104
Vegetables	60	0.5	12

Desserts:

	C	F	Cb
Cheesecake	280	15	31
Chocolate Cake	330	17	44
Flan	230	7	35
Strawberry Shortcake	290	15	37

Note: Yoshinoya Beef Bowl Restaurants are based in California.

Zoup!® (Aug '07)

Soups: Per Cup (8 fl.oz)

	C	F	Cb
Chicken Potpie	200	8	21
Cream of Broccoli	160	11	12
Fire Roasted Tomato Bisque	290	22	22
Ginger Butternut Squash	240	15	28
Jamaican Bay Gumbo	120	2.5	20
New England Clam Chowder	200	5	22
Seafood Bisque	150	6	12
Tomato Spinach/Rice; Tom. Chili, avg.	100	3	19
Vegetable Bounty	90	1.5	33
Vegetarian Split Pea	140	1.5	25
White Chkn Chili; Chkn Chowder, avg.	160	3	23
Other varieties, average	140	7	17

Paninis:

	C	F	Cb
Turkey Club, ½ sandwich	470	28	22
Italian Chicken, ½ sandwich	370	21	23
Smoked Ham and Swiss, ½ s'wich	190	8	18

Bread: Per Piece (2 oz)

	C	F	Cb
Extra Low-Carb French, 2 oz	105	2	7
Extra Multigrain, 2 oz	190	4	30
Extra Sourdough, 2 oz	170	1.5	31

Zero's Subs® (Aug '07)

Oven Baked Subs (6")
(Includes cheese, lettuce, tomato, onions, oil & vinegar)

	C	F	Cb
BLT	410	19	48
BLT, no Mayo	330	12	43
Cosmo Vegetarian	470	23	46
Cosmo Deluxe	490	25	48
Grinder	560	31	48
Grinder, Multigrain	560	32	50
Ham & Cheese	440	19	44
Meatball & Cheese	565	30	50
without Cheese	465	22	50
Pepperoni & Cheese	545	31	42
without Cheese	345	15	41
Roast Beef & Cheese	460	19	45
The Club	515	23	44
Tuna & Cheese	520	26	47
Turkey & Cheese	455	17	44

12" Size Subs: Double the figures for 6" size

6" Subs From The Grill

	C	F	Cb
Grilled Veggie	395	14	52
Hot Italian Sausage & Cheese	665	37	45
Philly Chicken & Cheese	400	10	48
w. Mushrooms/Green Peppers	500	21	50
without Cheese	330	4	47

Notes on Cholesterol

- **Cholesterol** is a white waxy substance produced mainly by our liver. It is also found in animal food products. Plant foods have no cholesterol.

- **Cholesterol is essential to life.** It is a structural part of every body cell wall and is the building block for vitamin D, sex hormones, and bile acids which help in the digestion of dietary fats.

- **The body makes sufficient cholesterol** for its needs and does not rely on cholesterol in the diet. Dietary fats have a major influence on blood cholesterol levels - more so than dietary cholesterol.

- **A high blood cholesterol increases** the risk of atherosclerosis - the thickening of arteries that can reduce or block blood flow to the heart muscle, brain, eyes, kidneys, sex organs and other body parts.

  This in turn increases the risk of heart attack, attack, stroke, blindness, kidney failure, impotence and other blood circulatory problems.

  Other risk factors which increase the risk of atherosclerosis include high blood pressure, smoking, obesity and diabetes (uncontrolled).

BLOOD CHOLESTEROL

CHECK YOUR RISK!

Total Cholesterol Level (mg/dl) ▼		Risk of Heart Attack ▼
240 and above	~	High Risk
200 - 239	~	Borderline/High
Below 200	~	Desirable

♥ **Know your cholesterol level, particularly if there is a family history of heart disease or stroke. If level is high, see your doctor.**

♥ **All adults should have their cholesterol, HDL and triglycerides tested at least every 5 years.**

▲ **Atherosclerosis can clog arteries and impede blood flow to the heart muscle or other body organs.**

▼ **A thrombus (blood clot) can form on unstable, festering athero- sclerotic plaque and rapidly block blood flow. A heart attack or stroke can result.**

HEART ATTACK WARNING SIGNALS

Many victims die before reaching the hospital by ignoring warning signals and delaying medical help. Symptoms vary and commonly include:

- **Chest pain**, vice-like squeezing or burning sensation in centre of the chest or between the shoulder blades, or in the mid-back. It may even feel like severe indigestion.

- **Pain** may spread to shoulders, neck, jaw or arms

- **Other signs**, with or without pain, include: sweating, (often cold, clammy) nausea, dizziness, shortness of breath, irregular pulse, anxiety

If you experience any of the above symptoms call for IMMEDIATE medical help. Every minute counts.
Call 911 *or your emergency number*

Fats & Cholesterol Guide

The amount and type of dietary fat has the greatest influence on blood cholesterol levels.

Fats in food are a mixture of 3 basic types: saturated, monounsaturated, and polyunsaturated. Animal fats are mainly saturated while plant oils and fish oils are mainly mono- and polyunsaturated.

Saturated fats have subgroups known as long chain, medium chain, and short chain fats. Most of the long chain fats raise blood cholesterol, and increase the risk of blood clots and thrombosis leading to artery blockage.

Long chain saturated fats are found mainly in full-cream milk, cheese, butter, cream, fatty meats and sausages, and processed foods.

Monounsaturated fats tend to more selectively lower 'bad' LDL-cholesterol and maintain the protective 'good' HDL-cholesterol in the bloodstream - but only if they replace saturated fats in the diet.

Foods rich in monounsaturates include canola and olive oils, canola margarine, peanuts, and avocados.

Polyunsaturated fats consist of two main classes. **Omega-6** polyunsaturates tend to lower blood cholesterol. Rich sources include safflower, sunflower and corn oils.

Omega-3 polyunsaturated fats can lower blood cholesterol, and also confer extra benefits by lowering blood triglycerides and reducing the risk of thrombosis, heart arrhythmias, and artery spasm.

Best practical omega-3 sources include canola oil and margarine, soybean oil and fish. (See adjoining chart)

A balanced intake of the two omega classes is important for optimal health. Slightly increasing omega-3 intake helps attain a more ideal balance. Adequate vitamin E intake is also important.

> *All fats are high in calories and need to be limited for weight control.*

DIETARY FATS COMPARISON

Legend: ■ Saturated Fat   ▢ Monounsaturated Fat
Polyunsaturated Fats: ▢ Linoleic (Omega-6)   ■ Alpha Linolenic (Omega-3)

OILS — PERCENTAGE CONTENT

Oil	Saturated	Monounsaturated	Linoleic (Omega-6)	Alpha Linolenic (Omega-3)
CANOLA OIL	7	63	20	10
LINSEED/FLAX OIL	9	19	17	55
SAFFLOWER OIL	9	14	77	
GRAPESEED OIL	10	22	68	
SUNFLOWER OIL	11	23	66	
CORN OIL	14	32	52	2
OLIVE OIL	14	76		10
SOYBEAN OIL	15	23	54	8
PEANUT OIL	19	45	34	2
COTTONSEED OIL	26	16	58	
PALM OIL	51	39	10	

SPREADS & FATS

Saturated Fat includes 'Trans Fats'   ▢ WATER CONTENT

Spread/Fat	Saturated	Monounsaturated	Linoleic	Alpha Linolenic	Water
LIGHT MARGARINE	14	14	21		51
CANOLA MARGARINE	18	45	12	6	19
POLYUNSATURATED MARG	24	20	36		20
BUTTER	57	18	2		24
LARD	41	47			12
BEEF FAT	44	37		4	15

GOOD SOURCES OF OMEGA-3 FATS

Plant Sources — Omega-3 Fats (Grams)

Canola Oil, 1 Tbsp, ½ fl.oz	1.5g
Flaxseed Oil, 1 Tbsp	8g
Soybean Oil, 1 Tbsp	1.2g
Canola Margarine, 1 Tbsp, ½ oz	1g
Soybeans, cooked, ½ cup, 4 oz	0.5g
Walnuts, ½ oz	0.5g

FISH - *Per 4 oz Serving*

High Content: Salmon (Chinook), Tuna, **3g**
Trout (Lake), Sardines, Herring, Mackerel **3g**

Medium Content:
  Salmon, (Pink/Red/Coho), 4 oz **2g**

Fair Content: *Per 4 oz Serving*

Bass, Catfish, Cod, Grouper, Hake, Halibut, Kingfish, Perch, Pollock, Shark, Trout (Rainbow), Tuna, Crab, Oysters, Blue Mussels, Shrimp, Squid } **0.5-1g**

How Much Is Needed?

As little as 1-2 grams daily of omega-3 fats may benefit general health. High doses of fish-oil supplements should only be taken as directed by your doctor.

Dietary Cholesterol

Cholesterol in food varies in its effect on blood cholesterol level (BCL) from person to person. Much depends on the amount and type of fat, and fiber eaten at the same meal.

Any elevating effect of dietary cholesterol on BCL is more likely to occur when the diet is high in saturated fat. Little elevation, if any, generally occurs when dietary fats are balanced in favor of monounsaturated and polyunsaturated fats (including omega-3 fats).

For example, while fish does contain cholesterol, the omega-3 fats can prevent any increase in BCL. Conversely, a meal containing no cholesterol but rich in saturated fat, may result in a significant increase in BCL.

Consequently, the need to be overly concerned about dietary cholesterol is being de-emphasized in favor of the approach of limiting total fat, saturated fat, and trans fats in particular – and substituting unsaturated fats.

The liver usually cuts back its own cholesterol production in response to cholesterol in the diet. Many people can consume normal amounts of high-cholesterol foods without concern.

However, it is difficult to identify just who is at risk - the so-called 'hyper-responders' - and because over 50% of Americans have a BCL above ideal levels, the **American Heart Association** advises all Americans to be prudent and limit their cholesterol intake to less than 300mg daily – as well as adopting a heart-healthy diet.

This limitation still allows the inclusion of most foods that are regularly eaten – even the overly-maligned egg.

Eggs contain a modest 5 grams of fat per large egg of which barely 2 grams are saturated, the rest being mono- and polyunsaturated.

By comparison, a cup of whole milk has 8g fat of which almost 5g is saturated.

CHOLESTEROL COUNTER

Cholesterol is found only in foods of animal origin. Plant foods contain no cholesterol.
AHA recommends limiting dietary cholesterol to less than 300mg/day.

	Chol mg
Meat - Average all types:	
Lean Meat, cooked, 4 oz	70
Fatty Meat, cooked, 4 oz	105
Fat, thick strip, 2 oz	35

Note. While lean meat and fat have similar amounts of cholesterol, choose lean meat to limit fat intake.

	Chol mg
Chicken/Turkey, average, 4 oz	90
Organ Meats: Liver, fried, 4 oz	500
Brains, beef, pan fried, 3 oz	1700
Sausages: Frankfurter, 1.5 oz	25
Salami, 2 slices, 2 oz	40
Bacon: 3 slices, cooked, 1 oz	20
Fish: Fish fillets, average, ckd, 4 oz	70
Tuna/Salmon, canned, 3 oz	30
Scallops, 9 medium, 3 oz	30
Shrimp, 12 large, raw, 3 oz	130
Oysters, raw, 6 medium, 3 oz	45
Lobster, Crab, raw, 3 oz	80
Eggs (Chicken), 1 large	210
1 medium	180
Egg White, *Egg Beaters*	0
Milk/Yogurt: Whole, 1 cup, 8 fl.oz	35
1% Milk, 1 cup	10
Skim/Non-fat, 1 cup	0
Soy Milk, Tofu, Tempeh	0
Cheese: Natural/Hard/Cream, 1 oz	30
Cottage, lowfat, 4 oz	5
Ricotta, part skim, 4 oz	25
Fats: Butter, 2 Tbsp, 1 oz	60
Margarine, Oils (vegetable)	0
Mayonnaise, 1 Tbsp	10
Cream: Heavy, whipping, 2 T, 1 oz	40
Half & Half/Sour, 2 Tbsp, 1 oz	10
Icecream: Regular, ½ cup, 4 fl.oz	30
Fruit, Vegetables, Avocados	0
Nuts, Seeds, Grains	0
Coffee, Tea, Soda, Beer, Wine	0

For Comprehensive Food Listings ~ see CalorieKing.com

Blood Cholesterol ~ Diet Hints

DIETARY HINTS TO LOWER BLOOD CHOLESTEROL

1. **Maintain a healthy weight.**
   If overweight, lose weight with a low-fat meal plan and daily exercise.

2. **Reduce saturated fat intake by:**
   (a) eating less dairy fat. Choose low-fat or fat-reduced varieties of milk, yogurt, soy drinks, cheese, and ice cream.

   (b) replacing saturated fats with fats and oils rich in monounsaturated and polyunsaturated fats. Choose vegetable oils such as canola, olive, sunflower and soybean. Avoid solid frying fats.

   Take Control and *Benecol* (spreads) contain plant stanol esters which can lower total and LDL cholesterol.

   (c) eating less fat from meat and poultry. Choose lean cuts of meat and skinless chicken. Go easy on luncheon meats, salamis and fatty sausages. Enjoy fish.

   (d) eating less saturated and trans fats from baked and fried fast-foods. Avoid deep-fried foods. Avoid donuts, cakes, pastries and cookies unless made with healthier fats and oils.

3. **Increase your 'soluble' fiber intake.**
   Foods rich in 'soluble' fiber include dried beans, baked beans, lentils, chick peas, hummus, nuts, seeds, psyllium seed husks and psyllium fiber supplements. Oat bran, rice bran and barley are also useful, as are fruit, veggies and avocados.

4. **Eat more soy bean products** such as: soy drinks, tofu, tempeh (cultured soy beans), soy flour and soy vegetarian foods. Soy protein in place of animal protein can significantly decrease high blood cholesterol levels as well as 'bad' LDL-cholesterol and blood triglycerides – 'good' HDL-cholesterol is maintained. For best results, eat at least 25g of soy protein per day (from 3-4 servings).

5. **Eat more fruit and vegetables and whole grains** in place of high-fat foods. Aim for 2 fruits and 5 servings of vegetables per day. They also contain valuable antioxidants. The fat of avocados (and most nuts) is mainly unsaturated and can lower blood cholesterol levels.

6. **Limit cholesterol to 300mg per day.**
   (Extra Notes ~ See Previous Page)

7. **Avoid brewed unfiltered coffee** (espresso; plunger-style). Several cups per day may raise blood cholesterol. American-style filtered coffee is fine.

8. **Spread your food intake over the day.**
   Have 5-6 small meals per day rather than just 2-3 large meals. Nibbling, versus gorging, favors lower blood cholesterol.

ALCOHOL - WINE

Alcohol is a mixed bag. Moderate amounts of 1-2 drinks daily appear to reduce the risk of heart attack and ischaemic stroke in older persons.

However, larger amounts increase the risk of high blood pressure, obesity, heart failure and hemorrhagic stroke; and can aggravate hypertriglyceridemia - as well as many other health hazards. *(See Alcohol Guide – Page 166)*

The speculative benefits of moderate alcohol intake have been overstated in the media. The overriding harmful effects of excess alcohol do not allow its recommendation for any aspects of health promotion.

Fruit, Vegetables & Tea Also Protect:
Red wine and red grapes (more so than white) contain antioxidants which may help protect cholesterol in the blood from becoming oxidized. Many fruits, vegetables, grains, nuts and tea also contain protective antioxidants.

How Fats Affect Blood Flow

Fats in the diet affect more than blood cholesterol levels. They can also strongly influence blood clot formation and thrombosis, as well as blood flow and ultimate oxygen delivery to body parts and organs.

While advanced atherosclerosis can impede blood flow to the heart and other organs, it is thrombosis (complete blockage by blood clots) or arterial spasm which commonly results in a heart attack or stroke.

Plant and fish oils rich in omega-3 fats lessen the risk of blood clots, thrombus formation, and artery spasm by reducing platelet stickiness and adhesion to artery walls. This reduces the risk of atherosclerotic plaque becoming unstable and reactive.

Omega-3 fats also improve blood flow by reducing blood viscosity and increasing the flexibility of red blood cells (RBC) that need to flex and twist on themselves in order to squeeze through tiny narrow capillaries often half their diameter.

A diet high in saturated fats has the opposite effect by stiffening RBC membranes and increasing blood viscosity, thereby hindering blood flow. The stiffening of the RBC membrane also reduces its ability to release vital oxygen to body cells and take up carbon dioxide.

Stiff red blood cells may also form aggregates that resembles coin stacks. In narrow blood vessels, this further impedes blood flow and impairs oxygen release from the much-lessened surface area of red blood cell membranes exposed to blood. (Smoking, lack of exercise, and stress can have similar adverse effects on thrombosis, red blood cell flexibility, and blood flow.)

▲ **Picture of Healthy Blood Flow**

Flexible red blood cells twist and slide through tiny capillaries - often half the diameter of red blood cells.

▲ **A Not-So-Healthy Picture!**

Red blood cells have lost their flexibility and ability to twist and slip through capillaries. They are stacked up, thereby impeding blood flow.

A diet high in saturated fats can contribute to this picture - as can smoking, lack of exercise, and stress.

Fiber Guide

Introduction

Fiber is the general term for those parts of **plant** food that we cannot digest (although bacteria in the large bowel partly digests fiber through fermentation). It is not found in foods of animal origin (meats, dairy products).

Fiber promotes intestinal health, bowel regularity, can benefit diabetes and blood cholesterol levels, and may help prevent colon cancer. High-fiber foods also assist weight control.

Most Americans don't eat enough fiber - less than 20 grams/day - instead of a healthier **25 to 35 grams/day.**

Fiber promotes good health, and better control of diabetes and cholesterol.

'An apple a day keeps the doctor away.'
... it just might!

Types of Fiber

Plant foods contain a mixture of different fibers in varying proportions. Insoluble and soluble fiber categories are based on their solubility in water. All types of fiber are beneficial to the body.

◆ Insoluble fibers (cellulose, hemi-celluloses, lignin) make up the structural parts of plant cell walls.

   Best food sources are wheat bran, corn bran, rice bran, whole-grain cereals and breads, dried beans and peas, nuts, seeds, and the skins of fruits and vegetables.

These fibers absorb many times their own weight in water. They create a soft bulk and hasten the passage of waste products through the intestines.

They promote bowel regularity, and aid in the prevention and treatment of uncomplicated forms of **constipation**, **diverticulosis and hemorrhoids.**

The risk of colon cancer may also be reduced by fiber's diluting effect of potentially harmful substances.

◆ Soluble fibers (pectin, gums, mucilages) are found mainly within plant cells, soy milk (whole bean) and products.

Types of Fiber (Cont)

Best Sources of Soluble Fiber: Fruits and vegetables, oat bran, barley, dried beans and peas, prunes, psyllium and flax seed.

These fibers form a gel which slows both stomach emptying and the absorption of sugars from the intestines. **This helps to control blood sugar levels.**

Weight control is also aided by the slower emptying of the stomach and the feeling of **fullness provided by soluble fiber.**

Some soluble fibers can lower **blood cholesterol** by binding bile acids and excreting them. More body cholesterol must then be broken down to supply bile acids for emulsification of dietary fats. **Rice bran, while not high in soluble fiber, can also lower blood cholesterol.**

◆ Resistant starch is that part of starchy foods (approx. 10%) which is tightly bound by fiber and resists normal digestion. Friendly bacteria in the large bowel ferment and change the resistant starch into short-chain fatty acids, which are important to bowel health and may protect against colon cancer.

Starchy foods include bread, cereals, rice, pasta, potatoes and legumes.

Fiber & Weight Control

Fiber can assist weight control in several ways. Fiber-rich foods such as fresh fruit and vegetables, potatoes and whole-grain bread contain few calories for their large volume (due to their low-fat, high-water content).

Their bulk fills the stomach and satisfies the appetite much earlier than fiber-depleted foods. The extra chewing time also contributes to satiety, and gives the stomach time to register a feeling of fullness. Excessive calories are less likely to be consumed.

Fiber-depleted foods and drinks are more concentrated in calories; e.g. fats, sugar, candy, soft drinks, fruit juices, alcohol. They require little or no chewing. Large amounts with excessive calories can be consumed before the appetite is satisfied.

Example: Whereas one fresh apple might satisfy our appetite, an apple juice drink with the equivalent sugars and calories of 2-3 apples does little to satisfy the appetite. (See illustration below.)

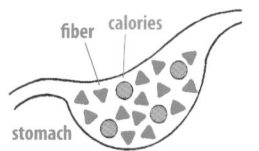

High-fiber foods fill the stomach. Fewer calories are consumed.

fiber   calories

stomach

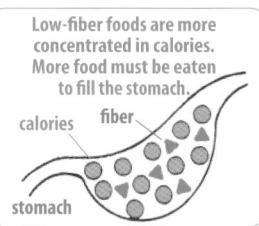

Low-fiber foods are more concentrated in calories. More food must be eaten to fill the stomach.

calories   fiber

stomach

EFFECTS OF REMOVING FIBER FROM FOOD

2-3 pieces of fresh fruit produces 1 glass of fruit juice. The removal of fiber concentrates the sugar and calories.

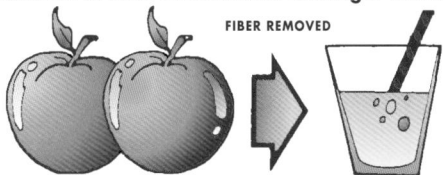

FIBER REMOVED

Fresh Fruit		Fruit Juice
High Fiber	←	Negligible Fiber
Low Calorie Density	←	High Calorie Density
Long Eating Time	←	No Eating Time (Drink)
Satisfies Hunger	←	Does Not Satisfy Hunger
Sugar Slowly Absorbed	←	Sugar More Quickly Absorbed
Less Insulin Required	←	More Insulin Required

Fiber Guide - Constipation

Constipation

Constipation can reasonably be defined as a failure to have a bowel movement at least every second day – and just as importantly, without straining or pain.

Typically, stools are too hard, too narrow and too small.

The **main cause** is simply a lack of dietary fiber. Other contributing factors include insufficient fluids, too little exercise, emotional stress, gastrointestinal disease, lack of proper dentition to chew high-fiber foods, and some medications (e.g. some antacids, antidepressants, pain medications).

Note: Check with your doctor to rule out any underlying medical problem – especially if you have a change in bowel habits in middle-age or later years.

DESIRABLE FIBER INTAKE

Adults: 25-35gm per day
Children (under 18): Age + 5gm
Example: 6-year old (6 + 5)=11gm

SAMPLE FOOD QUANTITIES
For 35 Grams of Fiber/Day

	Fiber
Breakfast Cereal (higher-fiber)	5g
plus 4 slices whole-grain Bread	6g
plus 3 servings fresh Fruit	9g
plus 1 medium Potato (w. skin)	
or 1 cup Brown Rice	4g
or ½ cup whole-grain Pasta	
plus 3-4 servings Veggies/Salad	6g
plus 1 cup Bean Soup	
or ¼ cup Baked/Soy Beans	
or ½ cup Corn/Peas/Lentils	5g
or 1¼ oz Almonds (natural)	
or 3 medium Figs	

HINTS TO INCREASE FIBER AND AVOID CONSTIPATION

① **Breakfast is an important** contributor to daily fiber intake. Eat high-fiber breakfast cereals (bran-based cereals, oatmeal etc.). Add 1-2 tablespoons of unprocessed bran.

Dried fruits, chopped nuts, soy grits, and seeds are also excellent additions to cereals.

Note: A gradual increase in fiber will prevent bloating, gas or pain. People intolerant to bran may benefit from psyllium-based fiber supplements and cereals.

② **Drink adequate water daily.** Fiber works by absorbing many times its own weight in water.

③ **Eat whole-grain breads,** or fiber-enriched breads. They have over double the fiber of regular white bread.

④ **Enjoy fruit as fresh fruit** with skins rather than as fruit juice. Enjoy whole-grain pasta, barley, brown rice, nuts and seeds.

⑤ **Eat more vegetables,** salads and legumes – especially cooked dried beans, baked beans, lentils, potatoes with skins, avocado, broccoli, brussels sprouts, cabbage, carrots, celery, and peas.

⑥ **Add bran** (barley/rice/wheat) or soy grits to soups, casseroles, yogurt, desserts, cookies, cakes. Also use whole-meal flour or soy flour in place of white flour. Use nuts, seeds, and ground linseed.

⑦ **Snack** on fresh or dried fruits, carrot or celery sticks, popcorn, nuts or seeds, whole-grain crackers, high-fiber bars (low-fat). Limit amounts if overweight.

⑧ **Exercise regularly** to strengthen abdominal muscles and stimulate the gut. Keep up water intake, especially in warm weather.

⑨ **Avoid** indiscriminate and regular use of harsh laxatives. They can overstimulate the intestinal muscles and may make normal bowel activity impossible. It may take several weeks to restore normal bowel function.

Fiber Guide

Fiber ~ Fiber (grams)

Breakfast Cereals (Cont)   **Fiber**

Kashi: GoLEAN Cereal, 1 cup, 1.8 oz	10
GoLEAN Crunch!, 1 cup, 1.9 oz	8
GoLEAN Bars, avg. (1)	4
Good Friends: Original, 1 cup, 1.9 oz	12
Cinna-Raisin Crunch, 1 cup, 1.8 oz	8
Heart to Heart, ¾ cup, 1.2 oz	5
7 Whole Grain Pilaf, ½ cup, cooked, 5 oz	6
7 Whole Grain Puffs, 1 cup, 0.7 oz	1
Quaker: Cap'n Crunch, ¾ cup, 1 oz	1
100% Natural Granola, avg., ½ cup, 1.8 oz	3
Crunchy Corn Bran, 1 cup, 1 oz	5
Life Cereal, ¾ cup, 1.1 oz	2
Oat Bran, ½ cup, 1.4 oz	6
Oatmeal, average, 1 packet	3
Post: 100% Bran, ⅓ cup, 1 oz	9
Alpha Bits, 1 cup, 1 oz	3
Blueberry Morning, 1 cup, 1.9 oz	2
Cocoa/Fruity Pebbles, 1 cup, 1 oz	3
Cranberry Almond Crunch, 1 cup, 1.8 oz	3
Fruit & Bran, 1 cup, 1.9 oz	6
Grape-Nuts, ½ cup, 2 oz	6
Great Grains, ⅔ cup, 1.9 oz	4
Honey Bunches of Oats, ¾ cup, 1.1 oz	2
Shredded Wheat & Bran, ½ cup, 2 oz	6

Breakfast Cereals   **Fiber**

General Mills:	
Basic 4, 1 cup, 2 oz	3
Cheerios (Honey Nut; Multigrain), 1 c., 1 oz	3
Multi-Bran Chex, 1 cup, 2 oz	7
Oatmeal Crisp Almond, 1 cup, 2 oz	4
Raisin Nut Bran, 1¼ cup, 2 oz	5
Total, average all types, ¾ cup, 1 oz	3
Wheat Chex, 1 cup, 2 oz	5
Wheaties ¾ cup, 1 oz	3
Health Valley:	
Amaranth Flakes, ¾ cup, 1 oz	4
Crunches & Flakes, ¾ cup, 1.9 oz	4
Fiber 7 Flakes, ¾ cup, 1 oz	4
Golden Flax, ¾ cup, 1.9 oz	6
Granola (Low-Fat), ⅔ cup 2 oz	6
Healthy Fiber Flakes, ¾ cup, 1.1 oz	4
Oat Bran Flakes, all types, 1 oz	3
Oat Bran O's, ¾ cup, 1 oz	3
Real Oat Bran, ½ cup, 1.7 oz	5
Kellogg's: All-Bran, ½ cup, 1.1 oz	10
All-Bran w. Extra Fiber, ½ cup, 1 oz	13
All-Bran Bran Buds, 1 cup, 1.1 oz	13
Corn Flakes, Fruit Loops, Smacks 1 cup, 1 oz	1
Cocoa/Rice Krispies Treats, 1¼ cup, 1 oz	0
Complete: Wheat Bran Flakes, ¾ c., 1 oz	5
Oat Bran Flakes, ¾ cup, 1.1 oz	4
Corn Pops, 1 cup, 1.1 oz	0.5
Cracklin'Oat Bran, ¾ cup, 1.7oz	6
Frosted Mini Wheats, 24 bisc., 2 oz	5
Granola w. Raisins, ⅔ cup, 2.1 oz	3
Nutri-Grain Cereal Bars, 1 bar, 1.3 oz	1
Raisin Bran, 1 cup, 2.1 oz	7
Smart Start, Healthy Heart, 1¼ cups, 2 oz	5
Product 19, 1 cup, 1.1 oz	1
Special K, 1 cup, 1.1 oz	0.5

Brans & Supplements

Oat Bran: 1 Tbsp (level)	1
⅓ cup, (5⅓ Tbsp), 1 oz	5
Rice Bran, raw. ¼ cup, 1 oz	6
Wheat Bran (unprocessed):	
Raw, 1 Tbsp	1.5
2 Tbsp (level), ¼ oz	3
¼ cup, (4 Tbsp), ½ oz	6
½ cup, 1 oz	12
Corn Germ: Toasted, ¼ cup, 1 oz	1
Wheat Germ: Raw, ¼ cup, 1 oz	4
Psyllium Seed Husks, 2 Tbsp	8
Metamucil, 1 dose	3.5

Hot Cereals, Oatmeal

Bulgur (cracked Wheat), ckd, 1 cup	8
Corn/Hominy Grits, dry, 3 Tbsp, 1 oz	0.5
Cream of Wheat, cooked, ¾ cup	
Oatmeal (uncooked ⅓ cup), ckd, ⅔ cup	3

Fiber Guide

Breads & Crackers | Fiber

Bread: White, 1 slice, 1 oz	0.6
Whole-wheat, 1 slice, 1 oz	1.5
Whole-grain, 1 slice, 1 oz	2
Rye, Pumpernickel, 1 oz	2
Bagel/Roll/Bun, 1 medium, 2 oz	1.5
Pita, whole wheat, 6½" pocket	4.5
Crackers: Graham, average, 2	0.4
Saltine, 4 crackers	0.4
Crispbreads (Rye), average, 2	4
Matzo 1 board, 1 oz	1
Rice Cakes, average, 1 cake	0.3
Tortilla: Regular, 6"	0.5
Whole-wheat, 6"	1.3

Barley, Pasta, Rice & Flours

Barley, pearled, raw, ¼ cup, 1.7 oz	8
Rice: White, cooked, 1 cup	0.6
Brown, cooked, 1 cup	3.5
Rice-A-Roni, average, 1 cup, prepared	1.5
Spaghetti/Noodles: Cooked, 1 cup	2
Whole-Wheat, cooked, 1 cup	4
Flour: Wheat, All-purpose, 1 cup, 4½ oz	3.5
Whole-Wheat, 1 cup, 4½ oz	15
Cornmeal, stone ground, 1 cup, 4½ oz	13
Carob Flour, 1 cup, 3½ oz	41
Rye Flour, 1 cup, 3½ oz	15
Soy Flour: Defatted, 1 cup, 3½ oz	17
Full-fat, raw, 1 cup, 3 oz	8
Soy Meal, defatted, 1 cup, 4½ oz	14

Frozen Entrees & Dinners

Average All Brands: Per Serving	
Beans/Chili base, average	6-10
Potato/Pasta base, average	4-6
Vegetable base, average	3
Meat/Chicken base, average	2-3
Pizzas, ¼ large, average	3
Vegetarian Soy Burgers, 1 pattie	4

Soups

Chicken Noodle, 1 cup	0.5
Tomato Soup, average, 1 cup	0.5
Vegetable Soup, average, 1 cup	3
Health Valley: Per 1 Cup Serving	
Black Bean; Minestrone	8
Tomato	1
5-Bean Vegetable; Lentil & Carrots	10
Mushroom Barley; Vegetable	4
Split Pea	5

Fast Foods & Restaurants | Fiber

Hamburgers: Small, average	1.5
Large/Whopper, average	2.5
Hot Dog, Regular	1.5
French Fries: Small serving, 2½ oz	2.5
Regular/Medium, 3½ oz	3.5
Chicken Nuggets, 6 pack	0.5
Chicken Sandwich, average	2
Taco, average	4
Sundaes, Shakes, Soft Drinks	0
Arby's: Baked Potato w. Broc. & Cheese	8
Roast Beef Sandwich, regular	2
Denny's: Grilled Chicken Salad, no bread	4
Classic Burger, no fries	4
Club Sandwich, no fries	4
Grilled Chicken Sandwich, no fries	4
Domino's (Classic): Vegi Feast, 1 sl. (12")	2
Hawaiian Feast, 1 slice, (12")	2
Pepperoni Feast, 1 slice (12")	2
McDonald's: Big Mac	3
Hamburger; Quarter Pounder	1
Egg McMuffin	2
Grilled Chicken Caesar Salad	3
McVeggie Burger on Wheat Bun	8
Pizza Hut: Per 1 Slice, Medium	
Pan Pizza: Cheese, Pepperoni	1
Supreme	2
Thin 'n Crispy, Supreme	2
Hand-Tossed, average all varieties	2
Subway: Sandwich, white roll, avg.	3
w. Honey Wheat Roll, average	3.2
Footlong w. Wheat Roll, average	8
Salads, average	4

Cakes, Cookies, Snack Bars

Apple/Fruit Pie, 1 serving, 4 oz	2
Cake: w. plain flour, 1 serving, 3.4 oz	1.5
w. whole-wheat flour, 1 serving	3
Carrot Cake, 1 serving, 1.2 oz	2
Cookies, oatmeal, (3 small/1 large)	1
Donuts, Medium, 1.7 oz	0.7
Fruit Cake, 1 serving, 1½ oz	2
Fig Bars, 1 cookie, ½ oz	0.7
Muffins, Oat Bran (2 small, 1 large), 4 oz	5
Granola Bars, average, 1 bar	2
Atkins Advantage Bars, average	7
Clif Bars, 2.5 oz	5
Curves, Chocolate Peanut Bar, 25g	5
Fi-Bar Chewy & Nutty 1 bar	5
Health Valley: Fruit/Granola Bars	3
Cereal Bars	1
Luna Bars, avg., 1.7 oz	3

Fiber Guide

Chocolate, Chips, Popcorn — Fiber

	Fiber
Cheese Balls/Curls/Twists	1
Chocolate, Hard Candy, 1 oz	0
Chocolate with nuts/fruit, 2 oz bar	1.5
Mars Bar, 1.8 oz	1
Potato Chips, corn chips, 1 oz	1
Popcorn, 3 cups	3
Pretzels, Twists (6)	1

Nuts, Seeds

	Fiber
Almonds: Natural, 25 kernels, 1 oz	3.5
Blanched (skins removed), 1 oz	3
Cashews, Filberts, Pecans, 1 oz	1.7
Peanuts, Mixed Nuts, Coconut, 1 oz	2.5
Peanut Butter, 2 Tbsp, 1 oz	2
Pistachio Nuts, dried, shelled, 1 oz	3
Walnuts, Black/English, dried, 1 oz	2
Seeds: Amaranth, 2½ Tbsp, 1 oz	3.5
Flax Seeds, 3 Tbsp, 1 oz	7
Psyllium Seed Husks, 5 Tbsp, 1 oz	20
Quinoa Seeds, 3 Tbsp, 1 oz	1.7
Sesame Seeds, whole, 1 oz	3.4
Sesame Butter/Tahini, 2 Tbsp, 1.1 oz	1.4
Sunflower kernels, ¼ cup, 1 oz	3.8
Teff Seeds, 1 oz	3.8

Fruit – Fresh

	Fiber
Apples: 1 medium, 5½ oz (whole)	
with skin + core	3.7
with skin, no core	3.2
without skin, no core	1.7
Apricots, 2 medium, 4 oz	1.5
Avocado, average, ½ medium	6.7
Banana, 1 medium, 6 oz (w. skin)	3
Blueberries, raw, ½ cup, 2½ oz	1.7
Cherries, sweet, raw, 8 fruits, 1.6 oz	1
Grapefruit, average, ½ fruit, 10 oz	1.4
Grapes, 1 medium bunch, seedless, 7 oz	2
Kiwifruit, 1 medium, 2.7 oz	2.3
Mango, 1 medium, 11 oz (whole)	1.6
Melons, Cantaloupe, ¼ (edible)	1
Nectarine, 1 medium, 4 oz	1.9
Olives, average all types, 7 jumbo, 2 oz	1.5
Oranges, 1 medium (7-8 oz w. skin)	
5½ oz (peeled)	3.8
Passionfruit, 2 medium, 2½ oz	5
Peaches, 1 large, 6 oz	2
Pears, raw, 1 medium, 6 oz	4.5
Pineapple, 1 slice, 3 oz	1.2
Plums, 2 medium, 4 oz	1.8
Strawberries, 6 medium/3 large, 2 oz	1
Watermelon, 4 oz (edible)	0.5

Fruit – Dried, Juice — Fiber

	Fiber
Dried Fruit: Apricots, 8 halves, 1 oz	2.2
Dates (3 med); Raisins (2 Tbsp), 1 oz	1.5
Figs, 3 medium, 1½ oz	5
Prunes, 4 medium, 1 oz	2
Fruit Juice: Orange/Apple etc, 1 glass	<0.5
Prune Juice, 1 c.	1.4
Carrot Juice, 8 oz	1.8

Vegetables

	Fiber
Asparagus, 4 medium spears	1.3
Bean Sprouts, ½ cup, 2 oz	1
Beans: Snap/Green, ½ cup, 2 oz	2
Baked Beans in Tom Sce, ½ c, 4½ oz	5
Dried Beans, ckd, average, ½ cup	7
Beets, ckd, slices, ½ cup, 3 oz	1.7
Broccoli, cooked, ½ cup, 3 oz	2.4
Brussels Sprouts, ckd, ½ cup, 3 oz	3.5
Cabbage: White, ckd, ½ cup, 2½ oz	1
Red, ckd, ½ cup, 2½ oz	2
Carrots, 1 medium (7½"), ½ cup, 3 oz	2.5
Cauliflower, cooked, 3 flowerets, 2 oz	1.5
Celery, raw, diced, 1 cup, 3½ oz	1.6
Chick Peas (Garbanzos), ckd, ½ c., 3 oz	6.5
Corn, kernels, ckd, ½ cup, 2½ oz	2.5
Cream-style, ½ cup, 4½ oz	1.5
Cucumber/Lettuce/Mushrooms, 2 oz	0.5
Eggplant, raw, sliced, ½ cup , 1½ oz	2
Lentils, cooked, ½ cup, 3½ oz	8
Mixed Vegetables, frozen, cooked, ½ cup	3
Onions, Raw, 1 medium, 4 oz	1.5
Spring Onions, chop., ¼ cup, 1 oz	0.7
Peas: Green, Raw, 2½ oz	3.7
Cowpeas (Black-eyed), ckd, ½ cup	10
Split Peas, ckd, ½ cup, 3½ oz	3
Peppers, sweet, raw, 1 large, 6 oz	3
Potatoes: 1 medium, with skin, 5 oz	4
without skin	2.5
½ cup mashed, 3½ oz	1.5
French Fries, small, 2.6 oz	3
Spinach, cooked, ½ cup, 3 oz	2.2
Squash: Summer, cooked, ½ cup, 3 oz	2.5
Winter, cooked, ½ cup, 3½ oz	2.4
Tomatoes: 1 medium, 4½ oz	1.5
Tomato Sauce, 1 cup	0.3
Soybean Products: Miso, ½ c., 5 oz	7.4
Tempeh, cooked, 1 piece, 3 oz	3
Tofu, ½ cup, 4.4 oz	0.4

Salads: Side Salad, average

	Fiber
Salads: Side Salad, average	1
Bean Salad, ½ cup	5
Coleslaw, ½ cup	1
Potato Salad, ½ cup	2

Protein Guide

General Notes

- **Protein has many important body functions.** It builds and repairs muscle, and is the basis of our body's organs, hormones, enzymes, and antibodies to fight infection.

- **Protein is also an emergency fuel** in the absence of sufficient carbohydrate and fats. For this reason, weight loss should be gradual so as to preserve protein levels in muscle, the heart and other body organs.

- **It is easy to obtain sufficient protein,** even if vegetarian. **Plant proteins are not inferior to animal proteins.** In fact, eating more soy and other plant proteins, and less animal protein, may help to build stronger bones and prevent osteoporosis, and may help to control blood cholesterol levels.

- **When changing to a vegetarian diet,** include soybeans, and other dried beans, soy milk drinks (calcium-enriched), lentils, tofu, tempeh, nuts and whole-grain breads and cereals. Milk, yogurt, cheese and eggs can enhance nutrient intake.

Protein & Muscle

- Although muscles are built of protein, protein is not a special fuel for working muscle cells – carbohydrates and fats are.

- In fact, a diet high in protein (and fat) and low in carbohydrate can significantly reduce the performance of endurance sports athletes. **Carbohydrate** is the best fuel for muscles exercised for long periods.

- Any **extra protein** required by athletes and body-builders can easily be obtained from the extra food eaten to satisfy hunger and energy needs.

- Remember, **excessive protein** intake will not build bigger muscles. Any excess is converted and stored as fat. Excess protein can also strain the kidneys, which excrete the waste products of protein metabolism.

Elderly people (and dieters) must eat sufficient food to ensure adequate protein intake.

Inadequate protein leads to a drop in immune response with greater susceptibility to illness and infections. Muscle strength and muscle mass also drop.

Protein needs are easily met with sensible eating. Athletes who eat enough food for their energy needs can obtain sufficient protein.

RECOMMENDED DAILY PROTEIN INTAKE ~ HEALTHY RANGE
(Lower figure is RDA)

		PROTEIN
Children:	1-3 yrs	13g-26g
	4-8 yrs	19g-38g
	9-13 yrs	34g-64g
Males:	14-18 yrs	52g-120g
	19+	56g-120g
Females:	14+	46g-110g
Pregnancy:		71g-120g
Breastfeeding:		71g-120g

Note: On lower-calorie diets, aim for higher amounts of protein within the Healthy Range.

Iron & Anemia Guide

- **Iron deficiency** is one of the most common nutritional deficiencies in women. The risk is increased in dieters who do not eat well-balanced meals. Chronic shortage of iron leads to anemia.

- **Women** between 11 and 50 years of age are at greater risk because of the monthly loss of menstrual blood. Pregnancy, growth, and endurance sports also demand extra iron.

- **In red blood cells,** iron combines with protein to form **hemoglobin** – the red pigment which carries oxygen in the blood. A lack of iron limits the production of hemoglobin and consequently the amount of vital oxygen delivered to body cells.

Note: A blood test will tell you if your Hb and Iron stores (ferritin) are adequate. (Iron stores can be low even when Hb is normal.)

- **Vitamin C** (in fruits/veggies/salads) enhances absorption of 'non-heme' iron in bread, cereals, milk, vegetables, nuts, eggs and iron supplements. Small amounts of meat, fish or poultry also help. (They contain 'heme' iron).

- **Iron absorption is lessened** by up to 60% when high calcium foods are consumed with iron-rich main meals. Tea, coffee, phytates (in bran) and oxalates lessen absorption of non-heme iron.

- **For infants to 1 year,** use iron-fortified milk/soy formula if not breast-feeding. Introduce iron-fortified baby cereals at 4-6 months.

Note: Iron deficiency in children (even without anemia), can result in lethargy, irritability, repeated infections, and developmental problems.

Iron Supplements

- **Most people** can obtain adequate iron from their diet. **A wide variety** of animal and plant foods contain iron. (See Iron Counter).

- **Iron supplements** are only recommended for women with heavy menstrual blood losses or during pregnancy (if tests show a low-iron status), endurance athletes with low blood ferritin (iron stores) and for persons with diagnosed anemia. Check with your doctor.

- While the 5 mg of iron in multi-vitamin/mineral supplements is safe for most people, large amounts can be toxic, (especially in persons with hemochromatosis iron-overload condition).

ANEMIA SYMPTOMS

Anemia reduces the amount of oxygen carried in the blood. The body tissues become starved of oxygen. Symptoms include:

- **Pale skin; brittle fingernails (may turn up into spoon shape)**
- **Excessive tiredness or fatigue**
- **Breathlessness**
- **Feeling of malaise and irritability**
- **Always feel cold**
- **Decrease in attention span**

Note: Other medical conditions may also cause similar symptoms. Check with your doctor.

A nutritious diet with adequate iron is important - particularly for women and athletes.

RECOMMENDED DAILY IRON INTAKE (mg)

			Iron
Infants (0-6 mths):			
	Breastfed	~	0.5mg
	Bottlefed	~	3mg
	6-12 mths	~	11mg
Children:	1-11 yrs	~	7-10mg
Males:	12-18 yrs	~	11mg
	19+ yrs	~	8mg
Females:	12-18 yrs	~	15mg
	19-50 yrs	~	18mg
	51+ yrs	~	8mg
	Pregnancy	~	27mg
	Breastfeeding	~	12-16mg

Pro ~ Protein (grams)   Iron ~ Iron (mg)

Meat

	Pro	Iron
Steak: Average all cuts, lean (no fat)		
Small (4 oz raw/3 oz ckd)	23	2.3
Medium (6 oz raw/4¼ oz ckd)	34	3.4
Large (10 oz raw/7¼ oz ckd)	57	5.7
Roast Beef, lean, 2 slices, 3 oz	24	2.5
Ground Beef patty, lean, ckd, 3 oz	21	2
Lamb chop, broiled, 3 oz	22	1.5
Liver, cooked, 3 oz	23	5.5
Veal cutlet, 1 medium	23	1
Pork, cooked, lean, 3 oz	24	1
Bacon, 3 medium slices	6	0.3
Ham, roasted, 2 pieces, 3 oz	18	1
Ham, luncheon, 2 slices, 1½ oz	7	0.3
Pastrami (Oscar Mayer), 3 sl., 1¾ oz	10	1.3
Sausages: Bologna, 2 sl., 2 oz	7	1
Braunschweiger, 2 sl., 2 oz	8	5.3
Pork link, thick, 2 oz	6	0.4
Frankfurter, 1⅓ oz	5	0.5
Salami, hard, 3 slices, 1 oz	7	0.5
Vegetarian (Boca Burger), 1 pattie	13	2

Chicken/Turkey (Without Skin)

	Pro	Iron
Chicken, ckd; Breast, Roasted, 4 oz	36	1.5
Leg/Thigh,Roasted, 2 oz	14	0.5
½ Whole Chicken	60	2.5
Drumstick, Roasted, 1 med., 3 oz	13	0.6
Turkey, cooked: Light meat, 3 oz	28	2
Dark meat, lean, 3 oz	24	2

Fish

	Pro	Iron
Fresh Fish: Per 4 oz, cooked		
Cod, Flounder/Sole, Pollock	28	0.5
Catfish, Haddock, Halibut, M/Mahi	28	1.3
Ocean Perch, Swordf., Orange Roughy	28	1.3
Canned Fish: Tuna, Light, 3 oz	25	1.5
White, 3 oz	23	0.5
Salmon, pink, 3 oz	17	0.7
Salmon, red, 3 oz	17	1
Sardines, 3 whole (3"), 1¼ oz	9	1
Anchovies, 1 can, 1½ oz	13	2
Shellfish: Crabmeat, 3 oz	17.5	0.7
Clams, raw, 4 large/9 sml, 3 oz	11	12
Crayfish, cooked, 3 oz	20	2.7
Lobster, cooked, 3 oz	17	0.5
Oysters, raw, 6 medium, 3 oz	7	5
Scallops, 2 lge/5 small, 1 oz	5	0.1
Shrimp, raw, 6 large, 1½ oz	8.5	1
Fish Products: Fish Sticks, 4 sticks	10	0.5
Fish Portions, in batter, 4 oz	13	0.6
Gefilte Fish, 1 medium ball, 2 oz	8	1

Eggs

	Pro	Iron
1 Large Egg, whole	6	0.7
Egg Yolk	3	0.7
Egg White	3	0
Omelet: Plain, 2 eggs	13	1.7
Ham & cheese	17	3
Egg Substitutes (liquid):		
Eggbeaters, 1 egg equiv.	4.5	1
Better 'n Eggs/Scramblers, ¼ cup, 2 oz	6	0.7

Milk, Yogurt, Icecream

	Pro	Iron
Milk: Whole/Lowfat/Skim, 8 fl.oz cup	8	0.1
Protein Enriched, 1 cup	10	0.1
Carb Countdown (2% or Fat Free), 1 c.	8	0
Chocolate Milk, 1 cup	8	0.6
Thick Shake, Chocolate, 10 oz	9	1
Vanilla, 10 oz	11	0.3
Soymilk (fortified), average, 1 cup	7	1
Yogurt: Plain, 6 oz	10	0.1
Fruit flavors: 6 oz	8	0.3
8 oz	11	0.5
Ice-Cream: Rich, ½ cup	2	0
Regular, Vanilla, ½ cup	2.5	0
Sherbet, ½ cup	1	0
Custard, baked, ½ cup	7	0.5

Cheese

	Pro	Iron
Hard Cheeses, average, 1 oz	7	0.2
4 oz piece	28	0.8
Cottage Cheese, ½ cup	13	0.3
Ricotta, part skim, ½ cup	14	1

Bread, Bagels, Biscuits

	Pro	Iron
Bread (w. enriched flour): 1 slice, 1 oz	2	1
4 thin slices, 4 oz	8	4
4 thick slices, 6 oz	1.2	6
Bagel, plain 2 oz	6	1.5
Biscuits, 1 oz	2	0.7
Pita Bread, 1 pita, 1½ oz	4	1
Pumpernickel, 1 slice, 1 oz	3	1

Infant/Baby Foods

	Pro	Iron
Infant Formula Milk:		
Enfamil/Gerber/Similac, 5 fl.oz		
Regular/Low Iron	2.2	0.2
With Iron	2.2	1.8
Isomil/Nursoy/ProSobee	3	1.8
Baby Cereals: Average All Brands		
Dry, 4 Tbsp, ½ oz	1	7
Jars (w. fruit), 4½ oz	1	7

Breakfast Cereals

	Pro	Iron
Hot Type, cooked:		
Bulgur, cooked, 1 cup, 5 oz	9	2
Oatmeal: Reg., non-fortified, 1 cup	6	1.5
Instant, fortified, avg., 1 pkt	4	8
Quaker, all flavors, ½ cup	5	18
McCann's, Steelcut, ¼ cup dry	4	18
Corn/Hominy Grits: Reg., 1 cup	3	1.5
Quaker: Reg., 3 Tbsp, 1 oz	2	0.8
Instant White, 1 packet	2	8
Cream of Wheat, 1 cup	4	10
Brands ~ Ready-To-Eat		
Arrowhead: Average all varieties, 1 oz	3	1
General Mills: Basic 4, 1 cup, 2 oz	4	4.5
Cheerios, Original, 1 cup, 1 oz	3	8
Cocoa Puffs, 1 cup, 1 oz	1	4.5
Kix, 1⅓ cups, 1 oz	2	8
Multi-Bran Chex, 1 cup, 2 oz	4	16
Country Corn Flakes, 1 cup, 1.2 oz	2	8
Total Raisin Bran, 1 cup, 2 oz	3	18
Wheaties ¾ cup, 1 oz	3	8
Health Valley: Oat Bran O's, ¾ cup, 1 oz	3	0.7
Amaranth Flakes, 1 cup, 1 oz	3	0.7
Bran Flakes w. Raisins, ¾ cup, 1.1 oz	3	0.7
Low-Fat Granola, ⅔ cup, 2 oz	5	1.4
Real Oat Bran Alm. Crunch, ½ cup, 1.7 oz	6	0.7
Golden Flax, ¾ cup, 1.9 oz	6	1
Kashi: Friends, 1 cup, 1.9 oz	5	1.8
GoLean Crunch!, 1 cup, 1.9 oz	9	1.8
7 Whole Grain Flakes, 1 c., 1.8 oz	4	1.4
Kellogg's: All-Bran: ½ cup, 1 oz	4	4.5
Complete Oat Flakes, ¾ cup, 1.1 oz	3	18
Cocoa Krispies, ¾ cup, 1 oz	1	4.5
Corn Flakes, 1 cup, 1 oz	2	8
Low-fat Granola w. Raisins ⅔ c., 2.1 oz	4	2
Product 19, 1 cup, 1 oz	2	18
Raisin Bran, 1 cup, 2 oz	5	4.5
Rice Krispies, 1¼ cup, 1.2 oz	2	9
Smart-Start Healthy Heart, 1.8 oz	6	4.5
Special K: Regular, 1 cup, 1.1 oz	7	8
Protein Plus, ¾ cup, 1 oz	10	8
Post: Raisin Bran, ⅔ cup, 2 oz	4	11
Grape Nuts, ½ cup, 2 oz	7	16
Quaker: Crunchy Corn Bran, 1 cup, 1 oz	2	8
100% Natural Granola, ½ cup, 1.7 oz	5	1.4
Life, ¾ cup, 1 oz	3	8
Cap'n Crunch, ¾ cup, 1 oz	1	4.5
Oat Bran, ½ cup, 1.4 oz	7	2.7

Brans & Wheatgerm

	Pro	Iron
Oat Bran, raw, 1 Tbsp	2	0.5
Rice Bran, raw, 2 Tbsp	1	1
Wheat Bran, unprocessed, 2 T.	1	1
Wheat Germ, 2 Tbsp, ½ oz	4	1.3

Grains & Flours

	Pro	Iron
Amaranth, ½ cup, 3.4 oz	14	7
Barley, ½ cup, 3.2 oz	12	2
Buckwheat Flour: Whole-groat, 1 cup	15	2.7
Carob Flour, 1 cup, 3.6 oz	5	3
Corn Flour, 1 cup, 4 oz	11	2
Corn Meal, 1 cup, 4½ oz	8	3.5
Flour: White, 1 cup, 5.6 oz	9	6
Whole-grain, 1 cup, 4¼ oz	16	5
Millet, whole-grain, 1 cup, 3½ oz	12	7
Rye Flour: Dark, 1 cup, 4½ oz	18	6
Light, 1 cup, 3½ oz	9	1
Soy Flour, full fat, 1 cup, 3 oz	29	5.5
Yeast: Active, dry, 1 Tbsp, ½ oz	5	1.5

Rice, Spaghetti, Macaroni

	Pro	Iron
Rice: Brown/White, average 1 cup cooked, 6½ oz	5	1
Spaghetti/Macaroni/Noodles (enriched):		
Cooked, 1 cup, 4½ oz	7	2
Canned: in Tomato Sauce, ½ cup	2	0.5
w. Meatballs, 1 cup, 8 oz	10	2
Macaroni & Cheese, 1 cup, 8.5 oz	8	1

Soups

	Pro	Iron
With Noodles/Vegetables, 1 c.	3	0.5
With Meat/Beans/Peas, 1 cup	8	1.5

Fruit

	Pro	Iron
Fresh/Canned:		
Average, all types 1 medium/2 small fruit	1	0.5
Avocado, ½ medium	2	1
Dried Fruit: Apricots, 8 halves, 1 oz	1	1.3
Dates, 6 dates, 2 oz	1.5	0.7
Figs, 4 medium figs, 2 oz	2	1.7
Prunes, 5 medium, 1½ oz	1	1
Raisins, 1 oz	1	0.7
Fruit Juice: Average, 1 cup	0.5	0.5
Prune Juice, 6 fl.oz	1	2.5
Tomato Juice, 1 cup, 8 fl.oz	1.5	1

King Kong was a vegetarian!

Protein & Iron Counter

Vegetables

	Pro	Iron
Beans: Snap/green, ½ cup, 2 oz	1	0.8
Dried: Average all types, cooked, ½ cup	7	2.5
Baked Beans, ½ cup 4½ oz	5	2
Bean Sprouts, mung, 1 cup, 4 oz	3	1
Broccoli, 3raw, ½ cup, 1½ oz	1.5	0.7
Cabbage; Cauliflower, raw, 1 c. 3 oz	1.5	0.6
Corn, raw, ½ cup kernels, 3 oz	2.5	0.3
1 ear trimmed to 3½"	2	0.4
Lentils, cooked, ½ cup, 3½ oz	9	3.3
Mushrooms, raw, ½ cup, sliced	1	0.3
Peas: Green, raw, ½ cup, 2½ oz	4	1.2
Split Peas, cooked, 1 cup, 7 oz	16	2.5
Potatoes, cooked:		
1 medium, with skin, 5 oz	3.3	2
without skin, 4 oz	2.3	1
French Fries, small, 2.6 oz	2	1
Potato Salad, ½ cup, 4 oz	3.5	2.5
Pumpkin, ½ cup mashed, 4.3 oz	1	1
Seaweed, kelp, 1 oz	<1	2.5
Spinach, cooked, ½ cup, 3 oz	2.7	3.5
Squash, ckd, all types, ½ cup	1	0.3
Tomatoes, 1 medium, 4½ oz	1	0.6
Vegetables, mixed, ckd, 1 cup	2.5	0.7
Soybeans, cooked, ½ cup, 3 oz	14	4.4

Tofu, Tempeh, Miso

	Pro	Iron
Tofu, raw, firm, ½ cup, 4½ oz	10	1.5
Tempeh, ½ cup, 3 oz	16	2
Miso, ½ cup, 5 oz	16	4
Miso Soup, 1 cup	3	0.4
Soybean Protein (TVP), 1 oz	18	3

Cakes, Pastries, Pies
(Made with enriched flour)

	Pro	Iron
Carrot w. cream cheese frosting, 4 oz	4	1.3
Cheesecake, 1 piece, 4 oz	6	0.5
Chocolate, 1 piece, 2 oz	2	2
Fruitcake, 1 piece, 3 oz	4	2
Plain, 1 piece, 3 oz	4	1.2
Croissant, plain, 2 oz	5	2
Danish Pastry, 1 pastry, 2¼ oz	4	1.3
Donuts, average, 2 oz	4	1.2
Muffins, average, 1 med., 1½ oz	3	1
Pancakes, 4" diam., two, 2 oz	4	1
Pies: Fruit, 1 piece, 5½ oz	4	1.5
Pecan, 1 piece, 5 oz	7	4.5
Puddings, average, ½ cup, 4½ oz	4	0.3
Waffles, 1 large, 2½ oz	7	1.5

Peanut Butter

	Pro	Iron
Regular: 2 Tbsp, 1.1 oz	8	0.5
Peter Pan Plus, 2 Tbsp, 1.1 oz	8	4.5

Sugar, Honey, Jam

	Pro	Iron
Sugar: White	0	0
Brown, 1 Tbsp	0	0.3
Molasses: Light/Medium, 1 Tbsp	0	1
Blackstrap, 1 Tbsp, ¾ oz	0	3
Corn Syrup, 1 Tbsp, ¾ oz	0	1
Honey, Jams, Jelly	0	0.2

Candy, Chocolate, Carob

	Pro	Iron
Candy, sugar-based	0	0
Chocolate: Plain, 2 oz bar	4	0.8
with nuts, 2 oz bar	6	0.8
Carob, plain, 2 oz	6	0.7

Cookies, Crackers, Chips

	Pro	Iron
Cookies, average, 4 cookies	2	1
Crackers, Graham, 2½" sq., (2)	1	0
Rice Cakes, average, one	1	0
Corn/Potato Chips, 1 oz	2	0.3
Nuts: Almonds, shelled, 20-25 nuts	6	1
Brazil Nuts, 7-8 medium nuts, 1 oz	4	1
Cashews, 12-16 nuts, 1 oz	5	1.5
Macadamias, 1 oz	2	0.5
Peanuts, dry rsted, 40 nuts, 1 oz	6	0.6
Pecans, 24 halves, 1 oz	2	0.5
Walnuts, 15 halves, 1 oz	4	0.7
Seeds: Sesame Seeds, dry, 1 Tbsp	2	0.6
Pumpkin Kernels, dry, hulled, 1 oz	7	4.2
Sunflower Seeds, dried, hulled, 1 oz	6	2
Tahini, 1 Tbsp, ½ oz	2.5	1.4

Granola & Food/Protein Bars

	Pro	Iron
Granola Bars, average, 1 bar, 2 oz	2	0.5
Atkins Advantage Bar, avg., 2.1 oz	20	1.8
Balance Bars, Original, 1.76 oz	14	4.5
Bariatrix Proti-Bars (1), 1.4 oz	15	0.7
Dr Soy Protein Bars, 1.76 oz	11	18
GeniSoy Bar, 1.5 oz	14	4.5
Jenny Craig Bars, 1.8 oz	4	3.6
Met-Rx "Big 100", 3.5 oz	27	7.2
Myoplex Carb Sense Bar, 2.5 oz	26	2
Planters Carb Well Bar, 1.2 oz	6	1
PowerBar: Harvest	10	4.5
Performance Bar, 2.3 oz	10	6.3
ProteinPlus, 1 bar, avg., 2.75 oz	24	8
Slim-Fast Optima Diet Bar, 1 oz	2	1.4
Special K:		
Protein Meal Bar, 1.6 oz	10	1.8
Protein Snack Bar, 0.9 oz	4	0.7

Nutritional & High Protein Drinks

	Pro	Iron
Atkins Shakes, 11 fl.oz can	18	2.7
Boost Ready To Drink, 8 oz can	10	3.5
Carnation Instant Breakfast, 10 oz	13	4.5
Curves Protein Drink, 2 scoops, dry	15	18
Ensure Plus, 8 oz can	13	2.3
GeniSoy Shake, 1 scoop, 1.2 oz	14	3.6
Kashi GoLean Shake, 2 scoops, 2.1 oz	21	2.7
Met-Rx RTD 40	40	4.5
Myoplex, Original Nutrition Shake, 1 pkt	42	5.4
Optifast 800, made-up, 8 oz	14	3.6
Resource (Novartis) Standard, 8 fl.oz	15	4.5
Revival Soy, Plain, 58g pkt	20	3
Slim-Fast Shakes, 325 ml can	10	3.6
High Protein, 1 can	15	6.3
Special K₂0 Protein Water, 16 fl.oz	5	0
Usana Soyamax, 2 scoops, 1 oz	24	6
Walgreens Slim For Less, 11 oz can	10	2.7
Weider Mass 1000, 4 scoops, 7 oz	34	6

Coffee, Tea, Soda

Coffee, Coffee Substitutes, 1 cup, 8 fl.oz	0	0
Coffee w. 2 oz milk, 1 cup, 8 fl.oz	2	0
Caffe latte, large, 16 fl.oz	12	0
Cappuccino, large, 16 fl.oz	8	0
Frappuccino, average, 16 fl.oz	6	0
Tea (all types); Soft Drinks/Soda	0	0
Hot Chocolate (all milk), 1 cup, 8 fl.oz	8	1.2

Beer, Wine, Spirits

Beer, 12 fl.oz	1	0
Wines, red/white, 1 glass	0	0.4
Spirits/Liquor	0	0

Fast-Foods/Burgers

For extra listings ~ see CalorieKing.com

Pancakes: Average all outlets, 3	8	2
Shakes, Chocolate, 16 fl.oz	12	0.4
Sundaes: Average all outlets	7	0.3
Arby's: Roast Beef Sandwich, reg.	21	3.6
Chicken Club Salad	32	3.8
Roast Beef Sandwich, Super	21	3.8
Burger King: Whopper S/wich	28	5.4
Bacon Double Cheeseburger	33	4.5
BK Big Fish Sandwich	24	4.5
Carl's Jr: Famous Star Hamburger	24	2
Bacon Swiss Crispy Chicken	35	2
Charbroiled Chicken Club Sandwich	40	3
Super Star Hamburger	41	3

Fast Foods/Burgers (Cont)

	Pro	Iron
Domino's Pizza: Deep Dish (12")		
Cheese, 2 slices	16	2
Pepperoni, Sausage, Ham, 1 slice	11	2
Extravaganza, 1 slice	18	2.4
KFC: Original, Breast	37	1
Crispy Strips, 3 strips	29	1.8
Snacker, Regular	15	2.7
McDonald's: Big Mac	25	4
Cheeseburger	15	3
Chicken McNuggets (6)	15	1
Crispy Chicken Classic Burger	27	3
Filet-O-Fish	15	2
Grilled Chicken Caesar Salad	30	2
Hamburger	12	3
Quarter Pounder w. Cheese	29	5
French Fries: Small, 2.6 oz	3	0.4
Large, 6 oz	6	1
Salads w. Chicken, average	30	3
Thick Shake, average, 16 fl.oz	13	0
Breakfast: Egg McMuffin	18	3
Bacon, Egg & Cheese McGriddles	19	2
Ham, Egg & Cheese Bagel	27	4
Sausage McMuffin w. Egg	21	3
Pizza Hut: *Per Medium, 1 slice*		
Fit n' Delicious, Ham/Pineapple	8	1
Hand Tossed, Pepperoni	12	1.5
Pan Pizzas, average	14	2
Thin 'n Crispy, Supreme	12	1
Subway (6" Subs): Roast Beef	19	6
Cheese Steak	29	8
Meatball Marinara	24	7
Roast Chicken Breast	24	4
Subway Club	24	6
Sweet Onion Chicken Teriyaki	24	4
Taco Bell: Bean Burrito	13	2.7
Chicken Quesadilla	28	1.8
Chicken/Steak Enchirito	21	1.8
Gordita Baja Beef	13	2.7
Steak Burrito Supreme	18	2.7
Taco Supreme	9	1
Tostado	11	1.5
Wendy's: Old Fashioned Single Burger	25	4.5
Club Frescata Sandwich	22	3.6
Hamburger (Kid's Meal)	15	3.6

High Blood Pressure

High Blood Pressure

Many American adults have hypertension (high blood pressure), and are unaware of it. It is generally symptomless, so **have your blood pressure checked annually** – particularly if it runs in the family.

Untreated hypertension overworks the heart, damages arteries and promotes atherosclerosis. This in turn greatly increases the risk of heart disease, stroke, blindness, kidney disease and impotence. The earlier hypertension is detected, the sooner it can be brought under control.

HYPERTENSION DAMAGES ARTERIES & PROMOTES ATHEROSCLEROSIS

STROKE (Brain) Artery blockage or rupture

NECK ARTERIES Artherosclerosis can limit blood flow to brain

HEART ATTACK Coronary artery blockage

BLOOD PRESSURE CLASSIFICATION

For Adults Age 18 & Older ~ Not Acutely Ill or on Medication (American Heart Association)

	DIASTOLIC		**SYSTOLIC**
Normal ➤	Below 80	and	Below 120
Prehypertension ➤	80-89	or	120-139
Hypertension:			
Stage 1 ➤	90-99	or	140-159
Stage 2 ➤	100 or more	or	160 or more

Treating Hypertension

Prehypertension (in the chart above) means you don't have high blood pressure now but are likely to develop it in the future.

You can take steps to lessen the risk by adopting healthy lifestyle habits.

- reducing sodium intake
- eating adequate fruit and vegetables
- losing weight if overweight
- limiting alcohol to 2 drinks or less daily
- quitting smoking
- exercising regularly, managing stress.

Stage 1 hypertension can often be treated with the above lifestyle changes.

Stage 2 hypertension usually requires drug therapy. However, salt restriction, abstaining from alcohol, and the above lifestyle changes will improve the success of drug therapy, and enable smaller drug doses to be prescribed.

STROKE

KNOW THE WARNING SIGNS!

If you notice one or more of these signs, **call your doctor immediately**. They may be signalling a possible stroke or transient ischemic attack:

- **Sudden weakness** or numbness in your face, arm, or leg on one side of your body.

- **Sudden dimness**, blurring or loss of vision, particularly in one eye.

- **Loss of speech**, or trouble talking or understanding speech.

- **Sudden severe headache** - 'a bolt out of the blue' - with no apparent cause.

- **Unexplained dizziness**, unsteadiness or a sudden fall, especially if accompanied by any of the other symptoms.

Salt & Sodium

- **Sodium is a mineral element** most commonly found in salt (sodium chloride). It also occurs naturally in much smaller amounts in animal and plant foods, and water – normally sufficient for our needs without having to add salt to our diet.

- **Sodium is required** for nerve and muscle function, as well as to balance the amount of fluid in our tissues and blood.

  Sodium acts like a sponge to attract and hold fluids in body tissues.

- **Excess sodium** can cause water retention, and increase the risk of developing hypertension. Very high salt intake may also increase the risk of stomach cancer.

- **Too little sodium** may cause low blood pressure (hypotension), and decrease blood flow to the heart, brain and kidneys - especially during exercise. (A certain blood volume is required to sustain the blood pressure needed for adequate blood flow in the capillaries.)

Salt-Sensitive Persons

- **Normally, our kidneys** excrete excess dietary sodium. The thirst we feel after a salty meal is the body calling for water to dilute the sodium, and enable the kidneys to flush out excess sodium.

- **However, 'salt - sensitive' persons** (up to 50% of adults) tend to retain excess sodium (above approximately 3000mg daily) instead of excreting it. Such persons are more likely to develop hypertension and would benefit most from sodium restriction. Assume you are susceptible if there is a family history of hypertension.

- **Although not everyone will benefit, all Americans are being asked to moderate their salt and sodium intake** as a public health measure – particularly because so many do not know whether or not they have hypertension, and also because we do not know just who is salt-sensitive.

SAFE SODIUM LEVELS

The American Heart Association recommends a **maximum sodium intake of 2300mg per day** for adults with normal blood pressure. However, people who consume less than 1500mg sodium have the lowest blood pressure levels.

Persons with hypertension and kidney ailments are usually restricted to as little as **1000mg sodium per day**. Your doctor will discuss the correct sodium level for you.

Persons with Menière's Disease (chronic attacks of vertigo, dizziness, hearing loss, imbalance), often benefit from lower sodium intake of less than 2000mg/day, as well as even distribution of food and fluids over the day (to prevent fluctuations in body fluids and pressure in the inner ear). Also avoid caffeine and MSG. Limit sugar and alcohol.

further info: www.CalorieKing.com

FINDING HIDDEN SODIUM

On average, **less than one third of our sodium intake comes from the salt shaker.**
The rest is hidden in processed foods that have salt added during manufacture.

Sodium compounds added to food or medicinals can also contribute significant sodium.

Sodium bicarbonate in particular is widely used in antacid tablets (such as Alka Seltzer) and powders. Sodium bicarbonate contains 27% sodium by weight. Each gram contributes 270mg sodium. Large amounts of sodium can be unwittingly consumed – up to 600mg per tablet. (See Antacids ~ Page 293)

Example: 2 Alka-Seltzer Tablets = 1000mg sodium

Other sodium compounds include monosodium glutamate (MSG), sodium ascorbate, sodium nitrite, and sodium citrate.

ALCOHOL DANGER

Excessive alcohol intake contributes to hypertension. Susceptible persons should limit alcohol intake to 1-2 drinks per day.

Salt Sodium Guide

Sodium accounts for only 40% of the weight of salt (sodium chloride). Examples:
1 gram (1000mg) Salt has 400mg Sodium
1 teaspoon (5g) Salt has 2000mg Sodium

HINTS TO REDUCE SODIUM

- **Watch the salt shaker.** Start with an easy 50% cut in sodium by using Lite Salt (*Morton*) or *Cardia* Salt. Then gradually cut back until you can leave the salt shaker off the table.

- **Taste your food before salting.** Use the pepper shaker (small holes) for more controlled sprinkling of salt.

- **Choose low-sodium,** sodium-free, and reduced-sodium products in place of regular salted products.

- **Check food labels for sodium levels.** FDA Guidelines for sodium descriptors are:
  - **Reduced Sodium:** At least 25% less sodium than the original product
  - **Low Sodium:** 140 mg or less/serving
  - **Very Low Sodium:** 35mg or less/serving
  - **Sodium Free:** Less than 5mg/serving
  - **No Salt Added:** Made without the salt added, but still contains the sodium that is a natural part of the food

- **Use reduced-sodium breads,** butter and margarine. Regular varieties contain up to 2% salt. This is considered high in view of their significant contribution to our diet.

- **Go easy on condiments and sauces** such as ketchup, mustard, soy sauce and spaghetti sauces, as well as salad dressings. Use low-sodium varieties.

- **Limit pizzas and salty fast-foods.** Check *CalorieKing.com* food database.

- **Avoid salty snack foods** such as potato chips, corn chips, salted nuts, pretzels and cheesy-flavored snacks. **Choose unsalted** popcorn, nuts or seeds. Eat more fruit.

- **Don't salt children's food** to your taste.

- **Limit or avoid antacids and saline powders with** sodium bicarbonate (such as *Alka-Seltzer*). They are high in sodium.

FOODS HIGH IN SODIUM

- Cheese, Butter, Margarine
- Pickles, Sauerkraut, Olives
- Condiments, Sauces
- Salad Dressings
- Canned vegetables/salads/beans
- Deli Salads (with dressing)
- Frozen/Packaged Meals/Entrees
- Soups: Canned/dry; bouillon cubes
- Meats: Ham, bacon, sausage, luncheon meats, smoked meats
- Canned Fish (in brine/salt)
- Sea Salt, Garlic/Celery Salt
- Snack Foods (potato chips, pretzels)
- Tomato Juice (Canned), V8 Vegetable Juice
- Fast Foods: Pizza, Burgers, Chicken
- *Alka-Seltzer* Antacid

MODERATE SODIUM

- Bread (Reduced Salt)
- Meat, Fish, Poultry - Unprocessed
- Milk, Yogurt, Soy Drinks, Eggs
- Peanut Butter
- Breakfast Cereals (less than 200mg/serving)
- Chocolate Candy, Fruit/Nut Bars
- *Reduced Sodium & Low Sodium* Products

FOODS LOW IN SODIUM

- Products labelled *Very Low Sodium*, or *Sodium Free*
- Fresh fruits and vegetables
- Canned and Dried Fruits
- Potatoes, Rice, Pasta
- Dried Beans & Lentils, Tofu
- Nuts & Seeds (unsalted)
- Corn & Popcorn (unsalted)
- Pepper, Spices, Herbs
- Jam, Honey, Syrup
- Candy, Gum
- Hard & Jelly Candy
- Coffee, Tea, Alcohol
- Fresh Fruit Juices, Water

The American Heart Association recommends a sodium intake of **less than 2300mg/day**

Milk & Dairy Products

	Sodium
Milk: Whole/lowfat/skim, average	
1 cup, 8 fl.oz	120
Whole, low sodium, 1 cup	5
Choc Milk (Hershey's), 1 cup	130
Soy Milk, 8 fl.oz	30
Buttermilk, cultured, 8 fl.oz	250
Dry/Powder, skim, ¼ cup, 1 oz	110
Yogurt, with fruit average, 8 oz	130
Cheese: Blue, 1 oz	330
Parmesan, 1 oz	450
Kraft Cheddar, 2% milk, 1 oz	230
Philadelphia Cream Cheese, 1 oz	90
Process Cheese., average,1 oz	430
Swiss, 1 oz	40
Cottage Cheese, ½ cup, 4 oz	450
Ricotta Cheese, ½ cup, 4 oz	150

Icecream, Frozen Yogurt

Icecream, average,½ cup	50
Frozen Yogurt, ½ cup	50

Fats/Oils

Butter/Margarine:	
Regular, 2 Tbsp, 1 oz	230
Unsalted, reg., 2 Tbsp, 1 oz	5
Mayonnaise, aver., 2 Tbsp, 1 oz	160
Oils/Lard/Dripping	0
Cream, average, 1 Tbsp	6
Coffee-Mate: Powdered, 1 tsp	2
Liquid, 1 Tbsp	5

Eggs

Whole, 1 large	70
Omelet, 2 egg, plain	220
w. cheese	400
Egg Beaters (Fleischmann's), ¼ cup	115

Meats

Meat, average all types, cooked	
(Beef/Lamb/Veal/Pork), 4 oz	80
Corned Beef, cooked, 3 oz	800
Bacon, cooked, 2 slices, ½ oz	270
Ham, 3 oz	1100

Chicken & Turkey

Chicken/Turkey, cooked, unsalted, 4 oz	80
Stuffing Mixes, average., ½ cup	500

Sodium ~ **Sodium (mg)**

Sausages & Meats

	Sodium
Bologna, 1 oz	280
Frankfurter, 2 oz	640
Ham, chopped, ¾ oz slice	290
Liverwurst (Braunschweiger), 1 oz	320
Pepperoni, 5 slices, 1 oz	570
Salami, cooked, 1 oz	350
dry/hard, 1 oz	600
Sausage, 1 oz link	220
Pork, 2 oz patty	260
Turkey Roll, 1 oz	160

Fish: Fresh Fish, average, plain

Cooked, 4 oz (no bone)	60
Broiled w. butter, 4 oz	150
Breaded & fried, 4 oz	320
Fish fillets, batter-dipped 3 oz	350
Fish sticks, 1 oz stick	160
Gefilte Fish (w. broth), 1 pce, 1½ oz	220
Herring, pickled, 2 pces, 1 oz	260
Lobster, meat only, 4 oz	180
Oysters, fresh, 6 med., 3 oz	95
Salmon: Canned, 3 oz	460
No Salt Added, 3 oz	65
Smoked fish, average, 3 oz	650
Tuna: Canned, 3 oz	330
No Added Salt, 3 oz	40

Entrees & Meals

Frozen Meals, average	600-900
Lean Cuisine, average	700
Stouffer's, average	580
Dinners, average	900-1200
Side Dishes, average	400-600
Pizza, frozen, ¼ large, 6 oz	800-1200
Microwave Cup Meals	900-1200
Cup O'Noodles, average	1500

Fast-Foods & Restaurants

Cheeseburger	750
Chicken Dinner (3 piece)	2200
Chicken Nuggets w. Sauce	800
Fish/Chicken Sandwich	1000
French Fries, small, 2½ oz	150
Hamburger: Regular	500
Large with cheese	1100
Hot Dog (Frankfurter)	800
Pizza, 2 medium slices	1200
Shake, chocolate	250
Taco	400

Extra Listings ~ see CalorieKing.com

Sodium Counter

Sodium ~ Sodium (mg)

	Sodium
Soups: Condensed, 1 c., 8 oz	800-1000
Low Sodium	70
Chicken Noodle, 1 cup	900
Bouillon Cube, average	950
Cup-A-Soup: Average	850
Lite, average	450
Soup Mixes, average, 1 cup	900

Condiments, Sauces, Dressings

A-1 Sauce, 1 Tbsp	280
Barbecue Sauce, 1 Tbsp	130
Bragg Liquid Aminos, 1 tsp	220
Chili Sauce, 1 Tbsp	230
Ketchup: Tomato, 1 Tbsp	180
Low Sodium, 1 Tbsp	20
Mayonnaise, 1 Tbsp	80
Mustard, 1 tsp	70
Pizza Sauce, ½ cup	700
Salad Dressings, 2 Tbsp, 1 oz	160-400
Spaghetti Sauce, ½ cup	500
Soy Sauce: 1 Tbsp	900
Lite *(Kikkoman),* 1 Tbsp	600
Sweet & Sour, ½ cup	250
Tabasco, 1 tsp	25
Vinegar, Lemon Juice	0
Worcestershire, 1 Tbsp	200
Tomato: Sauce, 1 cup	1200
Paste/Puree (salted), ½ cup	1000
No Salt Added, ½ cup	25

Salt & Salt Substitutes

Table Salt: 1 teaspoon, 6g	2400
Single Serve package, 1 g	400
Cardia Salt, 1 teaspoon	1080
Lite Salt *(Morton),* 1 teaspoon, 6g	1200
Morton Salt Substitute	5
No Salt **Salt Substitute,** 1 teaspoon	5
Garlic/Seasoned Salt 1 teaspoon, 4g	1300
Sea Salt, 1 teaspoon, 5g	2250

Seasonings, Herbs & Spices

Baking Powder, 1 tsp, 3g	340
Baking Soda (Sodium bicarb), 1 tsp, 3g	810
Accent (Flavor Enhancer), 1 tsp	600
Chili Powder, 1 tsp, 3g	25
Curry Powder	0
Lemon Pepper *(Lawry's),* 1 tsp	340
Meat Tenderizer, 1 tsp, 5g	1750
MSG (Monosodium glutamate), 5g	500
Mrs Dash (Herb/Spice Blend), 1 tsp	1
Pepper, Mustard (dry), 1 tsp	1
Yeast, Nutritional, 1 Tbsp	10

Breakfast Cereals

Kellogg's:

	Sodium
All-Bran, ½ cup, 1 oz	80
Oatbran Flakes, ¾ cup, 1 oz	210
Corn Flakes, 1 cup, 1 oz	200
Just Right, ¾ cup, 2 oz	240
Mini Wheats Frosted, 24 bisc., 1.8 oz	5
Health Valley Cereals, 1 serving	5
Quaker: Cap'n Crunch, ¾ cup, 1 oz	200
Crunchy Corn Bran, ¾ cup, 1 oz	230
100% Natural Granola, ½ cup, 1 oz	15
Puffed Rice/Wheat, 2 cups, 1 oz	1
General Mills: Total, ¾ cup, 1 oz	190
Oatmeal: Regular, ¾ cup	1
Instant *(Quaker),* ⅔ cup (1 pkt)	270

Breads, Bagels, Crackers

Bread: Average all types, 1 oz	140
Low Sodium, 1 oz	10
Bagels: Plain, 2 oz	200
Sara Lee, 3 oz	500
Biscuits, average, 1 oz	180
Bun/Roll, 1 medium, 1½ oz	200
Crackers: Saltine, 2 crackers	70
Low Salt *(Premium),* 2	25
Graham, 2 regular	50
Croissant, average, 2 oz	280
Rice Cakes, average	25
Ry-Krisp Crispbread, Sesame, 2	100

Cookies, Cakes, Desserts

Cookies: Average, 2-3 cookies, 1 oz	100
Mrs Fields', average, 2½ oz	180
Baked Custard, ½ cup	100
Brownie, ¼ oz piece	75
Cake, average, 3 oz piece	250
Cinnamon Sweet Roll, 2 oz	250
Danish, Apple	250
Donut, average	150
Muffins: 1 medium, 2 oz	150
Pancakes, 3 x 4"	360
Pie, average ⅙ of 9" pie	300
Pudding: Average, ½ cup	160
Jell-O (Mix), Instant, ½ cup	400
Waffles:	
Home-made, 7", 2½ oz	350
Frozen: Average, 1¼ oz	260
Aunt Jemima, avg, 2½ oz	565

Sodium Counter

Fruit & Juices	Sodium
Fresh Fruit, average all types, 1 serving	1
Dried/Canned Fruit, ½ cup	1
Fruit Juice: Fresh, sqz'd, 6 fl.oz	1
Commercial, aver. 6 fl.oz	20
Carrot Juice (Ferraro's), 8 fl.oz	230
Tomato Juice (Campbell's), 6 fl.oz	570
Low Sodium (No Salt Added)	20
V8 Vegetable (Campbell's), 6 fl.oz	600
(No Salt Added), 6 fl.oz	45

Vegetables	
Fresh/Frozen (No Salt Added): *Per 1/2 Cup*	
Asparagus, Bean Sprouts, Corn	3
Beets, Carrots, Celery, ½ cup	40
Broccoli, Cabbage, Cauliflower	10
Cucumber, Green Beans, Mushroom, Okra	3
Onions, Peas, Potato, Pumpkin, Squash	3
Peppers, Hot Chili, raw, each	3
Spinach, Turnips, ½ cup, ckd	40
Tomato, 1 medium, 5 oz	10
Canned: Asparagus, 4 spears	300
Beans, baked in tomato sauce	450
Beets, ½ cup, 3 oz	240
Corn Kernels, ½ cup, 3 oz	190
Creamed, ½ cup, 4½ oz	330
Mushrooms w. butter sce, 2oz	550
Peas, ½ cup, 3 oz	250
Sauerkraut, ½ cup, 4 oz	750

Pickles, Olives	
Olives, pickled: Green, 1 large	90
Ripe/black, 1 large	40
Pickles: Bread & Butter, 4 sl., 1 oz	200
Dill, 1 pickle, 2½ oz	900
Sweet, 1 gherkin, ½ oz	130

Soybean Products	
Miso (Soy Paste), ¼ c., 2½ oz	2500
Soybean Protein Isolate, 1 oz	280
Tempeh, ½ cup, 3 oz	5
Tofu, average, ½ cup, 4 oz	5

Jam, Honey, Syrups	
Jam/Jelly, 1 Tbsp	2
Honey/Maple Syrup, 1 Tbsp	1
Log Cabin Syrup, 1 fl.oz	35
Lite, 1 fl.oz	90

Peanut Butter	
Peanut Butter, regular, 1 Tbsp	70
Unsalted, 1 Tbsp	1

Snacks, Nuts	Sodium
Cheese Balls/Curls, 1 oz	280
Corn/Tortilla Chips, average, 1 oz	220
Granola bars, average, 1 bar	80
Nuts: Plain, unsalted, 1 oz	1
Lightly salted, 1 oz	80
Salted or Honey Roasted, 1 oz	160
Popcorn: Plain (unsalted), 1 cup	1
Flavored, average, 1 cup	60
Salt added, 1 cup	180
Potato Chips: Plain, 1 oz	160
Flavored, average, 1 oz	250
Pretzels, regular, 3, 1 oz	450

Candy, Chocolate	
Chocolate, milk, 1 oz	30
Carob Milk Bar, 1 oz	55
Fudge, chocolate, 1 oz	55
Candy Bars, average, 1½ oz	60
Hard Candy, Jelly Beans, 1 oz	10
Licorice, 1 oz	30

Beverages, Alcohol	
Coffee (& Substitutes), Tea, 1 cup	1
Cocoa, dry, plain, 1 Tbsp	0
Mix, average, 1 envelope	120
Quik (Nestle), 2 tsp	35
Soft Drinks, average, 8 fl.oz	20
Mineral Water, Perrier, 8 fl.oz	5
Gatorade Thirst Quencher, 8 fl.oz	110
Water: Average, 1 cup, 8 fl.oz	5
Drier regions, 1 cup	20+
Alcohol: Beer, average, 12 fl.oz	15
Wines, average, 4 fl.oz	10
Spirits (distilled), 1½ fl.oz	1

Antacids – Alka-Seltzer	Sodium
Alka-Seltzer (Per Tablet):	
Alka-Seltzer P.M., 1 tablet	500
Original (Light Blue Box)	570
Extra Strength (Dark Blue Box)	590
Flavored Lemon/Lime & Cherry	500
Antacid (yellow Box)	310
Gelatine Capsule, 1	0
Alka-Mints, chewable	0
Bromo Seltzer, ¾ capful	760
Rolaids, all types	0
Tums, Regular/Extra Strength	0
Sodium Bicarbonate (27% sodium), 1g	270

Index A - B

FAST-FOOD RESTAURANTS INDEX
~ SEE PAGE 183 ~

FAST-FOODS INDEX
~ PAGE 183 ~

Index H - L

Index P - S

FAST-FOOD RESTAURANTS INDEX
~ SEE PAGE 183 ~

Index U - Z